# 44

## Update in Intensive Care and Emergency Medicine

Edited by J.-L. Vincent

E. Abraham   M. Singer (Eds.)

# Mechanisms of Sepsis-Induced Organ Dysfunction and Recovery

With 48 Figures and 22 Tables

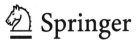 Springer

*Series Editor*

Prof. Jean-Louis Vincent
Head, Department of Intensive Care
Erasme University Hospital
Route de Lennik 808, 1070 Brussels
Belgium
jlvincen@ulb.ac.be

*Volume Editors*

Edward Abraham, MD
University of Colorado
Health Sciences Center
Division Pulmonary & Critical Care
Medicine
E. Ninth Avenue 4200
80262 Denver, CO
USA

Mervyn Singer, MD
University College Hospital
Bloomsbury Institute of Intensive
Care
Division Medicine
Gower Street, WC1E 6BT
London
United Kingdom

ISSN  0933-6788

ISBN  978-3-540-30157-8  Springer Berlin Heidelberg New York

Library of Congress Control Number: 2006929196

Springer is a part of Springer Science+Business Media
springer.com

© Springer-Verlag Berlin Heidelberg 2007

Editor: Dr. Ute Heilmann, Heidelberg, Germany
Desk Editor: Meike Stoeck, Heidelberg, Germany
Typesetting and production: LE-TEX Jelonek, Schmidt & Vöckler GbR, Leipzig, Germany
Cover design: WMX Design, Heidelberg, Germany
Printed on acid-free paper    27/3100/YL – 5 4 3 2 1 0

# Table of Contents

# Contributors

Abraham E
Department of Medicine
University of Alabama
1530 3rd Ave S
Birmingham, AL 35294-0012
USA

Adib-Conquy M
UP Cytokines & Inflammation
Institut Pasteur
28 rue Dr Roux
75015 Paris
France

Aird WC
Molecular Medicine
Beth Israel Deaconess Medical Center
RW-663
330 Brookline Avenue
Boston, MA 02215
USA

Annane D
Service de Réanimation
Hospital Raymond Poincaré
104 Boulevard Raymond Poincaré
92380 Garches
France

Bellingan G
Center for Respiratory Research
University College London
Rayne Institute
University St
London, WC1E 6JJ
United Kingdom

Billiar TR
Department of Surgery
University of Pittsburgh School of Medicine
20 Lothrop Street

Presbyterian Hospital F1200
Pittsburgh, PA 15213
USA

Bongers T
Division of Metabolic and Cellular Medicine
School of Clinical Science
Duncan Building, UCD
University of Liverpool
Liverpool, L69 3GA
United Kingdom

Bromberg Z
Department of Anesthesia
and Critical Care Medicine
Hadassah Hebrew University School
of Medicine
Jerusalem 91120
Israel

Calandra T
Infectious Diseases Service
Department of Medicine
Centre Hospitalier Universitaire Vaudois
1011 Lausanne
Switzerland

Carré J
Wolfson Institute of Biomedical Research
University College of London
Gower Street
London, WC1E 6BT
United Kingdom

Cavaillon JM
UP Cytokines & Inflammation
Institut Pasteur
28 rue Dr Roux
75015 Paris
France

*Chambers RC*
Center for Respiratory Research
The Rayne Institute
5 University Street
London, WC1E 6JJ
United Kingdom

*Cristofaro PA*
Infectious Diseases Division
Memorial Hospital of RI
111 Brewster Street
Pawtucket, RI 02860
USA

*Czura CJ*
Laboratory of Biomedical Science
North Shore-LIJ Research Institute
350 Community Dr.
Manhasset, NY 11030
USA

*Davis IC*
Department of Anesthesiology
University of Alabama
1530 3rd Avenue South
Birmingham, AL 35294
USA

*De Backer D*
Department of Intensive Care Medicine
Erasme University of Brussels Hospital
Route de Lennik 808
1070 Brussels
Belgium

*Deutschman CS*
Department of Anesthesiology
and Critical Care Medicine
University of Pennsylvania School of Medicine
Dulles 781A/HUP
3400 Spruce Street
Philadelphia, PA 19104-4283
USA

*Elbers PWG*
Department of Anesthesiology,
Intensive Care and Pain Management
St. Antonius Hospital
Koekoekslaan 1
Postbus 2500
3430 EM Nieuwegein
Netherlands

*Evans TW*
Department of Intensive Care Medicine
Royal Brompton Hospital
Sydney Street
London, SW3 6 NP
United Kingdom

*Fink MP*
Departments of Critical Care Medicine,
Surgery, Pharmacology and Pathology
University of Pittsburgh School of Medicine
Room 616 Scaife Hall
3550 Terrace Street
Pittsburgh, PA 15261
USA

*Friedman SG*
Laboratory of Biomedical Science
North Shore-LIJ Research Institute
350 Community Drive
Manhasset, NY 11030
USA

*Griffiths RD*
Division of Metabolic and Cellular Medicine
School of Clinical Science
Duncan Building, UCD
University of Liverpool
Liverpool, L69 3GA
United Kingdom

*Guidoux C*
Service de Réanimation
Hospital Raymond Poincaré
104 Boulevard Raymond Poincaré
92380 Garches
France

*Hagimoto N*
Pulmonary Research Labs, 151L
VA Puget Sound Medical Center
1660 S. Columbian Way
Seattle, WA 98108
USA

*Howell DCJ*
Center for Respiratory Research
The Rayne Institute
5 University Street
London, WC1E 6JJ
United Kingdom

Ince C
Clinical Physiology
Academic Medical Center
Meibergdreef 9
1105 AZ Amsterdam
Netherlands

Jeyabalan G
Department of Surgery
University of Pittsburgh School of Medicine
20 Lothrop Street
Presbyterian Hospital F1200
Pittsburgh, PA 15213
USA

Kaech C
Infectious Diseases Service
Department of Medicine
Centre Hospitalier Universitaire Vaudois
1011 Lausanne
Switzerland

Kellum JA
Department of Critical Care Medicine
615 Scaife Hall
University of Pittsburgh
3550 Terrace Street
Pittsburgh, PA 15261
USA

Kumar A
Section of Critical Care Medicine
Health Sciences Center, GE706
820 Sherbrooke St
Winnipeg, Manitoba R3A 1R9
Canada

Lang JD Jr
Department of Anesthesiology
University of Alabama
1530 3rd Avenue South
Birmingham, AL 35294
USA

Langouche L
Department of Intensive Care Medicine
Katholieke Universiteit Leuven
Herestraat 49
3000 Leuven
Belgium

Laurent GJ
Center for Respiratory Research
The Rayne Institute
5 University Street
London, WC1E 6JJ
United Kingdom

Lee JW
Department of Medicine and Anesthesia
Cardiovascular Research Institute
University of California
505 Parnassus Avenue
San Francisco, CA 94143-0624
USA

Lemiale V
Medical Intensive Care Unit
Groupe Hospitalier Cochin –
St Vincent de Paul
René Descartes University – Paris V
27 rue du Faubourg St Jacques
75679 Paris Cedex 14
France

Levi M
Academic Medical Center
Department of Internal Medicine
Meibergdreef 9, Room G2-130
1105 AZ Amsterdam
Netherlands

MacCallum NS
Department of Intensive Care Medicine
Royal Brompton Hospital
Sydney Street
London, SW3 6NP
United Kingdom

Malam Z
Sepsis Research Laboratory
St. Michael's Hospital
4th Floor Bond Wing, Rm. 4-007
30 Bond Street
Toronto, ON M5B 1W8
Canada

Marshall JC
Sepsis Research Laboratory
St. Michael's Hospital
4th Floor Bond Wing, Rm. 4-007
30 Bond Street
Toronto, ON M5B 1W8
Canada

Martin TR
Pulmonary Research Labs, 151L
VA Puget Sound Medical Center
1660 S. Columbian Way
Seattle, WA 98108
USA

Matalon S
Department of Anesthesiology
University of Alabama
1530 3rd Avenue South
Birmingham, AL 35294
USA

Matthay MA
Department of Medicine and Anesthesia
Cardiovascular Research Institute
University of California
505 Parnassus Avenue
San Francisco, CA 94143-0624
USA

Matute-Bello G
Pulmonary Research Labs, 151L
VA Puget Sound Medical Center
1660 S. Columbian Way
Seattle, WA 98108
USA

McArdle A
Division of Metabolic and Cellular Medicine
School of Clinical Science
Duncan Building, UCD
University of Liverpool
Liverpool, L69 3GA
United Kingdom

Meisel C
Institute of Medical Immunology
Universitätsmedizin Charité Campus Mitte
Schumanstrasse 20/21
10117 Berlin
Germany

Mira JP
Medical Intensive Care Unit
Groupe Hospitalier Cochin –
St Vincent de Paul
René Descartes University – Paris V
27 rue du Faubourg St Jacques
75679 Paris Cedex 14
France

Moncada S
Wolfson Institute of Biomedical Research
University College of London
Gower Street
London, WC1E 6BT
United Kingdom

Opal SM
Infectious Diseases Division
Memorial Hospital of RI
111 Brewster Street
Pawtucket, RI 02860
USA

Parrillo JE
Cardiovascular and Critical Care Services
Cooper University Hospital
One Cooper Plaza
Camden, NJ 08103
United States

Pugin J
Department of Intensive Care Medicine
University Hospital
Rue Micheli-du-Crest
1211 Geneva 14
Switzerland

Quinlan GJ
Department of Intensive Care Medicine
Royal Brompton Hospital
Sydney Street
London, SW3 6 NP
United Kingdom

Raghavan M
Department of Critical Care Medicine
615 Scaife Hall
University of Pittsburgh
3550 Terrace Street
Pittsburgh, PA 15261
USA

Rooyackers O
Dept of Anesthesiology
and Intensive Care Medicine
K32
Karolinska University Hospital Huddinge
14186 Stockholm
Sweden

Sharshar T
Service de Réanimation
Hôpital Raymond Poincaré
104 Boulevard Raymond Poincaré
92380 Garches
France

Singer M
Bloomsbury Institute
of Intensive Care Medicine
Wolfson Institute of Biomedical Research
University College London
Gower Street
London, WC1E 6BT
United Kingdom

Texereau J
Cochin Institute of Molecular Genetics
Groupe Hospitalier Cochin –
St Vincent de Paul
René Descartes University – Paris V
27 rue du Faubourg St Jacques
75679 Paris Cedex 14
France

Tracey KJ
Laboratory of Biomedical Science
North Shore-LIJ Research Institute
350 Community Dr.
Manhasset, NY 11030
USA

Tsung A
Department of Surgery
University of Pittsburgh School of Medicine
20 Lothrop Street
Presbyterian Hospital F1200
Pittsburgh, PA 15213
USA

Van den Berghe G
Department of Intensive Care Medicine
Katholieke Universiteit Leuven
Herestraat 49
3000 Leuven
Belgium

van der Poll T
Academic Medical Center
Department of Internal Medicine
Meibergdreef 9, Room G2-130
1105 AZ Amsterdam
Netherlands

Vanhorebeek I
Department of Intensive Care Medicine
Katholieke Universiteit Leuven
Herestraat 49
3000 Leuven
Belgium

Venkataraman R
Department of Critical Care Medicine
615 Scaife Hall
University of Pittsburgh
3550 Terrace Street
Pittsburgh, PA 15261
USA

Vincent JL
Department of Intensive Care Medicine
Erasme University of Brussels Hospital
Route de Lennik 808
1070 Brussels
Belgium

Volk HD
Institute of Medical Immunology
Universitätsmedizin Charité Campus Mitte
Schumanstrasse 20/21
10117 Berlin
Germany

Weiss YG
Department of Anesthesiology
and Critical Care Medicine
University of Pennsylvania School of Medicine
Dulles 781A/HUP
3400 Spruce Street
Philadelphia, PA 19104-4283
USA

Wernerman J
Dept of Anesthesiology and Intensive Care
Medicine
K32
Karolinska University Hospital Huddinge
14186 Stockholm
Sweden

Wiersinga WJ
Academic Medical Center
Department of Internal Medicine
Meibergdreef 9, Room G2-130
1105 AZ Amsterdam
Netherlands

# Common Abbreviations

| | |
|---|---|
| ALI | Acute lung injury |
| APACHE | Acute physiology and chronic health evaluation |
| ARDS | Acute respiratory distress syndrome |
| BAL | Bronchoalveolar lavage |
| CNS | Central nervous system |
| DIC | Disseminated intravascular coagulation |
| HMGB | High mobility group box protein |
| ICAM | Intercellular adhesion molecule |
| ICU | Intensive care unit |
| IFN | Interferon |
| IL | Interleukin |
| IL-1ra | Interleukin-1 receptor antagonist |
| LPS | Lipopolysaccharide |
| MAPK | Mitogen-activated protein kinase |
| MHC | Major histocompatibility complex |
| MOF | Multiple organ failure |
| NF-κB | Nuclear factor-kappa B |
| NO | Nitric oxide |
| NOS | Nitric oxide synthase |
| PAF | Platelet activating factor |
| PMN | Polymorphonuclear leukocyte |
| ROS | Reactive oxygen species |
| SIRS | Systemic inflammatory response syndrome |
| TGF | Transforming growth factor |
| TLR | Toll-like receptor |
| TNF | Tumor necrosis factor |

# Setting the Scene

J.L. Vincent

## Introduction - What is the Cause of Death in Multiple Organ Failure?

Multiple organ failure (MOF) is a common cause of death in intensive care unit (ICU) patients [1]. But what are the mechanisms underlying the development of MOF? Why, when we can support many of the individual organs, e.g., the kidneys with extracorporeal renal support, the lungs with mechanical ventilation, etc., do we all too often end up withholding/withdrawing these life-supporting therapies when we feel that there is no chance of recovery, or more precisely that the "multiple organ failure" state has become irreversible.

Early therapy of patients with sepsis is associated with improved outcomes [2,3] and worsening organ function early in the course of disease is associated with worse outcomes. Lopes Ferreira et al. [4] reported that worsening organ dysfunction, as assessed by an increasing sequential organ failure assessment (SOFA) score in the first 48 hours was associated with a mortality rate of at least 50% regardless of the baseline SOFA sore. More recently, we reviewed the time course of organ failure in two placebo-controlled sepsis clinical trials with Eli-Lilly and Co [5]. We found that improved cardiovascular, renal, or respiratory organ function within the first 24 hours following development of sepsis-induced organ dysfunction was associated with increased survival. Improved understanding of the mechanisms underlying the development of organ dysfunction and MOF may enable us to develop therapies targeted at preventing or limiting the early events associated with later development of fatal organ dysfunction, and hence improve outcomes. In this chapter, we will briefly explore some of the possible mechanisms involved in the terminality and irreversibility of organ failure.

## The Role of Tissue Hypoxia

The lack of oxygen availability to the cell is perhaps the most obvious cause of organ failure, typically occurring in a patient with decreased blood flow as a result of advanced cardiovascular failure. Cells are able to withstand considerable reductions in oxygen concentration, but with prolonged or severe hypoxia, mechanisms are put into place to prevent oxygen depletion and to maintain cellular ATP levels and avoid cell death [6]. Various strategies are employed including increasing glycolysis to produce ATP and upregulating vascular endothelial growth factor (VEGF) which stimulates angiogenesis and hence oxygen delivery. Many of these mechanisms are controlled by the transcription factor, hypoxia-inducible factor (HIF)-1$\alpha$ which accumulates in hypoxia as its degradation is inhibited and its transcription is activated [7]. Activation of HIF during hypoxia results in the expression of glycolytic enzymes, membrane glucose transporters, VEGF, and erythropoietin, and many other genes involved in oxygen homeostasis and cell survival [7]. HIF-1 is also involved in coordinating the immune response to bacterial infection with effects on nitric oxide (NO) production and tumor necrosis factor (TNF)-$\alpha$ [8]. Although the role of HIF-1 in hypoxia is now relatively well understood, the mechanisms by which cells sense oxygen concentrations and the presence of hypoxia remain undefined. Potential candidates include prolyl hydroxylases and the mitochondria [9]. Whatever the underlying mechanisms, hypoxia can have deleterious effects locally. In the alveolar epithelium, for example, hypoxia impairs transepithelial sodium and fluid transport, may increase apoptosis, and disturbs tight junctions [6].

## The Role of Cellular Alterations

Hypoxia is not the only phenomenon involved in cell death and organ dysfunction. Patients may die with normal or high cardiac output, normal or high mixed venous oxygen saturation (SvO$_2$), although admittedly these are surrogate measures of local tissue hypoxia. Nevertheless, increased tissue oxygen tensions have been found in animals and patients with sepsis [10,11], suggesting that the problem may be with the way in which cells use available oxygen rather than (or in addition to) the actual oxygen availability. Cellular hibernation may also play a role. Hibernation is a process whereby cells down-regulate oxygen consumption, energy requirements, and ATP demand, a potentially protective mechanism in hypoxia and ischemia, which may become pathologic if the threat is prolonged. This has been shown to occur in myocardial cells during hypoxia, ischemia and sepsis, and it is interesting to speculate that hibernation may also occur in cells of other organs [12].

### The Role of the Mitochondrion

The role of the mitochondrion has been debated for decades, and these cellular 'power plants' are now believed to play a central role in cell and organ damage during various disease processes [13]. Mitochondrial oxidative phosphorylation is responsible for over 90% of oxygen consumption and ATP generation [14], and the respiratory chain is inhibited by reactive oxygen and nitrogen species that are produced in large quantities in sepsis. Endotoxin injection in cats caused liver mitochondrial injury with damage to the inner and outer mitochondrial membranes [15]. In rats, intraperitoneal injection of endotoxin reduced diaphragm mitochondrial oxygen consumption and selective components of the electron transport chain, resulting in diminished electron flow, ATP formation and proton pumping [16]. The incubation of human umbilical vein endothelial cells in

serum from patients with septic shock was associated with depressed mitochondrial respiration and reduced cellular ATP levels, effects which were attenuated by
pre-treatment with a NO synthase (NOS) inhibitor or a blocker of poly(ADP-ribose)
synthase [17]. In a clinical study, Brealey et al. [14] reported that mitochondrial
dysfunction in skeletal muscle was associated with increased shock severity and
mortality in patients with sepsis and MOF.

## The Role of Necrosis and Apoptosis

Cells can die in one of two ways – necrosis or apoptosis. In necrosis, cells die
as the result of exposure to a physiological stress, with cellular swelling and dis-
integration – this has been termed cellular 'murder' as the cell is an unwilling
participant [18]. Apoptosis, or programmed cell death, on the other hand, has
been described as cell 'suicide' as the cell is actively involved in its own death [18].
Apoptosis can be physiologic or pathologic and occurs via two main pathways.
The first, the extrinsic pathway, is initiated by the activation of cell death receptors,
e.g., Fas and TNF receptors 1 and 2, which results in the activation of caspase
8, which activates other caspases, ultimately leading to the cleavage of DNA and
membrane lysis. The other pathway, the intrinsic pathway, involves the release of
pro-apoptotic substances from mitochondria, leading to the activation of caspase
3 [19]. Increased apoptosis has been demonstrated in lung, liver, spleen, kidney
and myocardium in animal models of septic or endotoxic shock [20,21]. Human
serum from patients with septic shock can activate apoptosis in human cardiomyocytes [22], and human studies of septic shock have suggested increased apoptosis
primarily in cells of the immune system although intestinal epithelial cells have also
been implicated [23,24]. A number of factors can delay apoptosis, including the
pro-inflammatory cytokines interleukin (IL)-1, IL-8, TNF and interferon (IFN)-γ.

## The Role of pH

The role of pH is complex. Although acidosis was long considered as harmful, work
in the seventies showed that it may, in fact, have more protective than detrimental
effects. Acidosis may occur as a result of increases in arterial $PCO_2$ (respiratory
acidosis) or from a variety of organic or inorganic fixed acids (metabolic acidosis). Metabolic acidosis occurs wherever there is inadequate oxygen delivery to
support energy metabolism and the most vulnerable organs are those that have
the highest energy requirements, e.g., the brain and the kidney. Within organs,
different cell types will be affected differently by acidosis as they have different
energy requirements. Importantly, arterial pH may not reflect cellular pH, and
the underlying cause of the acidosis may be more important than the acidosis
itself [25]. Several studies have documented the effects of decreased extracellular
pH on the synthesis and release of inflammatory mediators, especially TNF and
NO [26,27]. Because protein function is sensitive to the $[H^+]$ of its environment,
an increase in arterial $[H^+]$ might be expected to have important detrimental effects on a host of bodily functions [28]. Lowering the arterial pH has been shown

to cause a decrease in cardiac contractility, and a decrease in the responsiveness of adrenergic receptors to circulating catecholamines. Nevertheless, experimental data suggest that acidosis can be protective; a low pH delays the onset of cell death in isolated hepatocytes exposed to anoxia [29] and to chemical hypoxia [30], and acidosis during reperfusion limits myocardial infarct size [31]. In addition, many patients with acute respiratory distress syndrome (ARDS) or status asthmaticus are now treated with permissive hypercapnia or hypercapnic acidosis, in which hypercapnia and acidemia are tolerated to avoid alveolar overdistention, and this therapy has been associated with a reduced 28-day mortality in patients with acute lung injury (ALI) or ARDS [32].

## Role of Oxygen Free Radicals

Oxygen free radicals have been widely studied and it is well established that they can be very cytotoxic. Under normal physiological conditions, a homeostatic balance exists between the formation of reactive oxygen species and their removal by endogenous antioxidant scavenging compounds. Oxidative stress occurs when this balance is disrupted by excessive production of reactive oxygen species, including superoxide, hydrogen peroxide and hydroxyl radicals, and/or by inadequate antioxidative defences including superoxide dismutase (SOD), catalase, vitamins C and E, and reduced glutathione (GSH) [33]. Oxidative stress causes damage to DNA, cellular proteins, and lipids. It also affects cellular calcium metabolism. Uncontrolled rises in intracellular free calcium can result in cell injury or death. Damage to DNA strands can occur directly by free radicals in close proximity to the DNA or indirectly, for example, by impairing production of protein needed to repair DNA. Free radicals can attack fatty acid side chains of intracellular membranes and lipoproteins causing lipid peroxidation. The products of lipid peroxidation can further damage membrane proteins, disrupting membrane integrity. In health, a balance of the reduction and oxidation (redox) of free radicals is maintained by endogenous antioxidant systems present extra- and intracellularly. Primary antioxidants prevent oxygen radical formation, whether by removing free radical precursors or by inhibiting catalysts, e.g., glutathione peroxidase and catalase. Secondary antioxidants react with reactive oxygen species which have already been formed, either to remove or inhibit them, e.g., vitamins C and E [33]. Anti-oxidant therapies have been proposed as treatment for a wide variety of diseases and conditions associated with cell death and organ dysfunction, from aging to arthritis to Alzheimer's disease, but despite the harmful effects of oxygen free radicals, they are an important component of mitochondrial respiration, prostaglandin production, and host defence. It is possible that excessive anti-oxidant administration may have negative effects. Clinical trials of various antioxidants, including N-acetylcysteine, in sepsis have given conflicting results but none has been associated with increased survival [34, 35]. The precise role of anti-oxidant therapies thus remains undetermined.

## The Role of Nitric Oxide

The place of NO in cellular death and organ dysfunction is very complex! NO has many molecular targets and can have both beneficial and detrimental effects on many organ systems in sepsis [36]. Many of the effects of NO are mediated by the activation of guanylyl cyclase, resulting in the formation of guanosine monophosphate (cGMP). The reaction of NO with oxygen or superoxide can result in the formation of reactive nitrogen and oxygen species that can damage the cells. Particularly important is the reaction of NO with the superoxide ion, generating peroxynitrite, that can damage cell DNA, although NO may also protect cells from oxidative damage by scavenging oxygen free radicals and inhibiting oxygen free radical production [37].

## The Role of Carbon Monoxide

Carbon monoxide and NO share a number of common characteristics, including involvement in vasodilation, bronchodilation, and platelet anti-aggregating effects [38]. Like NO, carbon monoxide binds to the heme moieties of hemoproteins, and at high concentrations induces tissue hypoxia. Some activities of carbon monoxide are mediated by cGMP, while others involve mitogen-activated protein kinase (MAPK) and other undefined pathways. Carbon monoxide possesses anti-inflammatory actions including the down-regulation of TNF, IL-1 and IL-6, and augmentation of IL-10 [39]. Carbon monoxide is produced in the body from heme degradation catalyzed by heme oxygenases (HO). HO-1 activity is increased by lipopolysaccharide (LPS) [40]. In animal models of ALI/ARDS [41] and in patients with ARDS, HO-1 levels were raised in bronchoalveolar lavage fluid and lung biopsy tissue [42]. HO-1 has been shown to have anti-inflammatory, antiapoptotic, and antiproliferative effects, with salutary effects in diseases as diverse as atherosclerosis and sepsis [43]. HO-1 and its major downstream product, carbon monoxide, are generally believed to have primarily cytoprotective effects [44]: Rats exposed to hyperoxia in the presence of a low concentration of carbon monoxide (250 ppm) exhibit less lung injury than control rats exposed to oxygen alone [45]; in mice, carbon monoxide protects against ischemic lung injury [46]; in mouse-to-rat cardiac transplants exogenous carbon monoxide suppressed graft rejection, associated with inhibition of platelet aggregation, thrombosis, myocardial infarction, and apoptosis [47]; and carbon monoxide pretreatment in a pig model of LPS-induced ALI improved the derangement in pulmonary gas exchange, reduced the development of disseminated intravascular coagulation (DIC) and completely suppressed serum levels of IL-1, while augmenting the anti-inflammatory cytokine IL-10, and blunted the deterioration of kidney and liver function [48]. However, given the known toxic effects of higher doses of carbon monoxide further research is needed before carbon monoxide moves into the clinical arena.

## Other Pathways

There are multiple other potential pathways involved in the cellular alterations that lead to organ dysfunction, many of which remain to be discovered. Some examples include: leptin with reduced leptin levels contributing to a decreased host response [49]; bombesin/gastrin-releasing peptide (GRP), which is secreted by activated macrophages and may be involved in the control of central nervous system and gastrointestinal system functions, cancer growth and immune cell regulation [50]; and glycogen synthase kinase (GSK)-3, a serine-threonine protein kinase, inhibition of which attenuated the renal dysfunction, hepatocellular injury, pancreatic injury and neuromuscular injury induced by endotoxemia in the rat [51].

## Immune Dysregulation

Cytokines like TNF are essential to protect ourselves from microbial invasion, but at the same time can be the cause of organ damage. TNF administration in animals can reproduce all the elements of MOF, with shock, ARDS, coagulation abnormalities, etc. [52]. The roles of some cytokines, e.g., TNF and IL-1, have been well demonstrated as promoting the inflammatory response. However, almost in parallel with the surge of pro-inflammatory mediators, there is a rise in anti-inflammatory substances, e.g., IL-10, the result being a state of immunoparalysis (or 'monocyte hyporesponsiveness') [53]. During sepsis, monocyte/macrophage desensitization may result from depletion of protein kinase C$\alpha$ [54].

Apart from the key cytokines, multiple other mediators and cells play a role in the immune dysregulation that leads to organ dysfunction. For example, transforming growth factor (TGF)-$\beta$ plays an important role in the development of ALI [55]. Other mediators are released later, like high mobility group box 1 (HMGB1) and macrophage migration inhibitory factor (MIF) [56, 57]. The neutrophil is an important cell, playing a critical role in host defence, but also releasing a number of toxic products including reactive oxygen species, proteases, and eicosanoids [58].

As techniques become available that can assess and monitor the immune status better, the effects of immune dysregulation on organ function and outcomes will become clearer.

## The Role of Fever

Although attempts are often made to reduce fever, fever may be protective. In a mouse model of Gram-negative pneumonia, fever was associated with increased neutrophil accumulation, pro-inflammatory cytokine release, and pulmonary endothelial and epithelial injury [59]. Antipyretic therapy may contribute to worse outcomes, with Schulman et al. [60] suggesting an increased risk of infections and increased mortality rates in trauma patients treated to maintain body temperature less than 38.5 °C as compared to those in whom anti-pyretic treatment was not initiated until a temperature of 40 °C. Hypothermia may increase the risk of infection with subsequent organ dysfunction, and this may account for the disappointing results of induced hypothermia in severe head trauma [61].

## Influence of Organ Systems

### The Role of the Endothelium

The endothelium is a vast organ lining all the organs and may, therefore, represent a link to account for the development of MOF. Endothelial cells are involved in a range of vascular activities including vasoconstriction and vasodilation, thrombosis and fibrinolysis, atherosclerosis, angiogenesis, and inflammation. Damage to the pulmonary vascular endothelium occurs in patients with ARDS [62] and endothelial damage has been implicated in many other disease processes leading to organ dysfunction, although the mechanisms underlying these alterations are still largely undefined. Microvascular abnormalities have been well described in sepsis with reduced vessel density and fewer perfused small vessels [63]. Insufficient availability of sphingosine 1-phosphate, a potent barrier enhancing lipid produced by numerous cell types including platelets, can participate in alterations in vascular permeability leading to vascular leakage and compromised endothelial integrity [64]. The availability of growth factors is very important to normal endothelial function, and decreased availability of VEGF may contribute to capillary leak syndrome, even though its overexpression may be deleterious [65]. The release of endothelial progenitor cells, involved in the repair of damaged vasculature, into the circulation is associated with improved survival in patients with ALI [66]. Angiotensin may also play a role in endothelial dysfunction [67], and adrenomedullin may help stabilize endothelial barrier function [68]. Markers like endocan (endothelial cell specific molecule-1) are associated with disease severity in sepsis, and may be useful in monitoring endothelial dysfunction [69].

### The Role of Coagulation Abnormalities

Many patients with organ failure develop coagulation abnormalities secondary to DIC. Teleogically, this reaction aims at reducing the spread of an infection. Coagulation abnormalities are related to the development of organ failure and the severity of organ dysfunction [70]. The mechanisms underlying this again remain largely unknown, although microvascular thrombosis has been suggested to play a role. Thrombin, levels of which are increased in sepsis, can impair alveolar fluid clearance and increase endothelial permeability [71]. A number of studies have documented a complex interplay between the coagulation response and the inflammatory response, hence the suggestion that anti-coagulation may limit the severity of organ failure. Studies have shown the be reficial effects of activated protein C (APC, drotrecogin alfa [activated]) [72], but these have not been demonstrated conclusively for antithrombin [73] or tissue factor pathway inhibitor (TFPI) [74]. Further investigation reveals that even though these three agents are all natural anti-coagulants, they have different modes of action. The mode of action of APC is very complex, largely mediated by the endothelial PC receptor (EPCR) [75]. Recent studies have even suggested that APC derivatives may be developed that keep the beneficial cytoprotective effects but have a reduced anticoagulant action [76].

## The Role of the Epithelium

The epithelium also plays an important role in the pathophysiology of lung injury and other disease processes [77]. Derangements in the formation or function of tight junctions in epithelial cells may be a key factor leading to lung, liver, gut, and perhaps kidney dysfunction in conditions such as sepsis and ALI [78]. Epithelial apoptosis may also play an important role [79].

## The Role of the Gut

While the gut has long been proposed as the motor of organ failure [80], this remains a hypothesis, although splanchnic hypoperfusion may contribute to immunosuppression [81]. Many studies have focused on the role of vasoactive agents on the distribution of blood flow [82], but the clinical implications of these findings are still questionable. Perhaps the most compelling evidence supporting the gut theory is the protective effects of selective digestive decontamination (SDD) [83].

## The Role of the Brain

Much is mediated by the brain and nervous systems, and brain death can induce profound disturbances in endocrine function and an intense inflammatory reaction [84]. Brain injury may alter bone metabolism following trauma [85] and massive head trauma can also exacerbate lung injury [86]. Neuroimmunological pathways have recently been identified, which may be influenced by nutrition [87].

## The Role of the Endocrine System

The importance of relative adrenal insufficiency has been underlined recently [88], as has the role of hyperglycemia [89]. Acute, even transient, hyperglycemia can significantly alter innate immunity and result in immunosuppressive effects [90]. Exposure to glucose-rich solutions has been associated with increased neutrophil apoptosis although this may have been due to the increased osmolarity [91]. Hyperglycemia can increase the expression of adhesion molecules on leukocytes as well as on endothelial cells [92], and may also contribute to permeability alterations by increasing endothelial glycocalyx permeability [93]. Van den Berghe and colleagues recently showed that tight blood sugar control can provide endothelial protection and limit hepatic mitochondrial damage [94, 95]. Insulin itself may have anti-inflammatory effects, by inhibition of nuclear-factor-kappa B (NF-$\kappa$B) and stimulation of inhibitor kappa B (I-$\kappa$B) [96]. Insulin can also increase high-density lipoproteins (HDL).

## Interorgan Interplay

We have discussed these organ systems separately, but clearly complex interactions exist between organs. For example, endotoxin-induced lung injury requires interaction with the liver. In an experimental piglet preparation, Siore et al. noted that endotoxemia caused pulmonary vasoconstriction and neutrophil sequestration but not lung injury in isolated lungs; for cytokine release, oxidant stress and lung injury to occur, the presence of the liver was necessary [97].

## Therapeutic Interventions – the Iatrogenic Component

Various interventions that have been used in intensive care medicine have, in fact, been found to have negative effects in some patients (Table 1). For example, therapies instituted with the intent of raising oxygen delivery ($DO_2$) to supranormal levels may have had deleterious effects [98]. Mechanical ventilation with excessive tidal volumes may result in harmful effects not only on the lungs [99] but also on other organs, by the release of pro-inflammatory mediators [100]. Mechanical ventilation per se may promote bacterial growth [101]. Inotropic agents with beta-adrenergic properties can have immunosuppressive effects, and, likewise, anesthetic and sedative agents may influence a patient's immunity [102]. Propofol, a commonly used sedative agent, may have anti-inflammatory effects, anti-arrhythmic drugs may have pro-arrhythmic effects, and diuretics may alter renal function [103].

Table 1. Some potentially iatrogenic effects and their mechanisms

| Potentially iatrogenic effect | Mechanism |
| --- | --- |
| Excessive tidal volumes | Pro-inflammatory effects on the lung and remote organs |
| Excessive use of inotropic agents | Excessive increase in cardiac work, immunosuppressive effects |
| Parenteral nutrition | Hyperglycemia, risk of infections |
| Excessive sedation | Prolonged alteration in consciousness, immunosuppression |
| Antipyretic agents | Decreased immune response |
| Blood transfusions | Errors, immunomodulation |

## Conclusion

The mechanisms underlying MOF are complex and intertwined. Cellular alterations combine with immune dysregulation and individual organ factors to produce tissue dysfunction and death. What or if there is a final common element in this process remains to be determined. In addition, all these factors are influenced by genetic factors, with increased risks of developing disease and associated organ dysfunction dependent in part on genetic makeup. The pre-existing degree of inflammatory stimulation may also influence the development of sepsis [104]. Clearly there is much we do not know about how the various mechanisms are triggered and then work together to their MOF endpoint, but new insights and inroads are being made on an almost daily basis. With these developments comes the exciting challenge of converting the science into clinical strategies that can assist in preventing or reversing organ dysfunction.

## References

1. Gajewska K, Schroeder M, de Marre F, et al (2004) Analysis of terminal events in 109 successive deaths in a Belgian intensive care unit. Intensive Care Med 30:1224–1227
2. Rivers E, Nguyen B, Havstad S, et al (2001) Early goal-directed therapy in the treatment of severe sepsis and septic shock. N Engl J Med 345:1368–1377
3. Vincent JL, Bernard GR, Beale R, et al (2005) Drotrecogin alfa (activated) treatment in severe sepsis from the global open-label trial ENHANCE. Crit Care Med 33:2266–2277
4. Lopes Ferreira F, Peres Bota D, Bross A, et al (2001) Serial evaluation of the SOFA score to predict outcome. J A M A 286:1754–1758
5. Levy MM, Macias WL, Vincent JL, et al (2005) Early changes in organ function predict eventual survival in severe sepsis. Crit Care Med 33:2194–2201
6. Jain M, Sznajder JI (2005) Effects of hypoxia on the alveolar epithelium. Proc Am Thorac Soc 2:202–205
7. Schumacker PT (2005) Hypoxia-inducible factor-1 (HIF-1). Crit Care Med 33:S423–S425
8. Peyssonnaux C, Datta V, Cramer T, et al (2005) HIF-1alpha expression regulates the bactericidal capacity of phagocytes. J Clin Invest 115:1806–1815
9. Lahiri S, Roy A, Baby SM, et al (2005) Oxygen sensing in the body. Prog Biophys Mol Biol
10. Boekstegers P, Weidenhofer S, Kapsner T, et al (1994) Skeletal muscle partial pressure of oxygen in patients with sepsis. Crit Care Med 22:640–650
11. Rosser DM, Stidwill RP, Jacobson D, et al (1995) Oxygen tension in the bladder epithelium rises in both high and low cardiac output endotoxemic sepsis. J Appl Physiol 79:1878–1882
12. Levy RJ, Piel DA, Acton PD, et al (2005) Evidence of myocardial hibernation in the septic heart. Crit Care Med 33:2752–2756
13. Hubbard WJ, Bland KI, Chaudry IH (2004) The role of the mitochondrion in trauma and shock. Shock 22:395–402
14. Brealey D, Brand M, Hargreaves I, et al (2002) Association between mitochondrial dysfunction and severity and outcome of septic shock. Lancet 360:219–223
15. Crouser ED, Julian MW, Huff JE, et al (2004) Abnormal permeability of inner and outer mitochondrial membranes contributes independently to mitochondrial dysfunction in the liver during acute endotoxemia. Crit Care Med 32:478–488

16. Callahan LA, Supinski GS (2005) Downregulation of diaphragm electron transport chain and glycolytic enzyme gene expression in sepsis. J Appl Physiol 99:1120–1126
17. Boulos M, Astiz ME, Barua RS, et al (2003) Impaired mitochondrial function induced by serum from septic shock patients is attenuated by inhibition of nitric oxide synthase and poly(ADP-ribose) synthase. Crit Care Med 31:353–358
18. Sedlak TW, Snyder SH (2006) Messenger molecules and cell death: therapeutic implications. JAMA 295:81–89
19. Kiechle FL, Zhang X (2002) Apoptosis: biochemical aspects and clinical implications. Clin Chim Acta 326:27–45
20. McDonald TE, Grinman MN, Carthy CM, et al (2000) Endotoxin infusion in rats induces apoptotic and survival pathways in hearts. Am J Physiol Heart Circ Physiol 279:H2053–H2061
21. Hiramatsu M, Hotchkiss RS, Karl IE, et al (1997) Cecal ligation and puncture (CLP) induces apoptosis in thymus, spleen, lung, and gut by an endotoxin and TNF-independent pathway. Shock 7:247–253
22. Kumar A, Kumar A, Michael P, et al (2005) Human serum from patients with septic shock activates transcription factors STAT1, IRF1, and NF-kappaB and induces apoptosis in human cardiac myocytes. J Biol Chem 280:42619–42626
23. Hotchkiss RS, Swanson PE, Freeman BD, et al (1999) Apoptotic cell death in patients with sepsis, shock, and multiple organ dysfunction. Crit Care Med 27:1230–1251
24. Coutinho HB, Robalinho TI, Coutinho VB, et al (1997) Intra-abdominal sepsis: an immuno-cytochemical study of the small intestine mucosa. J Clin Pathol 50:294–298
25. Kellum JA, Song M, Li J (2004) Science review: extracellular acidosis and the immune response: clinical and physiologic implications. Crit Care 8:331–336
26. Bellocq A, Suberville S, Philippe C, et al (1998) Low environmental pH is responsible for the induction of nitric-oxide synthase in macrophages. Evidence for involvement of nuclear factor-kappaB activation. J Biol Chem 273:5086–5092
27. Heming TA, Dave SK, Tuazon DM, et al (2001) Effects of extracellular pH on tumour necrosis factor-alpha production by resident alveolar macrophages. Clin Sci (Lond) 101:267–274
28. Gehlbach BK, Schmidt GA (2004) Bench-to-bedside review: treating acid-base abnormalities in the intensive care unit - the role of buffers. Crit Care 8:259–265
29. Bonventre JV, Cheung JY (1985) Effects of metabolic acidosis on viability of cells exposed to anoxia. Am J Physiol 249:C149–C159
30. Gores GJ, Nieminen A-L, Wray BE, et al (1989) Intracellular pH during "chemical hypoxia" in cultured rat hepatocytes. Protection by intracellular acidosis against the onset of cell death. J Clin Invest 83:386–396
31. Kitakaze M, Takashima S, Funaya H, et al (1997) Temporary acidosis during reperfusion limits myocardial infarct size in dogs. Am J Physiol 272:H2071–H2078
32. Kregenow DA, Rubenfeld GD, Hudson LD, et al (2006) Hypercapnic acidosis and mortality in acute lung injury. Crit Care Med 34:1–7
33. Macdonald J, Galley HF, Webster NR (2003) Oxidative stress and gene expression in sepsis. Br J Anaesth 90:221–232
34. Spapen HD, Diltoer MW, Nguyen DN, et al (2005) Effects of N-acetylcysteine on microalbuminuria and organ failure in acute severe sepsis: results of a pilot study. Chest 127:1413–1419
35. Ortolani O, Conti A, De Gaudio AR, et al (2000) The effect of glutathione and N-acetylcysteine on lipoperoxidative damage in patients with early septic shock. Am J Respir Crit Care Med 161:1907–1911
36. Vincent JL, Zhang H, Szabo C, et al (2000) Effects of nitric oxide in septic shock. Am J Respir Crit Care Med 161:1781–1785
37. Clancy RM, Leszczynska-Piziak J, Abramson SB (1992) Nitric oxide, an endothelial cell relaxation factor, inhibits neutrophil superoxide anion production via a direct action on the NADPH oxidase. J Clin Invest 90:1116–1121

38. Morse D, Choi AM (2005) Heme oxygenase-1: from bench to bedside. Am J Respir Crit Care Med 172:660–670
39. Otterbein LE, Bach FH, Alam J, et al (2000) Carbon monoxide has anti-inflammatory effects involving the mitogen-activated protein kinase pathway. Nat Med 6:422–428
40. Camhi SL, Alam J, Otterbein L, et al (1995) Induction of heme oxygenase-1 gene expression by lipopolysaccharide is mediated by AP-1 activation. Am J Respir Cell Mol Biol 13:387–398
41. Zegdi R, Fabre O, Lila N, et al (2003) Exhaled carbon monoxide and inducible heme oxygenase expression in a rat model of postperfusion acute lung injury. J Thorac Cardiovasc Surg 126:1867–1874
42. Mumby S, Upton RL, Chen Y, et al (2004) Lung heme oxygenase-1 is elevated in acute respiratory distress syndrome. Crit Care Med 32:1130–1135
43. Morse D, Choi AM (2002) Heme oxygenase-1: the "emerging molecule" has arrived. Am J Respir Cell Mol Biol 27:8–16
44. Jin Y, Choi AM (2005) Cytoprotection of heme oxygenase-1/carbon monoxide in lung injury. Proc Am Thorac Soc 2:232–235
45. Otterbein LE, Mantell LL, Choi AM (1999) Carbon monoxide provides protection against hyperoxic lung injury. Am J Physiol 276:L688–L694
46. Fujita T, Toda K, Karimova A, et al (2001) Paradoxical rescue from ischemic lung injury by inhaled carbon monoxide driven by derepression of fibrinolysis. Nat Med 7:598–604
47. Sato K, Balla J, Otterbein L, et al (2001) Carbon monoxide generated by heme oxygenase-1 suppresses the rejection of mouse-to-rat cardiac transplants. J Immunol 166:4185–4194
48. Mazzola S, Forni M, Albertini M, et al (2005) Carbon monoxide pretreatment prevents respiratory derangement and ameliorates hyperacute endotoxic shock in pigs. FASEB J 19:2045–2047
49. Matarese G, Moschos S, Mantzoros CS (2005) Leptin in immunology. J Immunol 174:3137–3142
50. Dal Pizzol F, Di Leone LP, Ritter C, et al (2006) Gastrin-releasing peptide receptor antagonist effects on an animal model of sepsis. Am J Respir Crit Care Med 173:84–90
51. Dugo L, Collin M, Allen DA, et al (2005) GSK-3beta inhibitors attenuate the organ injury/dysfunction caused by endotoxemia in the rat. Crit Care Med 33:1903–1912
52. Van der Poll T, Bueller HR, ten Cate H, et al (1990) Activation of coagulation after administration of tumor necrosis factor to normal subjects. N Engl J Med 322:1622–1626
53. Sfeir T, Saha DC, Astiz M, et al (2001) Role of interleukin-10 in monocyte hyporesponsiveness associated with septic shock. Crit Care Med 29:129–133
54. von Knethen A, Tautenhahn A, Link H, et al (2005) Activation-induced depletion of protein kinase C alpha provokes desensitization of monocytes/macrophages in sepsis. J Immunol 174:4960–4965
55. Wesselkamper SC, Case LM, Henning LN, et al (2005) Gene expression changes during the development of acute lung injury: role of transforming growth factor beta. Am J Respir Crit Care Med 172:1399–1411
56. Yang H, Tracey KJ (2005) High mobility group box 1 (HMGB1). Crit Care Med 33:S472–S474
57. Leng L, Bucala R (2005) Macrophage migration inhibitory factor. Crit Care Med 33:S475–S477
58. Marshall JC (2005) Neutrophils in the pathogenesis of sepsis. Crit Care Med 33:S502–S505
59. Rice P, Martin E, He JR, et al (2005) Febrile-range hyperthermia augments neutrophil accumulation and enhances lung injury in experimental gram-negative bacterial pneumonia. J Immunol 174:3676–3685
60. Schulman CI, Namias N, Doherty J, et al (2005) The effect of antipyretic therapy upon outcomes in critically ill patients: a randomized, prospective study. Surg Infect (Larchmt) 6:369–375
61. Clifton GL, Miller ER, Choi SC, et al (2001) Lack of effect of induction of hypothermia after acute brain injury. N Engl J Med 344:556–563

62. Ware LB, Matthay MA (2000) The acute respiratory distress syndrome. N Engl J Med 342:1334–1349
63. De Backer D, Creteur J, Preiser JC, et al (2002) Microvascular blood flow is altered in patients with sepsis. Am J Respir Crit Care Med 166:98–104
64. McVerry BJ, Peng X, Hassoun PM, et al (2004) Sphingosine 1-phosphate reduces vascular leak in murine and canine models of acute lung injury. Am J Respir Crit Care Med 170:987–993
65. Mura M, Dos Santos CC, Stewart D, et al (2004) Vascular endothelial growth factor and related molecules in acute lung injury. J Appl Physiol 97:1605–1617
66. Burnham EL, Taylor WR, Quyyumi AA, et al (2005) Increased circulating endothelial pro-genitor cells are associated with survival in acute lung injury. Am J Respir Crit Care Med 172:854–860
67. Imai Y, Kuba K, Rao S, et al (2005) Angiotensin-converting enzyme 2 protects from severe acute lung failure. Nature 436:112–116
68. Brell B, Hippenstiel S, David I, et al (2005) Adrenomedullin treatment abolishes ileal mucosal hypoperfusion induced by Staphylococcus aureus alpha-toxin – an intravital microscopic study on an isolated rat ileum. Crit Care Med 33:2810–016
69. Scherpereel A, Depontieu F, Grigoriu B, et al (2006) Endocan, a new endothelial marker in human sepsis. Crit Care Med 34:532–537
70. Dixon B, Santamaria J, Campbell D (2005) Coagulation activation and organ dysfunction following cardiac surgery. Chest 128:229–236
71. Vadasz I, Morty RE, Olschewski A, et al (2005) Thrombin impairs alveolar fluid clearance by promoting endocytosis of Na+,K+-ATPase. Am J Respir Cell Mol Biol 33:343–354
72. Bernard GR, Vincent JL, Laterre PF, et al (2001) Efficacy and safety of recombinant human activated protein C for severe sepsis. N Engl J Med 344:699–709
73. Warren BL, Eid A, Singer P, et al (2001) Caring for the critically ill patient. High-dose antithrombin III in severe sepsis: a randomized controlled trial. J A M A 286:1869–1878
74. Abraham E, Reinhart K, Opal S, et al (2003) Efficacy and safety of tifacogin (recombinant tissue factor pathway inhibitor) in severe sepsis: a randomized controlled trial. J A M A 290:238–247
75. Macias WL, Yan SB, Williams MD, et al (2005) New insights into the protein C pathway: potential implications for the biological activities of drotrecogin alfa (activated). Crit Care 9 Suppl 4:S38–S45
76. Mosnier LO, Gale AJ, Yegneswaran S, et al (2004) Activated protein C variants with normal cytoprotective but reduced anticoagulant activity. Blood 104:1740–1744
77. Matthay MA, Robriquet L, Fang X (2005) Alveolar epithelium: role in lung fluid balance and acute lung injury. Proc Am Thorac Soc 2:206–213
78. Fink MP, Delude RL (2005) Epithelial barrier dysfunction: a unifying theme to explain the pathogenesis of multiple organ dysfunction at the cellular level. Crit Care Clin 21:177–196
79. Martin TR, Hagimoto N, Nakamura M, et al (2005) Apoptosis and epithelial injury in the lungs. Proc Am Thorac Soc 2:214–220
80. Carrico CJ, Meakins JL, Marshall JC, et al (1986) Multiple organ failure syndrome. Arch Surg 121:196–208
81. Holland J, Carey M, Hughes N, et al (2005) Intraoperative splanchnic hypoperfusion, in-creased intestinal permeability, down-regulation of monocyte class II major histocom-patibility complex expression, exaggerated acute phase response, and sepsis. Am J Surg 190:393–400
82. De Backer D, Creteur J, Silva E, et al (2003) Effects of dopamine, norepinephrine, and epinephrine on the splanchnic circulation in septic shock: Which is best? Crit Care Med 31:1659–1667
83. de Jonge E, Schultz MJ, Spanjaard L, et al (2003) Effects of selective decontamination of the digestive tract on mortality and the acquisition of resistant bacteria in intensive care patients. Lancet 362:1011–1016

84. Lopau K, Mark J, Schramm L, et al (2000) Hormonal changes in brain death and immune activation in the donor. Transpl Int 13 Suppl 1:S282–S285
85. Trentz OA, Handschin AE, Bestmann L, et al (2005) Influence of brain injury on early posttraumatic bone metabolism. Crit Care Med 33:399–406
86. Lopez-Aguilar J, Villagra A, Bernabe F, et al (2005) Massive brain injury enhances lung damage in an isolated lung model of ventilator-induced lung injury. Crit Care Med 33:1077–1083
87. Luyer MD, Greve JW, Hadfoune M, et al (2005) Nutritional stimulation of cholecystokinin receptors inhibits inflammation via the vagus nerve. J Exp Med 202:1023–1029
88. Annane D, Sebille V, Charpentier C, et al (2002) Effect of treatment with low doses of hydrocortisone and fludrocortisone on mortality in patients with septic shock. J A M A 288:862–871
89. Van den Berghe G, Wouters P, Weekers F, et al (2001) Intensive insulin therapy in the critically ill patient. N Engl J Med 345:1359–1367
90. Turina M, Fry DE, Polk HC, Jr. (2005) Acute hyperglycemia and the innate immune system: clinical, cellular, and molecular aspects. Crit Care Med 33:1624–1633
91. Catalan MP, Reyero A, Egido J, et al (2001) Acceleration of neutrophil apoptosis by glucose-containing peritoneal dialysis solutions: role of caspases. J Am Soc Nephrol 12:2442–2449
92. Altannavch TS, Roubalova K, Kucera P, et al (2004) Effect of high glucose concentrations on expression of ELAM-1, VCAM-1 and ICAM-1 in HUVEC with and without cytokine activation. Physiol Res 53:77–82
93. Zuurbier CJ, Demirci C, Koeman A, et al (2005) Short-term hyperglycemia increases endothelial glycocalyx permeability and acutely decreases lineal density of capillaries with flowing red blood cells. J Appl Physiol 99:1471–1476
94. Vanhorebeek I, de Vos R, Mesotten D, et al (2005) Protection of hepatocyte mitochondrial ultrastructure and function by strict blood glucose control with insulin in critically ill patients. Lancet 365:53–59
95. Langouche L, Vanhorebeek I, Vlasselaers D, et al (2005) Intensive insulin therapy protects the endothelium of critically ill patients. J Clin Invest 115:2277–2286
96. Dandona P, Aljada A, Mohanty P, et al (2001) Insulin inhibits intranuclear nuclear factor kappaB and stimulates IkappaB in mononuclear cells in obese subjects: evidence for an anti-inflammatory effect? J Clin Endocrinol Metab 86:3257–3265
97. Siore AM, Parker RE, Stecenko AA, et al (2005) Endotoxin-induced acute lung injury requires interaction with the liver. Am J Physiol Lung Cell Mol Physiol 289:L769–L776
98. Hayes MA, Timmins AC, Yau EH, et al (1994) Elevation of systemic oxygen delivery in the treatment of critically ill patients. N Engl J Med 330:1717–1722
99. The ARDS Network (2000) Ventilation with lower tidal volumes as compared with traditional tidal volumes for acute lung injury and the acute respiratory distress syndrome. N Engl J Med 342:1301–1308
100. Ranieri VM, Suter PM, Tortorella C, et al (1999) Effect of mechanical ventilation on inflammatory mediators in patients with acute respiratory distress syndrome: a randomized controlled trial. J A M A 282:54–61
101. Charles PE, Etienne M, Croisier D, et al (2005) The impact of mechanical ventilation on the moxifloxacin treatment of experimental pneumonia caused by Streptococcus pneumoniae. Crit Care Med 33:1029–1035
102. Ploppa A, Kiefer RT, Nohe B, et al (2006) Dose-dependent influence of barbiturates but not of propofol on human leukocyte phagocytosis of viable Staphylococcus aureus. Crit Care Med 34:478–483
103. Mehta RL, Pascual MT, Soroko S, et al (2002) Diuretics, mortality, and nonrecovery of renal function in acute renal failure. J A M A 288:2547–2553
104. Yende S, Tuomanen EI, Wunderink R, et al (2005) Preinfection systemic inflammatory markers and risk of hospitalization due to pneumonia. Am J Respir Crit Care Med 172:1440–1446

# The Inflammatory Response

# Genetics and Severe Sepsis

J. Texereau, V. Lemiale, and J.-P. Mira

## Introduction

Despite significant advances in understanding the molecular basis of host-pathogen relationships and associated immunological responses, severe sepsis remain a problem world-wide, associated with multiple organ dysfunctions and elevated mortality [1]. Annually, more than 100,000 people in the USA die from septic shock, the most severe form of sepsis, which thereby represents the most common cause of death in the intensive care unit (ICU). Morbidity and mortality of severe sepsis are usually ascribed to incorrect or delayed diagnosis, inadequate antimicrobial therapy and underlying illnesses [2,3]. More recently, the host-specific immune response has been shown to be another important determinant of outcome of infectious diseases [4]. Genetically-determined differences in immune responses might explain why some people get sick and die when they encounter a pathogen whereas others stay perfectly healthy. The aim of this chapter is to review current knowledge regarding genetic variability associated with increased susceptibility to severe sepsis with emphasis on selected polymorphisms associated with a poor outcome. More extensive reviews have been recently published [4–9].

## Rationale for Genetics in Sepsis and Infectious Diseases

The influence of genetic factors in determining susceptibility and resistance to severe infectious diseases has long been suspected. Numerous reports in animal models, ethnic groups, familial cases, twin and adoptee studies have definitively proved the importance of genetics in severe infections [10].

The use of animal models, which mimic human severe sepsis, is important in elucidating the molecular mechanisms of sepsis. Genetic factors differentiate inbred strains, and epigenetic factors elicit variations within a strain. In this regard, the prevalence of genetic strain differences, contributing to susceptibility to microbial infections has been well recognized in rodents. These models, essentially mice, are genetically well defined and may be easily genetically-modified (using genetically-engineered strains such as knock-outs) to demonstrate the physiological importance of a suspected gene [4,11,12]. The interest in studies of mice lies in the fact that nearly all of the murine genes involved in the response to sepsis have human homologs. Analysis of susceptibility to certain infectious diseases in mice has led to the mapping and identification of candidate genes for human studies. Hence, some groups have shown that Toll-like receptor 2 (TLR2) knock-out mice do not respond to *Staphylococcus aureus* infection. After bacterial challenge, these mice have decreased production of cytokines, increased concentration of bacteria in blood and kidneys, and a higher mortality rate than wild-type mice [13,14]. Similarly, whe ninfected by *Mycobacterium tuberculosis*, TLR2 knock-out mice have deficient bacterial clearance and develop chronic pneumonia [15]. Interestingly, similar susceptibility to *S. aureus* infection and tuberculosis have been reported in human populations carrying TLR2 polymorphisms [16–20]. Identification of the effects in such human states validates the use of murine knockout models to identify key pathways controlling predisposition to infection.

Studies in twins have also provided arguments for 'genetically programmed' susceptibility to infection, when homozygous twins who have the same genome are compared with heterozygous twins who are genetically different. Such studies clearly demonstrate that, in case of infection of the first twin, the risk for the second one to be infected by the same pathogen was higher for homozygous pairs versus heterozygous pairs [21–23].

Estimates of genetic predisposition, independent of environmental effects, have been obtained also from adoptee studies. Sorensen et al. [24] reported a large study of etiologies of premature death in 1,000 families with children adopted early in life. Adoptees with a biological parent who died before the age of 50 from an infectious disease had a 5.8-fold increase in the relative risk of dying from an infection. In contrast, the death of an adoptive parent from an infectious cause had no significant effect on the adoptee's risk of such a death, clearly indicating that host genetic factors are major determinants of susceptibility to infectious diseases [24].

## Genetic Predisposition to Severe Sepsis: Mendelian or Non-Mendelian Genetics?

Genetic predisposition to severe sepsis may be either a monogenic or a complex multifactorial disorder.

### Single Gene Defects

In monogenic diseases, mutation in a single gene is necessary and sufficient to produce the clinical phenotype. More than 100 rare major genetic defects of the immune system have been identified [25–31]. They are most commonly associated with unusual and recurrent bacterial infections detected in childhood. Recent genetic defects have been shown to be responsible for lethal tuberculosis or severe bacterial infections [27]. Thus, predisposition to rare and atypical mycobacteria (*M. cheloniae, M. fortuitum, M. avis*) or disseminated Bacille Calmette-Guerin (BCG) vaccine infections have been described in children that lack either chain of interferon-gamma (IFN-γ) IFN-γ receptor or the interleukin (IL)-12 receptor [32]. Single gene defects provide valuable insights into the molecular and cellular basis of host immunity against specific pathogens.

Even a single mutated locus may generate a large spectrum of phenotypes in terms of disease severity. Cystic fibrosis is a classical example of such a monogenic trait with more than 1,000 identified mutations in the cystic fibrosis transmembrane conductance regulator (*CFTR*) gene [33]. Each of these mutations has been associated with the development of clinical signs of cystic fibrosis, but large variations in the severity of the phenotype exist for each genotype. Indeed, modifying the effects of other genes may result in marked variations in the symptoms of patients with the same disease [34].

## Complex Multifactorial Disorders

Common diseases, such as diabetes, asthma or hypertension, are thought to result from a combination of diverse genetic and environmental factors [35]. Genetic predisposition to severe sepsis is also considered to be a non-Mendelian disease [10]. These complex diseases differ dramatically from illnesses associated with single-gene defects. The complexity of common diseases results from the fact that penetrance (the frequency at which a genotype gives rise to a disease) is highly variable. Hence, even if an identical twin has a multi-factorial disease, the second twin may not develop the trait.

Additional definitions are necessary to understand the molecular basis of genetic predisposition to severe sepsis. A *polymorphism* is a region of the genome that varies between individual members of a population and is present in more than 1% of the population. A *single nucleotide polymorphism* (SNP) is a polymorphism caused by the change of a single nucleotide. The difference may be an inversion (G to C or A to T), a transition (G/C to A/T or inverse), an insertion or a deletion of one base. Most genetic variations between individual humans are believed to be due to SNPs, but other variants are important, such as duplicate genes or repeat DNA sequences. Humans carry two sets of chromosomes, one from each parent. Equivalent genes in the two sets might be different, because of SNPs or other polymorphisms. An *allele* is one of the two (or more) forms of a particular gene. A particular combination of alleles or sequence variations that are closely linked on the same chromosome is named *haplotype*.

Complex diseases, such as sepsis, are characteristically caused by interacting genetic and environmental determinants. To identify genes that might confer susceptibility or resistance to severe sepsis, different approaches may be used depending on historical evidence, ease of recruiting study populations, and cost of genotyping [36]. Currently, most studies in the field of sepsis are association genetic studies. These involve a binary disease trait (such as development of septic shock, acute respiratory distress syndrome [ARDS], multiple organ failure [MOF], or mortality) and a functional gene with two alleles. They require an adequate number of unrelated individuals to have been typed for the gene of interest and classed as having, or not having, the trait and have to fulfill all recommended criteria from published guidelines [37, 38].

The validity of genetic association studies relies on basic rules [39]. Studied populations have to be homogeneous: allele frequencies and frequency-dependent measures like linkage disequilibrium can only be estimated accurately from properly identified and sampled populations. Control groups should be in Hardy-Weinberg equilibrium. Sample design is crucial and an adequate study size and study power are also necessary to exclude false conclusions. Definition of the phenotype is a key issue in the design of any genetic study whose goal is to detect gene(s) involved in the course of the disease. For example, selecting more severely ill septic patients without significant comorbidities may help to identify the candidate genes responsible for septic shock. Inclusion of patients with severe co-morbidities or who received treatment that can contribute to mortality, such as inappropriate antibiotics, can lead to false negative studies. Despite these limitations, association study design is simple and provides high power to detect common genetic variants that confer susceptibility to sepsis. However, interpretation of their results is complex (Table 1).

**Table 1.** Interpretations of genetic association studies

1) Significant association:
  a) True positive association
    Variant is causal
    Variant is in linkage disequilibrium with causal variant
  b) False positive association
    False positive due to multiple testing
    False positive due to systematic genotyping error
    False positive due to population stratification or other confounder

2) Reasons for lack of replication
  a) Original report is a false positive
  b) False negative
    Phenotypes differ across studies
    Study populations differ in genetic or environmental background
    Replication study is under powered

## Genetic Polymorphisms in Severe Sepsis and Septic Shock

Antimicrobial host defense is a complex process that relies both on innate and adaptive components [40, 41]. The generation of a large repertoire of antigen-recognition receptors and immune memory, hallmarks of acquired immunity, depends on the presence of an efficient innate immunity. Hence, innate immunity represents the first-line of host defense necessary to limit infection in the early hours after pathogen invasion and controls adaptive immune responses. Early protection against microorganisms involves three mechanisms: 1) recognition of the pathogen; 2) phagocytosis and elimination of invading microorganisms; and 3) development of an inflammatory response necessary for resolution of the infection. Each step of this immune reaction may be affected by gene polymorphisms of individual components of the immune system which lead to susceptibility or resistance to infection and have been associated with organ failure and/or risk of death [42].

## Gene Polymorphisms Altering Pathogen Recognition (Table 2)

Table 2. Gene polymorphisms modifying pathogen recognition receptors

| Gene | Polymorphisms | Type of Infection |
|---|---|---|
| MBL | Codon 52, 54, 57 | Respiratory infections, meningococcal disease, pneumococcal disease, sepsis in ICU |
| Fc-γRIIA | H131R | Meningococcal disease, pneumococcal disease, SARS infection, cerebral malaria |
| CD14 | C159T | Septic shock |
| TLR5 | | Legionnaire's disease |
| TLR4 | D299G | Gram negative sepsis, malaria |
| TLR2 | R753Q | Gram positive sepsis, Borrelia sepsis, tuberculosis, Leprosy |
| CCR5 | CCR5-Δ32 | HIV-1 'resistance' |

Throughout evolution, innate immunity has developed a very efficient system that recognizes invariant molecular constituents of infectious agents called pathogen-associated molecular patterns (PAMPs) [40]. This system of detection is currently referred to as pattern recognition receptors (PRR) and can be divided into three classes: 1) soluble receptors, such as mannose binding lectin (MBL) and the components of the complement system; 2) endocytic receptors, such as Fcγ receptors and scavenger receptors (including MARCO and DC-SIGN); and 3) and signaling receptors such as TLR and nucleotide-binding oligomerization domain (NOD) receptors. Almost all of these receptors have functional polymorphisms that have been associated with increased susceptibility to severe infections primarily through decreased clearance of pathogens. However, only MBL and CD14 variants are potentially associated with the severity of, and mortality from, septic shock.

## Mannose Binding Lectin

MBL is a member of the collectin family of proteins. This calcium-dependent plasma lectin binds to sugars and possibly endotoxin on microbial surfaces, and then activates complement, acting as a so-called ante-antibody [9]. MBL can also directly act as an opsonin and bind to specific receptors expressed on the cell surface of various cell types, including monocytes, thereby potentiating TLR responses.

Thus, MBL clearly appears to be a pluripotent molecule of the innate immune system.

For maximal efficacy, proteins of the innate immune system have to be present at physiologically significant levels. The concentrations of MBL in human plasma are genetically determined and are profoundly reduced by either structural gene mutations or by promoter gene polymorphisms [43]. Three different alleles, resulting in structurally variant proteins, have been identified in codons 52, 54 and 57 of the exon 1 of the MBL gene. Structural variants within the MBL gene are common, with frequencies ranging between 0.11 and 0.29, and reduce complement activation independent of the MBL plasma level. Whereas MBL deficiencies can be explained by these three mutations, these structural gene mutations do not explain why MBL serum levels vary so widely between individuals. Genetic variations have also been detected in the promoter region of the MBL gene. These variations have been reported to control the plasma levels of structurally normal MBL [43]. In particular, G to C inversions at position −550 or −221 in the promoter region are associated with varying expression levels of MBL. Furthermore, these SNPs are always linked with the structural variants in most populations creating relevant haplotypes. As an example, the median serum concentrations of MBL for Caucasians were found to be 1,630 ng/ml for wild-type genotype; 358 ng/ml in patients heterozygous for the codon 54 mutation; and 10 ng/ml in patients homozygous for the codon 54 mutation.

A large number of studies have attempted to define the role of MBL in predisposing to severe infection [9]. Hibberd et al. reported a large cohort of patients with meningococcal disease admitted to a pediatric ICU and a second cohort of children who had survived meningococcal disease in the UK [44]. Both studies showed a clear association between MBL polymorphisms and susceptibility to meningococcal disease, with an odds ratio (OR) of 6.5 for the homozygous patients in the hospital study and of 4.5 in the national study. Heterozygous patients were also at increased risk of meningococcal infection, but to a lesser degree since the OR ranged from 1.7 in the hospital study to 2.2 in the national study. Using the population attributable fraction assessment, it is possible to calculate that gene variants could account for as many as a third of meningococcal disease cases. Similarly in the UK, adult patients homozygous for MBL structural variants, who represent about 5% of northern Europeans and North Americans, have a substantially increased risk of developing invasive pneumococcal disease [45]. Furthermore, in 272 prospectively monitored critically ill patients with systemic inflammatory response syndrome (SIRS), the presence of MBL variant alleles was associated with the development of sepsis, severe sepsis, and septic shock. An increased risk of fatal outcome was observed in patients carrying variant alleles [46]. All these data show that genetic variants contributing to inadequate MBL levels play an important role in the susceptibility of critically ill patients to the development and progression of severe sepsis and confer a substantial risk of fatal outcome.

## Fcγ Receptor Polymorphism and Encapsulated Bacteria Infections

Antibodies, antibody receptors, and complement are essential components in defense against invasive encapsulated bacteria (*S. pneumoniae, Haemophilus influenzae, Neisseria meningitidis*). Fcγ receptors are located on the phagocytic cell surface, bind the Fc region of IgG, and mediate binding, phagocytosis, and destruction of bacteria opsonized with IgG. Certain genetically determined variations of IgG receptors on neutrophils (FcγIIa, FcγIIIb) as well as monocytes and macrophages (FcγIIa, FcγIIIa) are associated with reduced binding of antibodies and an increased risk of bacteremia and meningitis. In a study of 50 surviving meningococcal disease patients, 183 first-degree relatives of patients with meningococcal disease, and 239 healthy controls, the combination of low affinity polymorphisms of FcγIIa, FcγIIIa, and FcγIIIb was present significantly more often in relatives of patients than in the healthy control group [47]. Moreover, the distribution of FcγIIa and FcγIIIa differed between patients presenting with sepsis and those presenting with meningitis.

## LPS Complex Receptor

Lipopolysaccharide (LPS) recognition by TLR4 on the cell surface is achieved in cooperation with several protein components, including LPS-binding protein (LBP), CD14, and MD-2, and leads to the activation of nuclear transcription factors, such as nuclear factor-kappa B (NF-κB) [40]. Modulation of cytokine expression as a result of the initial host–microbial interaction is important in the pathophysiology of sepsis. TLR4, CD14, and MD-2 have been reported to have polymorphic sites associated with altered functioning of the LPS receptor complex and with susceptibility to severe sepsis [27,48].

In 2000, Arbour et al. identified two polymorphisms of the TLR4 gene (Asp299Gly and Thr399Ile), associated with hyporesponsivness to inhaled LPS in humans [49]. In 2002, Lorenz and colleagues studied the association between these two mutations and the outcome of patients with septic shock. First, these authors genotyped 91 patients with septic shock and 73 healthy controls. They found that the TLR4 Asp299Gly allele was present exclusively in patients with septic shock and also that patients with the TLR4 Asp299Gly/Thr399Ile co-mutation had a higher prevalence of Gram-negative infections [50]. Other studies have confirmed this result and shown that these variants are associated with mortality in SIRS [51]. Interestingly, these two frequent SNPs showed no association with susceptibility to, or severity of, meningococcal disease, although rare TLR4 mutations have been implicated in meningococcal susceptibility [52]. Despite these reports and the central role played by TLR4 in the development of Gram-negative sepsis, additional controlled studies, with increased numbers of patients are required to determine whether TLR4 SNPs are associated with risk or severity of Gram-negative sepsis.

The CD14 gene contains a promoter polymorphism (–159C/T) that has been reported to modulate both the density of CD14 expression on the membrane of monocytes and circulating levels of soluble CD14. CD14-159C/T polymorphisms have been reported to be associated with susceptibility to septic shock and with the mortality rate from this condition [53–55]. However, evidence against this association has been found in trauma patients with severe sepsis as a secondary complication [56]. As mentioned above, the disparity in the results from these studies may be due to study differences, including the number of patients analyzed, the types of patients included (trauma, pneumonia, surgery), and heterogeneity in the patient populations (ethnicity or co-morbidities).

## Gene Polymorphisms Modifying the Inflammatory Immune Response

The inflammatory reaction is an essential component of host defense mechanisms. Inflammation is tightly regulated by mediators that initiate and maintain the inflammatory process as well as others required for its resolution [57]. Cytokines are key protein regulators of inflammation. These small proteins, with molecular weights ranging from 8 to 40 kDa, are primarily involved in host response to infection and inflammation. Cytokines initiate and orchestrate immune reactions as local and/or systemic intercellular regulatory factors. Within minutes of an infectious challenge, pro-inflammatory cytokines, such as tumor necrosis factor (TNF)-α, IL-1, and IL-6, are secreted leading to strong activation of monocytes, chemokine-recruited polymorphonuclear cells, and endothelial cells. This initial pro-inflammatory state is followed by release of anti-inflammatory cytokines, such as IL-10, and inhibitory proteins, such as IL-1 receptor antagonist (IL-1ra), which are able to suppress the expression or actions of pro-inflammatory cytokines, chemokines, or adhesion molecules. Both pro-inflammatory and anti-inflammatory cytokines co-exist in infected sites and in the bloodstream in markedly increased amounts. Their relative concentrations correlate with the severity and the outcome of septic shock [40, 57, 58].

In humans, most cytokine genes are polymorphic and there is increasing evidence that the host's cytokine production is genetically determined [59]. Since most cytokines are not expressed spontaneously and have to be synthesized *de novo* in response to pathogens, functional promoter variants of their genes can have dramatic consequences. Hence, genetic variability of cytokines underlies the complexity of interindividual differences in the immune response to microbial invasion.

## Pro-inflammatory Cytokines: TNF-α

TNF-α is a pro-inflammatory cytokine with a central role in many inflammatory diseases, including severe sepsis and septic shock. TNF may be produced by many different cell types and is one of the first mediators to appear in response to a diverse range of infectious stimuli. Once secreted, TNF-α elicits a wide spectrum of immune and inflammatory responses responsible for fever, shock, and tissue injury, and induces the release of additional inflammatory mediators, including other cytokines, nitric oxide (NO), and free oxygen radicals, and up-regulates adhesion molecule expression. Neutralization of TNF production by anti-TNF antibodies or in TNF-knock-out mice has been associated with increased mortality in several models of infection, demonstrating that TNF is a critical mediator of host defense against infection [60]. However, TNF may cause severe pathology when produced in excess. *In vivo* injection of TNF produces clinical manifestations mimicking those observed after injection of bacteria. Hemodynamic disturbances and mortality have been shown to be correlated with TNF plasma levels. Hence, excessive production of TNF may be associated with tissue injury, shock, and death due to an imbalance between pro-inflammatory and anti-inflammatory cytokines.

Given TNF's role as a central element in the host defense response, its production has to be tightly regulated to preserve cellular homeostasis. Interestingly, marked inter-individual variability in TNF production in response to different stimuli has been reported in healthy subjects. Since the TNF response to infection is partly regulated at the transcriptional level, TNF promoter polymorphisms have been the subject of intense research and are probably the most extensively studied of all cytokines involved in sepsis pathophysiology (more than 25 publications).

Two polymorphisms in the TNF-α locus have been linked to variability in TNF production. The first TNF-α polymorphism consists of a G (called TNF1) to A (called TNF2) 308 base pairs upstream from the transcriptional start of *TNFA*. TNF2 was associated with higher TNF-α secretion than TNF1. The second TNF-α polymorphism is located within the *TNFB* gene, but still affects TNF-α synthesis. It was identified in 1991 by Pociot et al. who reported a biallelic *NcoI* restriction enzyme fragment length polymorphism (RFLP) in the TNF gene locus that was associated with increased TNF-α production [61]. This site has been mapped to the first intron of the LT gene (*TNFB*) at position +250 and allows the definition of two alleles, TNFB1 and TNFB2. The latter does not possess the *NcoI* RFLP and seems to be associated with increased TNF-α plasma concentrations. The precise mechanisms underlying this result remain unclear; the *NcoI* polymorphism may not be directly related to TNF production, but rather serve as a major histocompatibility complex (MHC) marker because of its location in the class III region of the MHC. Significant linkage disequilibrium between the two TNF SNPs has been reported with almost all individuals homozygous for TNFB2 (high TNF producer) also being homozygous for TNF1 (low TNF producer), adding some complexity to the final schema of TNF production [62].

Both TNF2 and TNFB2 polymorphisms have been associated with greater severity and worse outcome in a variety of infectious diseases. For example, TNF2 was described as an independent risk factor for cerebral malaria in large case-control studies of African populations [63]. Homozygosity for the TNF2 allele is associated with a relative risk of 6.8 for death or severe neurological sequelae due to cerebral malaria. A strong association has also been reported between TNF polymorphisms and mucocutaneous leishmaniasis, scarring trachoma, lepromatous leprosy, nephropathia epidemica, and with death from meningococcal disease, severe meliodosis, community-acquired pneumonia, and septic shock [64]. In septic shock, the TNF2 allele increases the risk of death by 3.7 fold even after controlling for age and severity of illness [65]. TNF2 is also clearly associated with increased mortality from sepsis in neonates and ventilated, very low birth weight infants [66]. However, other studies have failed to demonstrate associations between either TNF2 or TNFB2 and mortality [67]. This discordance may arise, at least in part, from methodological problems such as incorrect genotype assignment and differences in study populations or inclusion and exclusion criteria [68].

## Anti-inflammatory Cytokine SNPs: IL-10

Sepsis induces an initial pro-inflammatory response followed by an important release of anti-inflammatory cytokines (IL-4, IL-10, IL-13) responsible for a down-regulation of humoral and cellular immunity that has been called immunoparalysis or compensatory anti-inflammatory response syndrome (CARS). Genetic polymorphisms responsible for uncontrolled and intense CARS may have the same dramatic consequences on outcome from sepsis as an overwhelming inflammatory response.

IL-10 is expressed and secreted by a variety of cell types, including T and B cells, monocytes/macrophages, and epithelial cells, usually after an activation stimulus such as infection. It suppresses the function of macrophages (down-regulation of Th1 cytokines) and indirectly inhibits the activity of B cells. High IL-10 production also inhibits IFN-γ expression and delays clearance of intracellular pathogens, such as Chlamydia [69]. The potent anti-inflammatory effects of IL-10 indicate that this cytokine might play a crucial role in both the resolution and pathogenesis of severe sepsis and septic shock. Concentrations of IL-10 correlate with the severity of the inflammatory response as assessed by the APACHE score, MOF, or death [70,71]. The risk of fatal outcome from meningococcal disease is increased in families with high IL-10 production. Although both genetic and non-genetic factors contribute to IL-10 production, twin studies suggest that genetics could account for up to 75% of the variability in IL-10 production [72,73].

The human IL-10 gene demonstrates several polymorphisms resulting in interindividual differences in cytokine production. Within the IL-10 proximal promoter, two CA-repeat microsatellites, and three SNPs at −1,082 (G/A), −819 (C/T), −592 (C/A) upstream of the transcription start site, have been reported [69]. More SNPs in the distal IL-10 promoter have been identified recently with either a high- or a low IL-10 production phenotype, thereby creating eight distal promoter haplotypes [74]. *In vitro*, the IL10-1082G polymorphism has been associated with high IL-10 production by lymphocytes. Within the Mandikas ethnic group, the IL10-1082G homozygous genotype is significantly more common among trachoma patients than controls (odds ratio 5.1; confidence interval, 1.24–24.2; $p = 0.009$) [75]. In contrast, the IL10-1082G allele appears to be more common in persons with mildly symptomatic or asymptomatic Epstein-Barr Virus (EBV) diseases than in patients with EBV infections requiring hospitalization [76]. These findings suggest that high IL-10 producers are partially protected from severe EBV infection and show clearly that changes at the level of a given cytokine do not exert the same effects on all infectious agents. This may explain why the results from genetic association studies of IL-10 polymorphisms in sepsis are contradictory.

The IL-10 −1,082 G/G genotype, which is linked with greater expression of IL-10, has been associated with higher severity scores and worse outcome in patients with community-acquired pneumonia [77]. Similarly, another IL-10 polymorphism (the −592 A allele, associated with low levels of IL-10) was associated with death both in patients with sepsis and in critically ill patients without sepsis [78]. In that study, although the IL-10 −1,082 allele frequencies were significantly different between cases and controls at admission to an ICU, no association was observed between the IL-10 −1,082 allele and the risk of death from sepsis. Recently, a new IL-10 haplotype, −592C/734G/3367G, has been associated with increased mortality and organ dysfunction in critically ill patients with sepsis secondary to a pulmonary source of infection, but not in similarly ill patients with extrapulmonary sepsis [79]. Overall, the data suggesting a role for genetic variation in the IL-10 gene on death due to severe sepsis remain inconsistent.

## Hemostatic Gene Polymorphisms and Severe Sepsis

The inflammatory response observed during severe sepsis leads to a strong activation of coagulation and fibrinolysis. However, early increases in the anticoagulant tissue plasminogen activator are rapidly followed by sustained elevations in plasminogen-activator-inhibitor-1 (PAI-1) leading to a prolonged antifibrinolytic and a net procoagulant state. Activation of coagulation together with inhibition of fibrinolysis are responsible for the development of fibrin deposition and microthrombi that cause extensive endothelial damage associated with MOF [57]. High plasma concentrations of PAI-1 have been associated with an adverse outcome in patients with sepsis and septic shock [8]. Several polymorphisms have been described within the human PAI gene, which is located on chromosome 7, including a common single-base-pair polymorphism (four or five guanine bases) in the promoter region of the gene, 675 bp upstream of the transcriptional start site (4G/5G). The 4G allele (or deletion polymorphism) has been associated with higher plasma concentrations of PAI-1. Individuals homozygous for the 4G allele have higher basal and inducible concentrations of PAI-1 than those with one or two copies of the 5G allele that contains an additional G at location −675 of the PAI-1 promoter gene (insertion polymorphism) [52]. In addition to its antifibrinolytic properties, the 4G PAI-1 variant also seems to influence pro-inflammatory cytokine production. The 4G/4G patients not only had higher PAI-1 concentrations, but also demonstrated significantly higher plasma levels of TNF-$\alpha$ and IL-1 compared to the other genotypes [80]. Emonts et al. confirmed, in a population of 175 children with meningococcal disease and 226 controls, that those with the 4G/4G genotype had significantly higher PAI-1 concentrations compared to those with the 4G/5G or 5G/5G genotype (1051 [550-2440] versus 370 [146-914] ng/ml, $p < 0.0001$). In addition, the 4G/4G patients had an increased relative risk of death (2.0; 95% CI 1.0–3.8) [52]. Three studies reported similar results, indicating that the PAI-1 'deletion' promoter polymorphism influences the prognosis of meningo-coccal disease and severely injured patients [80–82]. The latter study investigated the relationship between outcome from severe trauma and the PAI-1 genotype; it found that 58% of injured patients with the 4G/4G genotype died, whereas only 28% with the heterozygous genotype 4G/5G and 15% of patients with genotype 5G/5G did not survive [80].

## Perspectives and Conclusions

Severe sepsis is a complex multifactorial and polygenic disorder that is thought to result from an interaction between an individual's genetic makeup, co-morbidities (such as diabetes mellitus, obesity, cardiac failure), and environmental factors, such as the invasive microorganism responsible for the infection. In recent years, several studies have correlated genetic variations with the risk of, or outcome from, severe sepsis. However, the results of these studies are too inconsistent to enable useful conclusions to be drawn. This inconsistency can be attributed to the heterogeneity of the selected patients, the methods used to select cases and controls, study sizes, the genetic (racial) makeup of the populations studied, and the variability of the microorganisms causing the infections. As more and more polymorphisms are reported, the real multigenic scope of severe sepsis will emerge, and the polymorphisms present in an individual will have increasingly complex clinical implications. The development of technologies that allow high-throughput, fast, and low-cost genotyping will lead to greater insights into host susceptibility at the level of the individual patient.

Genetic markers are not like most biological markers that have wide ranges of values that overlap in people with and without a disease; rather, they are either present or absent. However, the interactions between environmental effects and the molecular mechanisms that influence outcome from sepsis remain poorly understood. An inherited predisposition to sepsis may remain clinically silent until an additional environmental factor occurs. Large-scale association studies that examine many polymorphisms simultaneously are required to allow reliable predictions to be made concerning the risks incurred by genetic factors in severe infection.

As genetic screening to evaluate the individual risk factors for infectious diseases becomes available, insights into the molecular interaction between a pathogen and its host will reveal novel molecular targets for drugs or vaccines. Increased understanding of molecular medicine will shift clinical practice from empirical treatment to therapy based on specific cellular mechanisms of infectious disease. Such approaches are already used in oncology, in which genetic testing can clearly identify persons at high risk, allowing for targeted intervention while sparing the personal and economic cost of unnecessary intervention in those who do not carry a relevant mutation. Detection of the genetic differences which affect drug response, commonly referred to as pharmacogenomics, may also result in further classification of diseases, and consequently, the development of 'personalized' therapies.

Another important consequence of the development of genomics will be to begin incorporating genetic markers into severity scores and the design of clinical trials. A diagnosis that lacks sufficient power often results in treatment failure. Other factors such as the genetic characteristics of the host (polymorphisms in genes regulating drug bioavailability or in genes regulating production of the target) can also contribute to a heterogeneous response to therapy in a group of patients. Genetic screening and improved understanding of host–pathogen interactions will allow selection of the best treatment option for a given patient.

The last, but not the least important, point to consider concerns the ethical implications of research on the human genome. When the Human Genome Project was launched in 1990, a parallel program named ELSI (Ethical, Legal, and Social Implications) was established, to identify the various consequences of genetic information being available. Among its goals, ELSI includes practical ethical issues, such as preparation of guidelines for clinicians and enhancing public awareness of the ethical issues related to the human genome project. Whereas research into the genetic predisposition to severe sepsis could have beneficial effects, it also carries with it important ethical issues, such as the use of presymptomatic screening, as well as possible subsequent social discrimination due to 'at-risk polymorphisms'. Genetic data should not be used to predict outcomes or limit treatments; rather, identification of high-risk patients should help us to look for new preventive and therapeutic interventions for those who need them most [83, 84].

## References

1. Martin GS, Mannino DM, Eaton S, Moss M (2003) The epidemiology of sepsis in the United States from 1979 through 2000. N Engl J Med 348:1546–1554
2. Alberti C, Brun-Buisson C, Burchardi H, et al (2002) Epidemiology of sepsis and infection in ICU patients from an international multicentre cohort study. Intensive Care Med 28:108–121
3. Angus DC, Linde-Zwirble WT, Lidicker J, Clermont G, Carcillo J, Pinsky MR (2001) Epidemiology of severe sepsis in the United States: analysis of incidence, outcome, and associated costs of care. Crit Care Med 29:1303–1310
4. De Maio A, Torres MB, Reeves RH (2005) Genetic determinants influencing the response to injury, inflammation, and sepsis. Shock 23:11–17
5. Arcaroli J, Fessler MB, Abraham E (2005) Genetic polymorphisms and sepsis. Shock 24:300–312
6. Dahmer MK, Randolph A, Vitali S, Quasney MW (2005) Genetic polymorphisms in sepsis. Pediatr Crit Care Med 6:S61–73
7. Texereau J, Chiche JD, Taylor W, Choukroun G, Comba B, Mira JP (2005) The importance of Toll-like receptor 2 polymorphisms in severe infections. Clin Infect Dis 41 (Suppl 7):S408–415
8. Texereau J, Pene F, Chiche JD, Rousseau C, Mira JP (2004) Importance of hemostatic gene polymorphisms for susceptibility to and outcome of severe sepsis. Crit Care Med 32:S313–319
9. Worthley DL, Bardy PG, Mullighan CG (2005) Mannose-binding lectin: biology and clinical implications. Intern Med J 35:548–555
10. Frodsham AJ, Hill AV (2004) Genetics of infectious diseases. Hum Mol Genet 13 Spec No 2:R187–194

11. Hernandez-Valladares M, Naessens J, Iraqi FA (2005) Genetic resistance to malaria in mouse models. Trends Parasitol 21:352–355

12. Stewart D, Fulton WB, Wilson C, et al (2002) Genetic contribution to the septic response in a mouse model. Shock 18:342–347

13. Knuefermann P, Sakata Y, Baker JS, et al (2004) Toll-like receptor 2 mediates Staphylococcus aureus-induced myocardial dysfunction and cytokine production in the heart. Circulation 110:3693–3698

14. Takeuchi O, Hoshino K, Kawai T, et al (1999) Differential roles of TLR2 and TLR4 in recognition of gram-negative and gram-positive bacterial cell wall components. Immunity 11:443–451

15. Drennan MB, Nicolle D, Quesniaux VJ, et al (2004) Toll-like receptor 2-deficient mice succumb to Mycobacterium tuberculosis infection. Am J Pathol 164:49–57

16. Ben-Ali M, Barbouche MR, Bousnina S, Chabbou A, Dellagi K (2004) Toll-like receptor 2 Arg677Trp polymorphism is associated with susceptibility to tuberculosis in Tunisian patients. Clin Diagn Lab Immunol 11:625–626

17. Bochud PY, Hawn TR, Aderem A (2003) Cutting edge: a Toll-like receptor 2 polymorphism that is associated with lepromatous leprosy is unable to mediate mycobacterial signaling. J Immunol 170:3451–3454

18. Kang TJ, Chae GT (2001) Detection of Toll-like receptor 2 (TLR2) mutation in the lepromatous leprosy patients. FEMS Immunol Med Microbiol 31:53–58

19. Lorenz E, Mira JP, Cornish KL, Arbour NC, Schwartz DA (2000) A novel polymorphism in the toll-like receptor 2 gene and its potential association with staphylococcal infection. Infect Immun 68:6398–6401

20. Ogus AC, Yoldas B, Ozdemir T, et al (2004) The Arg753GLn polymorphism of the human toll-like receptor 2 gene in tuberculosis disease. Eur Respir J 23:219–223

21. Lin WJ, Wang CC, Lo WT, Chu ML, Lee CM (2005) Dizygotic twins discordant for early-onset Citrobacter koseri and group B streptococcal sepsis. J Formos Med Assoc 104:367–369

22. Malaty HM, Engstrand L, Pedersen NL, Graham DY (1994) Helicobacter pylori infection: genetic and environmental influences. A study of twins. Ann Intern Med 120:982–986

23. Simonds B (1957) The collection of 300 twin index cases for a study of tuberculosis in twins and their families. Acta Genet Stat Med 7:42–47

24. Sorensen TI, Nielsen GG, Andersen PK, Teasdale TW (1988) Genetic and environmental influences on premature death in adult adoptees. N Engl J Med 318:727–732

25. Wang JE (2005) Can single nucleotide polymorphisms in innate immune receptors predict development of septic complications in intensive care unit patients? Crit Care Med 33:695–696

26. Yuan FF, Tanner J, Chan PK, et al (2005) Influence of FcgammaRIIA and MBL polymorphisms on severe acute respiratory syndrome. Tissue Antigens 66:291–296

27. Puel A, Yang K, Ku CL, et al (2005) Heritable defects of the human TLR signalling pathways. J Endotoxin Res 11:220–224

28. Picard C, Casanova JL (2005) Novel primary immunodeficiencies. Adv Exp Med Biol 568:89–99

29. de Vries E (2001) Immunological investigations in children with recurrent respiratory infections. Paediatr Respir Rev 2:32–36

30. Cunningham-Rundles C, Ponda PP (2005) Molecular defects in T- and B-cell primary immunodeficiency diseases. Nat Rev Immunol 5:880–892

31. Casanova JL, Fieschi C, Bustamante J, et al (2005) From idiopathic infectious diseases to novel primary immunodeficiencies. J Allergy Clin Immunol 116:426–430

32. Casanova JL, Abel L (2002) Genetic dissection of immunity to mycobacteria: the human model. Annu Rev Immunol 20:581–620

33. Rowe SM, Miller S, Sorscher EJ (2005) Cystic fibrosis. N Engl J Med 352:1992–2001

34. Drumm ML, Konstan MW, Schluchter MD, et al (2005) Genetic modifiers of lung disease in cystic fibrosis. N Engl J Med 353:1443–1453

35. Hirschhorn JN (2005) Genetic approaches to studying common diseases and complex traits. Pediatr Res 57:74R–77R
36. Burton PR, Tobin MD, Hopper JL (2005) Key concepts in genetic epidemiology. Lancet 366:941–951
37. Cooper DN, Nussbaum RL, Krawczak M (2002) Proposed guidelines for papers describing DNA polymorphism-disease associations. Hum Genet 110:207–208
38. Hattersley AT, McCarthy MI (2005) What makes a good genetic association study? Lancet 366:1315–1323
39. Vitali SH, Randolph AG (2005) Assessing the quality of case-control association studies on the genetic basis of sepsis. Pediatr Crit Care Med 6:S74–77
40. Ulevitch RJ, Mathison JC, da Silva Correia J (2004) Innate immune responses during infection. Vaccine 22 (Suppl 1):S25–30
41. Vivier E, Malissen B (2005) Innate and adaptive immunity: specificities and signaling hierarchies revisited. Nat Immunol 6:17–21
42. Lin MT, Albertson TE (2004) Genomic polymorphisms in sepsis. Crit Care Med 32:569–579
43. Garred P, Larsen F, Seyfarth J, Fujita R, Madsen HO (2006) Mannose-binding lectin and its genetic variants. Genes Immun 7:85–94
44. Hibberd ML, Sumiya M, Summerfield JA, Booy R, Levin M (1999) Association of variants of the gene for mannose-binding lectin with susceptibility to meningococcal disease. Meningococcal Research Group. Lancet 353:1049–1053
45. Roy S, Knox K, Segal S, et al (2002) MBL genotype and risk of invasive pneumococcal disease: a case-control study. Lancet 359:1569–1573
46. Garred P, J JS, Quist L, Taaning E, Madsen HO (2003) Association of mannose-binding lectin polymorphisms with sepsis and fatal outcome, in patients with systemic inflammatory response syndrome. J Infect Dis 188:1394–1403
47. van der Pol WL, Huizinga TW, Vidarsson G, et al (2001) Relevance of Fcgamma receptor and interleukin-10 polymorphisms for meningococcal disease. J Infect Dis 184:1548–1555
48. Schroder NW, Schumann RR (2005) Single nucleotide polymorphisms of Toll-like receptors and susceptibility to infectious disease. Lancet Infect Dis 5:156–164
49. Arbour NC, Lorenz E, Schutte BC, et al. (2000) TLR4 mutations are associated with endotoxin hyporesponsiveness in humans. Nat Genet 25:187–191
50. Lorenz E, Mira JP, Frees KL, Schwartz DA (2002) Relevance of mutations in the TLR4 receptor in patients with gram-negative septic shock. Arch Intern Med 162:1028–1032
51. Child NJ, Yang IA, Pulletz MC, et al (2003) Polymorphisms in Toll-like receptor 4 and the systemic inflammatory response syndrome. Biochem Soc Trans 31:652–653
52. Emonts M, Hazelzet JA, de Groot R, Hermans PW (2003) Host genetic determinants of Neisseria meningitidis infections. Lancet Infect Dis 3:565–577
53. Sutherland AM, Walley KR, Russell JA (2005) Polymorphisms in CD14, mannose-binding lectin, and Toll-like receptor-2 are associated with increased prevalence of infection in critically ill adults. Crit Care Med 33:638–644
54. Gibot S, Cariou A, Drouet L, Rossignol M, Ripoll L (2002) Association between a genomic polymorphism within the CD14 locus and septic shock susceptibility and mortality rate. Crit Care Med 30:969–973
55. D'Avila LC, Albarus MH, Franco CR, et al (2006) Effect of CD14 -260C>T polymorphism on the mortality of critically ill patients. Immunol Cell Biol 84:342–348
56. Heesen M, Bloemeke B, Schade U, Obertacke U, Majetschak M (2002) The -260 C->T promoter polymorphism of the lipopolysaccharide receptor CD14 and severe sepsis in trauma patients. Intensive Care Med 28:1161–1163
57. Adrie C, Alberti C, Chaix-Couturier C, et al (2005) Epidemiology and economic evaluation of severe sepsis in France: age, severity, infection site, and place of acquisition (community, hospital, or intensive care unit) as determinants of workload and cost. J Crit Care 20:46–58
58. Ulloa L, Tracey KJ (2005) The "cytokine profile": a code for sepsis. Trends Mol Med 11:56–63

59. Haukim N, Bidwell JL, Smith AJ, et al (2002) Cytokine gene polymorphism in human disease: on-line databases, supplement 2. Genes Immun 3:313–330
60. Dinarello CA (2003) Anti-cytokine therapeutics and infections. Vaccine 21 (Suppl 2):S24–34
61. Pociot F, Molvig J, Wogensen L, et al (1991) A tumour necrosis factor beta gene polymorphism in relation to monokine secretion and insulin-dependent diabetes mellitus. Scand J Immunol 33:37–49
62. Heesen M, Kunz D, Bachmann-Mennenga B, Merk HF, Bloemeke B (2003) Linkage disequilibrium between tumor necrosis factor (TNF)-alpha-308 G/A promoter and TNF-beta NcoI polymorphisms: Association with TNF-alpha response of granulocytes to endotoxin stimulation. Crit Care Med 31:211–214
63. Gimenez F, Barraud de Lagerie S, Fernandez C, Pino P, Mazier D (2003) Tumor necrosis factor alpha in the pathogenesis of cerebral malaria. Cell Mol Life Sci 60:1623–1635
64. Imahara SD, O'Keefe GE (2004) Genetic determinants of the inflammatory response. Curr Opin Crit Care 10:318–324
65. Mira JP, Cariou A, Grall F, et al (1999) Association of TNF2, a TNF-alpha promoter polymorphism, with septic shock susceptibility and mortality: a multicenter study. JAMA 282:561–568
66. Hedberg CL, Adcock K, Martin J, Loggins J, Kruger TE, Baier RJ (2004) Tumor necrosis factor alpha – 308 polymorphism associated with increased sepsis mortality in ventilated very low birth weight infants. Pediatr Infect Dis J 23:424–428
67. Gordon AC, Lagan AL, Aganna E, et al (2004) TNF and TNFR polymorphisms in severe sepsis and septic shock: a prospective multicentre study. Genes Immun 5:631–640
68. Peters DL, Barber RC, Flood EM, Garner HR, O'Keefe GE (2003) Methodologic quality and genotyping reproducibility in studies of tumor necrosis factor -308 G->A single nucleotide polymorphism and bacterial sepsis: implications for studies of complex traits. Crit Care Med 31:1691–1696
69. Scumpia PO, Moldawer LL (2005) Biology of interleukin-10 and its regulatory roles in sepsis syndromes. Crit Care Med 33:S468–S471
70. Neidhardt R, Keel M, Steckholzer U, et al (1997) Relationship of interleukin-10 plasma levels to severity of injury and clinical outcome in injured patients. J Trauma 42:863–870
71. Friedman G, Jankowski S, Marchant A, Goldman M, Kahn RJ, Vincent JL (1997) Blood interleukin 10 levels parallel the severity of septic shock. J Crit Care 12:183–187
72. Kremer Hovinga JA, Franco RF, Zago MA, Ten Cate H, Westendorp RG, Reitsma PH (2004) A functional single nucleotide polymorphism in the thrombin-activatable fibrinolysis inhibitor (TAFI) gene associates with outcome of meningococcal disease. J Thromb Haemost 2:54–57
73. de Craen AJ, Posthuma D, Remarque EJ, van den Biggelaar AH, Westendorp RG, Boomsma DI (2005) Heritability estimates of innate immunity: an extended twin study. Genes Immun 6:167–170
74. Gibson AW, Edberg JC, Wu J, Westendorp RG, Huizinga TW, Kimberly RP (2001) Novel single nucleotide polymorphisms in the distal IL-10 promoter affect IL-10 production and enhance the risk of systemic lupus erythematosus. J Immunol 166:3915–3922
75. Mozzato-Chamay N, Mahdi OS, Jallow O, Mabey DC, Bailey RL, Conway DJ (2000) Polymorphisms in candidate genes and risk of scarring trachoma in a Chlamydia trachomatis-endemic population. J Infect Dis 182:1545–1548
76. Helminen ME, Kilpinen S, Virta M, Hurme M (2001) Susceptibility to primary Epstein-Barr virus infection is associated with interleukin-10 gene promoter polymorphism. J Infect Dis 184:777–780
77. Gallagher PM, Lowe G, Fitzgerald T, et al (2003) Association of IL-10 polymorphism with severity of illness in community acquired pneumonia. Thorax 58:154–156
78. Lowe PR, Galley HF, Abdel-Fattah A, Webster NR (2003) Influence of interleukin-10 polymorphisms on interleukin-10 expression and survival in critically ill patients. Crit Care Med 31:34–38

79. Wattanathum A, Manocha S, Groshaus H, Russell JA, Walley KR (2005) Interleukin-10 haplo-type associated with increased mortality in critically ill patients with sepsis from pneumonia but not in patients with extrapulmonary sepsis. Chest 128:1690–1698
80. Menges T, Hermans PW, Little SG, et al (2001) Plasminogen-activator-inhibitor-1 4G/5G promoter polymorphism and prognosis of severely injured patients. Lancet 357:1096–1097
81. Geishofer G, Binder A, Muller M, et al (2005) 4G/5G promoter polymorphism in the plasminogen-activator-inhibitor-1 gene in children with systemic meningococcaemia. Eur J Pediatr 164:486–490
82. Haralambous E, Hibberd ML, Hermans PW, Ninis N, Nadel S, Levin M (2003) Role of functional plasminogen-activator-inhibitor-1 4G/5G promoter polymorphism in suscepti-bility, severity, and outcome of meningococcal disease in Caucasian children. Crit Care Med 31:2788–2793
83. Cariou A, Chiche JD, Charpentier J, Dhainaut JF, Mira JP (2002) The era of genomics: impact on sepsis clinical trial design. Crit Care Med 30:S341–348
84. Bashyam MD, Hasnain SE (2003) The human genome sequence: impact on health care. Indian J Med Res 117:43–65

# Cell Signaling Pathways of the Innate Immune System During Acute Inflammation

S.M. Opal and P.A. Cristofaro

## Introduction

The innate immune response has evolved in multi-cellular organisms to initiate a coordinated host response to microbial challenge. A breach across the integument of the metazoan host by a potential microbial pathogen represents an immediate threat to the viability of the host. Rapid recognition of danger signals and an orchestrated antimicrobial host response are of vital importance in a world cove red with microorganisms. In vertebrate species, the innate immune system is the primary immediate host defense system in response to foreign invaders. These early, non-clonal, innate immune signaling events also prime the highly specific, adaptive immune response.

Many of the critical elements that constitute the early recognition and signaling networks of innate immunity have recently been identified. These phylogenetically ancient pattern recognition receptors (PRR) can be traced back hundreds of millions of years and antedate the evolutionary separation between plants, invertebrates and vertebrate species [1,2]. The highly conserved nature of these signaling mechanisms attests to their quintessential survival value. A fuller appreciation of these early signaling pathways should provide insights into how to protect vulnerable patients with congenital and acquired immune defects. An understanding of the molecular mechanisms underlying innate immune activation should also provide new treatment options for patients who manifest deleterious systemic immune reactions from infectious and non-infectious inflammatory states. Disordered immune responses from inappropriate cell signaling events underlie a diverse array of inflammatory states such as Crohn's disease [3], arthrosclerosis [4], asthma [5], rheumatoid arthritis [6], and psoriasis [7]

The fundamental detection strategy for the cellular elements of innate immunity was formulated by Janeway and colleagues [8,9]. Detection of non-self molecular patterns of highly conserved structures intrinsic to microorganisms is the central signaling mechanism of innate immunity. The discovery of the Toll-like receptors (TLRs) over the past decade [10] and advances in defining the early events of complement-mediated phagocytosis [11] have linked theory with the actual structural elements of cell signaling. While acute inflammatory events provide an essential role in early recognition and clearance of microbial pathogens, the same system left unchecked, or activated inappropriately by endogenous molecules, results in disordered inflammation injurious to the host.

Under resting conditions, the cellular elements of innate immunity (neutrophils, monocyte/macrophage cell types and natural killer [NK] cells) are maintained in a quiescent, inhibitory state. This is mediated, in part, by continued expression of intracellular phosphatases that remove signal inducing phosphate-linked amino acids from signal transducer proteins [12]. These phosphatases are induced by specialized regions found within the intracellular domains on ubiquitous immunoglobulin-like and lectin-like superfamily receptors. These endogenous and constitutively expressed receptors recognize major histocompatibility complex (MHC) class I antigens found under physiologic conditions on nearly all normal cells. Specialized regions of these receptors are called immunoreceptor tyrosine-based inhibitory motifs (ITIMs). Under basal conditions these phosphatases maintain innate immune cells in an inactive state. As soon as non-self, microbial pattern molecules are recognized, networks of newly activated kinases rapidly overwhelm these inhibitory influences, and cellular activation rapidly ensues.

## A Survey of the Currently Recognized Pattern Recognition Receptors

Nuesslein-Volhard and Wieschaus first described the Toll receptor as a type 1 transmembrane receptor that controls dorsal-ventral polarity during embryogenesis in *Drosophila* flies in 1991 [13]. It was quickly realized that this same receptor played an essential role in antimicrobial defense in adult flies. Toll-deficient flies are exquisitely susceptible to fungal infection but not bacterial infection [10]. Analogous structures were shown to exist throughout the plant and animal kingdom with remarkable homologies to the previously characterized interleukin-1 (IL-1) signaling pathways [8,10,14]. It is now evident that a number of human Toll homologs (known as Toll-like receptors or TLRs) exist and function as pattern recognition molecules. They sense conserved elements expressed by microbial pathogens and alert the host to the presence of this critical danger signal [8, 10]. The central elements comprising the pattern recognition system of the human innate immune system are enumerated in Table 1.

There are 10 recognized human TLRs and numerous associated co-receptors and adaptor molecules that make up the TLR family. The highly conserved and homologous nature of the TLR system and the IL-1 signaling pathways are depicted in Fig. 1 [15–19].

TLR share a common intra-cellular domain with the type one IL-1 receptor. This conserved region is termed the Toll/IL-1R (TIR) domain [14]. The TIR domain, when activated by the surface receptor, initiates an enzyme cascade involving MyD88 (myeloid differentiation factor), IRAK 4 (IL-1 receptor associated kinase), TRAF6 (tumor necrosis factor [TNF] receptor associated factor), a series of MAP (mitogen-activated protein) kinases, IKK-1 (inhibitor κB kinase) and IKK-2. This network of signal activators eventually catalyzes the phosphorylation of IκB (inhibitor kappa B-cell). This phosphorylation reaction disassociates IκB from nuclear factor-kappa B (NF-κB), freeing the nuclear localization sequence of NF-κB

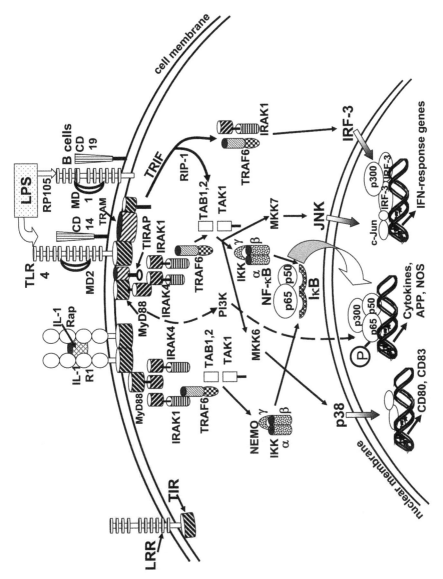

**Fig. 1.** The shared signaling pathways of human interleukin-1 (IL-1) and the Toll-like receptors (TLRs). LPS: lipopolysaccharide; IL-1Rap-interleukin-1 receptor associated protein; LRR: leucine rich repeat, TIR: Toll/interleukin receptor; MyD88: myeloid differentiation factor; TIRAP: Toll-interleukin receptor adapter protein; TRIF: TIR domain adapter inducing interferon-β; TRAM: TRIF related adaptor molecule; PI3K: phosphoinositide-3 kinase; IRAK: interleukin 1 receptor associated kinase; TRAF: tumor necrosis factor receptor associated factor; TAK: transforming growth factor associated kinase; RIP-1: receptor interacting protein; JNK: Janus N-terminal-linked kinase; IRF: interferon regulatory factor; IFN: interferon; IKK: IκB kinase; IκB: inhibitory subunit κB; NF-κB: nuclear factor-κB; NEMO: NF-κB essential modulator; TAB1,2: TAK binding protein 1 and 2; MKK: mitogen activated protein kinase kinase; APP: acute phase proteins; NOS: nitric oxide synthases. Other TLRs share similar intracellular pathways. (Adapted from [15] with permission)

**Table 1.** Toll-like receptors (TLRs), nucleotide oligomerization domain proteins (NODs) and other pattern recognition receptors and ligands

| TLR | Cell types | Likely natural ligands | Other possible ligands (comments) |
|---|---|---|---|
| CD14 | Myeloid cells | LPS, LTA, PGN, fungal antigens | Hyluronan |
| CR1, CR3 | Myeloid cells | Opsonized microbial antigens with C3bi | Immune complexes, C3 fixed human cells |
| Dectin- 1 | Myeloid | Beta-glucan from fungi | |
| TLR1 | Myeloid, T, B, natural killer cells | With TLR2- BLP, OSP of *Borrelia* spp. | |
| TLR2 | Myeloid, T cells, epithelial cells | PGN, BLP, MALP-2, LAM, LTA, OMP, HSV, β-glucan, GPI-linked parasite proteins | Leptospira LPS, fungal GXM, LPM, viral antigen, HMGB-1, Hyluronan |
| TLR3 | Epithelial cells, dendritic cells | Vral dsRNA | Some ssRNA viruses, schistosome RNAs |
| TLR4 | Myeloid, epithelial cells | LPS, RSV F protein, Candida antigens | HSP60, fibrinogen, Hyluronan, HMGB-1 |
| TLR5 | Myeloid, epithelial cells | Flagellin Gram+ or - bacteria | |
| TLR6 | Myeloid, dendritic cells | With TLR2-MALP-2, PGN | Fungal antigen-Zymosan |
| TLR7 | B cells, PDC | ssRNA (in mice) | imidazoquinolines |
| TLR8 | Myeloid | ssRNA (in humans) | imidazoquinolines |
| TLR9 | Epithelial cells, B cells, PDC | Unmethylated CpG motifs in bacterial DNA | Some DNA viruses |
| TLR10 | PDC, epithelial cells | Unknown, may form heterodimers with TLR2 | |
| TLR11 | Myeloid, uroepithelial cells | Uropathogenic bacteria and parasite proteins (mice) | (Human TLR11 gene is inactivated) |
| NOD1 | Epithelial cells | Diamino pimelate in PGN | Gram– PGN |
| NOD2 | Epithelial cells | Muramyl dipeptide in PGN | Gram+ and Gram- PGN |

LPS: lipopolysaccharide; LTA: lipoteichoic acid; PGN: peptidoglycan; OSP: outer surface protein; BLP: bacterial lipopeptide; MALP-2: macrophage activating lipopeptide; LAM: lipoarabinoman-nan; OMP: outer membrane protein; HSV: herpes simplex virus; GPI: glycosyl phosphatidylinos-itol; GXM: glucuronoxylomannan; LPM: lipophosphomannan; RSV: respiratory syncytial virus; PDC: plasmacytoid dendritic cells; HSP: heat shock protein; HMGB1: high mobility group box 1; CpG: cytidine-phosphate-guanosine; ds: double-stranded; ss: single stranded

to bind to the nuclear membrane and translocate to the nucleus. NF-κB along with other activators (see Fig. 1) initiates the transcription of inflammatory cytokines chemokines, acute phase proteins, and other host response elements [15].

The extracellular ectodomains of the TLRs are distinctly different from the IL-1 receptor. While the IL-1 receptor consists of a chain of loop-like immunoglobulin (Ig) domains, the TLR ectodomains exist as tubular structures composed of stacked leucine rich repeat (LRR) domains. Each TLR shares this LRR configuration but differs in the intrinsic binding region to their cognate, natural ligands [10].

Human genome searches for TIR domain homologs have identified ten TLRs. Mice have at least one additional TIR open reading frame, TLR-11, which recognizes uropathogenic bacteria. Human genome surveys thus far indicate that a stop codon is present in the open reading frame (ORF) of the candidate TLR11 gene, rendering it inactive [20]. The human TLR5 gene also contains a common polymorphism resulting in premature chain termination and gene inactivation. The location of these receptors in various tissues, their known natural ligands and principal functions are summarized in Table 1.

The nature of the primary ligands and basic arrangement of the TLRs within the cell or on the cell surface segregates the human TLRs into three groups. The TLRs that recognize protein ligands (TLR 2, 4 and 5) primarily reside on the external surface of human cells. TLRs 1, 2, 4, 6 and 10, along with their co-receptors and adaptor proteins (CD14 for TLR4 and TLR2, CD36 for TLR6, and MD2 for TLR4) recognize a variety of ligands including phospholipids, and glycopeptides. These receptors are located on the cell membrane with direct access to the extracellular environment. Another set of receptors (TLRs 3, 7, 8, 9) recognizes nucleic acid ligands. These TLRs are primarily found within the endosomal component following phagocytosis of microbial antigens. Intracellular signaling following engagement with pathogen-associated molecular patterns (PAMPs) within the cytosolic space is mediated by a related set of pattern recognition molecules known as the NODs (nucleotide binding oligomerization domain) (Table 1).

## The TLR2 Complex

TLR2 is a pivotal member of the TLR family that features the capacity to recognize the broadest array of exogenous ligands. TLR2 is expressed on many different cell types including immune effector cells and epithelial surfaces [16]. TLR2 is readily upregulated by a variety of inflammatory stimuli and stress hormones. It is markedly downregulated by vigorous exercise [15–17].

TLR2 is unique in that it partners with two different TLRs to form heterodimers as the functional elements for cell signaling. TLR2 pairs with TLR1 to engage the triacyl lipopeptides found in a large number of bacterial outer membranes (known as bacterial lipopeptide (BLP). TLR2-TLR6 heterodimers recognize (along with CD36) diacylated lipopeptides from *Mycoplasma* species, peptidoglycan from the outer membrane of most bacterial organisms, and zymosan, a cell wall component found in fungi [21, 22]. TLR2 also binds to the lipoteichoic acid of Gram-positive bacteria, lipoarabinomannan found in mycobacterial species, mannans found in the polysaccharide capsules of fungal pathogens, and glycosylphosphatidylinositol-linked products from protozoan pathogens [10,15,18,23,24]. Numerous viral proteins are also recognized by TLR2 [25, 26]. Thus, TLR2 and its signaling partners represent a highly versatile PRR complex that recognizes a wide spectrum of pathogens and their products.

TLR2-mediated signaling events appear to be primarily funneled through MyD88-dependent pathways. A MyD88-independent pathway may also exist with the use of a second adaptor known as TIRAP (Toll IL-1 receptor domain containing adaptor protein). TLR2 intracellular signaling is also facilitated by activation of phosphoinositide 3 kinase (PI3K) [10].

## TLR3

TLR3 recognizes double-stranded (ds) RNA found in some RNA viral genomes (i.e., reoviruses) and the standard immunostimulant poly I:C (polyinosine-polycytidylic acid) [10]. This TLR functions primarily within endosomes and induces an antiviral type 1 interferon (IFN) response to dsRNA viral pathogens and perhaps other non-viral pathogens. It shares an intracellular signaling pathway with TLR4 initiated by an adaptor protein known as TRIF (TIR domain adapter inducing IFN-$\beta$) [27]. This common signaling pathway may explain some of the similarities between severe systemic viral infections and the generalized inflammatory response to lipopolysaccharide (LPS).

TLR3 may actually be exploited by some viruses to gain access to host tissues. West Nile Virus (WNV) is a single-stranded RNA flavivirus but has dsRNA as part of its replication cycle. TLR3 deficient mice are less susceptible to WNV encephalitis [28]. The inflammatory response induced by TLR3-mediated cytokine generation promotes enhanced entry of WNV into the central nervous system (CNS) leading to severe encephalitis.

Recent studies indicate that TLR3 may recognize other RNA moieties besides double stranded RNA viruses. RNA particles from the eggs of the helminthic parasite *Schistosoma mansoni* activate NF-κB signaling in dendritic cells [29]. Schistosome eggs possess RNAse resistant dsRNA sequences that can activate TLR3. TLR3 deficient mouse strains have reduced host responses to schistosome eggs compared to wild type animals.

## TLR4

TLR4 is the LPS receptor on human immune effector cells. The currently recognized ligands for TLR4 are listed in Table 1 and the major components that mediate TLR4 signaling are illustrated in Figure 1. TLR4 has both MyD88-dependent and MyD88-independent pathways. In the MyD88 independent pathway, TRIF is activated through TLR4 and an adaptor molecule known as TRAM (TRIF related adaptor molecule). This pathway follows a similar cascade of intracellular signals as TLR3 resulting in the production of IFN-$\beta$ [19].

LPS is also a major stimulus for induction of septic shock from Gram-negative bacteria [8–10]. This TLR4 agonist is also implicated in reactive airways disease [5], inflammatory bowel disease [3], and a host of other inflammatory disease states including coronary artery disease [4]. Single-nucleotide polymorphisms (SNPs) in the coding region for the human TLR4 gene that result in reduced signaling, may be protective against atherosclerosis and coronary artery disease [30]. The statin, cholesterol-lowering drugs decrease TLR4 expression and downstream signaling in monocytes [31]. Much of the cardioprotective effects of this class of drugs may relate to its effects on TLR4 signaling and immune modulation rather than its effects on cholesterol metabolism. SNPs in the TLR4 gene have also been shown to lower the risk of acquiring *Legionella* infection [32]

LPS signaling is a complex and highly regulated process that rapidly affects the transcript frequency of over one thousand genes within hours of cell activation. The pattern recognition molecule CD14 receives the LPS ligand from a plasma carrier protein known as LPS binding protein (LBP). Since CD14 has no intracytoplasmic signaling domain, a co-receptor which spans the cell membrane is necessary for signaling. TLR4 are of critical importance as the membrane spanning signaling receptor for LPS. A third essential protein known as MD-2 [33], also lacking an intracellular domain, interacts with TLR4, CD14 and LPS to complete the cell membrane LPS signaling complex.

A second type of LPS receptor, RP105, has been found on B cells and plasmacytoid dendritic cells [10]. Its ectodomain, a series of leucine-rich repeats, is similar to the TLRs, but it lacks the intracellular TIR domain. It does possess a short cytosolic tail which contains an ITAM (immunoreceptor tyrosine based activation motif). The ITAM induces tyrosine phosphorylation motif which activates src kinases. Activation is dependent on MD-1, a protein similar to MD-2 [15, 21].

## TLR5

Bacterial flagellin proteins are highly conserved structures, and structural homology makes them a potential pattern recognition system for immune effector cells. Motility is an important virulence property of numerous bacterial pathogens, including Gram-negative bacteria (e.g., *Vibrio*, *Salmonella* and *Pseudomonas spp.*) and Gram-positive pathogens, such as *Listeria monocytogenes*. Flagellin monomers from both Gram-negative and Gram-positive bacteria are highly inflammatory and signal through TLR5 [34]. Purified flagellar proteins derived from bacterial cultures stimulate monocyte/macrophage cells in a TLR5-specific, CD14-independent manner.

Along epithelial surfaces, TLR5 is normally expressed on the basolateral surface rather than apical position. In this position, TLR5 can generate danger signals in response to invasive rather than commensal bacteria residing upon the luminal surface. TLR5-signaling generates a Th-2 biased immunity favoring secretory antibody secretion appropriate for gut mucosal immunity [35].

The role of TLR5 in human disease pathogenesis is incompletely understood. Complex interactions with other TLRs and other signaling receptors are noted with multiple pathogens in the gut, bronchial mucosal, and genitourinary tract [15]. A polymorphism in the TLR5 receptor confers increased susceptibility to Legionnaire's disease but not typhoid fever [36].

## TLR7 and TLR8

The natural ligands for TLR7 and TLR8 have recently been identified as single stranded (ss)RNA. There are numerous ssRNA viruses and TLR7/8 is instrumental in the activation of antiviral defenses such as type 1 IFN generation and other pro-inflammatory cytokines (IL-12, TNF) and chemokines (IFN-γ-inducible protein-10 [IP-10]) [37]. TLR7 is the primary ssRNA receptor in mice, while TLR8 plays the dominant role for ssRNA recognition in human cell lines. Both TLR7 and TLR8 require acidified endosomes for signal transduction. TLR7/8 recognizes both foreign and human ssRNA moieties (including 'self' mRNA or rRNA) when delivered to the endosomal compartment. This may have therapeutic implications as tumor RNA transfected dendritic cells are known to induce strong cytotoxic T cell responses in cancer immunotherapy treatments [15].

Small molecule agonists for TLR7/8 are already in clinical use as antiviral agents against papillomavirus-induced genital warts. The imidazone quinolines, imiquimod and resiquimod, are effective as immunoadjuvants in eliminating genital warts and a related compound loxoribine, also a TLR8 agonist, has anti-tumor activity [18].

## TLR9

TLR9 is the receptor for specific sequences found in both bacterial and viral DNA. Bacterial DNA stimulates pro-inflammatory cytokines, nitric oxide (NO) and MHC class II expression by macrophage/monocyte cell lines, promotes B cell activation, and induces a Th1 type cytokine response by T cells [10]. Unmethylated CpG motifs are widespread sequences in bacterial DNA, but these motifs are rarely found in human DNA. When these sequences do occur in mammalian DNA, they are usually modified by methylation. When unmethylated CpG sequences are flanked by two purines on the 5' side and two pyrimidines on the 3' end, they induce a strong pro-inflammatory signal for human immune effector cells. The specific sequence that is optimally recognized by human cells is GT-C-p-G-TT.

TLR9-deficient mutants have markedly impaired TNF-α, IL-12, IL-6 and IFN-γ responses to CpG motifs [38]. TLR9 knockout mice are refractory to lethal shock from synthetic oligonucleotides bearing unmethylated CpG motifs, which rapidly induce refractory hypotension and death in wild-type mice.

The intracellular signaling pathways induced by CpG DNA are CD14 independent, MyD88 dependent, and necessitate endocytosis of the CpG DNA-TLR9 complex. TLR9 ligation with CpG motifs strongly promotes B cell responses and a vigorous Th1 response to selected antigens, making TLR9 agonists potential targets for development as vaccine adjuvants [15].

# TLR10

The natural ligand and physiologic role of human TLR10 remains unclear. The mouse genome (but not the rat genome) lacks TLR10 and this has delayed the search to define the natural TLR10 ligands. Mice have a non-functional partial gene structure for TLR10 that has a retroviral insertion in the open reading frame (ORF) [39]. The human gene for TLR10 is located on the short arm of chromosome 4 in close proximity to the genes for TLR1 and TLR6, both known partners with TLR2. TLR10 can heterodimerize with either TLR1 or TLR2 and associate with MyD88 [40]. Polymorphisms in the TLR10 gene are strongly linked to asthma, suggesting a functional role in the detection of airway antigens.

# TLR11

TLR11 in the mouse appears to have a critically important role in recognition of urinary pathogens by uroepithelial cells [20], yet humans lack a functional homolog of TLR11. Perhaps the propensity of humans to develop urinary tract infection is explained by the loss of a functional TLR11. Murine TLR11 also functions as a pattern recognition sensor for a profilin-like protein isolated from *Toxoplasma gondii* and related proteins found in other clinically relevant protozoan pathogens including *Cryptosporidium parvum* and *Plasmodium spp* [41]. How these functions are compensated for in human immunology in the absence of TLR11 remains to be defined.

## The NOD Proteins

The cytosolic space has a related set of PRRs consisting of two major intracellular proteins known as NOD1 and NOD2. These proteins contain a N-terminal CARD (caspase recruitment domain) sequence, a central NOD core region, and a C-terminal leucine rich repeat region that functions as a PRR. NOD1 recognizes diamino-pimelate containing moieties found within the peptidoglycan of Gram-negative bacteria. NOD2 recognizes muramyl dipeptide, a ubiquitous structure found in the peptidoglycan of nearly all Gram-negative and Gram-positive bacteria [42].

These NOD proteins synergize with each other and with TLRs in activating the innate immune response to invasive bacterial pathogens. Deficiencies in TLR4 signaling appear to increase the risk of inflammatory bowel disease and variants of NOD2 have been highly linked to Crohn's disease [43]. Delayed or ineffective clearance of bacterial antigens from variants of TLR4 or NODs may contribute to a chronic inflammatory state within the gut mucosal surfaces characteristic of inflammatory bowel disease [3]. The signaling pathways that are activated by NOD proteins are incompletely understood but it is evident that NODs do not use MyD88 as an adapter molecule.

A specific phosphorylating enzyme known as RICK (receptor interacting serine/threonine kinase) is critical for NOD signaling. Many of the late signaling molecules for NF-κB nuclear translocation are shared by both TLRs and NODs.

## Coordination of TLR Signals in Response to Bacterial Pathogens

Multiple TLRs are available to detect the myriad of PAMPs available on bacterial pathogens. Figure 2 depicts the TLR and NOD structures that recognize molecular patterns expressed on Gram-positive pathogens. TLR2 is likely to be the key recognition receptor along with TLR5 for flagellated Gram-positive organisms. NOD2 is critically important in the detection of bacterial pathogens that have invaded into the intracellular space.

Gram-negative bacterial pathogens activate a markedly different set of genes in human immune effector cells than do Gram-positive organisms. These differences are related to a disparate array of TLRs and NODs that interact with Gram-negative molecular patterns (Fig. 3). TLR4 is the dominant receptor in the detection of Gram-negative pathogens as a result of LPS in the Gram-negative outer membrane. TLR4 is exquisitely sensitive to LPS within the cell microenvironment and immediately activates a network of signal transducing molecules. TLR2 also recognizes a number of molecular patterns expressed on Gram-negative pathogens [44]. TLR5 further contributes to cellular activation signals in response to flagellar antigens in motile strains of gram-negative bacteria. TLR9 adds activation signals from bacterial DNA within the endosomal compartment and both NOD1 and NOD2 recognize peptidoglycan components found in Gram-negative bacteria that escape detection and reach the cytosolic space.

## Coordination of TLR Signals in Response to Viral Pathogens

Signaling pathways differ significantly when viral pathogens, rather than bacterial organisms, invade the host. Depending on the viral genomic characteristics, viruses may signal via TLR3 (dsRNA viruses), TLR7/8 (ssRNA viruses), or TLR9 (DNA viruses). Numerous viral proteins may also signal via TLR2 including herpes viruses, influenza, and measles virus [25, 26]. The TLR2 signal pathway appears to be the dominant detection system when these viruses engage the susceptible host [45]. Remarkably, respiratory syncytial virus (RSV) F protein is recognized by TLR4 and appears to be the principal signaling receptor following RSV infection. Signaling pathways following recognition of viral or fungal pathogens are depicted in Fig. 4.

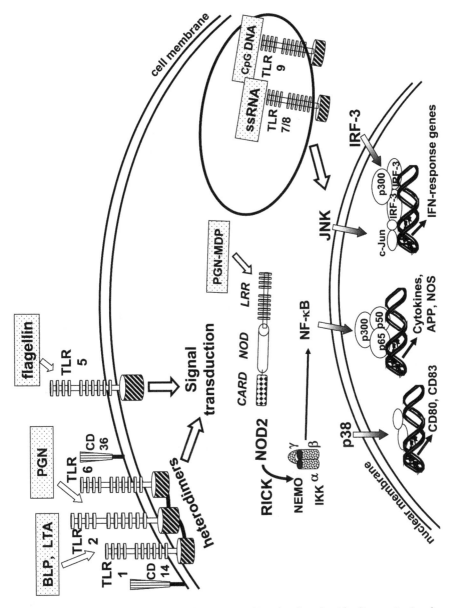

**Fig. 2.** The signaling pathways for Toll-like receptors (TLRs) and nucleotide oligomerization domains (NODs) upon exposure to Gram-positive bacterial pathogens. BLP: bacterial lipopeptide; LTA: lipoteichoic acid; PGN: peptidoglycan; CARD: caspase recruitment domain; LRR: leucine rich repeats; PGN: peptidoglycan; MDP: muramyl dipeptide; RICK: receptor interacting serine/threonine kinase; JNK: Janus N-terminal-linked kinase; IRF: interferon regulatory factor; IFN: interferon; IKK: IκB kinase; IκB: inhibitory subunit-κB; NF-κB: nuclear factor-κB; NEMO: NF-κB essential modulator; APP: acute phase proteins; NOS: nitric oxide synthases

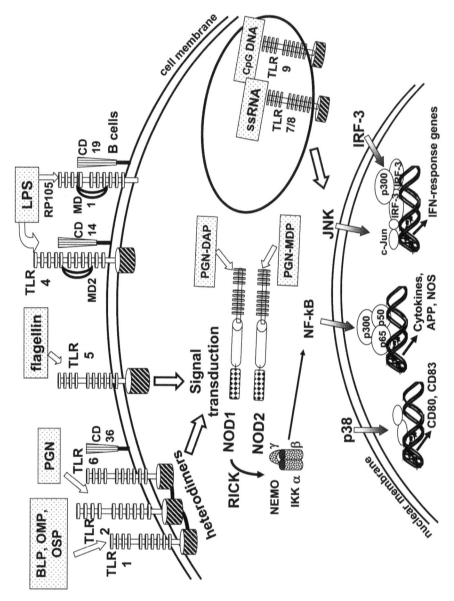

**Fig. 3.** Signaling pathways for Toll-like receptors (TLRs) and nucleotide oligomerization domains (NODs) upon exposure to Gram-negative bacterial pathogens. BLP: bacterial lipopeptide; OMP: outer membrane protein; OSP: outer surface protein; PGN: peptidoglycan; LPS: lipopolysaccharide; TIR: Toll/interleukin-1 receptor; DAP: diamino-pimelate; MDP: muramyl dipeptide; RICK: receptor interacting serine/threonine kinase; ssRNA: single-stranded RNA; CpG DNA: cytidine-phosphate-quanosine DNA; JNK: Janus N-terminal-linked kinase; IRF3: interferon regulatory factor; IFN: interferon; IKK: IκB kinase; NF-κB: nuclear factor-κB; NEMO: NF-κB essential modulator; APP: acute phase proteins; NOS: nitric oxide synthase

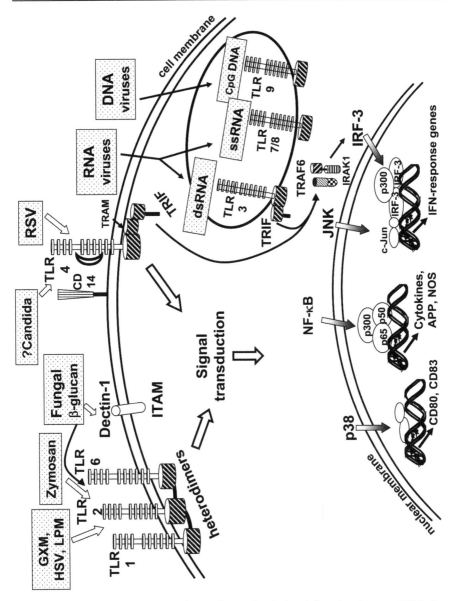

**Fig. 4.** Toll-like receptor (TLR) signaling pathways for viral and fungal pathogens. GXM: glucuronoxylomannan; HSV: herpes simplex virus; LPM: lipophosphomannan; RSV: respiratory syncytial virus; TRIF: TIR domain adapter inducing interferon-β; TRAM: TRIF related adaptor molecule; dsRNA: double-stranded RNA; ssRNA: single-stranded RNA; CpG DNA: cytidine-phosphate-quanosine DNA; IRAK: interleukin 1 receptor associated kinase; TRAF6: tumor necrosis factor receptor associated factor 6; JNK: Janus N-terminal-linked kinase; IRF3: interferon regulatory factor; IFN: interferon; NF-κB: nuclear factor-κB; APP: acute phase proteins; NOS: nitric oxide synthase

## Coordination of TLR Signals in Response to Fungal Pathogens

Fungal pathogens are detected by multiple PRRs including CD14, TLR2, TLR4, and TLR6 [23, 46]. Zymosan, a component of the fungal cell membrane, and multiple phospholipid and polysaccharide elements in the capsular structures of *Candida* and *Cryptococcus* spp. are recognized ligands for TLRs (see Fig. 4). Dectin-1 is a phagocytic receptor for beta-glucan, a unique polysaccharide intrinsic to the cell wall of fungi. It functions in concert with TLRs to orchestrate the initial host response to fungal pathogens [46]. TLR2-deficient mice exhibit increased susceptibility to *Aspergillus fumigatus* supporting the importance of TLR2 in fungal antimicrobial defense mechanisms [47].

TLR2 ligation by *C. albicans* elements may actually impair host defenses to this common fungal pathogen. TLR2-deficient mice are less susceptible to disseminated candidal infection than wild-type mice [48]. TLR2 signaling promotes IL-10 synthesis in candidiasis and contributes to the expansion of CD4+ CD25+ T re gulatory (Tre g cells. TLR2 deficie nt mice have a greate r apacity to eliminate *C. albicans*, as Treg cells impaired the candidacidal activity of activated macrophages. It is conceivable that *Candida* species have evolved substances like lipophosphomannan as a mechanism to subvert host defense systems by this form of TLR2 activation.

## Coordination of TLR Signals in Response to Parasitic Pathogens

The signaling events that follow exposure to potentially pathogenic protozoan and helminthic pathogens are poorly understood at present. It has been determined that some protozoa such as *Trypanosoma cruzi*, the etiological agent responsible for the Central and South American form of trypanosomiasis, may activate innate immune responses through engagement of TLR2 [24]. Glycosyl-phosphatidyl-inositol-linked peptides expressed by *T. cruzi* have been demonstrated to function as TLR2 ligands. Similar antigenic structures exist in other parasites and may serve a similar function in the host response to protozoan parasites.

TLR11 is of critical importance to parasite recognition in the murine system but no such TLR structure is found in humans [41]. These functions must be compensated for in the human immune system but the details of alternative recognition and signaling pathways have yet to be defined.

TLR3 detects partial dsRNA sequences found in the eggs of the widespread human pathogen *Schistosoma mansoni* [29]. Whether similar TLR3 ligands are found in other parasitic organisms has yet to be determined. The mechanisms by which parasites activate the innate immune system are under active basic and clinical investigation currently.

## The Contribution of the TLRs to Phagocytosis by Immune Effector Cells

Pattern recognition by the TLR and NOD systems of highly conserved molecules found on microbial pathogens is quite distinct from phagocytosis and intracellular killing of pathogens by phagocytic cells. Phagocytosis is an essential feature of innate immunity and is characteristic of neutrophils, monocyte/macrophage cell lines, and immature dendritic cells. Phagocytosis not only eliminates pathogens by oxidative and non-oxidative cidal actions, but it also initiates partial antigen digestion, processing, and presentation by innate immune cells. Immature dendritic cells are highly phagocytic. Activation by TLR signaling and/or active phagocytosis of microbial antigens induces dendritic cell maturation. Mature dendritic cells lose much of their phagocytic capacity but gain the ability to effectively present processed epitopes with co-stimulatory molecules for recognition by elements of the adaptive immune system [50].

TLR ligands are optimally presented as soluble, monomeric structures that are released from pathogens during growth or upon cell death. In contrast, phagocytic signals induced by cell surface scavenger receptors, complement receptors or immunoglobulin Fc receptors necessitate direct contact with the pathogen for active endocytosis to begin. A comparison of common and contrasting features of TLR events and phagocytic events are listed in Table 2.

Table 2. Comparison of signaling events between human TLRs and phagocytic receptors

| Property | Toll-like receptors (TLR 1–10) | Phagocytic receptors (CR3, Dectin-1, FcγR) |
|---|---|---|
| Preferred ligand type | Soluble | Particulate |
| Ligand expression | Released during microbial growth or cell lysis | Surface expressed on intact, viable microbes |
| Proximity to ligand source | May be distant | Must be local |
| Size of ligand | Small, monomeric | Large, often multimeric |
| Net inflammatory effect | Activates cytokines, chemokines and cellular recruitment, NET formation | Stimulates phagocytosis and intracellular killing |
| Extracellular processing and transfer | May need carrier proteins (LBP, CD14, MD2, etc) | May need antibody or complement (opsonization) |

CR3: complement receptor 3; FcγR: immunoglobulin crystallizable fragment gamma receptor; NET: neutrophil extracellular traps; LBP: lipopolysaccharide binding protein

The process of phagocytosis induces the synthesis of numerous genes whose products mediate actin formation, cell remodeling, phagosome formation, and proteolytic activity. TLRs are not directly involved in phagocytosis as TLR deficient cells show no evidence of impaired phagocytosis to the cognate ligand [50].

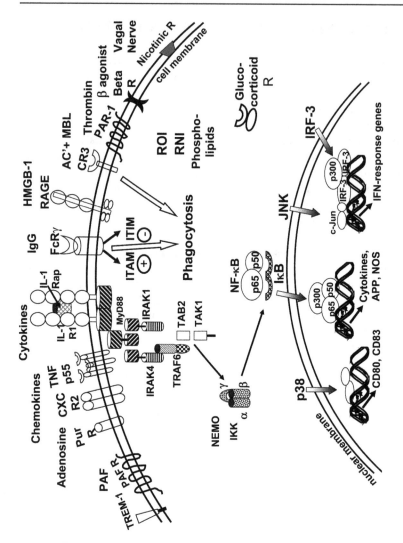

**Fig. 5.** Other signaling pathways that affect innate immune responses. Trem: triggering receptor expressed on myeloid cells; PAF: platelet activating factor; Pur R: purinergic receptor; CXC: cysteine-any amino acid-cysteine; TNF: tumor necrosis factor; IL: interleukin; IL-1Rap: interleukin-1 receptor associated protein; IgG: immunoglobulin G; FcγR: immunoglobulin crystallizable fragment gamma receptor; HMGB-1: high mobility group box-1; RAGE: receptor for advanced glycation end products; AC': alternative complement pathway; MBL: mannose binding lectin pathway; PAR: protease activated receptor; MyD88: myeloid differentiation factor; IRAK: interleukin 1 receptor associated kinase; TRAF6: tumor necrosis factor receptor associated factor 6; TAK-1: transforming growth factor associated kinase-1; TAB2: TAK binding protein 1 and 2; NEMO: NF-κB essential modulator; IFN: interferon; IKK: IκB kinase; IκB: inhibitory subunit κB; NF-κB: nuclear factor-κB; ITAM: immunoreceptor tyrosine based activation motif; ITIM: immunoreceptor tyrosine based inhibitory motif; ROI: reactive oxygen intermediates; RNI: reactive nitrogen intermediates; JNK: Janus N-terminal-linked kinase; IRF3: interferon regulatory factor; APP: acute phase proteins; NOS: nitric oxide synthase

## Conclusion

The discovery of the human TLRs over the past decade represents a major advance in our understanding of the cellular immunology of the early events of acute inflammation. This knowledge creates an opportunity to fundamentally understand the molecular details that initiate the acute inflammatory response. Integration of signaling events that follow engagement of the TLRs by microbial ligands in the presence of a myriad of modulating factors remains a major challenge. Some of those modulating features are enumerated in Fig. 5.

Some of the related events, such as TREM-1 [51] and phagocytic activation [52, 53], can significantly amplify TLR signaling. Other elements such as Fcγ II receptor activity, glucocorticoid receptors, or beta-adrenergic receptors may downregulate cell activation networks. Complex, polygenetic, direct and indirect, non-linear signaling circuits with positive and negative feedback loops exist in cell activation pathways. The magnitude of the cellular response to a given stimulus changes over time, with ligand dose, receptor density, cell type and baseline level of tissue responsiveness. Integration of this information will be critical if we are to intelligently utilize these data and optimize their clinical value in acute inflammatory states in the future.

## References

1. Hoffman JA, Reichhart JM (1997) Drosophila immunity. Trends Cell Biol 7:309–316
2. Whitham S, Dinesh-Kumar SP, Choi D, Hehl R, Corr C, Baker B. (1994) The product of the tobacco mosaic virus resistance gene N: similarity to toll and the interleukin-1 receptor. Cell 78:1101–1115
3. Franchimont D, Vermeire S, El Housni H, et al (2004) Deficient host-bacteria interactions in inflammatory bowel disease? The toll-like receptor (TLR)-4 Asp299gly polymorphism is associated with Crohn's disease and ulcerative colitis. Gut 53:987–992
4. Laberge M, Moore K, Freeman M (2005) Atherosclerosis and innate immune signaling. Ann Med 37:130–140
5. Redecke V, Hacker H, Datta SK, et al (2004) Cutting edge: activation of Toll-like receptor 2 induces a Th2 immune response and promotes experimental asthma. J Immunol 172:2739–2743
6. Pierer M, Rethage J, Seibl R, et al (2004) Chemokine secretion of rheumatoid arthritis synovial fibroblasts stimulated by Toll-like receptor 2 ligands. J Immunol 172:1256–1265
7. Baker B, Ovigne J, Powles A, et al (2003) Normal keratinocytes express Toll-like receptors (TLRs) 1,2 and 5: Modulation of TLR expression in chronic plaque psoriasis. Br J Dermatol 148:670–679
8. Janeway CA Jr, Medzhitov R (2002) Innate immune recognition. Annu Rev Immunol 20:197–216
9. Hoffman JA, Kafatos FC, Janeway CA, Ezekowitz RAB (1999) Phylogenetic perspectives in innate immunity. Science 284:1313–1317
10. Means TK, Golenbock DT, Fenton MJ (2000) The biology of Toll-like receptors. Cytokine Growth Factor Rev 11:219–232

11. Neth O, Jack DL, Dodds AW, et al (2000) Mannose-binding lectin binds to a range of clinically relevant microorganisms and promotes complement deposition. Infect Immun 62:688–693
12. Lanier LL (1998) NK cell receptors. Annu Rev Immunol 16:359–393
13. Stein D, Roth S, Vogelsang E, Nusslein-Volhard C (1991) The polarity of the dorsoventral axis in the Drosophila embryo is defined by an extracellular signal. Cell 65:725–735
14. Bowie A, O'Neill L (2000) The interleukin-1 receptor/Toll-like receptor superfamily: Signal generators for pro-inflammatory interleukins and microbial products. J Leukoc Biol 67:508–514
15. Cristofaro P, Opal SM (2006) Role of Toll like receptors in infection and immunity: clinical implications. Drugs 66:15–29
16. Weiss DS, Raupach B, Takeda K, et al (2004) Toll-like receptors are temporarily involved in host defense. J Immunol 172:4463–4469
17. Lancaster GI, Khan Q, Drysdale P, et al (2005) The physiological regulation of toll-like receptor expression and function in humans. J Physiol 563.3:945–955
18. Akira S, Takeda K (2004) Toll-like receptor signaling. Nat Rev Immunol 4:499–511
19. Kawai T, Akira S (2005) Toll-like receptor downstream signaling. Arthritis Res Ther 7:12–19
20. Zhang D, Zhang G, Hayden MS, et al (2004) A Toll-like receptor that prevents infection by uropathogenic bacteria. Science 303:1522–1526
21. Takeda K (2005) Evolution and integration of innate immune recognition systems: the Toll-like receptors. J Endotoxin Res 11:51–55
22. Hoebe K, Georgel P, Rutschmann S, et al (2005) CD36 is a sensor of diacylglycerides. Nature 433:523–527
23. Yauch LE, Mansour MK, Sholham S, et al (2004) Involvement of CD14, Toll-like receptors 2 and 4, and MyD88 in the host response to the fungal pathogen *Cryptococcus neoformans* in vivo. Infect Immun 72:5373–5383
24. Campos MA, Almeida IC, Takeuchi O, et al (2001) Activation of Toll-like receptor-2 by glycosylphosphatidylinositol anchors from a protozoan parasite. J Immunol 167:416–423
25. Bieback K, Lien E, Klagge IM, et al (2002) Hemagglutinin protein of wild-type measles virus activates Toll-like receptor 2 signaling. J Virol 76:8729–8736
26. Compton T, Kurt-Jones, EA, Boehme KW, et al (2003) Human cytomegalovirus activates inflammatory cytokine responses via CD14 and Toll-like receptor 2. J Virol 77:4588–4596
27. Fitzgerald KA, Rowe DC, Barnes BJ, et al (2003) LPS–TLR4 signaling to IRF-3/7 and NF-κB involves the toll adapters TRAM and TRIF. J Exp Med 198:1043–1055
28. Wang T, Town T, Alexopoulou L, et al (2004) Toll-like receptor 3 mediates West Nile virus entry into the brain causing lethal encephalitis. Nat Med 10:1366–1373
29. Aksoy E, Zouain CS, Vanhoutte F, et al (2005) Double-stranded RNAs from the helminth parasite Schistosoma activate TLR3 in dendritic cells. J Biol Chem 280:277–283
30. Ameziane N, Beillat T, Verpillat P, et al (2003) Association of the Toll-like receptor gene Asp299Gly polymorphism with acute coronary events. Arterioscler Thromb Vasc Biol 23:61–64
31. Methe H, Kim J, Kofler S, et al (2005) Statins decrease toll-like receptor 4 expression and downstream signaling in human CD14+ monocytes. Arterioscler Thromb Vasc Biol 25:1439–1445
32. Hawn T, Verbon A, Janer M, et al (2005) Toll-like receptor 4 polymorphisms are associated with resistance to Legionnaires' disease. Proc Natl Acad Sci 102:2487–2489
33. Viriyakosol S, Tobias PS, Kitchens RL, Kirkland TN (2001) MD-2 binds to bacterial lipopolysaccharide. J Biol Chem 276:38044–38051
34. Smith KD, Andersen-Nissen F, Hayashi K, et al (2003) Toll-like receptor 5 recognizes a conserved site on flagellin required for protofilament formation and bacterial motility. Nat Immunol 4:1247–1253
35. Ramos, H, Rumbo M, Sirard J (2004) Bacterial flagellins: mediators of pathogenicity and host immune responses in mucosa. Trends Microbiol 12:509–516
36. Dunstan S, Hawn T, Hue N, et al (2005) Host susceptibility and clinical outcomes in toll-like receptor 5-deficient patients with typhoid fever in Vietnam. J Infect Dis 191:1068–1071

37. Heil F, Hemmi H, Hochrein H, et al (2004) Specific recognition of single-stranded RNA via Toll-like receptor 7 and 8. Science 303:1526–1529
38. Hemmi H, Takeuchi O, Kawai T, et al (2000) A Toll-like receptor recognizes bacterial DNA. Nature 408:740–744
39. Hasan U, Chaffois C, Gaillard C, et al (2005) Human TLR10 is a functional receptor, expressed on B cells and plasmacytoid dendritic cells, which activates gene transcription through MyD88. J Immunol 174:2942–2960
40. Lazarus R, Raby BA, Lange C, et al (2004) Toll-like receptor 10 genetic variation is associated with asthma in two independent samples. Am J Respir Crit Care Med 170:594–600
41. Yarovinsky F, Zhang D, Anderson J, et al (2005) TLR11 activation of dendritic cells by a protozoan profiling-like protein. Science 308:1626–1629
42. Opitz B, Püschel A, Schmeck B, et al (2004) Nucleotide-binding oligomerization domain proteins are innate immune receptors for internalized *Streptococcus pneumoniae*. J Biol Chem 279:36426–36432
43. Lakatos P, Lakatos L, Szalay F, et al (2005) Toll-like receptor 4 and NOD2/CARD 15 mutations in Hungarian patients with Crohn's disease: phenotype-genotype correlations. World J Gastroenterol 11:1489–1495
44. Latz E, Franko J, Golenbock DT, et al (2004) *Haemophilus influenzae* Type b-outer membrane protein complex glycoconjugate vaccine induces cytokine production by engaging human Toll-like Receptor 2 (TLR2) and requires the presence of TLR2 for optimal immunogenicity. J Immunol 172:2431–2438
45. Finberg RW, Kurt-Jones EA (2004) Viruses and Toll-like receptors. Microb Infect 6:1356–1360
46. Levitz SM (2004) Interactions of Toll-like receptors with fungi. Microb Infect 6:1351–1355
47. Balloy V, Si-Tahar M, Takeuchi O, et al (2005) Involvement of Toll-like receptor 2 in experimental invasive pulmonary aspergillosis. Infect Immun 73:5420–5425
48. Netea MG, Sutmuller R, Herman C, et al (2004) Toll-like receptor 2 suppresses immunity against *Candida albicans* through induction of IL-10 and regulatory T cells. J Immunol 172:3712–3718
49. Ellerbroek PM, Ulfman LH, Hoepelman AI, et al (2004) Cryptococcal glucuronoxylomannan interferes with neutrophil rolling on the endothelium. Cell Microbiol 6:581–592
50. Underhill DM, Gantner B (2004) Integration of Toll-like receptor and phagocytic signaling for tailored immunity. Microb Infect 6:1368–1373
51. Gibot S (2005) Clinical review: Role of triggering receptor expressed on myeloid cells-1 during sepsis. Crit Care 9:485–489
52. Ravetch JV, Bolland S (2001) IgG Fc receptors. Annu Rev Immunol 19:275–290
53. Brinkmann V, Reichard U, Goosemann C, et al (2004) Neutrophil extracellular traps kill bacteria. Science 303:1532–1535

# Early-Onset Pro-inflammatory Cytokines

C. Kaech and T. Calandra

## Introduction

Cytokines are a key family of effector molecules that coordinate the innate and acquired host antimicrobial defense responses [1, 2]. The cytokine family of messenger molecules comprises tumor necrosis factor (TNF), the interleukins, the chemokines, the interferons, and the colony stimulating factors. The cytokines are small molecules (typically less than 30 kDa), whose expression is induced by infectious and inflammatory stimuli, but can also be constitutive. Two typical features of this class of mediators are pleiotropism (i.e., the capacity for a given cytokine to stimulate several cell types) and redundancy (i.e., the ability of different cytokines to exert similar effects). In addition, cytokines frequently stimulate each other's expression, which results in the production of a broad network of interacting molecules. They are released by a wide range of immune and non-immune cells and are key players in the pathogenesis of sepsis. Cytokines interact with specific receptors expressed on target cells and exert autocrine, paracrine, and endocrine activities. Pro-inflammatory cytokines recruit and activate cells of the immune system and induce the production of numerous mediators. They up-regulate the expression of the major histocompatibility complex (MHC) class I and II molecules and participate in the activation and proliferation of B and T lymphocytes. Anti-inflammatory cytokines, on the other hand, mitigate the inflammatory process either by inhibiting or by counteracting these effects.

## Tumor Necrosis Factor

TNF, a secreted 17 kDa cytokine produced by a broad range of cells, including myeloid cells (monocytes, macrophages, dendritic cells, and neutrophils), lymphotoxins $\alpha$ and $\beta$, and Fas ligand, belongs to a family of ligands that bind to a group of structurally related receptors, comprising the two TNF receptors, the lymphotoxin beta receptor (LT$\beta$R), and the TNF/nerve growth factor family (reviewed in [3]). TNF binds to the TNF type I receptor (TNFRI, also designated as p55-TNFR) and to the TNF type II receptor (TNFRII, also designated as p75-TNFR) that are co-expressed on many cells and tissues. TNF activates myeloid cells and triggers the synthesis of pro-inflammatory mediators such as cytokines (including TNF itself), eicosanoids, nitric oxide (NO), platelet activating factor (PAF), and free radicals. TNF recruits immune cells to inflammatory and infectious sites through induction of endothelial adhesion molecules and chemokines. TNF also plays an important role in the synthesis of hepatic acute phase proteins. It is a potent inducer of apoptosis of inflammatory cells, fibroblasts, and myocytes. TNF is a pyrogenic cytokine; it causes anorexia and can induce shock by decreasing vascular resistance, causing capillary leak and depressing myocardial function.

Upon cell activation by TNF, the p55-TNFR and the p75-TNFR are shed from the cell membrane and circulate as soluble molecules in the bloodstream [4, 5]. Soluble TNF receptors bind TNF and function as decoy receptors preventing cell activation. Shedding of TNF receptors is, therefore, a physiological mechanism whereby cells are protected from TNF overstimulation. However, binding of TNF to its soluble receptors may prolong its half-life, and TNF may be released from the receptor at a later stage of disease, as shown for p75-TNFR [6–9].

## Experimental Animal Models (Table 1)

The recognition of the critical role played by TNF as a proximal mediator in experimental endotoxemia and live bacterial infections was a major step forward in our understanding of the pathogenesis of sepsis. Infusion of TNF in animals mimicked the symptoms and signs of sepsis [10]. Subsequently, several groups of investigators have shown that anti-TNF antibodies confer protection against experimental sepsis induced by large amounts of microbial toxins (lipopolysaccharide [LPS], peptidoglycan, staphylococcal enterotoxin B, or toxic shock syndrome toxin 1). However, it is worth noting that the protective effects of anti-TNF antibodies were generally lost when therapy was started after exposure to microbial toxins. In contrast, in all but one study, TNFR deficient mice were not protected from endotoxemia. In models of systemic sepsis caused by live bacteria, the results obtained with anti-TNF antibodies have varied in function of the inoculum, of the microorganisms used, and of the site and severity of sepsis. Neutralization of TNF was protective in some, but not all models of Gram-negative or Gram-positive sepsis. In focal sepsis models and in models of sepsis caused by fungi or intracellular bacteria, inhibition of TNF profoundly impaired innate immune responses and resulted almost uniformly in increased morbidity and mortality.

Four chimeric fusion proteins comprised of either the extracellular portion of the p55- or p75-TNFR and of the Fc portion of human IgG1 or IgG3 (soluble p55-TNFR-IgG1, p55-TNFR-IgG3, p75-TNFR-IgG1, and p75-TNFR-IgG3) have been created. The TNF neutralizing activity of these constructs has been tested in mouse and baboon models of endotoxemia and sepsis. Prophylactic administration of soluble p55-TNFR-IgG constructs reduced mortality from endotoxic shock or Gram-negative sepsis. In some experiments, delayed administration of soluble p55-TNFR-IgG was protective. However, no protection was observed when soluble p75-TNFR-IgG constructs were used.

**Table 1.** Evaluation of the role of TNF, IL-1, and IL-6 in animal models of endotoxemia and sepsis. Adapted from [2] with permission

| Animal Model | Treatment or Condition | Effect on Mortality |
|---|---|---|
| *Endotoxemia* | | |
| Low dose LPS, | anti-TNF, TNF ko, | Beneficial |
| with D-galactosamine | p55-TNFR-IgG1/3, p55-TNFR ko | |
| | p75-TNFR-IgG3, p75-TNFR ko | No effect |
| High dose LPS | anti-TNF, p55-TNFR-IgG1 | Beneficial |
| | p55-TNFR ko, p75-TNFR ko, IL-6, | No effect |
| | IL-6 ko | |
| | IL-1ra | Beneficial // No effect |
| Very high dose LPS | anti-TNF | No effect |
| | | |
| *Gram-positive cell walls* | | |
| *or exotoxins* | | |
| Peptidoglycan (*S. pneumoniae*) | anti-TNF | Beneficial |
| Staphylococcal enterotoxin B | anti-TNF, IL-6 | Beneficial |
| Toxic shock syndrome toxin 1 | anti-TNF | Beneficial |
| | | |
| *Systemic bacterial sepsis* | | |
| *E. coli* i.v. | anti-TNF, p55-TNFR-IgG1/3, | Beneficial |
| | IL-1 ra | |
| | p75-TNFR-IgG1, anti-IL1-β | No effect |
| | IL-6 ko | Harmful |
| *K. pneumoniae* i.v. | anti-TNF | No effect |
| *S. aureus* i.v. | anti-TNF | Beneficial |
| | TNF ko | Harmful |
| *S. epidermidis* i.v. | IL-1 ra | Benefical |
| *S. pyogenes* i.v. | anti-TNF | No effect |

ko: knockout

## Clinical Studies

The pivotal role played by TNF in experimental sepsis and the fact that elevated concentrations of TNF were detected in the circulation of septic patients, served as the basis of adjunctive anti-TNF therapy in patients with severe sepsis and septic shock [11–13]. Eight clinical trials of anti-TNF monoclonal antibodies have been performed in more than 6,000 patients with severe sepsis or septic shock (reviewed in [2]). There was no significant difference in mortality between patients treated with placebo and patients treated with anti-TNF antibodies in these trials. In a subgroup analysis of one trial, anti-TNF therapy led to a significant reduction of mortality in patients with elevated interleukin (IL)-6 serum levels (defined as IL-6 > 1,000 pg/ml) [14]. When the results of these eight studies are pooled, anti-TNF therapy is associated with a 2.9% absolute reduction in mortality (36.7% *vs.* 39.6%) [2]. However, one should always be cautious with this kind of crude meta-analysis, as patients' characteristics and prognostic factors may differ between the two pooled treatment groups.

Table 1. (continued)

| *Focal bacterial sepsis* | | |
|---|---|---|
| Cecal ligation puncture | anti-TNF | No effect // Harmful |
| *E. coli* peritonitis | anti-TNF, p55-TNFR ko | No effect |
| | IL-6 ko | Harmful |
| *N. meningitidis* peritonitis | anti-TNF | Beneficial |
| *S. pneumoniae* peritonitis | p55-TNFR ko | Harmful |
| | p55-TNFR-IgG3, p75-TNFR ko | No effect |
| group B streptococci peritonitis | anti-TNF | No effect |
| *P. aeruginosa* pneumonia | anti-TNF | Harmful |
| *K. pneumoniae* pneumonia | p55-TNR-IgG1 | Harmful |
| *S. pneumoniae* pneumonia | anti-TNF, IL-6 ko | Harmful |
| *K. pneumoniae* s.c. | IL-1ra | Harmful |
| group B streptococci s.c. | IL-6 | Beneficial |
| *P. aeruginosa* p.o. | anti-TNF | Beneficial |
| *Intracellular and fungal infections* | | |
| *S. typhimurium* | anti-TNF | Harmful |
| *L. monocytogenes* | anti-TNF, TNF ko, p55-TNFR ko, IL-6 ko | Harmful |
| | p75-TNFR ko | No effect |
| | IL-6 | Beneficial |
| *M. tuberculosis* | IL-6 ko | Harmful |
| *C. trachomatis* | anti-TNF | Harmful |
| *C. albicans* | anti-TNF, TNF ko | Harmful |
| *C. neoformans* | TNF ko | Harmful |

The efficacy and safety of the soluble p55- and p75-TNFR-IgG fusion proteins were evaluated in three clinical trials including a total of 1927 patients (reviewed in [2]). In the first of these trials, a statistically significant, dose-dependent increase in mortality was observed in 141 patients with septic shock who had been treated with three doses of soluble p75-TNFR-IgG1 [15]. Mortality was 30% in patients treated with placebo or low-dose p75-TNFR-IgG1, and 48% and 53% in patients treated with medium or high doses of p75-TNFR-IgG1, respectively. It is possible that the increased mortality observed in the high dose p75-TNFR-IgG1 treatment group was related to a detrimental effect of prolonged neutralization of TNF. In the other two studies, patients with severe sepsis or septic shock were randomized to receive either a single dose of p55-IgG1 or placebo [16,17]. A reduction in mortality approaching significance was observed in a prospectively defined subgroup of patients with severe sepsis or early septic shock, but not in patients with refractory septic shock.

## Interleukin-1

The IL-1 gene family comprises seven members, of which three (IL-1α, IL-1β, and IL-1ra) have been investigated in septic patients (reviewed in [18]). IL-1α and IL-1β are agonists, whereas IL-1ra is a receptor antagonist. Synthesized as a 31 kDa precursor protein (pro-IL-1α), IL-1α is a biologically active membrane-bound cytokine. In contrast, IL-1β is a secreted cytokine produced by enzymatic cleavage of a cytoplasmic precursor protein (pro-IL-1β). A cysteine protease called the IL-1β-converting enzyme (ICE), also known as caspase-1, is responsible for the cleavage of pro-IL-1β. There are three IL-1 receptor chains. When IL-1 binds to the ubiquitously expressed type I receptor (IL-1RI), a complex is formed which then binds to the IL-1 receptor accessory protein (IL-1R-AcP), resulting in a high affinity signal transducing heterodimer. The type II receptor (IL-1RII) functions as a decoy receptor for IL-1β, as binding of IL-1 to IL-1RII, which is devoid of an intracellular signal transducing domain, does not trigger cell activation. IL-1 and TNF exert overlapping biological activities. IL-1ra, a naturally occurring specific receptor antagonist, is the third member of the IL-1 gene family. A variety of microbial products or pathogens (viruses, bacteria and yeasts) and IL-1 and TNF induce the production of IL-1ra. As its name suggests, IL-1ra competes with IL-1 by binding to the IL-1 type I receptor, but not to the IL-1R-AcP, therefore blocking the biological effects mediated by IL-1. Even when injected at high concentrations, IL1-ra does not have agonist activity.

## Experimental Animal Models (Table 1)

Administration of IL-1β in mice or rabbits induced a shock-like state [19,20]. Unlike TNF or p55-TNFR deficient mice, mice with deletion of the *IL-1β* gene were not resistant to the lethal effect of endotoxin, indicating that IL-1β is not an essential mediator of the systemic responses to LPS [21]. IL-1ra therapy improved survival in experimental models of endotoxemia, Gram-negative (*Escherichia coli*) and Gram-positive (*Staphylococcus epidermidis*) sepsis. However, IL-1ra only partially inhibited cytokine production induced by endotoxemia in baboons [22–24].

## Clinical Studies

Elevated concentrations of IL-1β and of IL-1ra have been detected in the circulation of patients with septic shock [12,13]. The concentrations of IL-1ra measured in septic patients are usually below 20 ng/ml, and much higher concentrations of IL-1ra are needed to block the binding of IL-1 to target cells. The impact of a 72-hour infusion of human IL-1ra on mortality of patients with severe sepsis and septic shock has been investigated in three clinical studies (reviewed in [2]). In a 99-patient phase II study, IL-1ra reduced day 28 mortality in a dose-dependent fashion (44% in the placebo group versus 32%, 25%, and 16% in the three IL-1ra treatment groups, respectively) [25]. However, two subsequent phase III clinical trials including 893 and 696 patients did not confirm the beneficial effects of IL-1ra [26,27]. In the first phase III trial, day 28 mortality was 31% and 29% in the two IL-1ra groups (1 and 2 mg/hour) and 34% in the placebo group [26]. A post-hoc analysis indicated that patients with a predicted mortality greater than 24%

did benefit from IL-1ra. However, a confirmatory phase III study was stopped for futility after an interim analysis as the mortality rates in the placebo group and IL-1ra group were 36% and 33%, respectively [27].

## Interleukin-6

IL-6 is considered to be a prototypic pro-inflammatory cytokine (reviewed in [28]). This postulate is based on the fact that IL-6, like TNF and IL-1, is produced abundantly after LPS exposure. IL-6 circulates in high concentrations in patients with acute infections, but unlike TNF and IL-1, IL-6 does not up-regulate the expression of pro-inflammatory effector molecules such as NO, prostaglandins, or adhesion molecules (such as intercellular adhesion molecule [ICAM]-1). Also unlike TNF and IL-1, administration of large doses of IL-6 does not cause shock. Moreover, IL-6 inhibits TNF, IL-1 and chemokine production *in vitro* and *in vivo* and might, therefore, also be considered to be an anti-inflammatory cytokine. IL-6 induces acute phase protein synthesis in hepatocytes and plays a key role in the differentiation of myeloid cells. IL-6 binds to the IL-6 receptor, composed of a ligand-binding chain (gp80) and a ubiquitously expressed signal transducing peptide (gp130).

### Experimental Animal Models (Table 1)

IL-6 is a marker of inflammation, but does not appear to be a critical cytokine of experimental shock induced by LPS or staphylococcal enterotoxin B. IL-6 was shown to play a beneficial role in the resolution of experimental sepsis caused by live bacteria, including intracellular pathogens.

### Clinical Studies

Of all the cytokines studied in patients with sepsis, severe sepsis, or septic shock, IL-6 is one of the best predictors of disease severity and patient outcome. In several studies, high levels of IL-6 were associated with an increased risk of fatal outcome [29–31]. IL-6 levels have thus been used as an enrolment criterion in sepsis trials [14,31].

## Interferon Gamma, Interleukin-12, and Interleukin 18

Interferon-gamma (IFNγ), IL-12, and IL-18 are three closely related cytokines. IFNγ, a 17 kDA protein produced primarily by activated T lymphocytes and natural killer (NK) cells, is induced upon exposure to microbial toxins (LPS and Gram-positive superantigenic exotoxins) (reviewed in [32]). IFNγ binds to a unique receptor. IFNγ exerts very powerful priming effects on monocytes and macrophages and enhances the microbicidal activity of macrophages. It upregulates the expression of the MHC class I and II molecules and of the Fc receptor and promotes the production of cytokines, hydrogen peroxide, and NO by cells exposed to pro-inflammatory stimuli.

IL-12 is a heterodimeric cytokine composed of two covalently linked subunits (p35 and p40) (reviewed in [33]). IL-12 is produced by myeloid cells (monocytes, macrophages, and dendritic cells) and B lymphocytes when exposed to microbial products or intracellular parasites. IL-12 binds to the IL-12 receptor, a member of the gp130-like cytokine receptor superfamily. It plays an important role in the initiation of the inflammatory response. One of its main effects is the upregulation of IFNγ production by NK and T cells. IL-12 also stimulates the proliferation of activated NK and T cells and sustains the ge ne ration of cytolytic T cells. Conve rsely, IFNγ promotes the release of IL-12 by macrophages, thereby inducing a critical positive feedback loop for the phagocytosis of microbial pathogens and for the differentiation of T cells.

Identified as an IFNγ-inducing factor, IL-18 is expressed by a broad range of cells (including macrophages, T and B cells) stimulated with microbial products (reviewed in [34]). Like IL-1β, IL-18 is produced as a precursor pro-IL-18 molecule and is processed to the mature bioactive IL-18 by enzymatic cleavage by ICE/caspase-1. Similarly to IL-12, IL-18 stimulates the production of IFNγ by NK and T cells. However, it first requires the upregulation of the IL-18 receptor by IL-12.

## Experimental Animal Models (Table 2)

IFNγ, IL-12, and IL-18 have been shown to be important cytokines of experimental endotoxemia. Treatment of endotoxemic mice with anti-IFNγ, anti-IL-12 or anti-IL-18 antibodies improves survival. Likewise, anti-IFNγ antibodies reduced mortality in animal models of *E. coli* sepsis, even when treatment was started after the onset of shock [35]. IL-18 knockout mice were protected from death induced by *S. aureus* sepsis. Inhibition of IFNγ, IL-12 or IL-18 had harmful effects in all but one model of focal sepsis and of sepsis caused by fungi or intracellular bacteria. In models of *E. coli* peritonitis, neutralization of IL-12 or IL-18 activity led to a decrease in bacterial clearance, faster dissemination of bacteria into the bloodstream, and more organ injury. However, anti-IL-12 and anti-IL-18 therapies did not have an impact on survival.

## Clinical Studies

Elevated concentrations of IFNγ, IL-12, and IL-18 are detected in the circulation of septic patients. HLA-DR expression and cytokine production by monocytes from septic patients improves after treatment with IFNγ [36,37]. Yet, since IFNγ-treated patients were compared to historical controls, it is difficult to assess the impact of IFNγ on patient outcome. Randomized, placebo-controlled studies are needed to determine whether IFNγ may improve the outcome of septic patients.

Table 2. Evaluation of the role of IFNγ, IL-12, IL-18, and MIF in animal models of endotoxemia and sepsis. Adapted from [2] with permission

| Animal Model | Treatment or Condition | Effect on Mortality |
|---|---|---|
| *Endotoxemia* | | |
| Low dose LPS, with D-galactosamine | anti-IFNγ | No effect |
| | IFNγR ko | Beneficial |
| Low dose LPS, priming with *P. acnes* | anti-IL-18, IL-18 ko | Beneficial |
| Low dose LPS, priming with BCG | anti-IL-12 | Beneficial |
| High dose LPS | anti-IFNγ, IFNγ ko, anti-IL-12, anti-IL-18, anti-MIF, MIF ko | Beneficial |
| *Gram-positive cell walls or exotoxins* | | |
| Staphylococcal enterotoxin B | MIF ko | Beneficial |
| Toxic shock syndrome toxin 1 | anti-MIF | Beneficial |
| *Systemic bacterial sepsis* | | |
| *E. coli* i.v. | anti-IFNγ | Beneficial |
| group B streptococci i.v. | anti-IL-12 | Harmful |
| *S. aureus* i.v. | IL-18 ko | Beneficial |
| *Focal bacterial sepsis* | | |
| Cecal ligation puncture | anti-IL-12 | Harmful |
| | anti-MIF | Beneficial |
| *E. coli* peritonitis | anti-IFNγ, anti-MIF | Beneficial |
| | anti-IL-12, IL-12 ko, IL-18 ko | No effect |
| *K. pneumoniae* pneumonia | anti-IL-12 | Harmful |
| *Intracellular and fungal infections* | | |
| *S. typhimurium* | anti-IFNγ, anti-IL-18 | Harmful |
| *L. monocytogenes* | anti-IFNγ, IFNγR ko | Harmful |
| *Y. enterocolitica* | anti-IFNγ, anti-IL-12, anti-IL-18 | Harmful |
| *M. tuberculosis, M. bovis* | IFNγ ko, IL-12 ko, IL-18 ko | Harmful |
| *C. neoformans* | IL-12 ko | Harmful |

ko: knockout

## Macrophage Migration Inhibitory Factor (MIF)

MIF has recently emerged as an important effector molecule of the host antimicrobial defense and stress responses [38]. Identified in the 1960s as a T cell cytokine [39,40], MIF was rediscovered in the early 1990s as a constitutively expressed cytokine released by endocrine cells (pituitary gland and adrenals) in a hormone-like fashion after exposure to endotoxin and stress [41–43]. Also released by cells of the myeloid lineage after stimulation with microbial products or with pro-inflammatory mediators [44], MIF acts in an autocrine, paracrine, and endocrine fashion to promote pro-inflammatory and immune responses. The biological activities ascribed to MIF (reviewed in [38]) include the upregulation of the expression of Toll-like receptor 4 (TLR4) to facilitate sensing of endotoxin-bearing bacteria and the maintenance of pro-inflammatory functions of macrophages through the inhibition of p53-dependent apoptosis. MIF also activates the extracellular signal-regulated kinase-1/2 (ERK-1/2) mitogen-activated protein kinase (MAPK) pathway and inhibits the activity of JAB1/CSN5, a co-activator of the activator protein 1 (AP-1). Glucocorticoids were observed to induce MIF release by immune cells, which then acts as a counter-regulator of the anti-inflammatory and immunosuppressive effects of glucocorticoids [43]. Recent data have shown that MAPK phosphatase 1 (MKP-1) is a critical target of MIF-glucocorticoid crosstalk [45]. Consistent with its modulatory effects on inflammatory and innate immune reactions, MIF has been implicated in the pathogenesis of severe sepsis and septic shock, acute respiratory distress syndrome (ARDS), rheumatoid arthritis, glomerulonephritis, and inflammatory bowel diseases (reviewed in [38]).

## Experimental Animal Models (Table 2)

MIF is an important mediator of experimental endotoxemia and sepsis. Co-administration of LPS and recombinant MIF increased mortality, while anti-MIF therapy or deletion of the *MIF* gene decreased the production of pro-inflammatory cytokines (such as TNF) and improved survival. Administration of recombinant MIF or anti-MIF antibodies exerted similar effects in experimental shock induced by Gram-positive toxins. Bacterial peritonitis models showed that concentrations of MIF increased at the primary site of infection and in the systemic circulation during sepsis. Neutralization of MIF activity with anti-MIF antibodies protected mice from lethal peritonitis induced by cecal ligation and puncture (CLP) or by intraperitoneal injection of *E. coli*. Of note, protection occurred even when treatment was delayed several hours after the onset of peritonitis [46]. Similar to what had been observed in the endotoxic shock model, improved survival was associated with a reduction in circulating TNF levels. Conversely, administration of recombinant MIF during the acute phase of sepsis potentiated mortality from *E. coli* peritonitis [46].

## Clinical Studies

Elevated serum levels of MIF have been detected in several studies of patients with severe sepsis or septic shock caused by Gram-negative or Gram-positive bacteria. Consistent with the notion that high levels of MIF are harmful in the context of an acute inflammation or infection, MIF levels were significantly higher in patients with septic shock than in patients with severe sepsis, or control patients and healthy subjects [46]. MIF concentrations were more elevated in non-survivors than in survivors and were correlated with levels of cortisol and IL-6.

## Conclusion

An abundant literature indicates that cytokines play an essential role in host innate anti-microbial defences and, therefore, in the pathogenesis of sepsis. Cytokines are key players in the initiation of the host inflammatory response and in the orchestration of the cellular and humoral responses needed to either wall off or eliminate invading microorganisms. Yet, deregulated cytokine responses can cause shock, organ failure, and death, indicating that tight control of cytokine production is critical to keep the immune response in check. In that respect, severe sepsis and septic shock can be viewed as clinical manifestations of failing innate immune responses.

In contrast to the promising results of cytokine-directed therapies obtained in pre-clinical sepsis models, clinical trials in patients with severe sepsis or septic shock have been largely disappointing. Many factors, including the enormous complexity of the sepsis syndrome only partially mimicked in experimental animal models, inappropriate dosing and timing of cytokine-directed therapy, heterogeneity of the target population, and limitations of outcome measures, may have contributed to these unsatisfactory clinical results (reviewed in [47]). Translation of basic research progress and of previous lessons learned in experimental animal models into future clinical investigations remains one of the major challenges of medical research in the twenty-first century.

*Acknowledgement.* Supported by grants from the Swiss National Science Foundation (3100-066972), the Bristol-Myers Squibb Foundation, the Leenaards Foundation, and the Santos-Suarez Foundation for Medical Research.

## References

1. Dinarello CA (2000) Proinflammatory cytokines. Chest 118:503–508
2. Calandra T, Bochud PY, Heumann D (2002) Cytokines in septic shock. Curr Clin Top Infect Dis 22:1–23
3. Hehlgans T, Pfeffer K (2005) The intriguing biology of the tumour necrosis factor/tumour necrosis factor receptor superfamily: players, rules and the games. Immunology 115:1–20
4. Spinas GA, Keller U, Brockhaus M (1992) Release of soluble receptors for tumor necrosis factor (TNF) in relation to circulating TNF during experimental endotoxinemia. J Clin Invest 90:533–536
5. Van Zee KJ, Kohno T, Fischer E, Rock CS, Moldawer LL, Lowry SF (1992) Tumor necrosis factor soluble receptors circulate during experimental and clinical inflammation and can protect against excessive tumor necrosis factor alpha in vitro and in vivo. Proc Natl Acad Sci U S A 89:4845–4849
6. Aderka D, Engelmann H, Maor YBC, Wallach D (1992) Stabilization of the bioactivity of tumor necrosis factor by its soluble receptors. J Exp Med 175:323–329
7. Evans TJ, Moyes D, Carpenter A, et al (1994) Protective effect of 55- but not 75-kD soluble tumor necrosis factor receptor-immunoglobulin G fusion proteins in an animal model of gram-negative sepsis. J Exp Med 180:2173–2179

8. Mohler KM, Torrance DS, Smith CA, et al (1993) Soluble tumor necrosis factor (TNF) receptors are effective therapeutic agents in lethal endotoxemia and function simultaneously as both TNF carriers and TNF antagonists. J Immunol 151:1548–1561
9. Moller B, Ellermann-Eriksen S, Storgaard M, Obel N, Bendtzen K, Petersen CM (1996) Soluble tumor necrosis factor (TNF) receptors conserve TNF bioactivity in meningitis patient spinal fluid. J Infect Dis 174:557–563
10. Tracey KJ, Beutler B, Lowry SF, et al (1986) Shock and tissue injury induced by recombinant human cachectin. Science 234:470–474
11. Waage A, Halstensen A, Espevik T (1987) Association between tumour necrosis factor in serum and fatal outcome in patients with meningococcal disease. Lancet 1:355–357
12. Girardin E, Grau G, Dayer J, Roux-Lombard P, Lambert PH (1988) Tumor necrosis factor and interleukin-1 in serum of children with severe infectious purpura. N Engl J Med 319:397–400
13. Calandra T, Baumgartner JD, Grau GE, et al (1990) Prognostic values of tumor necrosis factor/cachectin, interleukin-1, alpha-interferon and gamma-interferon in the serum of patients with septic shock. J Infect Dis 161:982–987
14. Panacek EA, Marshall JC, Albertson TE, et al (2004) Efficacy and safety of the monoclonal anti-tumor necrosis factor antibody F(ab')2 fragment afelimomab in patients with severe sepsis and elevated interleukin-6 levels. Crit Care Med 32:2173–2182
15. Fisher CJ, Agosti JM, Opal SM, et al (1996) Treatment of septic shock with the tumor necrosis factor receptor:Fc fusion protein. N Engl J Med 334:1697–1702
16. Abraham E, Glauser MP, Butler T, et al (1997) p55 tumor necrosis factor receptor fusion protein in the treatment of patients with severe sepsis and septic shock. A randomized controlled multicenter trial. JAMA 277:1531–1538
17. Abraham E, Laterre PF, Garbino J, et al (2001) Lenercept (p55 tumor necrosis factor receptor fusion protein) in severe sepsis and early septic shock: A randomized, double-blind, placebo-controlled, multicenter phase III trial with 1,342 patients. Crit Care Med 29:503–510
18. Dinarello CA (1998) Interleukin-1, interleukin-1 receptors and interleukin-1 receptor antagonist. Intern Rev Immunol 16:457–499
19. Okusawa S, Gelfand JA, Ikejima T, Connolly RJ, Dinarello CA (1988) Interleukin 1 induces a shock-like state in rabbits. Synergism with tumor necrosis factor and the effect of cyclooxygenase inhibition. J Clin Invest 81:1162–1172
20. Waage A, Espevik T (1988) Interleukin-1 potentiates the lethal effect of TNF-alpha/cachectin in mice. J Exp Med 167:1987–1992
21. Fantuzzi G, Zheng H, Faggioni R, et al (1996) Effect of endotoxin in IL-1β-deficient mice. J Immunol 157:291–296
22. Ohlsson K, Björk P, Bergenfeldt M, Hageman R, Thompson RC (1990) Interleukin-1 receptor antagonist reduces mortality from endotoxin shock. Nature 348:550–552
23. Alexander HR, Doherty GM, Buresh CM, Venzon DJ, Norton JA (1991) A recombinant human receptor antagonist to interleukin 1 improves survival after lethal endotoxemia in mice. J Exp Med 173:1029–1032
24. Fischer E, Marano MA, Van Zee KJ, et al (1992) Interleukin-1 receptor blockade improves survival and hemodynamic performance in Escherichia coli septic shock, but fails to alter host responses to sublethal endotoxemia. J Clin Invest 89:1551–1557
25. Fisher CJ, Jr., Slotman GJ, Opal SM, et al (1994) Initial evaluation of human recombinant interleukin-1 receptor antagonist in the treatment of sepsis syndrome: a randomized, open-label, placebo-controlled multicenter trial. Crit Care Med 22:12–21
26. Fisher CJ, Dhainaut JF, Opal SM, et al (1994) Recombinant human interleukin 1 receptor antagonist in the treatment of patients with sepsis syndrome: results from a randomized, double-blind, placebo-controlled trial. JAMA 271:1836–1843
27. Opal SM, Fisher CJ, Dhainaut JF, et al (1997) Confirmatory interleukin-1 receptor antagonist trial in severe sepsis: a phase III, randomized, double-blind, placebo-controlled, multicenter trial. Crit Care Med 25:1115–1124

28. Jones SA (2005) Directing transition from innate to acquired immunity: defining a role for IL-6. J Immunol 175:3463–3468
29. Calandra T, Gerain J, Heumann D, Baumgartner JD, Glauser MP, and the Swiss-Dutch J5 study group (1991) High circulating levels of interleukin-6 in patients with septic shock: evolution during sepsis, prognostic value, and interplay with other cytokines. Am J Med 91:23–29
30. Oberholzer A, Souza SM, Tschoeke SK, et al (2005) Plasma cytokine measurements augment prognostic scores as indicators of outcome in patients with severe sepsis. Shock 23:488–493
31. Reinhart K, Menges T, Gardlund B, et al (2001) Randomized, placebo-controlled trial of the anti-tumor necrosis factor antibody fragment afelimomab in hyperinflammatory response during severe sepsis: The RAMSES Study. Crit Care Med 29:765–769
32. Schroder K, Hertzog PJ, Ravasi T, Hume DA (2004) Interferon-gamma: an overview of signals, mechanisms and functions. J Leukoc Biol 75:163–189
33. Trinchieri G (2003) Interleukin-12 and the regulation of innate resistance and adaptive immunity. Nat Rev Immunol 3:133–146
34. Akira S (2000) The role of IL-18 in innate imunity. Curr Op Immunol 12:59–63
35. Lainee P, Efron P, Tschoeke SK, et al (2005) Delayed neutralization of interferon-gamma prevents lethality in primate Gram-negative bacteremic shock. Crit Care Med 33:797–805
36. Docke WD, Randow F, Syrbe U, et al (1997) Monocyte deactivation in septic patients: restoration by IFN-gamma treatment. Nat Med 3:678–681
37. Kox WJ, Bone RC, Krausch D, et al (1997) Interferon gamma-1b in the treatment of compensatory anti-inflammatory response syndrome. A new approach: proof of principle. Arch Intern Med 157:389–393
38. Calandra T, Roger T (2003) Macrophage migration inhibitory factor: a regulator of innate immunity. Nat Rev Immunol 3:791–800
39. Bloom BR, Bennett B (1966) Mechanism of a reaction in vitro associated with delayed-type hypersensitivity. Science 153:80–82
40. David J (1966) Delayed hypersensitivity in vitro: its mediation by cell-free substances formed by lymphoid cell-antigen interaction. Proc Natl Acad Sci USA 56:72–77
41. Bacher M, Meinhardt A, Lan HY, et al (1997) Migration inhibitory factor expression in experimentally induced endotoxemia. Amer J Pathol 150:235–246
42. Bernhagen J, Calandra T, Mitchell RA, et al (1993) MIF is a pituitary-derived cytokine that potentiates lethal endotoxaemia. Nature 365:756–759
43. Calandra T, Bernhagen J, Metz CN, et al (1995) MIF as a glucocorticoid-induced modulator of cytokine production. Nature 377:68–71
44. Calandra T, Bernhagen J, Mitchell RA, Bucala R (1994) The macrophage is an important and previously unrecognized source of macrophage migration inhibitory factor. J Exp Med 179:1895–1902
45. Roger T, Chanson AL, Knaup-Reymond M, Calandra T (2005) Macrophage migration inhibitory factor promotes innate immune responses by suppressing glucocorticoid-induced expression of mitogen-activated protein kinase phosphatase-1. Eur J Immunol 35:3405–3413
46. Calandra T, Echtenacher B, Roy DL, et al (2000) Protection from septic shock by neutralization of macrophage migration inhibitory factor. Nat Med 6:164–170
47. Marshall JC (2003) Such stuff as dreams are made on: mediator-directed therapy in sepsis. Nat Rev Drug Discov 2:391–405

# The Significance of HMGB1, a Late-Acting Pro-inflammatory Cytokine

E. Abraham

## Introduction

Multiple organ failure is a frequent occurrence after sepsis or multisystem accidental trauma associated with severe hemorrhage [1–4]. Acute lung injury (ALI), characterized by the accumulation of activated neutrophils into the lungs as well as epithelial and endothelial dysfunction that leads to the development of interstitial edema, is a common organ dysfunction in these clinical settings. Pro-inflammatory cytokines, such as tumor necrosis factor (TNF)-α and interleukin (IL)-1β, are increased in the lungs after blood loss, endotoxemia, or sepsis and appear to contribute to the development of ALI in this setting, but the mechanisms by which they induce ALI are incompletely characterized [5–7]. Although these same cytokines have been shown to participate in organ dysfunction and mortality associated with sepsis, recent data indicate that many of their actions may actually be through inducing the downstream release of high mobility group box 1 protein (HMGB1), a late acting pro-inflammatory mediator [8–18].

There are three HMGB chromosomal proteins: HMGB1 (previously known as HMG1), HMGB2 (previously HMG2), and HMGB3 (previously HMG4 or HMG2) [8, 10, 13, 19, 20]. HMGBs are composed of three different domains, including the homologous DNA binding boxes A and B, and the C-terminal domain [8–10, 13, 19, 21, 22]. The amino acid sequence within the HMGB family members exhibits 85% similarity, but the proteins have a distinctly different tissue expression pattern. HMGB1 is ubiquitously present in all vertebrate nuclei, but the expression of HMGB2 and HMGB3 is more restricted. HMGB2 is widely present during embryonic development, but is expressed only in the testes and lymphoid tissue of the adult mouse. HMGB3 expression is only present during embryogenesis.

HMGB1 is a 215 amino acid protein with a uniquely conserved sequence among species. Mouse HMGB1 differs from the human form by only two amino acids [10, 16,19,23]. HMGB1 deficient mice die within a few hours of birth, demonstrating the crucial role of this protein in cellular function. The two homologous DNA binding domains, HMGB boxes A and B, are each approximately 75 amino acids in length. The C terminal domain is highly negatively charged, consisting of a continuous stretch of glutamate or aspartate residues.

The truncated HMGB1 protein containing the B box motif is a potent inducer of TNF-α production in cultured macrophages [8, 13, 21, 22]. Similarly, synthesized B box protein also stimulates TNF-α release [8]. Affinity purified anti-B box antibodies inhibit TNF-α release induced by either full length HMGB1 or the B box protein, showing that the macrophage stimulating effects of HMGB1 are B box specific. *In vivo* experiments have also shown that the HMGB1 B box has pro-inflammatory effects. In particular, administration of the HMGB1 B box to lipopolysaccharide (LPS)-resistant C3H/HeJ mice was lethal and also significantly increased serum levels of TNF-α, IL-1β, and IL-6 [8]. Mice given anti-HMGB1 B box antibodies were significantly protected against lethal endotoxemia, indicating that selective inhibition of the HMGB1 B box decreases the toxicity of endogenous HMGB1 [8].

Unlike the B box of HMGB1, the A box does not stimulate pro-inflammatory cytokine production by cultured macrophages [8, 13, 21, 22]. In contrast, the A box functions as a competitive inhibitor of HMGB1. Such inhibitory actions of the HMGB1 A box are demonstrated by the fact that addition of the A box to macrophage cultures decreases HMGB1 induced release of IL-1β and TNF-α in a dose dependent manner and displaces $^{125}$I-labelled HMGB1 from macrophage binding [8]. The HMGB1 A box also has *in vivo* anti-inflammatory effects. In particular, administration of recombinant A box protein to mice subjected to sepsis induced by cecal ligation and puncture (CLP) improved survival [8]. Remarkably, injection of the A box of HMGB1 as late as 24 hours after cecal perforation still rescued mice from the lethal effects of sepsis [8].

HMGB1 appears to have two distinct functions in cellular systems. First, it has been shown to have an intracellular role as a regulator of transcription and, second, an extracellular role in which it promotes tumor metastasis and inflammation [8–10, 12, 19, 20, 24, 25]. Monocytes/macrophages stimulated by LPS, TNF-α, or IL-1 secrete HMGB1 [24, 26]. Addition of HMGB1 to monocytes in culture induces the release of TNF-α, IL-1α, IL-1β, IL-1 receptor antagonist (IL-1ra), IL-6, IL-8, macrophage inflammatory protein (MIP)-1α, MIP-1β, but not IL-10 or IL-12 [24, 26]. Activation of macrophages by HMGB1 occurs with delayed kinetics as compared to LPS-induced stimulation. For example, culture of macrophages with LPS results in increases in TNF-α that are apparent within less than one hour, whereas TNF-α synthesis after HMGB1 exposure only begins to occur after 2 hours and then persists for as long as 8 hours [12, 26]. In the in vivo setting, increases in circulating HMGB1 levels are found after serum TNF-α and IL-1β levels have returned to basal levels [8–12, 20, 26]. Administration of anti-HMGB1 antibodies decrease the severity of LPS induced ALI, even though pulmonary concentrations of pro-inflammatory cytokines, such as IL-1β or TNF-α, remain elevated [27]. Similarly, in septic mice with peritonitis, mortality can be reduced even if anti-HMGB1 antibodies are given as long as 24 hours after CLP [8, 28]. Such results indicate that HMGB1 is a late mediator of lethal inflammation, whose effects are independent of those of early acting pro-inflammatory mediators, such as TNF-α or IL-1β.

## HMGB1 and Sepsis

Serum concentrations of HMGB1 increase 8 to 32 hours after administration of LPS or TNF-α to mice [8, 26]. Systemic administration of purified recombinant HMGB1 is lethal in LPS sensitive C3H/HeN mice as well as in the LPS resistant C3H/HeJ mice, indicating that HMGB1 can mediate lethal toxicity in the absence of signal transduction by LPS [26]. These results also indicate that receptors other than the type 4 Toll-like receptor (TLR4), which is responsible for LPS-induced cellular activation, are involved in the inflammatory response initiated by HMGB1.

Administration of anti-HMGB1 antibodies protects mice from LPS-induced lethality even if the therapy is delayed several hours, and is administered after the appearance of the early pro-inflammatory cytokine response [8, 12, 13, 26]. Similarly, anti-HMGB1 antibodies can improve survival of mice subjected to peritonitis induced by CLP, even if administered 24 hours after the initiation of the septic insult [28].

In patients with severe sepsis, serum HMGB1 levels are increased, and the highest levels were initially reported to be present in non-survivors [26]. However, more recent studies have brought the relationship between HMGB1 levels and outcome from sepsis into question. In particular, although Sunden-Cullberg et al. found persistent increases in circulating HMGB1 levels in septic patients, there was no apparent relationship between HMGB1 levels and mortality in that study [29].

An important question is the mechanism through which HMGB1 may contribute to organ dysfunction and lethality in sepsis. Interestingly, there is evidence that HMGB1 itself does not cause hypotension, but rather may induce organ dysfunction through its effects on the epithelium and, in particular, through producing epithelial dysfunction that results in interstitial edema [15, 21]. Such findings are somewhat surprising, given the ability of HMGB1 to induce macrophages to produce TNF-α, which itself causes profound hypotension.

In addition to being secreted by activated macrophages, HMGB1 is also released into the extracellular milieu when cells die by necrosis, but not when cellular death occurs through apoptosis, when it remains bound to chromatin [23, 25]. In this respect, HMGB1 appears to function as a true 'danger signal', indicating when cells meet a fate that results in unexpected death. While enhanced apoptosis, particularly of lymphocytes and epithelial cells, is found in sepsis [30], the presence of increased circulating HMGB1 levels in this setting may also reflect enhanced rates of cell death by necrosis, a hypothesis that will require confirmation in future experiments.

## HMGB1, Hemorrhage, and Burns

As with sepsis, persistent elevations in serum HMGB1 levels are present in humans after life threatening hemorrhage, with increases occurring within the first 24 hours after the onset of blood loss and then continuing for more than 72 hours [31].

Of note, serum levels of HMGB1 after hemorrhage, up to 70 µg/l, are similar to those found in severe sepsis. Additionally, increased HMGB1 expression is found in experimental burn injury models [32]. In those thermal injury experiments, significant correlations were found between pulmonary HMGB1 expression and MPO activity, suggesting a role for HMGB1 in burn-induced ALI.

Hemorrhage results in increased expression of multiple pro-inflammatory cytokines in the lungs, including TNF-α and IL-1β [33–39]. Because pro-inflammatory cytokines, including TNF-α, are known to stimulate the production of HMGB1 by macrophages, endothelial cells, and other cell populations [9, 10, 12, 24, 26, 40, 41], it seemed likely that hemorrhage would be associated with increased generation of HMGB1 in the lungs. Recent experiments in murine models of hemorrhage have confirmed increased pulmonary levels of HMGB1 in this setting [42]. Additionally, anti-HMGB1 antibodies decreased the severity of hemorrhage-induced ALI, demonstrating a role for HMGB1 in this pathophysiologic process.

## HMGB1 and Acute Lung Injury

Intratracheal administration of HMGB1 produces ALI, and antibodies against HMGB1 decrease LPS- or hemorrhage-induced lung edema and neutrophil accumulation [27, 42]. Anti-HMGB1 antibodies did not significantly reduce the levels of the pro-inflammatory cytokines TNF-α, IL-1β, or MIP-2 in LPS-induced ALI, indicating that HMGB1 occupies a more distal position in endotoxin-induced pro-inflammatory cascades. In addition, these results suggest that the previously described roles of early appearing pro-inflammatory cytokines, such as TNF-α and IL-1β, in inducing LPS and perhaps sepsis-induced ALI may not all have been due to direct effects, but rather to their ability to produce generation of HMGB1.

## Receptors for HMGB1 Include RAGE, TLR2, and TLR4

The receptor for advanced glycation end products (RAGE), a multiligand member of the immunoglobulin superfamily of cell surface molecules, interacts with HMGB1 and triggers activation of key cell signaling pathways [43–47]. Binding of HMGB1 to RAGE leads to neurite outgrowth and enhanced expression of plasminogen activator by macrophages [40, 48–53]. Although RAGE is a major receptor for HMGB1 in neural tissue and some malignant cells [44, 48–50, 54], this receptor appears to be less important in HMGB1 signaling among other cell populations. For example, incubation of microvascular endothelial cells with anti-RAGE antibodies only decreased HMGB1-induced IL-8 production by 14% and TNF-α production by 17% [40].

Because the pattern of kinase activation and release of pro-inflammatory cytokines induced by HMGB1 in macrophages is similar to that which occurs after incubation with the Gram-negative bacterial product LPS that interacts with TLR4 or with the Gram-positive products peptidoglycan or lipotechoic acid that interact with TLR2, it seemed possible that HMGB1 might interact with these same receptors. Subsequent experiments, using transfection of TLR2 or TLR4 into HEK cells that normally do not bear these receptors, as well as studies that directly examined the interaction of HMGB1 with TLR2 or TLR4 on macrophages, showed that HMGB1 does produce cellular activation through TLR2 and TLR4 [55]. Interestingly, RAGE appears to be less important than either TLR2 or TLR4 for macrophage stimulation by HMGB1 [56].

## Cellular Activation Pathways Induced by HMGB1

Interaction of bacterial products with TLR2 or TLR4 leads to enhanced nuclear translocation of nuclear factor kappa B (NF-κB), occurring through activation of the IKKα/β kinase complex. In neutrophils and macrophages, the p38 mitogen activated protein kinase pathway (p38 MAPK) as well as the phosphoinositide-3 kinase (PI3-K) pathways are also activated when signaling is induced through TLR2 and TLR4, and also appear to contribute to inducing nuclear translocation of NF-κB [57].

Since the primary signaling initiated by HMGB1 in neutrophils and macrophages occurs through TLR2 and TLR4, it is not surprising that exposure of these cell populations to HMGB1 produces nuclear translocation of NF-κB and activation of the p38 and PI3-K kinase pathways with patterns resembling those induced by LPS [40, 41, 56]. However, gene array studies show that the patterns of gene expression induced by LPS and HMGB1, although similar in many respects, also demonstrate significant differences, consistent with the use of receptors other than TLR4 by HMGB1 [41].

Signaling pathways involving cellular activation by HMGB1 are shown in Fig. 1.

## Release of HMGB1 from Necrotic Cells Triggers Inflammation

When cells die by necrosis rather than apoptosis, they lose their membrane integrity and release intracellular contents. Necrotic cell death is common in the setting of trauma and blood loss. HMGB1 is passively released by necrotic or damaged cells [23, 25]. Transgenic cells lacking HMGB1 (HMGB1 -/-) have greatly reduced ability to promote inflammation when they die by necrosis, showing that the release of HMGB1 by necrotic cell death can initiate inflammatory responses in neighboring cells [19, 25, 58]. In contrast, apoptotic cells do not release HMGB1 even after undergoing secondary necrosis, and fail to promote inflammation even if not cleared promptly by phogocytic cells. In apoptotic cells, HMGB1 remains bound to chromatin because of generalized underacetylation of histones. If chromatin deacetylation is prevented during the apoptosis process, HMGB1 is released into the intracellular space and can promote inflammation. The *in vivo* role of HMGB1

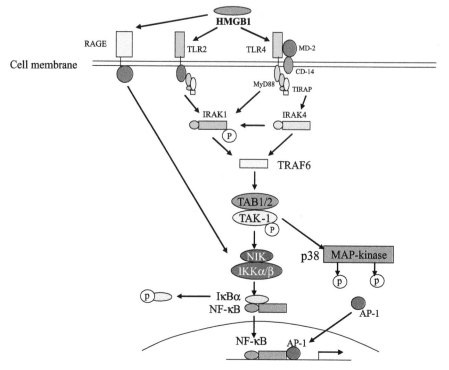

**Fig. 1.** Signaling pathways activated by high mobility group box protein 1 (HMGB1)

in mediating inflammation after cellular necrosis is shown in experiments where anti-HMGB1 antibodies reduce damage and inflammatory cell recruitment to the liver after acetaminophen-induced necrosis [25].

## Conclusion

HMGB1 is a novel late mediator of inflammatory responses that contributes to ALI and lethal sepsis. It appears to interact with at least three receptors, including RAGE, TLR2, and TLR4, potentially explaining the similarities in cellular activation induced by HMGB1 and bacterial products, such as LPS or peptidoglycan. However, the multiple receptors involved in HMGB1 signaling also provide insights into the differences in gene expression produced by cellular interaction with this mediator. Unlike the situation with classically described pro-inflammatory cytokines, such as TNF-α or IL-1β, where blockade is only effective in improving outcome from experimental sepsis if administered before or very early in the course of sepsis, inhibition of HMGB1 with specific antibodies or the HMGB1 A box sequence still reduces mortality even if performed up to 24 hours after the initiation of the septic insult. Such findings suggest that HMGB1 may be an appropriate therapeutic target in patients with sepsis or ALI, since it may participate in the pathogenesis of organ dysfunction and mortality even at later time points when such patients present for hospital or ICU admission.

*Acknowledgement.* This work was supported in part by NIH awards HL68743 and GM49222.

# References

1. Moore FA, Moore EE, Sauaia A (1997) Blood transfusion. An independent risk factor for postinjury multiple organ failure. Arch Surg 132:620–624
2. Sauaia A, Moore FA, Moore EE, et al (1994) Early predictors of postinjury multiple organ failure. Arch Surg 129:39–45
3. Sauaia A, Moore FA, Moore EE, Lezotte DC (1996) Early risk factors for postinjury multiple organ failure. World J Surg 20:392–400
4. Sauaia A, Moore FA, Moore EE, et al (1998) Multiple organ failure can be predicted as early as 12 hours after injury. J Trauma 45:291–301
5. Abraham E, Allbee J (1994) Effects of therapy with interleukin-1 receptor antagonist on pulmonary cytokine expression following hemorrhage and resuscitation. Lymphokine Cytokine Res 13:343–347
6. Abraham E, Coulson WF, Schwartz MD, Allbee J (1994) Effects of therapy with soluble tumour necrosis factor receptor fusion protein on pulmonary cytokine expression and lung injury following haemorrhage and resuscitation. Clin Exp Immunol 98:29–34
7. Abraham E, Jesmok G, Tuder R, et al (1995) Contribution of tumor necrosis factor-alpha to pulmonary cytokine expression and lung injury after hemorrhage and resuscitation. Crit Care Med 23:1319–1326
8. Andersson U, Erlandsson-Harris H, Yang H, Tracey KJ (2002) HMGB1 as a DNA-binding cytokine. J Leukoc Biol 72:1084–1091
9. Czura CJ, Tracey KJ (2003) Targeting high mobility group box 1 as a late-acting mediator of inflammation. Crit Care Med 31:S46–50
10. Czura CJ, Wang H, Tracey KJ (2001) Dual roles for HMGB1: DNA binding and cytokine. J Endotoxin Res 7:315–321
11. Ulloa L, Ochani M, Yang H, et al (2002) Ethyl pyruvate prevents lethality in mice with established lethal sepsis and systemic inflammation. Proc Natl Acad Sci USA 99:12351–12356
12. Wang H, Yang H, Czura CJ, et al (2001) HMGB1 as a late mediator of lethal systemic inflammation. Am J Respir Crit Care Med 164:1768–1773
13. Yang H, Wang H, Czura CJ, Tracey KJ (2002) HMGB1 as a cytokine and therapeutic target. J Endotoxin Res 8:469–472
14. Chen G, Ward MF, Sama AE, Wang H (2004) Extracellular HMGB1 as a proinflammatory cytokine. J Interferon Cytokine Res 24:329–333
15. Czura CJ, Yang H, Amella CA, Tracey KJ (2004) HMGB1 in the Immunology of Sepsis (Not Septic Shock) and Arthritis. Adv Immunol 84:181–200
16. Erlandsson Harris H, Andersson U (2004) Mini-review: The nuclear protein HMGB1 as a proinflammatory mediator. Eur J Immunol 34:1503–1512
17. Sadikot RT, Christman JW, Blackwell TS (2004) Molecular targets for modulating lung inflammation and injury. Curr Drug Targets 5:581–588
18. Wang H, Yang H, Tracey KJ (2004) Extracellular role of HMGB1 in inflammation and sepsis. J Intern Med 255:320–331

19. Muller S, Scaffidi P, Degryse B, et al (2001) New EMBO members' review: the double life of HMGB1 chromatin protein: architectural factor and extracellular signal. Embo J 20:4337–4340
20. Yang H, Wang H, Tracey KJ (2001) HMG-1 rediscovered as a cytokine. Shock 15:247–253
21. Sappington PL, Yang R, Yang H, et al (2002) HMGB1 B box increases the permeability of Caco-2 enterocytic monolayers and impairs intestinal barrier function in mice. Gastroenterology 123:790–802
22. Taudte S, Xin H, Bell AJ Jr, Kallenbach NR (2001) Interactions between HMG boxes. Protein Eng 14:1015–1023
23. Bustin M (2002) At the crossroads of necrosis and apoptosis: signaling to multiple cellular targets by HMGB1. Sci STKE 151:PE39
24. Andersson U, Wang H, Palmblad K, et al (2000) High mobility group 1 protein (HMG-1) stimulates proinflammatory cytokine synthesis in human monocytes. J Exp Med 192:565–570
25. Scaffidi P, Misteli T, Bianchi ME (2002) Release of chromatin protein HMGB1 by necrotic cells triggers inflammation. Nature 418:191–195
26. Wang H, Bloom O, Zhang M, et al (1999) HMG-1 as a late mediator of endotoxin lethality in mice. Science 285:248–251
27. Abraham E, Arcaroli J, Carmody A, et al (2000) HMG-1 as a mediator of acute lung inflammation. J Immunol 165:2950–2954
28. Yang H, Ochani M, Li J, et al (2004) Reversing established sepsis with antagonists of endogenous high-mobility group box 1. Proc Natl Acad Sci USA 101:296–301
29. Sunden-Cullberg J, Norrby-Teglund A, Rouhiainen A, et al (2005) Persistent elevation of high mobility group box-1 protein (HMGB1) in patients with severe sepsis and septic shock. Crit Care Med 33:564–573
30. Hotchkiss RS, Karl IE (2003) The pathophysiology and treatment of sepsis. N Engl J Med 348:138–150
31. Ombrellino M, Wang H, Ajemian MS, et al (1999) Increased serum concentrations of high-mobility-group protein 1 in haemorrhagic shock. Lancet 354:1446–1447
32. Fang WH, Yao YM, Shi ZG, et al (2002) The significance of changes in high mobility group-1 protein mRNA expression in rats after thermal injury. Shock 17:329–333
33. Le Tulzo Y, Shenkar R, Kaneko D, et al (1997) Hemorrhage increases cytokine expression in lung mononuclear cells in mice: involvement of catecholamines in nuclear factor-kappaB regulation and cytokine expression. J Clin Invest 99:1516–1524
34. Moine P, Shenkar R, Kaneko D, et al (1997) Systemic blood loss affects NF-kappa B regulatory mechanisms in the lungs. Am J Physiol 273: L185–192
35. Parsey MV, Tuder RM, Abraham E (1998) Neutrophils are major contributors to intra-parenchymal lung IL-1 beta expression after hemorrhage and endotoxemia. J Immunol 160:1007–1013
36. Shenkar R, Abraham E (1997) Hemorrhage induces rapid in vivo activation of CREB and NF-kappaB in murine intraparenchymal lung mononuclear cells. Am J Respir Cell Mol Biol 16:145–152
37. Shenkar R, Abraham E (1993) Effects of hemorrhage on cytokine gene transcription. Lymphokine Cytokine Res 12:237–247
38. Shenkar R, Coulson WF, Abraham E (1994) Hemorrhage and resuscitation induce alterations in cytokine expression and the development of acute lung injury. Am J Respir Cell Mol Biol 10:290–297
39. Shenkar R, Yum HK, Arcaroli J, et al (2001) Interactions between CBP, NF-kappaB, and CREB in the lungs after hemorrhage and endotoxemia. Am J Physiol Lung Cell Mol Physiol 281:L418–426
40. Fiuza C, Bustin M, Talwar S, et al (2003) Inflammation-promoting activity of HMGB1 on human microvascular endothelial cells. Blood 101:2652–2660

41. Park JS, Arcaroli J, Yum HK, et al (2003) Activation of gene expression in human neutrophils by high mobility group box 1 protein. Am J Physiol Cell Physiol 284:C870–C879
42. Kim JY, Park JS, Strassheim D, et al (2005) HMGB1 contributes to the development of acute lung injury after hemorrhage. Am J Physiol Lung Cell Mol Physiol 288:L958–L965
43. Bucciarelli LG, Wendt T, Rong L, et al (2002) RAGE is a multiligand receptor of the immunoglobulin superfamily: implications for homeostasis and chronic disease. Cell Mol Life Sci 59:1117–1128
44. Huttunen HJ, Fages C, Kuja-Panula J, et al (2002) Receptor for advanced glycation end products-binding COOH-terminal motif of amphoterin inhibits invasive migration and metastasis. Cancer Res 62:4805–4811
45. Schmidt AM, Yan SD, Yan SF, Stern DM (2001) The multiligand receptor RAGE as a progression factor amplifying immune and inflammatory responses. J Clin Invest 108:949–955
46. Sparatore B, Pedrazzi M, Passalacqua M, et al (2002) Stimulation of erythroleukaemia cell differentiation by extracellular high-mobility group-box protein 1 is independent of the receptor for advanced glycation end-products. Biochem J 363:529–535
47. Stern D, Du Yan S, Fang Yan S, Marie Schmidt A (2002) Receptor for advanced glycation endproducts: a multiligand receptor magnifying cell stress in diverse pathologic settings. Adv Drug Deliv Rev 54:1615–1625
48. Hori O, Brett J, Slattery T, et al (1995) The receptor for advanced glycation end products (RAGE) is a cellular binding site for amphoterin. Mediation of neurite outgrowth and co-expression of rage and amphoterin in the developing nervous system. J Biol Chem 270:25752–25761
49. Huttunen HJ, Fages C, Rauvala H (1999) Receptor for advanced glycation end products (RAGE)-mediated neurite outgrowth and activation of NF-kappaB require the cytoplasmic domain of the receptor but different downstream signaling pathways. J Biol Chem 274:19919–19924
50. Sajithlal G, Huttunen H, Rauvala H, Munch G (2002) Receptor for advanced glycation end products plays a more important role in cellular survival than in neurite outgrowth during retinoic acid-induced differentiation of neuroblastoma cells. J Biol Chem 277:6888–6897
51. Schmidt AM, Hori O, Cao R, et al (1996) RAGE: a novel cellular receptor for advanced glycation end products. Diabetes 45 (Suppl 3):S77–80
52. Taniguchi N, Kawahara K, Yone K, et al (2003) High mobility group box chromosomal protein 1 plays a role in the pathogenesis of rheumatoid arthritis as a novel cytokine. Arthritis Rheum 48:971–981
53. Parkkinen J, Raulo E, Merenmies J, et al (1993) Amphoterin, the 30-kDa protein in a family of HMG1-type polypeptides. Enhanced expression in transformed cells, leading edge localization, and interactions with plasminogen activation. J Biol Chem 268:19726–19738
54. Huttunen HJ, Kuja-Panula J, Rauvala H (2002) Receptor for advanced glycation end products (RAGE) signaling induces CREB-dependent chromogranin expression during neuronal differentiation. J Biol Chem 277:38635–38646
55. Park JS, Gamboni-Robertson F, He Q, et al (2005) High Mobility Group Box 1 protein (HMGB1) interacts with multiple Toll like receptors. Am J Physiol Cell Physiol 290:C917–924
56. Park JS, Svetkauskaite D, He Q, et al (2004) Involvement of Toll-like receptors 2 and 4 in cellular activation by High Mobility Group Box 1 protein. J Biol Chem 279:7370–7377
57. O'Neill LA (2002) Signal transduction pathways activated by the IL-1 receptor/toll-like receptor superfamily. Curr Top Microbiol Immunol 270:47–61
58. Bianchi ME, Beltrame M (2000) Upwardly mobile proteins. Workshop: the role of HMG proteins in chromatin structure, gene expression and neoplasia. EMBO Rep 1:109–114

# Nitric Oxide

J. Carré, M. Singer, and S. Moncada

## Introduction

Progression of sepsis to septic shock and multiple organ failure (MOF) is clinically characterized by (i) a hyperdynamic state with a high cardiac output; (ii) decreased vascular reactivity towards pressor agents, leading to vasodilatory shock despite adequate fluid resuscitation; (iii) myocardial depression (despite the often elevated cardiac output); and (iv) development of organ dysfunction. MOF carries a mortality of between 20–80%, with survival being inversely correlated to the number of dysfunctional organs [1]. Respiratory, cardiovascular, renal and hematological dysfunction are the most prevalent. The mechanisms underlying the pathogenesis of MOF remain to be fully elucidated but excess production of nitric oxide (NO) plays a central role.

Early indications of the involvement of nitrogen species during infection came from observations in the 1980s of elevated urinary nitrate levels in humans with diarrhea and fever [2]. Subsequently, urinary nitrate levels in rats treated with lipopolysaccharide (LPS, bacterial endotoxin) were found to correlate with the degree of fever [3]. Interest in the function of NO in the causation of septic shock escalated following the discovery of its role in vasorelaxation [4–6] and several reports of nitrate production by immune-stimulated macrophages (reviewed in [7]). As of December 2005, nearly 2,000 of the 72,000 PubMed listed abstracts citing 'NO' also contained the keyword 'sepsis'. Host production of NO has been modulated in a multitude of animal models and in clinical trials. Despite considerable interest in the use of NO synthase (NOS) inhibitors to reverse catecholamine-resistant septic shock, a phase III randomized, double-blind, placebo-controlled study was terminated prematurely because of increased mortality in the treatment group [8]. The conflicting results generated by these studies have heightened awareness of the cytopathic and cytoprotective roles that NO plays in sepsis and MOF. Significantly, the role of NO in the development of mitochondrial dysfunction, which appears to be a fundamental pathophysiological mechanism in the development of MOF, is being increasingly appreciated.

## Reactivity and Cellular Targets of NO and its Derivatives

### Direct Effects of NO

NO is a highly diffusible, lipophilic gas with a half-life of 6-10 seconds in aqueous environments. It can interact directly with ferrous iron in heme-containing proteins, resulting in either activation or inhibition of target proteins. A first target is the enzyme, soluble guanylate synthase (sGC). This enzyme is directly activated by NO binding to produce the second messenger molecule cGMP, resulting in a chain of events leading to NO-dependent vasorelaxation (Fig. 1). Second, NO competes with oxygen for the mitochondrial cytochrome c oxidase (complex IV), resulting in reversible inhibition of the complex at physiological NO concentrations [9–11]). Finally, activity of the family of NO synthase enzymes themselves is regulated by product-inhibition by NO [12].

### NO Derivatives and Their Molecular Targets

Although a free radical by virtue of possessing an uneven number of electrons, NO is relatively unreactive at physiological (nM) concentrations. Its reactivity increases at higher concentrations (low µM), such as would occur in biological membranes or upon inflammatory release of NO. In such cases, NO can react with molecular oxygen to generate nitrogen dioxide ($NO_2$) or dinitrogen trioxide ($N_2O_2$), or with superoxide ($O_2^-$) to yield peroxynitrite ($ONOO^-$). These derivatives can either nitrosylate and/or nitrate various molecules, including proteins and lipids. Reaction with thiol groups results in generation of nitrosothiols (see [7, 13] for review).

Peroxynitrite can react with various amino-acid side chains of different proteins, including mitochondrial enzymes ([14] reviewed in [15]), catalase, ion channels, receptors, cell signaling proteins, and transcription factors [16]. Additionally, while NO itself appears to inhibit the propagation of lipid peroxidation (by scavenging peroxyl radicals), the highly oxidizing peroxynitrite can react with unsaturated fatty acids and initiate lipid peroxidation directly, through scavenging of antioxidants, or by reaction with low-density lipoproteins (LDLs) [17]. Peroxynitrite can also shear DNA, thus causing recruitment and direct activation of poly(ADP-ribose) polymerase (PARP), an enzyme involved in DNA repair which may deplete $NAD^+$ stores (reviewed in [18]).

## Generation of Nitric Oxide: The Nitric Oxide Synthases

NO is primarily synthesized by the NOS family of proteins, by reaction of 1 mol of L-arginine with 1.5 mol NADPH and 2 mol of molecular oxygen to yield one mol each of L-citrulline and NO and 2 mol of water. There are three members of the family, numerically designated according to the order in which they were cloned:

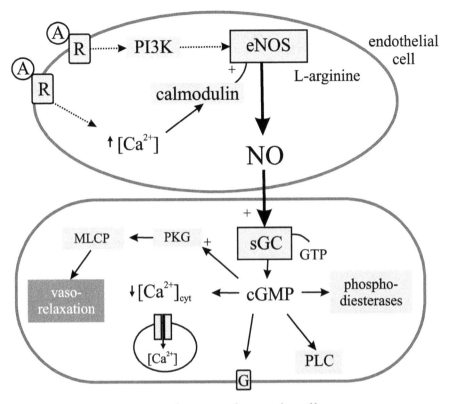

**Fig. 1.** Role of nitric oxide (NO) in cGMP-mediated vasorelaxation and in platelets. Endothelial cell activation by interaction of agonist (A, e.g., bradykinin, acetylcholine, insulin, estrogen) with cell-surface receptors (R), results in transient calcium-dependent and/or phosphoinositol-3-kinase (PI3)-dependent activation of eNOS. The NO produced rapidly diffuses into vascular smooth muscle cells (VSM) (and other nearby cells including platelets), where it activates soluble guanylate cyclase (sGC) directly, elevating cGMP levels. cGMP has numerous targets in different cells (arrows), including ion-channels, receptors (G), phosphatases, kinases, phospholipase C (PLC) and phosphodiesterases. In the VSM, cGMP acts on calcium channels and on myosin light-chain phosphatase (MLCP) *via* protein kinase G (PKG). In this way, the myosin contractile apparatus is dephosphorylated and desensitized to calcium, resulting in relaxation. In platelets, NO stimulates cGMP-mediated decreases in cytosolic $Ca^{2+}$ which, in combination with prostaglandins, prevent platelet activation and aggregation by negative regulation of, for example, glycoproteinIIb/IIIa receptors

NOS1 (neuronal, or nNOS), NOS2 (inducible, or iNOS) and NOS3 (endothelial or eNOS). Additionally, the existence of a mitochondrial isoform (mtNOS) has been proposed [19,20]. Each NOS isoform is dimeric and requires several cofactors and prosthetic groups: heme, tetrahydropterin, NADPH, FAD, FMN and calmodulin. Characteristics of the three NOS isoforms that have been identified are outlined in Table 1.

**Table 1.** Expression and regulatory aspects of nitric oxide synthase (NOS) isoforms

| Isoform | expression | regulation |
|---------|-----------|-----------|
| nNOS (NOS1) | neurons (CNS, PNS), skeletal muscle, some blood vessels, pulmonary epithelium, gastrointestinal and genitourinary systems | • *constitutive expression*<br>• *transcriptional activation*: ischemic preconditioning, wounding<br>• *regulation of enzyme activity*: receptor agonists affecting calcium/calmodulin; NO (feedback inhibition) |
| iNOS (NOS2) | *induced* in activated macrophages, neutrophils, monocytes, eosinophils, hepatocytes, vascular smooth muscle, epithelium, endothelium, myocytes, fibroblasts, osteoblasts *constitutive expression*: intestinal, bronchial & renal tubular endothelium | • *some constitutive expression*<br>• *transcriptional activation*: immunoactivation (LPS, interferon γ, TNF-α, IL-1); shear stress, L-arginine<br>• *transcriptional downregulation*: steroids; NO; heat shock response<br>• *protein activity*: calcium-independent |
| eNOS (NOS3) | vascular endothelium, blood platelets, cardiomyocytes | • *constitutive expression*<br>• *transcriptional activation*: shear stress, rho kinase pathways<br>• *post-transcriptional*: mRNA stability<br>• *enzyme activity*: receptor agonists affecting calcium/ calmodulin; NO (feedback inhibition); HSP90 |

CNS: central nervous system; PNS: peripheral nervous system; LPS; lipopolysaccharide; TNF: tumor necrosis factor; IL: interleukin; HSP: heat shock protein

Whereas iNOS has been classically viewed as the inducible NOS isoform (expressed in response to immunoactivation), with nNOS and eNOS as constitutively expressed isoforms, it is becoming apparent that all three isoforms are subject to regulation at the level of expression (Table 1) [21, 22]. Both eNOS and nNOS produce briefly elevated (pM to low nM) physiological concentrations of NO in response to $Ca^{2+}$ transients. NO produced under these conditions serves to act as a neurotransmitter (nNOS), as a signaling molecule (eNOS), and as a physiological regulator of cellular functions such as mitochondrial respiration (reviewed in [23]). On the other hand, expression of iNOS occurs over several hours and results in sustained synthesis of elevated levels of NO (high nM to low μM).

Mechanistic and regulatory characteristics of specific NOS isoforms are complex (reviewed in [24]). The different enzymes may be physiologically regulated to varying extents by local NO concentration and oxygen tension. Some of the physiological consequences of NOS isoform activity are discussed below.

## Cellular Effects of NO

### Vasorelaxant Effect

Vasorelaxation was one of the first physiological effects of NO to be described [4–6] (reviewed in [25]). Stimulation of the calcium/calmodulin-dependent eNOS isoform by factors such as endothelial shear stress or exogenous vasodilators (e.g., acetylcholine, histamine, bradykinin) releases picomolar levels of NO in the endothelium through transient rises in endothelial $Ca^{2+}$. NO rapidly diffuses to the vascular smooth muscle where it binds and activates sGC to generate cGMP. Amongst its key actions, this second messenger mediates uptake of $Ca^{2+}$ into the sarcoplasmic reticulum which, in turn, promotes vasorelaxation and also inhibits platelet aggregation and leukocyte adhesion (Fig. 1). Thus, through its effects on the vascular system, NO is intricately involved in modulating oxygen delivery to tissues.

### NO and the Immune Response

In response to stimuli such as endotoxin, interferon (IFN)-γ or expression of Toll-like receptors, various cells of the innate immune response system (including macrophages, neutrophils, vascular endothelial cells, and hepatocytes) release a host of inflammatory mediators, including cytokines such as tumor necrosis factor (TNF)-α and interleukin (IL)-1β, chemokines, clotting factors, proteases, and NO. The latter is produced due to an induction of the iNOS isoform that occurs *via* a nuclear factor-kappa B (NF-κB)-dependent transcription pathway in response to cytokine stimulation [26,27]. Induction of iNOS expression is inhibited by glucocorticoids [28]. Interestingly, NF-κB activation and the induction of iNOS in murine macrophages has been found to be significantly dependent on the activity of constitutive eNOS, in part *via* an sGC and cGMP-dependent mechanism [29].

### Effects of NO on Mitochondria

Mitochondria provide the majority of the cell's energy requirement in the form of ATP; furthermore, mitochondria are known to play a role in defining cell fate. NO affects mitochondrial function through the following interdependent mechanisms: (i) inhibition of mitochondrial respiration (both reversible and irreversible); and (ii) increasing concentrations of reactive oxygen intermediates (Fig. 2).

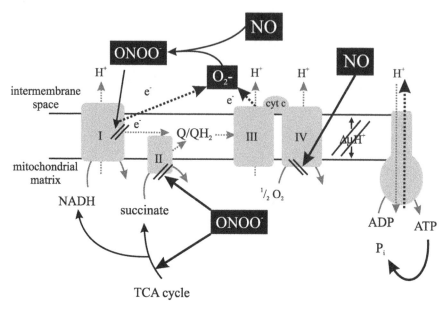

**Fig. 2.** Effects of nitric oxide (NO) on mitochondrial respiration. The respiratory chain, housed in the inner mitochondrial membrane, couples the energy released from oxidation of NADH- or FADH$_2$-linked substrates to the pumping of protons (H$^+$) across the membrane (gray arrows). The resulting membrane potential $\Delta\psi$ (and $\Delta$pH) is used to drive both the synthesis of ATP by F$_0$F$_1$ATPase, and the transport of ions and proteins into the mitochondrial matrix. Proton pumping is performed by the action of three protein complexes: NADH dehydrogenase complex (Complex I); the *bc*1 complex (Complex III) and cytochrome *c* oxidase complex (Complex IV). The effects of NO mitochondrial respiration are indicated with thick black arrows (see text for details) and comprise (i) inhibition of respiratory chain and tricarboxylic acid (TCA) cycle leading to (ii) decreased ATP synthesis, (iii) increased ROS production and (iv) gradual depolarization of the mitochondrial inner membrane. Depending on the extent to which it occurs, dissipation of $\Delta\psi$ may lead to hydrolysis of ATP by the ATPase, disruption of ion transport and calcium homeostasis, and persistent mitochondrial permeability transition

## Inhibition of mitochondrial respiration

At physiological concentrations of tissue oxygen (approximately 30 µM) NO is a potent, reversible inhibitor of cytochrome c oxidase (mitochondrial respiratory complex IV) [9–11] (reviewed in [23,30]), with half-maximal inhibition occurring at 60 nM [9]. This inhibition may represent a physiological means of regulation of respiration by influencing the affinity of cytochrome c oxidase for oxygen (see [31]). The source of NO for potential regulation of mitochondrial respiration remains uncertain. Although relatively short-lived, the highly diffusible and lipophilic nature of NO means that non-mitochondrial or even transcellular generation of NO may be sufficient to affect mitochondria. Under hypoxic conditions, NO outcompetes O$_2$, thus increasing the sensitivity of cytochrome c oxidase to NO inhibition [9,30,32].

Increasing concentrations of reactive oxygen intermediates

Interaction of NO with complex IV of the respiratory chain can result in leakage of electrons leading to the formation of superoxide, thus increasing the release of reactive oxygen species (ROS) by the respiratory chain. Under these conditions, the formation of peroxynitrite may be favored. Persistent exposure of cells or mitochondria to elevated NO leads to the formation of peroxynitrite, resulting in replacement of the reversible inhibition of complex IV by an irreversible inhibition of respiration at respiratory complex 1 (NADH dehydrogenase) (see [14]) and probably other sites such as aconitase (a tricarboxylic cycle enzyme) and GAPDH. In addition to increasing the production of ROS by blocking the electron transfer chain, peroxynitrite-induced inhibition of defense mechanisms (e.g., catalase, mitochondrial MnSOD) further exacerbates oxidative stress (see [14]; reviewed in [15,30]). Peroxynitrite can be scavenged by high concentrations of antioxidants, such as glutathione and ascorbic acid, which can decrease the extent of mitochondrial damage. Consequently, insufficient antioxidant capacity (which may occur when ROS production is high) will result in lasting detrimental effects on mitochondrial respiration. Mitochondrial dysfunction induced by prolonged exposure to elevated NO or peroxynitrite is becoming increasingly implicated in a number of pathological states, including sepsis (below) [33].

## Apoptosis and Necrosis

NO has been shown either to stimulate or prevent apoptosis, depending on the cell type and conditions. At physiological levels, NO may protect cells including cardiomyocytes, hepatocytes, thymocytes, and lymphocytes from apoptosis by inhibition of executor proteins including the caspase family of proteases, regulation of receptor or $Ca^{2+}$ channel activity, and upregulation of protective proteins such as Bcl-2, heme oxygenase and heat-shock proteins. On the other hand, NO participates in apoptosis of some cortical neurons and macrophages, while prolonged exposure to NO, such as occurs in inflammation, can result in increased apoptosis by several mechanisms including increasing Fas death receptor expression and down-regulation of apoptotic-inhibitor proteins. At the mitochondrial level, activation of apoptotic factors and disruption of $Ca^{2+}$ homeostasis by NO or peroxynitrite leads to an increase in mitochondrial membrane permeability and the subsequent release of cytochrome c (reviewed in [15,18,34]). NO-induced oxidation of lipids can also lead to apoptosis.

Necrosis may be induced in cells when ATP levels decrease to the extent that plasma membrane ion pumps fail, depolarization occurs, and cells swell and rupture due to loss of ion homeostasis. With prolonged exposure to NO, inhibition of mitochondrial respiration or, possibly, excess activation of the NAD-depleting DNA repair protein PARP, necrosis may ensue when demand for ATP cannot be met by glycolysis. By contrast, apoptotic pathways require a certain amount of ATP, so this process is prevented under conditions of severe ATP depletion, resulting in a necrotic mode of cell death.

## Mitochondrial Biogenesis

Although mitochondria carry their own DNA, this encodes less than 5% of the proteins located in this organelle. The majority are encoded by the nucleus and imported into the mitochondria using protein translocation machinery. The peroxisome proliferator-activated receptor-γ coactivators, PGC-1α and PGC-1β, appear to play a key role by triggering expression of the transcription factors NRF-1 and NRF-2. These factors regulate expression of nuclear-encoded mitochondrial respiratory proteins and proteins involved in expression of the mitochondrial genome. NO stimulates mitochondrial biogenesis in various cell types through cGMP-mediated activation of PGC-1α [35].

## Measurement of NO Production

Although a NO-sensitive electrode has been employed in some *in vitro* studies, it is inherently difficult to directly measure concentrations of NO produced in animal models or in patients, due to the relatively short half-life of this gas. Rates of NO production can be measured indirectly *in vitro* in tissue sample homogenates by the rate of transfer of radiolabel from [$^3$H]-L-arginine to [$^3$H]-L-citrulline. Most commonly, experimental and clinical studies assess the concentration of the NO breakdown products, $NO_3^-$ and $NO_2^-$ (often collectively referred to as NOx) in plasma or urine. The extent to which determinations of plasma or urinary NOx are a true reflection of NO production may be limited by the existence of renal failure, plasma protein levels, the type of food intake, and the half-life of the NOx species. Also, the reactions of NO described above result in the formation of other products, for example nitrotyrosine and nitrosothiols, which are not detected by this method [36]. Furthermore, while plasma NOx can be a useful indicator of altered NO metabolism, rates of production and accumulated concentrations of NO and its derivatives are likely to vary significantly between different tissues and organs during the progression of sepsis.

## NO Production in Sepsis

### Overproduction of NO

Large increases in NOx are frequently observed in rodent models of endotoxic shock or sepsis. However, in studies involving larger animals and patients, increases in plasma NOx concentrations occur to a much lesser extent. Plasma NOx concentrations in control patients are typically reported to be between 14 and 40 µM [36–39]. A 3.5-fold increase in plasma NOx was reported in septic patients with hypotension [39], and 6- to 8-fold increases during recurrent episodes of shock [36]. Arnalich et al. [38] noted that the peak increase in NOx (6-fold) occurred after several hours. An inverse correlation was found between plasma NOx and mean arterial pressure (MAP) [37]. Further correlations have been reported between plasma NOx and low systemic vascular resistance (SVR), high endotoxin levels [40,41] and cardiac output [40].

NOx levels are also elevated in tissues from septic patients. Brealey et al. [42] reported a 2- to 4-fold increase in NOx levels in skeletal muscle biopsies taken from patients with septic shock, which correlated with severity of illness assessed by norepinephrine requirements and the sequential Organ Failure Assessment (SOFA). Annane et al. [37] found that rates of [$^3$H]-citrulline synthesis (an indirect measure of NO production) were dramatically increased in skin, muscle, fat (> 70-fold) and arteriolar tissues (> 1,200-fold) compared to normal tissue.

In summary, NO over-production appears to be characteristic of patients with sepsis and MOF. The degree of overproduction appears to be less than that seen in rodents, but an equivalent effect is seen on blood pressure, cardiac output and illness severity.

## Sources of NO in Sepsis: Involvement of the Different NOS Isoforms

In rodent models of endotoxic shock, high levels of iNOS protein expression have been found in lung, liver, spleen, and duodenum, as well as kidney, thymus, ileum, and heart [27,43]. It is interesting to note that total NOS activity is high in the brains of LPS-treated rats, whilst iNOS is barely detectable [43], suggesting activation of the constitutive enzyme in this tissue. In rodents, it appears that a rapid increase in NO production by calcium-sensitive constitutive NOS is followed after 2-6 hours by a more sustained expression and activity of iNOS.

In human sepsis, expression of specific NOS isoforms varies in different tissues. Induction of iNOS, concomitant with a downregulation of the constitutive isoforms, has been demonstrated in some septic tissues, including vascular smooth muscle. A reciprocal relationship between eNOS and iNOS expression has been documented *in vitro* during inflammation [44], whilst a similar observation has been made between nNOS and iNOS expression and activity in skeletal muscle of septic patients [45]. A correlation between disease severity, a reduction in contractility of rectus abdominis muscle, and the level of iNOS protein in this tissue has been reported [45]. In post-mortem samples of brain taken from septic patients, Sharshar et al. noted that, whilst iNOS expression was barely detectable in neurons and microglial cells, endothelial iNOS expression was significant and correlated with the extent of apoptosis in the autonomic centers [46].

Earlier, a localized, rather than widespread, upregulation of iN OS had been suggested in tissues of patients with necrotizing fasciitis; activity of iNOS was limited to the nidus of infection in muscle, fat and artery, with approximately 70-fold increases in iNOS activity in putresecent tissues compared to normal muscle or fat tissue, and a > 1,200-fold increase in the aorta [37].

## Effects of NO in Sepsis-induced MOF

### NO and the Circulatory System

#### Decreased Systemic Vascular Resistance and Vascular Hyporeactivity

NO is implicated in vasodilatory shock by both cGMP-dependent and independent mechanisms [25,47]. The major effect of NO is likely to be mediated by sustained activation of sGC and the vasorelaxant mechanism depicted in Fig. 1. However, cGMP also activates calcium-dependent and ATP-dependent plasma membrane potassium channels ($K_{Ca}$ and $K_{ATP}$), allowing potassium efflux from the cell. Prolonged channel activation would lead to hyperpolarization of the plasma membrane, inhibition of voltage-gated calcium channels and decreased cytosolic calcium content, further contributing to vasorelaxation and promoting a hyporeactive response of the systemic vasculature to catecholamines. The contribution of this latter mechanism to the vasodilation and vascular hyporeactivity of septic shock has not been fully evaluated; however the $K_{ATP}$ channel is being increasingly implicated. This is the result of observations such as those demonstrating that sulfonylurea inhibitors of this channel result in a significant increase in MAP and SVR in endotoxic shock and other shock states (reviewed in [47]). Besides the loss of vascular tone, endothelial permeability is also compromised in sepsis, resulting in tissue edema and increased flux of circulating factors to the extravascular compartments.

#### Myocardial Depression

Myocardial depression is frequently found in fluid-resuscitated septic patients, despite the presence of a persistent hyperdynamic state. Although the cause of myocardial depression in sepsis is not fully understood, it is likely that the condition is not simply due to hypoperfusion and ischemia, and circulating depressant substances, including TNF-$\alpha$, IL-1$\beta$ and NO, appear to be involved [48]. Increases in iNOS expression correlating with cardiovascular depression were initially demonstrated in a model of septic shock in the rat [49]. This finding was later confirmed in isolated cardiac myocytes [50]. These observations, which have since been confirmed in other laboratories, indicate that NO plays a central role in sepsis-associated cardiac dysfunction, similar to that which it plays in producing vasodilation in septic shock.

Myocardial depression in septic patients is thought to involve both NO-independent adrenergic signaling defects and a stimulation of myocardial eNOS activity by cytokines and other circulating factors, producing cGMP-dependent loss of systolic contractile force and enhanced diastolic relaxation. As the inflammatory response is sustained, myocardial iNOS is expressed. In combination with sGC activation, NO may also be involved at this stage in adrenoreceptor dysfunction [48]. Whether in the late stages of septic shock depletion of L-arginine, and therefore low NO, plays a role in cardiac depression (as has been suggested by the experiments of Price et al. [51]) remains to be established.

# NO and Metabolism

## A Subsequent Bioenergetic Shutdown?

The concept of NO-mediated inhibition of mitochondrial function in septic organs is now firmly established. At the physiological level, an elevation in tissue oxygen tension ($PO_2$) is observed in sepsis (reviewed in [52]), in contrast to other shock states where tissue hypoxia occurs. Thus, whilst some maldistribution of microvascular blood flow undoubtedly occurs [53], tissue oxygenation in fluid-resuscitated, pressor-treated patients does not appear to be compromised. Two large clinical trials designed to optimize tissue oxygen delivery in patients with established MOF failed to demonstrate benefit [54, 55], and a later retrospective analysis concluded that, despite improved oxygen delivery, non-survivors displayed a lesser ability to increase tissue oxygen consumption following inotropic stimulation [56].

Although, at the biochemical level, alterations in mitochondrial function in human sepsis and in animal models have been described over the last 40 years (see [52, 57] for reviews), the mechanisms by which this may occur have only become apparent following the observations which indicated that persistent inhibition of complex IV by NO leads to a sequence of events including generation of ROS, depletion of glutathione, and subsequent inhibition of complex I [14]. In a recent study of septic patients, non-survivors exhibited depressed levels of skeletal muscle ATP and phosphocreatine, while ATP levels were significantly increased in survivors compared to controls [42]. An inverse correlation between tissue NOx levels and mitochondrial complex I activity or levels of reduced glutathione was seen [42]. Similar results were subsequently found in liver and muscle in a long-term resuscitated rat model of MOF [58], whilst reversible inhibition of complex IV by NO was observed in endotoxin- and IFN-induced aortic inflammation in the rat [59].

NO-dependent depression of mitochondrial respiration is thus clearly an important contributory factor to organ dysfunction in sepsis to such an extent that tissues obtained from iNOS knockout animals injected with endotoxin do not show impaired respiration [60]. Yet despite the decrease in ATP levels seen in severe long-term animal models and human non-survivors, cell death is not a significant feature in most failed organs (discussed below). Furthermore, organ recovery does not appear to be limited by the regenerative capacity of the tissue. It appears probable that where glycolysis is able to compensate for the decrease in mitochondrial ATP production and maintain cell viability (see [30]), the likelihood of organ recovery is increased. Whether the bioenergetic depression observed in organ failure represents an adaptive response analogous to hibernation would be worth investigating since, as recently suggested [61], a metabolic shutdown would increase the chances of cell (and organ) survival.

Hypoxia, Mitochondrial Metabolism, and Cell Death

In situations where microcirculatory disruption does lead to localized tissue hypoxia, it is likely that the effects of NO are detrimental to the survival of the cell. Direct competitive inhibition of respiration by NO will be enhanced at low oxygen tensions and ROS production increased. Peroxynitrite formation and irreversible inhibition of the respiratory chain and other mitochondrial enzymes will be favored. Under these conditions, ATP levels may decrease to an extent that glycolysis can no longer maintain cell viability, and cell death may become a feature. Indeed, hypoxia is known to sensitize mitochondria to inhibition by NO in both isolated inflamed aorta [62,63] and in activated macrophages [64], resulting in increased necrosis [62].

Differential regulation of neutrophil and lymphocyte apoptosis is a feature of sepsis. Neutrophils, the shortest-lived cells in the body, are normally constitutively apoptotic. In sepsis, however, delayed apoptosis of these cells has been observed. Conversely, more extensive apoptosis has been observed in lymphocytes, intestinal epithelium, and spleen [65]. While the mechanism for dysregulated apoptosis in the immune system is unclear, glucocorticoids and NO have been implicated [66].

## Pharmacological Modulation of NO Levels in Sepsis

Modulation of NO levels can be achieved pharmacologically in a number of ways (Table 2).

## Modulation of NOS Protein Expression

Expression of iNOS protein can be induced by the presence of toxic bacterial components, such as endotoxin, and by the presence of pro-inflammatory cytokines, such as TNF-$\alpha$, IL-1, and IL-6, and by the presence of its substrate, L-arginine. A meta-analysis of five prospective, randomized trials found that low-dose glucocorticoid treatment has a beneficial effect on survival and shock reversal [67]. It is unclear to what extent these findings reflect effects on NOS activity or, indeed, other immune-linked consequences of glucocorticoid administration.

## Inhibition of NOS Isoforms

NO production can be inhibited directly by a number of agents (Table 2). Effectors that prevent interaction of NOS with its substrate (such as L-arginine analogs or other amino-acid derivatives, e.g., L-NAME, L-NMMA) are often poorly selective for different NOS isoforms. A number of agents that are highly selective for iNOS have been identified, including 1400W, GW274150 and GW273629 [68] (Table 2). Partially selective inhibition of NOS can also be achieved with citrulline analogs, including L-thiocitrulline (eNOS, nNOS) and S-methyl-L-citrulline (nNOS) [22].

**Table 2.** Examples of pharmacological modulators of NO. Highly selective iNOS inhibitors are marked *

| Selectivity/type of agent | examples |
| --- | --- |
| **Non-selective NOS inhibitors** | |
| L-arginine analogs | L-NNA (L-NA; N-nitro-L-arginine); |
| | L-NAA (N-amino-L-arginine); |
| | L-NMMA (546C88; |
| | $N^G$-methyl-L-arginine-hydrochloride); |
| | L-NAME (N-nitro-L-arginine methyl ester) |
| **Partially-selective NOS inhibitors** | |
| L-citrulline analogs | L-thiocitrulline (eNOS, nNOS); |
| | S-methyl-L-citrulline (nNOS) |
| **Selective iNOS blockers** | |
| *gene expression* | glucocorticoids |
| *enzyme activity:* | |
| amino acid derivatives | L-NIL (L-N6-(1-iminoethyl)-lysine); |
| | GW274150 |
| | ((S)-2-amino-1-iminoethylamino)-5-thioheptanoic acid)* |
| amidines | ONO-1714* |
| guanidines | aminoguanidine; |
| | 2-mercaptoethylguanidine |
| isothioureas | AE-TIU (aminoethyl-isothiourea); |
| | S-methylisothiourea |
| bis-isothioureas | 1400W (N-3-aminomethyl-benzylacetamidine)* |
| **Selective nNOS inhibitors** | |
| Indazoles | 7-NI (7-nitroindazole) |
| **Downstream effectors** | |
| soluble guanylate cyclase blockers | methylene blue; |
| | ODQ (1H-(1,2,4)oxadiazole(4,3-[alpha])quinoxalin-1-one) |
| NO scavengers | hemoglobin; albumin; methylene blue |
| NO donors | S-nitrosothiols, NONOates |

## Administration of L-arginine Analogs (Non-selective NOS Inhibitors)

Early use of NOS inhibitors as pharmacological agents appeared promising; application of L-arginine analogs in animal models and in small series of patients improved blood pressure and increased the SVR. Detrimental effects, however, were revealed in subsequent studies, such as decreases in cardiac output and increases in pulmonary vascular resistance [69–71].

A multicenter, randomized, placebo-controlled double-blind study of the non-selective NOS inhibitor L-NMMA (also known as 546C88) was carried out in patients with septic shock. Results of the phase II trial were promising: a decrease in plasma nitrate levels in the treatment group was associated with a decreased requirement for vasopressors, earlier shock resolution, and an improvement in vascular resistance [72,73]. However, the subsequent phase III trial was terminated prematurely due to an increase in 28-day mortality in the treatment group [8], with a higher proportion of deaths from cardiac dysfunction related to pulmonary hypertension. The reasons for this finding are not clear; however, high doses of the compound may have led to excessive vasoconstriction and further mismatch of the circulation, increasing the severity of shock. Alternatively, the non-selective nature of the inhibition of NOS by 546C88 (which affects both iNOS and eNOS) may have abrogated not only the deleterious effect of iNOS-derived NO, probably due to peroxynitrite generation, but at the same time any protection afforded by NO generated by the constitutive enzyme. Rather overlooked was the *post hoc* finding that patients given low doses ($\leq$ 5 mg/kg/h) of the drug actually showed a significant survival benefit [8].

On the basis that totally inhibiting NO release is harmful, and to elucidate the roles of different NOS isoforms, the use of selective iNOS inhibitors (e.g., 1400W and ONO-1714) has been employed in a number of rodent studies of endotoxemia and bacteremia (see [16]). In many cases, the effects of selective iNOS inhibition have improved the responsiveness of the cardiovascular system to pressors without the negative effects seen with non-selective inhibitors, presumably by permitting some continued function of eNOS. To date, however, patient studies with selective iNOS inhibitors have not been reported.

## Use of Soluble Guanylate Cyclase (sGC) Inhibitors

Attempts have been made to target cGMP-mediated effects of NO specifically by modulation of sGC activity. Since the first preliminary report of its use in patients [74], methylene blue, a non-specific inhibitor of sGC, has been shown in a number of rodent models and small human studies to improve vascular contractility and decrease hypotension in septic shock. A small-scale randomized pilot study of septic patients receiving an infusion of methylene blue reported an increase in blood pressure, a decrease in catecholamine requirements, but no rise in pulmonary vascular resistance [75]. However, no significant improvements in organ function were seen and platelet counts decreased.

Methylene blue is now known to possess other pharmacological actions, including inhibition of NOS, generation of oxygen radicals, and inhibition of potassium channels. A more specific and potent inhibitor of sGC, 1H-(1,2,4)oxadiazole(4,3-[alpha])quinoxalin-1-one (ODQ), has been used in a limited number of studies of septic shock. Zingarelli et al. [76] reported increased survival in LPS-treated mice while Zacharowski et al. [77] found that pre-treatment with ODQ prior to the induction of sepsis decreased organ dysfunction and improved histology in their rat model.

The extent to which sGC-induced cGMP-dependent processes represent a useful therapeutic target in MOF remains unclear at present. Given that targeting sGC affects the actions of both constitutive and inducible forms of NOS, the potential for disruption of these processes by inhibiting sGC emphasizes the need for caution when applying non-selective inhibition of divergent pathways.

Many questions remain unanswered, for example, the effective concentration of these pharmacological agents in different tissues (and organelles), and the degree of NOS inhibition both overall and for individual isoforms. It may be the case that a non-selective, partial inhibition of NOS isoforms provides an improved outcome or that selective inhibition of iNOS may prove beneficial. It should be stressed that evidence is currently lacking for both of these possibilities and further study is warranted.

## Conclusion

Over the last ten years or so, a role of NO in sepsis and MOF has been established. A number of studies have been performed in animals and in patients in which the generation of NO in sepsis has been pharmacologically manipulated. While improvements in hemodynamics have generally been reported, to date none of these investigations has clearly demonstrated improved organ function or outcomes in human sepsis.

It is becoming increasingly clear that NO mediates both cytoprotective and cytopathic roles in sepsis. However, much remains to be elucidated in terms of how NO mediates these effects and also whether the consequences of NO are causative or reactive to organ dysfunction. Future therapies, better targeted towards selectively inhibiting iNOS, will no doubt help to clarify this question. In addition, it is possible that targeting downstream effects of NO, such as mitochondrial dysfunction or promoting mitochondrial biogenesis, may emerge as possible approaches to the management of this complex and widespread condition.

*Acknowledgement.* We would like to thank Annie Higgs for critical reading of the manuscript.

## References

1. Weycker D, Akhras KS, Edelsberg JMD, Angus DCM, Oster G (2003) Long-term mortality and medical care charges in patients with severe sepsis. Crit Care Med 31:2316–2323
2. Hegash E, Shiloah J (1982) Blood nitrates and infantile methemoglobinemia. Clin Chim Acta 125:107–115
3. Wagner DA, Young VR, Tannenbaum SR (1983) Mammalian nitrate biosynthesis: incorporation of $^{15}NH_3$ into nitrate is enhanced by endotoxin treatment. Proc Natl Acad Sci USA 80:4518–4521
4. Furchgott RF, Zawadzki JV (1980) The obligatory role of endothelial cells in the relaxation of arterial smooth muscle by acetylcholine. Nature 288:373–376
5. Palmer RMJ, Ferrige AG, Moncada S (1987) Nitric oxide release accounts for the biological activity of endothelium-derived relaxing factor. Nature 327:524–526
6. Ignarro LJ, Buga GM, Wood KS, Byrns RE, Chaudhuri G (1987) Endothelium-derived relaxing factor produced and released from artery and vein is nitric oxide. Proc Natl Acad Sci USA 84:9265–9269

7. Moncada S, Palmer RM, Higgs EA (1991) Nitric oxide: physiology, pathophysiology, and pharmacology. Pharmacol Rev 43:109–142
8. Lopez A, Lorente JA, Steingrub J, et al (2004) Multiple-center, randomized, placebo-controlled, double-blind study of the nitric oxide synthase inhibitor 546C88: Effect on survival in patients with septic shock. Crit Care Med 32:21–30
9. Brown GC, Cooper C (1994) Nanomolar concentrations of nitric oxide reversibly inhibit synaptosomal respiration by competing with oxygen at cytochrome oxidase. FEBS Lett 356:295–298
10. Cleeter MWJ, Cooper JM, Darley-Usmar VM, Moncada S, Schapira AHV (1994) Reversible inhibition of cytochrome c oxidase, the terminal enzyme of the mitochondrial respiratory chain, by nitric oxide : Implications for neurodegenerative diseases. FEBS Lett 345:50–54
11. Schweizer M, Richter C (1994) Nitric oxide potently and reversibly deenergizes mitochondria at low oxygen tension. Bioch Biophys Res Comm 204:169–175
12. Assreuy J, Cunha FQ, Liew FY, Moncada S (1993) Feedback inhibition of nitric oxide synthase activity by nitric oxide. Br J Pharmacol 108:833–837
13. Hughes MN (1999) Relationships between nitric oxide, nitroxyl ion, nitrosonium cation and peroxynitrite. Biochim Biophys Acta 1411:263–272
14. Beltran B, Orsi A, Clementi E, Moncada S (2000) Oxidative stress and S-nitrosylation of proteins in cells. Br J Pharmacol 129:953–960
15. Brown GC, Borutaite V (2002) Nitric oxide inhibition of mitochondrial respiration and its role in cell death. Free Rad Biol Med 33:1440–1450
16. Feihl F, Waeber B, Liaudet L (2001) Is nitric oxide overproduction the target of choice for the management of septic shock? Pharmacol Therap 91:179–213
17. Hogg N, Kalyanaraman B (1999) Nitric oxide and lipid peroxidation. Biochim Biophys Acta 1411:378–384
18. Murphy MP (1999) Nitric oxide and cell death. Biochim Biophys Acta 1411:401–414
19. Ghafourifar P, Richter C (1997) Nitric oxide synthase activity in mitochondria. FEBS Lett 418:291–296
20. Giulivi C, Poderoso JJ, Boveris A (1998) Production of NO by mitochondria. J Biol Chem 273:11038–11043
21. Stuehr DJ (1999) Mammalian nitric oxide synthases. Biochim Biophys Acta 1411:217–230
22. Dudzinski DM, Igarashi J, Greif D, Michel TM (2006) The regulation and pharmacology of endothelial nitric oxide synthases. Ann Rev Pharmacol Toxicol 46:235–276
23. Brown GC (1999) Nitric oxide and mitochondrial respiration. Biochim Biophys Acta 1411:351–369
24. Stuehr DJ, Santolini J, Wang ZQ, Wei CC, Adak S (2004) Update on mechanism and catalytic regulation in the NO synthases. J Biol Chem 279:36167–36170
25. Moncada S, Higgs AE (2006) The discovery of nitric oxide and its role in vascular biology. Br J Pharmacol 147:S193–S201
26. Cavaillon JM, Adib-Conquy M (2005) Monocytes/macrophages and sepsis. Crit Care Med 33:S504–S509
27. Titheradge MA (1999) Nitric oxide in septic shock. Biochim Biophys Acta 1411:437–455
28. Radomski MW, Palmer RMJ, Moncada S (1990) Glucocorticoids inhibit the expression of an inducible, but not the constitutive, nitric oxide synthase in vascular endothelial cells. Proc Natl Acad Sci USA 87:10043–10047
29. Connelly L, Jacobs AT, Palacios-Callender M, Moncada S, Hobbs AJ (2003) Macrophage endothelial nitric-oxide synthase autoregulates cellular activation and pro-inflammatory protein expression. J Biol Chem 278:26480–26487
30. Moncada S, Erusalimsky JD (2002) Does nitric oxide modulate mitochondrial energy generation and apoptosis? Nat Rev Mol Cell Biol 3:214–220
31. Brown GC (2001) Regulation of mitochondrial respiration by nitric oxide inhibition of cytochrome c oxidase. Biochim Biophys Acta 1504:46–57

32. Palacios-Callender M, Quintero M, Hollis VS, Springett RJ, Moncada S (2004) Endogenous NO regulates superoxide production at low oxygen concentrations by modifying the redox state of cytochrome c oxidase. Proc Natl Acad Sci USA 101:7630–7635
33. Duchen MR (2004) Mitochondria in health and disease: perspectives on a new mitochondrial biology. Mol Aspects Med 25:365–451
34. Almeida A, Almeida J, Bolanos JP, Moncada S (2001) Different responses of astrocytes and neurons to nitric oxide: The role of glycolytically generated ATP in astrocyte protection. Proc Natl Acad Sci USA 98:15294–15299
35. Nisoli E, Clementi E, Paolucci C, et al (2003) Mitochondrial biogenesis in mammals: the role of endogenous nitric oxide. Science 299:896–899
36. Strand OA, Leone A, Giercksky KE, Kirkeboen KA (2000) Nitric oxide indices in human septic shock. Crit Care Med 28:2779–2785
37. Annane D, Sanquer S, Sebille V, et al (2000) Compartmentalised inducible nitric-oxide synthase activity in septic shock. Lancet 355:1143–1148
38. Arnalich F, Hernanz A, Jimenez M, et al (1996) Relationship between circulating levels of calcitonin gene-related peptide, nitric oxide metabolites and hemodynamic changes in human septic shock. Reg Peptides 65:115–121
39. Evans T, Carpenter A, Kinderman H, Cohen J (1993) Evidence of increased nitric oxide production in patients with the sepsis syndrome. Circ Shock 41:77–81
40. Gomez-Jimenez J, Salgado A, Mourelle M, et al (1995) L-arginine: Nitric oxide pathway in endotoxemia and human septic shock. Crit Care Med 23:253–258
41. Ochoa JB, Udekwu AO, Billiar TR, et al (1991) Nitrogen oxide levels in patients after trauma and during sepsis. Ann Surg 214:621–626
42. Brealey D, Brand M, Hargreaves I, et al (2002) Association between mitochondrial dysfunction and severity and outcome of septic shock. Lancet 360:219–223
43. Hayashi Y, Abe M, Murai A, et al (2005) Comparison of effects of nitric oxide synthase (NOS) inhibitors on nitrite/nitrate levels and tissue NOS activity in septic organs. Microbiol Immunol 49:139–147
44. MacNaul K, Hutchinson N (1993) Differential expression of iNOS and cNOS mRNA in human vascular smooth muscle and endothelial cells under normal and inflammatory conditions. Bioch Biophys Res Comm 196:1330–1334
45. Lanone S, Mebazaa A, Heymes C, et al (2001) Sepsis is associated with reciprocal expressional modifications of constitutive nitric oxide synthase (NOS) in human skeletal muscle: Down-regulation of NOS1 and up-regulation of NOS3. Crit Care Med 29:1720–1725
46. Sharshar T, Gray F, de la Grandmaison GL, et al (2003) Apoptosis of neurons in cardiovascular autonomic centres triggered by inducible nitric oxide synthase after death from septic shock. Lancet 362:1799–1805
47. Landry DW, Oliver JA (2001) The pathogenesis of vasodilatory shock. N Engl J Med 345:588–595
48. Kumar A, Krieger A, Symeoneides S, Kumar A, Parrillo JE (2001) Myocardial dysfunction in septic shock: Part II. Role of cytokines and nitric oxide. J Cardiothor Vasc Anesth 15:485–511
49. Schulz R, Nava E, Moncada S (1992) Induction and potential biological relevance of a $Ca^{2+}$-independent nitric oxide synthase in the myocardium. Br J Pharmacol 105:575–580
50. Brady AJ, Poole-Wilson PA, Harding SE, Warren JB (1992) Nitric oxide production within cardiac myocytes reduces their contractility in endotoxemia. Am J Physiol 263:H1963–H1966
51. Price S, Mitchell JA, Anning PB, Evans TW (2003) Type II nitric oxide synthase activity is cardio-protective in experimental sepsis. Eur J Pharmacol 472:111–118
52. Singer M, Brealey D (1999) Mitochondrial dysfunction in sepsis. Biochem Soc Symp 66:149–166
53. De Backer D, Creteur J, Preiser JC, Dubois MJ, Vincent JL (2002) Microvascular blood flow is altered in patients with sepsis. Am J Respir Crit Care Med 166:98–104
54. Hayes MA, Timmins AC, Yau E, Palazzo M, Hinds CJ, Watson D (1994) Elevation of systemic oxygen delivery in the treatment of critically ill patients. N Engl J Med 330:1717–1722

55. Gattinoni L, Brazzi L, Pelosi P, et al (1995) A trial of goal-oriented hemodynamic therapy in critically ill patients. N Engl J Med 333:1025–1032
56. Hayes MA, Timmins AC, Yau EH, Palazzo M, Watson D, Hinds CJ (1997) Oxygen transport patterns in patients with sepsis syndrome or septic shock: influence of treatment and relationship to outcome. Crit Care Med 25:926–936
57. Crouser ED (2004) Mitochondrial dysfunction in septic shock and multiple organ failure. Mitochondrion 4:729–741
58. Brealey D, Karyampudi S, Jacques TS, et al (2004) Mitochondrial dysfunction in a long-term rodent model of sepsis and organ failure. Am J Physiol 286:R491–R497
59. Borutaite V, Matthias A, Harris H, Moncada S, Brown GC (2001) Reversible inhibition of cellular respiration by nitric oxide in vascular inflammation. Am J Physiol 281:H2256–H2260
60. Orsi A, Rees DD, Beltran B, Moncada S (2000) Physiological regulation and pathological inhibition of tissue respiration by nitric oxide in vivo. In: Moncada S, Gustafsson LE, Wiklund NP, Higgs EA (eds) The Biology of Nitric Oxide, Part 7. Portland Press, London, pp: 35
61. Singer M, De Santis V, Vitale D, Jeffcoate W (2004) Multiorgan failure is an adaptive, endocrine-mediated, metabolic response to overwhelming systemic inflammation. Lancet 364:545–548
62. Mander P, Borutaite V, Moncada S, Brown GC (2005) Nitric oxide from inflammatory-activated glia synergizes with hypoxia to induce neuronal death. J Neurosci Res 79:208–215
63. Borutaite V, Moncada S, Brown GC (2005) Nitric oxide from inducible nitric oxide synthase sensitizes the inflamed aorta to hypoxic damage via respiratory inhibition. Shock 23:319–323
64. Frost MT, Wang Q, Moncada S, Singer M (2005) Hypoxia accelerates nitric oxide-dependent inhibition of mitochondrial complex I in activated macrophages. Am J Physiol 288:R394–R400
65. Hotchkiss RS, Swanson PE, Freeman BD, et al (1999) Apoptotic cell death in patients with sepsis, shock, and multiple organ dysfunction. Crit Care Med 27:1230–1251
66. Perl M, Chung CS, Ayala A (2005) Apoptosis. Crit Care Med 33 (Suppl):S526–S529
67. Minneci PC, Deans KJ, Banks SM, Eichacker PQ, Natanson C (2004) Dose-dependent effects of steroids on survival rates and shock during sepsis: a meta-analysis. Ann Intern Med 141:47–56
68. Alderton WK, Angell ADR, Craig C, et al (2005) GW274150 and GW273629 are potent and highly selective inhibitors of inducible nitric oxide synthase in vitro and in vivo. Br J Pharmacol 145:301–312
69. Lorente JA, Landin L, Renes E, et al (1993) L-arginine pathway in the sepsis syndrome. Crit Care Med 21:759–767
70. Petros A, Lamb G, Leone A (1994) Effects of a nitric oxide synthase inhibitor in humans with septic shock. Cardiovasc Res 28:34–39
71. Avontuur JAMM, Nolthenius RPT, van Bodegom JWM, Bruining HAM (1998) Prolonged inhibition of nitric oxide synthesis in severe septic shock: A clinical study. Crit Care Med 26:660–667
72. Bakker JMD, Grover R, McLuckie A, et al (2004) Administration of the nitric oxide synthase inhibitor NG-methyl-L-arginine hydrochloride (546C88) by intravenous infusion for up to 72 hours can promote the resolution of shock in patients with severe sepsis: Results of a randomized, double-blind, placebo-controlled multicenter study. Crit Care Med 32:1–12
73. Watson D, Grover R, Anzueto A, et al (2004) Cardiovascular effects of the nitric oxide synthase inhibitor NG-methyl-L-arginine hydrochloride (546C88) in patients with septic shock: Results of a randomized, double-blind, placebo-controlled multicenter study. Crit Care Med 32:13–20
74. Schneider F, Lutun P, Hasselmann M, et al (1992) Methylene blue increases systemic vascular resistance in human septic shock. Intensive Care Med 18:309–311
75. Kirov M, Evgenov O, Evgenov N, et al (2001) Infusion of methylene blue in human septic shock: A pilot, randomized, controlled study. Crit Care Med 29:1860–1867

76. Zingarelli B, Hasko G, Salzman A, Szabo C (1999) Effects of a novel guanylyl cyclase inhibitor on the vascular actions of nitric oxide and peroxynitrite in immunostimulated smooth muscle cells and in endotoxic shock. Crit Care Med 27:1701–1707
77. Zacharowski K, Berkels R, Olbrich A, et al (2001) The selective guanylate cyclase inhibitor ODQ reduces multiple organ injury in rodent models of Gram-positive and Gram-negative shock. Crit Care Med 29:1599–1608

# Involvement of Reactive Oxygen and Nitrogen Species in the Pathogenesis of Acute Lung Injury

S. Matalon, I.C. Davis, and J.D. Lang Jr

## Introduction

Lung injury can present with different signs and symptoms and emanate from a variety of etiologies. However, whether it is the acute respiratory distress syndrome (ARDS) or other forms of lung injury, inflammatory stimuli giving rise to the generation of reactive oxygen species (ROS) and reactive oxygen-nitrogen species (RNS) contribute to lung pathophysiology [1]. These species, generated by activated inflammatory cells, circulating enzymatic generators (such as xanthine oxidase) and multiple other sources, damage the alveolar and capillary endothelia, lung surfactant and connective tissue contributing to the formation of non-cardiogenic pulmonary edema, the development of the multiple organ dysfunction syndrome (MODS) and death.

## Formation of Oxidative and Nitrosative Species

### Reactive Oxygen Species

ROS implicated in pulmonary pathophysiology include superoxide anions ($\cdot O_2^-$), hydrogen peroxide ($H_2O_2$), hydroxyl radical ($\cdot OH$), and hypochlorous acid (HOCl) (Fig. 1). Superoxide anion generation has been demonstrated from a number of biological sources. An important enzymatic source of superoxide is nicotinamide adenine dinucleotide phosphate oxidase (NADPH oxidase) which catalyzes a one-electron reduction of molecular oxygen to form $\cdot O_2^-$. NADPH oxidase is vital for yielding ROS in phagocytic cells that inhabit the lung (e. g., macrophages and polymorphonuclear cells) where these species play a role in host defense mechanisms that target killing and removal of invading microorganisms. It is not surprising then that a variety of systems are present to prevent and/or limit oxidative tissue injury. Four types of superoxide dismutase (SOD) catalyze the conversion of two moles of $\cdot O_2^-$ to $H_2O_2$, which is then converted to water by catalase and glutathione peroxidase (Fig. 1). Copper (Cu) and zinc (Zn) SODs (CuZn) are present in the cytosol, while manganese (Mn) SOD is found in the mitochondria. An extracellular form of SOD (ECSOD) has also been identified and may play an important role in converting extracellular $\cdot O_2^-$ to $H_2O_2$ as well as in controlling blood pressure by modulating the reaction of $\cdot O_2^-$ with NO.

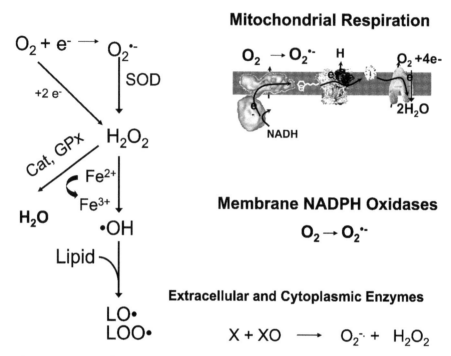

**Fig. 1.** Generation of reactive oxygen intermediates by the incomplete reduction of oxygen in the mitochondria, cytoplasm and cell membrane and extracellular space. $O_2$: oxygen; $\cdot O_2^-$: superoxide radical; $H_2O_2$: hydrogen peroxide; $\cdot OH$: hydroxyl radical; SOD: superoxide dismutase; Cat: catalase; GPx: glutathione peroxidase, LO$\cdot$, LOO.: lipid peroxides; X: xanthine; XO: xanthine oxidase; NADH: nicotinamide adenine dinucleotide; NADPH: nicotinamide adenine dinucleotide phosphate. From [37] with permission

In newborns, ECSOD exists both intracellularly and extracellularly and plays an important role in intracellular antioxidant defenses.

## Production of Nitric Oxide and Reactive Nitrogen Species

Nitric oxide (NO) synthases (NOS) catalyze the formation of NO and L-citrulline from L-arginine, and oxygen via a 5-electron redox reaction that also involves cofactors including NADPH, FAD and tetrahydrobiopterin. Various forms of NOS have been identified: NOS-1 or neuronal NOS (nNOS), NOS-2 or inducible NOS (iNOS), and NOS-3 or endothelial NOS (eNOS). nNOS and eNOS are expressed constitutively, and their activity is regulated largely by changes in intracellular $Ca^{2+}$ concentration. Although previous studies claimed that iNOS was not constitutively expressed, more recent findings show expression of iNOS in inflammatory cells and lung tissue of humans and mice under baseline conditions (Fig. 2) [2] with significant upregulation of mRNA, protein, and activity following exposure to

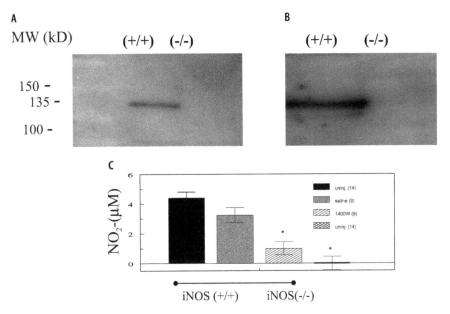

Fig. 2. iNOS is present and active under basal conditions in C57BL/6 mouse lungs. Representative western blots of (A) azygous lobes and (B) ATII cells isolated from iNOS(+/+) and iNOS(-/-) mice. Equal amounts of proteins were separated on a 7.5% SDS-PAGE, transferred to polyvinyldidene difluoride membranes, followed by probing with anti-mouse iNOS antibody, and then anti-rabbit horseradish peroxidase (HRP) conjugate as the secondary antibody, and finally developed by enhanced chemiluminescence (ECL) reagents. These measurements were repeated with proteins derived from five different mice with identical results. (C) Nitrite levels in the BAL of iNOS (+/+) and iNOS(-/-) mice. Some of the iNOS (+/+) mice were injected with either saline or 1400W. All mice were euthanized and their lungs were lavaged with sterile saline. $NO_3^-$ was first converted to $NO_2^-$ with *Escherichia coli* reductase and concentrations of $NO_2^-$ were measured using fluorescence utilizing 2,3-diaminonaphthalene (DAN). Values are means ± SEM. The number of samples for each group is shown in parentheses. *$p < 0.01$ as compared to the uninjected iNOS (+/+) value. From [2] with permission

cytokines and LPS. A form of NOS also has been identified in the mitochondria and may play an important role in regulating mitochondrial function.

Reactive nitrogen species (RNS) are a variety of nitrogen containing molecules that are typically derived via nitric oxide (NO) reactions. Those implicated in pulmonary pathology include peroxynitrite ($ONOO^-$), nitrogen dioxide ($NO_2$), and nitroxyl (HNO) which can be formed via NO-reactions as discussed below but also through environmental exposure and inhalation (Fig. 2) [3]. Peroxynitrite is formed by the rapid reaction of NO with superoxide and when protonated (addition of $H^+$), will decompose into $NO_2^-$ and ·OH, as well as nitrate ($NO_3^-$). These species may the ninte act with each othe r as well as with $O_2$ or ROS, forming higher oxides of nitrogen which may oxidize thiols, nitrate aromatic amino acids, most notably tyrosines, nitrosate and glutathionylate cysteines and oxidize a variety of amino acids including methionine and cysteines (Table 1). Myeloperoxidase

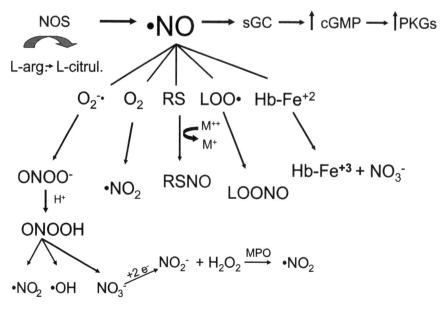

**Fig. 3.** Generation of reactive nitrogen species. Nitric oxide synthases (NOS) catalyze the formation of nitric oxide (NO) and L-citrulline from L-arginine. NO either binds to the heme center of soluble guanylate cyclase (sGC) leading to increased production of guanosine 3',5'-cyclic monospate (cGMP) and activation of cGMP-dependent protein kinases (PKGs), binds to oxygenated hemoglobin (Hb-Fe$^{+2}$) to form nitrate (NO$_3^-$) or interacts with superoxide ($\cdot$O$_2^-$), molecular oxygen (O$_2$), thiols (RS), or lipid peroxides (LOO$\cdot$) to form various intermediates. ONOO-: peroxynitrite; ONOOH: peroxynitrous acid; $\cdot$NO$_2$: nitrogen dioxide; RSNO: nitrosothiols; LOONO: nitrated unsaturated fatty acids; OH: hydroxyl radicals; NO$_2^-$: nitrite; MPO: myeloperoxidase; M: metal. From [37] with permission

(MPO), present in pulmonary neutrophils and secreted during their activation, catalyzes the production of nitrating, oxidizing and chlorinating species from H$_2$O$_2$, chloride and nitrite (Fig. 3).

Nitrite has also emerged as a key player in supporting NO-formation during hypoxemia and tissue ischemia, and in this context protects against reperfusion injury. Moreover, nitrite reactions *in vivo* also lead to diverse NO-dependent protein adducts including S-nitrosothiols and C-/N-nitrosamines, underscoring the rich biochemical interplay between distinct RNS and ROS. The therapeutic potential for this inorganic anion in replenishing NO during low oxygen states has also been demonstrated in the lung, with inhalation of nitrite reversing pulmonary hypertension in a manner analogous to inhaled NO. A key difference between nitrite and NO, however, was the lack of rebound hypertension upon withdrawing inhaled nitrite.

Table 1. Actions of reactive nitrogen species. From [37] with permission

| Signal Transduction | |
| --- | --- |
| Activation of cGMP/PKG | Vessel relaxation<br>Bronchodilation<br>Modification of ion channel function<br>Inhibition of platelet aggregation |
| cGMP-independent | Activation of NF-κb; MAPkinases |
| S-thiolation<br>S-nitrosation | NMDA, PKC, adenylate cyclase, complex I, cardiac ryanodine receptor, L-type calcium channels, GPx + others, Caspase-3, p21ras, CFTR |
| **Interactions/modifications** | |
| Binding to heme protein metal centers | Inhibition of protein and DNA synthesis<br>Inhibition of mitochondria respiration and ATP production<br>Increased methemoglobin levels<br>Deactivation of NOS<br>Enzyme inhibition (lipooxygenase, cyclooxygenase; ribonucleotide reductase) |
| **Post-translational modifications** | |
| Nitration | Proteins: Cerulsoplasmin; SP-A; transferrin; albumin; α1-protease inhibitor; actin; α1-antichymotrypsin; MnSOD β-chain fibrinogen<br>Lipids |
| Oxidation/deamination | Lipids, sulfhydryls, DNA base |

## Reactive Oxygen/Nitrogen Species as Signaling Molecules

Formation of RNS is related to the inflammatory environment within the lung at specific points in time, which has the potential to generate noxious concentrations of products detrimental to lung function. Production of NO in the lung serves as an important regulator of local functions, including airway tone, pulmonary vascular tone, mucin secretion, ciliary function, and ion channel activity. A number of studies have demonstrated that transcriptional factors (e.g., OxyR [4, 5]), ion channels (e.g., olfactory cyclic nucleotide-gated channel [6]) and enzymes can be activated or regulated by RNS via redox-based modifications of specific thiols within these proteins.

## Thiols

NO-derived species, such as nitrosonium ion ($NO^+$), $N_2O_3$ and $ONOO^-$ may react with thiols to form nitroso-thiols (RS-NO) [7]. Micromolar concentrations of

S-nitrosoglutathione have been detected in the airway fluid of normal subjects and significantly higher levels were observed in the lungs of patients with pneumonia or during inhalation of 80 ppm NO [8]. Formation of RS-NO adducts stabilizes NO, decreasing its cytotoxic potential while maintaining its bioactive properties. ·NO can also be transported on cysteine residues of hemoglobin which may facilitate efficient delivery of oxygen to tissues [9]. Nitrosylation of the N-methyl-D-aspartate (NMDA) receptor in the brain leads to decreased calcium transport and neuroprotection [10]. On the other hand, ·NO-induced S-nitrosylation of glyceraldehyde-3-phosphate dehydrogenase stimulated the apparent auto-ADP ribosylation and inhibited enzymatic activity [11]. It is important to note that the direct reaction of ·NO with thiol groups is unbalanced and can only occur in the presence of a strong electron acceptor.

## Activation of Protein Kinases

NO binds to the heme group of soluble guanylate cyclase (sGC) leading to an increase in cGMP levels. Many effects of cGMP are mediated by various isoforms of cGMP-dependent protein kinase which phosphorylate various substrate proteins, thereby reducing intracellular $Ca^{+2}$ and causing smooth muscle relaxation. NO-mediated increases in cGMP levels also decrease platelet aggregation and adhesion of neutrophils to endothelial cells, thus reducing oxidant load [12]. At lower concentrations, RNS function as signaling molecules (Table 1) regulating fundamental cellular activities such as cell growth and adaptation responses; at higher concentrations they can induce significant cellular injury, apoptosis, and death.

## Activation of Nuclear Factor-kappa B (NF-κB)

Among the most important transcription factors responsive to ROS during inflammation and oxidant stress is NF-κB, a transcriptional regulating protein. NF-κB is one member of a ubiquitously expressed family of *Rel*-related transcription factors. This is a family of structurally related eukaryotic transcription factors that are involved in the control of a vast array of processes, including immune and inflammatory responses, growth, development, and apoptosis. The production of ROS, cytokines, or other inflammatory stimuli can activate NF-κB and induce gene expression, eliciting a response generally observed to be pro-inflammatory in nature [13].

## Intracellular $Ca^{+2}$, PKC and MAPK

Evidence also indicates that ROS lead to an increase in intracellular calcium concentrations which correlate with endothelial permeability [14]. Some observations suggest that $Ca^{2+}$ influx occurs through membrane $Ca^{2+}$ channels that are regulated by ·OH generation. Myosin light chain kinase phosphorylation also increases when endothelial cells are treated with $H_2O_2$, suggesting that endothelial contraction may play an essential role in oxidant-induced endothelial barrier dysfunction. It appears that an important fundamental requirement for vascular endothelial permeability is the activation of endothelial contraction.

Additional signaling molecules, such as protein kinase C (PKC), mitogen-activated protein kinase (MAPK), tyrosine kinases and Rho GTPases appear vital in mediating endothelial barrier dysfunction. PKC (a family of serine/threonine protein kinases consisting of at least 12 isoforms) is activated in response to oxidants and increases endothelial permeability. In guinea pig lungs [15] pretreated with H-7 ( a non-specific PKC inhibitor acting on the catalytic site of the enzyme), there was no increase in the pulmonary capillary filtration coefficient in response to perfusion of $H_2O_2$. Increases in pulmonary microvascular permeability were accompanied by reorganization of actin cytoskeleton, a process inhibited by PKC inhibitors. The exact mechanism(s) for the role PKC plays in endothelial barrier function is complex but appears due to activation of ROS and probably involves only a few select PKC isoforms. The MAPK pathway is activated by ROS and is an important mediator of cellular responses to oxidant stress. The ERK (extracellular signal-regulated kinases), JNK (c-JUN $NH_2$-terminal kinase), and p38 cascades all contain the same series of three kinases. A MEK kinase phosphorylates and activates a MAPK, and then MEK phosphorylates and activates a MAPK. Various ROS, most notably $H_2O_2$, have been demonstrated to mediate endothelial injury via stimulation of ERK pathways. This $H_2O_2$-mediated action was inhibited by PD-98059, an ERK kinase (MEK) inhibitor. Furthermore, both ROS and RNS induce a variety of actions that are potentially detrimental and include abnormal cell differentiation/proliferation, apoptosis, and DNA damage, with the ERK pathway implicated as playing the predominant role.

## Adhesion Molecules

ROS have been shown to promote cellular and molecular events that result in enhanced aggregation and adhesion of leukocytes to endothelium. Prominent inflammatory participants emanating from these investigations include ICAM-1 (intercellular adhesion molecule-1) and selectins (a family of transmembrane molecules, expressed on the surface of leukocytes and activated endothelial cells involved in enhancing leukocyte-endothelial interactions). Investigations in diverse models using a variety of oxidant-generating systems (such as hypoxanthine/xanthine oxidase, $H_2O_2$, or prolonged hyperoxia) have demonstrated consistent increases in ICAM-1 and P-selectin expression in the vascular endothelium, which promote leukocyte adhesion. Interestingly, expression of these biomolecules is not uniform throughout the vasculature.

## Functional Consequences of Protein Nitration *In Vitro*

### Surfactant Protein-A (SP-A)

Protein nitration and oxidation by ROS and RNS *in vitro* have been associated with the diminished function of a variety of crucial proteins. Considerable levels of protein-associated nitrotyrosine ($\sim 400-500$ pmol/mg protein), as well as nitrated SP-A were present in pulmonary edema fluid from patients with either acute lung injury (ALI)/ARDS or hydrostatic pulmonary edema, and in bronchoalveolar lavage (BAL) fluid of patients with ARDS [16]. *In vitro* studies have indicated that nitrated SP-A loses its ability to enhance the adherence of *Pneumocystis carinii* to rat alveolar macrophages. Thus, nitration of SP-A may be one factor responsible for the increased susceptibility of patients with ARDS to nosocomial infections. The use of inhaled NO in patients with ARDS was shown to increase both 3-nitrotyrosine and 3-chlorotyrosine (an index of neutrophil activation) concentrations compared to comparable patients who did not receive inhaled NO.

### Current In Vivo Evidence Implicating RNS and ROS as Contributors to Lung Injury

Toxicity from oxygen-nitrogen metabolites released by stimulated neutrophils, macrophages and other cells has been proposed as one of the significant mechanisms of lung injury. One of the initial studies published described the effects of inflammation on alpha-1-proteinase inhibitor ($\alpha$-1-PI), which was found to be inactivated in BAL fluid samples from patients with ARDS [17]. This contrasted to plasma samples from the same patients which retained > 90% $\alpha$-1-PI activity. The activity of $\alpha$1-PI IN BAL fluid could be restored by the reducing agent, dithiothreitol, implicating oxidants generated in BAL as being responsible for its loss of function. Shortly after this study, a different group measured expired fractions of $H_2O_2$, a more stable membrane permeable and volatile oxidant [18]. These samples were collected in patients with normal lungs undergoing elective surgery and critically ill patients suffering from acute hypoxemic respiratory failure. Expired breath condensates of $H_2O_2$ were observed to be significantly greater in patients suffering from acute hypoxemic respiratory failure and focal pulmonary infiltrates than those without pulmonary infiltrates, indirectly implicating increased oxidation. Interestingly, $H_2O_2$ concentrations were greatest in patients with head injury and sepsis, whether pulmonary infiltrates were present or not. This unexpected finding suggested the participation of oxidants in sepsis and other forms of vital organ injury, such as in brain trauma.

Further studies have continued to create a solid foundation that implicates oxidant generation as a significant contributor to inflammatory-mediated lung injury. In fact, in one of the most recent studies, levels of plasma hypoxanthine, a key cofactor that accumulates during intervals of hypoxia leading to the production of $O_2^-$ and $H_2O_2$, were found to be significantly elevated in patients with ARDS [19].

However, the highest concentrations occurred in patients who did not survive, implicating oxidative damage as an influential contributor to mortality. Higher levels of nitrate and nitrite were also noted in the BAL fluid of patients with ARDS as compared to those of normal volunteers, as well as in the edema fluid of patients with either ARDS or cardiogenic pulmonary edema (Fig. 4) [20, 21].

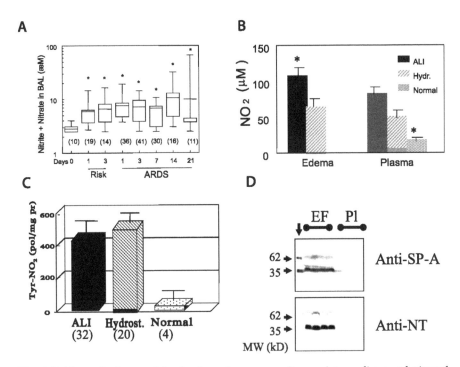

Fig. 4. Evidence for increased levels of reactive oxygen-nitrogen intermediates and nitrated proteins in the bronchoalveolar lavage (BAL), edema fluid (EF), and plasma (Pl) of patients with ARDS and hydrostatic pulmonary edema. (A) Nitrate and nitrite concentration in BAL from normal volunteers (NL), patients at-risk for ARDS (RISK), and patients with established ARDS (ARDS) studied at sequential times. The horizontal axis shows the patient group and the day on which the BAL was performed. (n) = number of subjects in each group. The data are presented as box plots showing the 10th, 25th, 75th, and 90th percentiles and the median. (*) $p < 0.005$ vs. normal subjects (From [20] with permission). (B) Nitrate and nitrite in pulmonary edema fluid and plasma samples from patients with acute lung injury (ALI), patients with hydrostatic edema (hydr.), and normal volunteers. Numbers in parenthesis are sample numbers. Values are means $\pm$ SEM (from [16] with permission). (C) Levels of nitrated proteins (measured by ELISA) in the plasma of patients with ALI, hydrostatic edema (hydrost) as well as normal volunteers (normal). Values are means $\pm$ SEM (n = number of patients or volunteers) (data adapted from [16] with permission). (D) Nitration of surfactant protein A (SP-A) in pulmonary edema fluid samples from ALI/ARDS patients. SP-A was immunoprecipitated from EF or Pl from four patients with ALI/ARDS. Immunoprecipitated SP-A was probed with polyclonal antibodies to SP-A (anti-SP-A) or nitrotyrosine (anti-NT). Nitrated SP-A was detected in the pulmonary edema fluid but not in the plasma of all patients. Vertical arrow shows purified human SP-A from a patient with alveolar proteinosis. Notice the lack of nitration in the control sample. From [16] with permission

Substantial evidence supports the notion that ROS and RNS are injurious to the pulmonary epithelium in a number of pathological conditions. Induction of immune complex alveolitis in rat lungs results in increased alveolar epithelial permeability, which is associated with the presence of NO decomposition products in the BAL fluid [22]. Moreover, alveolar instillation of the NOS inhibitor, N (G)-monomethyl-L-argnine, ameliorates NO production and alveolar epithelial injury [22]. Infection with pathogens such as *Bordetella pertussis* and influenza is associated with significant increases in NO production [23] and animals infected with *Bordetella pertussis* demonstrated a significant reduction in NO production with NOS inhibition.

## The 'Good' Side of NO

Although formation of $ONOO^-$ can result in tissue damage, NO can ameliorate tissue injury by several mechanisms. As mentioned above, NO increases steady state levels of cGMP resulting in vasodilation, and decreased platelet and neutrophil adhesion to endothelium, thereby reducing cell-mediated inflammatory damage. Additional anti-inflammatory mechanisms include downregulation of the NF-κB pathway. The reaction of NO with $\cdot O_2^-$ reduces steady-state levels of $O_2^-$ and limits $H_2O_2$ buildup, which may be especially important under conditions favoring $O_2^-$-dependent hydroxyl radical formation. Finally, by scavenging lipid radical species, such as alkoxyl (LO·) and peroxyl (LOO·) radicals, NO can inhibit oxidant-induced membrane and lipoprotein oxidation and terminate chain radical propagation reactions. These reactions may be of particular importance, since NO concentrates in lipophilic cellular compartments. However, species resulting from the reaction of NO with lipid peroxides may themselves have biological activity which could be either pro- or anti-inflammatory.

## Inhaled NO and ARDS: An ongoing debate

NO initially appeared to possess ideal properties for a selective pulmonary artery vasodilator in patients suffering from ALI/ARDS. In theory, selective pulmonary vasodilation would act on the endothelial surface of the lung to produce regional vasodilation in ventilated lung units, with the net effect being improved $PaO_2/FiO_2$ ratios and reduced pulmonary artery pressures. In a review of inhaled NO compared to placebo or no therapy administered to patients with acute hypoxemic respiratory failure, it was concluded that inhaled NO produced only moderate improvements in oxygenation and demonstrated no reduction in patient ventilator days or mortality [24]. However, there is agreement that oxygenation generally improves for 24–36 hours, which under certain clinical circumstances and combined with alternative treatment strategies, may lend itself to a multimodal approach to treatment in an individual patient with ALI/ARDS. Potential pitfalls of the recent clinical studies using inhaled NO in the treatment of patients suffering from inflammatory–mediated lung injury include: (1) Oxygenation may have very little to do with survival in patients suffering from inflammatory-mediated lung injury (as very few patients die of refractory hypoxemia); (2) benefits may have been masked by the negative effects of ventilator-induced lung injury (VILI); (3) long-term inhalation of NO may damage the lung by increasing steady state concentrations of RNS/ROS and thus overshadow their acute physiologic benefit; (4) inhaled NO may have been applied too late after the onset of injury since most enrollment occurred up to 72 hrs after patients presented with ALI. Currently, the only recognized and FDA-approved application for inhaled NO is for the treatment of hypoxic respiratory failure of the term and near-term newborn.

## Hypercapnia: An Example of a Radical Quandary?

The effect of carbon dioxide ($CO_2$) in excess (hypercapnia) and its impact on the generation of ROS/RNS is generating increased clinical interest. Due to the relatively higher concentration of $CO_2$ in plasma (1.2 mM), the majority of $ONOO^-$ generated in biological fluids will react with $CO_2$ to form the nitrosoperoxycarbonate anion ($O=N-OOCO_2^-$) [25, 26]. These species are more likely to nitrate and less likely to oxidize proteins. Thus, hypercapnia may either protect or enhance oxidant injury. For example, hypercapnia augmented LPS-induced injury across fetal alveolar epithelial cells *in vitro* [27] and rabbit lungs *in vivo* [28]. On the other hand, hypercapnia and acidosis decreased the inactivation of pulmonary surfactant by plasma proteins [29]. Thus, the precise mechanisms and consequences of hypercapnia are still unknown.

### Therapies to Attenuate RNS/ROS-Mediated Lung Injury

While the direct measurement of oxidants poses problems, monitoring of antioxidant concentrations and/or oxidant-antioxidant balance can also be assessed. For instance, levels of selected antioxidants, including plasma ascorbate, a major plasma antioxidant, were significantly decreased in patients with ongoing ARDS when compared to healthy controls [30]. In addition, ubiquinol, a key lipid-soluble antioxidant residing in the membranes of the mitochondria, was significantly decreased in patients suffering from ARDS. Interestingly, α-tocopherol, another plasma antioxidant, was unchanged. In a series of separate experiments, after plasma from a healthy donor was incubated with activated polymorphonuclear cells (PMNs), rapid oxidation of ascorbate was observed. The ubiquinol concentration slowly and steadily decreased over time, whereas α-tocopherol levels remained virtually unchanged. Glutathione (GSH), which is the most abundant non-protein thiol, is also an important antioxidant, especially for reducing $H_2O_2$ and HOCl, which are produced by activated neutrophils. Recently, samples of BAL fluid and epithelial lining fluid were analyzed for GSH in ten patients with ARDS and found to be decreased when compared to healthy controls [31]. Administration of N-acetylcysteine to patients with ARDS significantly improved oxygenation, pulmonary mechanics, and increased total plasma GSH concentrations [31]. Catalase, a scavenger of $H_2O_2$, was found to increase in patie rts with sepsis with and without the eventual progression to ARDS [32]. Interestingly, GSH peroxidase activity was unchanged when compared between control subjects, septic patients without ARDS, and septic patients with ARDS. Additional studies [33] have confirmed that in sepsis and lung injury, antioxidant responses are significantly elevated when compared to control patients. Recently, eight patients with ARDS receiving 'standardized' total parenteral nutrition were compared to 17 healthy individuals, on standard diets without vitamin or trace element supplementation, in an attempt to assess the influence of micronutrients on the oxidative system [34]. Plasma antioxidants and antioxidant enzyme systems were measured at baseline and on days 3 and 6. In addition, the lipid peroxidation product, malondiadehyde (MDA), superoxide anion, and $H_2O_2$ were measured over the same time points. Plasma levels of α-tocopherol, ascorbate, β-carotene, and selenium were reduced when compared to controls. MDA was significantly increased and was observed to increase significantly over the 6-day interval. The authors concluded that in patients with ARDS, the antioxidant systems are severely compromised, and there is evidence of progressive oxidant stress, as per the steady increase in MDA. Thus, administration of 'standardized' total parenteral nutrition seems inadequate to compensate for the increased requirement for antioxidants in ARDS.

In a contrasting study [35], when patients with ARDS were entered into a prospective, multicentered, double-blind, randomized controlled trial comparing a specialized enteral formulation (Oxepa®) containing fish oil (eicosapentanoic acid), borage seed oil (γ-linoleic acid), and elevated antioxidants (vitamin A, α-tocopherol, ascorbate, and β-carotene) versus an isonitrogenous, isocaloric standard diet, beneficial anti-inflammatory effects were observed, which translated into a reduction in mechanical ventilator days, a decreased length of stay in the ICU, and a reduction in new organ failure. When administered over a 4–7 day interval, the formulation significantly increased the $PaO_2/FiO_2$ ratio, decreased the production of neutrophils in BAL fluid, and decreased the total cell count in the BAL fluid. Oxidants and antioxidants *per se* were not directly measured, but a decrease in pulmonary inflammation with reduced neutrophil adhesion and oxidant production was observed. In a subsequent study conducted retrospectively by the same group [31], enteral feeding with the same formulation (Oxepa®) resulted in decreased BAL fluid interleukin (IL)-8 and leukotriene $B_4$ levels, together with a trend towards decreased BAL fluid total protein and neutrophils.

Albumin also has potential antioxidant ability, as a consequence of an exposed thiol group (Cys 34). Quinlan et al. [36] therefore, administered 25 g of albumin solution every 8 hours for a total of 9 doses to patients meeting criteria for ARDS and compared them to a placebo group. In this cohort of patients, supplementation with albumin increased total plasma albumin concentrations and decreased plasma protein carbonyls ( a marker of protein oxidation). Positive correlations were found between albumin and plasma thiol concentrations, and thiols and antioxidant capacity. This result was not observed in the placebo group.

## Conclusion

Reactive oxygen and nitrogen intermediates, produced by the interaction of NO with partially reduced oxygen species, affect lung function and homeostasis in a variety of different ways. They act as signaling agents and play an essential role in pathogen killing. On the other hand, they may contribute to tissue injury by upregulating genes responsible for the production of inflammatory mediators and by directly nitrating and oxidizing proteins, events known to adversely affect critical functions. A significant challenge to defining their role in lung injury results from their short biological half-lives, and lack of sensitive detection techniques, and the difficulty in deciphering the relevance of the various substrate concentrations to a particular measured response. Thus, many questions relating to the chemical, physiological, pathobiological, and clinical consequences of ROS and RNS generation remain unanswered. Therapeutic strategies, such as enhanced anti-inflammatory and antioxidant therapies are in their infancy in the clinical arena. Hence, this discussion of what is known leads one to realize how much is *not* known with regard to the role of RNS/ROS in lung injury.

## References

1. Gow AJ, Farkouh CR, Munson DA, Posencheg MA, Ischiropoulos H (2004) Biological significance of nitric oxide-mediated protein modifications. Am J Physiol Lung Cell Mol Physiol 287:L262–L268
2. Hardiman KM, McNicholas-Bevensee CM, Fortenberry J, et al (2004) Regulation of amiloride-sensitive Na(+) transport by basal nitric oxide. Am J Respir Cell Mol Biol 30:720–728
3. Bruckdorfer R (2005) The basics about nitric oxide. Mol Aspects Med 26:3–31
4. Kim SO, Merchant K, Nudelman R, et al (2002) OxyR: a molecular code for redox-related signaling. Cell 109:383–396
5. Georgiou G (2002) How to flip the (redox) switch. Cell 111:607–610
6. Broillet MC (2000) A single intracellular cysteine residue is responsible for the activation of the olfactory cyclic nucleotide-gated channel by NO. J Biol Chem 275:15135–15141
7. Gaston B, Drazen JM, Loscalzo J, Stamler JS (1994) The biology of nitrogen oxides in the airways. Am J Respir Crit Care Med 149:538–551
8. Gaston B, Reilly J, Drazen JM, et al (1993) Endogenous nitrogen oxides and bronchodilator S-nitrosothiols in human airways. Proc Natl Acad Sci USA 90:10957–10961
9. Jia L, Bonaventura J, Stamler JS (1996) S-nitrosohaemoglobin: a dynamic activity of blood involved in vascular control. Nature 380:221–226
10. Lipton SA, Choi YB, Sucher NJ, Pan ZH, Stamler JS (1996) Redox state, NMDA receptors and NO-related species. Trends Pharmacol Sci 17:186–187
11. Molina yVL, McDonald B, Reep B, et al (1992) Nitric oxide-induced S-nitrosylation of glyceraldehyde-3- phosphate dehydrogenase inhibits enzymatic activity and increases endogenous ADP-ribosylation. J Biol Chem 267:24929–24932.
12. Kubes P, Suzuki M, Granger DN (1991) Nitric oxide: an endogenous modulator of leukocyte adhesion. Proc Natl Acad Sci USA 88:4651–4655
13. Janssen-Heininger YM, Persinger RL, Korn SH, et al (2002) Reactive nitrogen species and cell signaling: implications for death or survival of lung epithelium. Am J Respir Crit Care Med 166:S9–S16

14. Vepa S, Scribner WM, Parinandi NL, English D, Garcia JG, Natarajan V (1999) Hydrogen peroxide stimulates tyrosine phosphorylation of focal adhesion kinase in vascular endothelial cells. Am J Physiol 277:L150–L158
15. Johnson A, Phillips P, Hocking D, Tsan MF, Ferro T (1989) Protein kinase inhibitor prevents pulmonary edema in response to H2O2. Am J Physiol 256:H1012–H1022
16. Zhu S, Ware LB, Geiser T, Matthay MA, Matalon S (2001) Increased levels of nitrate and surfactant protein a nitration in the pulmonary edema fluid of patients with acute lung injury. Am J Respir Crit Care Med 163:166–172
17. Gole MD, Souza JM, Choi I, et al (2000) Plasma proteins modified by tyrosine nitration in acute respiratory distress syndrome. Am J Physiol Lung Cell Mol Physiol 278:L961–L967
18. Sznajder JI, Fraiman A, Hall JB, et al (1989) Increased hydrogen peroxide in the expired breath of patients with acute hypoxemic respiratory failure. Chest 96:606–612
19. Quinlan GJ, Lamb NJ, Tilley R, Evans TW, Gutteridge JM (1997) Plasma hypoxanthine levels in ARDS: implications for oxidative stress, morbidity, and mortality. Am J Respir Crit Care Med 155:479–484
20. Sittipunt C, Steinberg KP, Ruzinski JT, et al (2001) Nitric oxide and nitrotyrosine in the lungs of patients with acute respiratory distress syndrome. Am J Respir Crit Care Med 163:503–510
21. Zhu S, Basiouny KF, Crow JP, Matalon S (2000) Carbon dioxide enhances nitration of surfactant protein A by activated alveolar macrophages. Am J Physiol Lung Cell Mol Physiol 278:L1025–L1031
22. Mulligan MS, Hevel JM, Marletta MA, Ward PA (1991) Tissue injury caused by deposition of immune complexes is L-arginine dependent. Proc Natl Acad Sci USA 88:6338–6342
23. Heiss LN, Lancaster JR Jr, Corbett JA, Goldman WE (1994) Epithelial autotoxicity of nitric oxide: role in the respiratory cytopathology of pertussis. Proc Natl Acad Sci USA 91:267–270
24. Lundin S, Mang H, Smithies M, Stenqvist O, Frostell C (1999) Inhalation of nitric oxide in acute lung injury: results of a European multicentre study. The European Study Group of Inhaled Nitric Oxide. Intensive Care Med 25:911–919
25. Berlett BS, Levine RL, Stadtman ER (1998) Carbon dioxide stimulates peroxynitrite-mediated nitration of tyrosine residues and inhibits oxidation of methionine residues of glutamine synthetase: both modifications mimic effects of adenylylation. Proc Natl Acad Sci U S A 95:2784–2789
26. Gow A, Duran D, Thom SR, Ischiropoulos H (1996) Carbon dioxide enhancement of peroxynitrite-mediated protein tyrosine nitration. Arch Biochem Biophys 333:42–48
27. Lang JD Jr, Chumley P, Eiserich JP, et al (2000) Hypercapnia induces injury to alveolar epithelial cells via a nitric oxide-dependent pathway. Am J Physiol Lung Cell Mol Physiol 279:L994–1002
28. Lang JD, Figueroa M, Sanders KD, et al (2005) Hypercapnia via reduced rate and tidal volume contributes to lipopolysaccharide-induced lung injury. Am J Respir Crit Care Med 171:147–157
29. Haddad IY, Holm BA, Hlavaty L, Matalon S (1994) Dependence of surfactant function on extracellular pH: mechanisms and modifications. J Appl Physiol 76:657–662
30. Cross CE, Forte T, Stocker R, et al.(1990) Oxidative stress and abnormal cholesterol metabolism in patients with adult respiratory distress syndrome. J Lab Clin Med 115:396–404
31. Pacht ER, Timerman AP, Lykens MG, Merola AJ (1991) Deficiency of alveolar fluid glutathione in patients with sepsis and the adult respiratory distress syndrome. Chest 100:1397–1403
32. Leff JA, Parsons PE, Day CE, et al (1992) Increased serum catalase activity in septic patients with the adult respiratory distress syndrome. Am Rev Respir Dis 146:985–989
33. Leff JA, Parsons PE, Day CE, et al (1993) Serum antioxidants as predictors of adult respiratory distress syndrome in patients with sepsis. Lancet 341:777–780
34. Metnitz PG, Bartens C, Fischer M, Fridrich P, Steltzer H, Druml W (1999) Antioxidant status in patients with acute respiratory distress syndrome. Intensive Care Med 25:180–185

35. Gadek JE, DeMichele SJ, Karlstad MD, et al (1999) Effect of enteral feeding with eicos-apentaenoic acid, gamma-linolenic acid, and antioxidants in patients with acute respiratory distress syndrome. Enteral Nutrition in ARDS Study Group. Crit Care Med 27:1409–1420
36. Quinlan GJ, Mumby S, Martin GS, Bernard GR, Gutteridge JM, Evans TW (2004) Albumin influences total plasma antioxidant capacity favorably in patients with acute lung injury. Crit Care Med 32:755–759l
37. Lang JD Jr, Davis JR, Patel I, Matalon S (2006) Oxidative and nitrosative lung injury. In: Fishma AP, Fishman JA, Grippi MA, Kaiser LB, Senior RM (eds) Fishman's Pulmonary Diseases and Disorders, 4th ed. McGraw-Hill, Columbus (in press)

# Heat Shock Proteins in Inflammation

Z. Bromberg, Y.G. Weiss, and C.S. Deutschman

## Introduction

From roundworms to mammals, living organisms have evolved strategies to permit survival in divergent environments. Evidence shows that some of these adaptive biological features are evolutionarily conserved; among these is heat acclimation. This phenomenon was described first as inducing physiological and biochemical adaptations to protect against extreme changes in environmental temperature [1]. This "heat shock response" is now accepted widely as a key mechanism to protect cells from untoward environmental perturbations [2].

The heat shock response was first identified in *Drosophila melanogaster* [3]. Early experiments showed that exposure to heat led to "chromosomal puffing" that correlated with a dramatic increase in the synthesis of a previously unrecognized group of proteins [3]. This finding was later extended to other eukaryotic organisms. These 'heat shock proteins' (HSPs) appeared to mediate a molecular mechanism that protected living cells from the untoward effects of heat [3]. Of these, one of the most widely studied is the 70 kDa HSP (HSP70). The genes encoding members of the HSP70 family are a key evolutionary adaptation that is conserved across species. The HSP70 gene is genetically simple, with a single exon and no introns, which permits rapid transcription and translation [4, 5]. Of the 70 kDa subfamily members, the inducible HSP72 is highly expressed during stress while the constitutive heat shock cognate protein (HSC)70 (also known as HSP73) is constitutively expressed, with basal levels present in the cytosol at most times [6].

Within the cytosol of eukaryotic cells, members of the 70 to 78 kDa subfamily of HSPs bind to and release both non-native protein aggregates and native proteins with incomplete or damaged tertiary structures [6]. In this sense, HSP70 family members act as molecular chaperones to 'guide' proteins to their ultimate fate–degradation, elimination, repair, or completion of the synthetic process. The chaperone's 'guiding' mechanism relies on recognition of hydrophobic regions of non-native proteins or unstructured back-bone regions of proteins. They promote the correct protein folding through cycles of substrate binding and release. This is regulated through a catalytic site by an energy-requiring ATPase dependent mechanism [3, 5, 7, 8].

Under environmental stress conditions, misfolded protein intermediates may accumulate. [9]. The self-association of non-native protein intermediates to nearby proteins may induce the formation of protein aggregates [10]. In contrast to mis-folding, aggregation is a highly cooperative inter-molecular process that strongly depends on the concentration of misfolded monomers. Aggregates may be com-posed of different oligomers over a wide distribution of sizes. The presence of these aggregates is common in a number of disease processes, including neurodegener-ative disorders such as Alzheimer's, Parkinson's, and Huntington's diseases. The exposure of hydrophobic protein domains to unaffected proteins or membranes may disrupt normal activity. For example, association of the hydrophobic region of a damaged protein with a neuronal cell membrane may change ion flux and alter function. HSP70 may prevent this and this may be a key mechanism by which HSPs limit or prevent intra-cellular pathological processes. This underscores the fundamental importance of the HSPs to normal living cells [11].

While this review will focus on HSP70, other subclasses among the HSPs play important roles. These are organized by their molecular size: HSP100, HSP90, HSP60, HSP40 (J-domain proteins) and small HSP families, such as HSP22/27 [12,13]. Most HSPs are constitutively and ubiquitously expressed molec-ular chaperones that guide the normal folding, intracellular disposition, and pro-teolytic turnover of many of the key regulators of cell growth and survival [14]. Thus, the protective process involves the interaction of many different HSPs. For example, HSP90, which comprises 1–2% of total cellular protein in non-stress conditions [15], supports meta-stable protein conformations and expresses a high affinity binding state to hormone receptors. This involves both HSP70, which par-ticipates in assembly of multiprotein complexes, and HSP40, a co-chaperone that stimulates HSP70 ATPase activity [14].

At the transcription level, HSPs, such as HSP70 and HSP90, are regulated by the activities of a family of heat shock transcription factors (HSF). One of these, HSF-1, normally is expressed in a negatively regulated state as an inert monomer in either the cytoplasm or nuclear compartments [16]. Upon exposure to a variety of stresses, HSF-1 trimerizes and accumulates in the nucleus. HSF-1 trimers bind DNA re gions called heat shock ele me nts (HSEs) with high affinity. Some small HSPs are transcribed constitutively due to multiple binding of low levels of HSF1 [16].

The great divergence in HSP70 expression explains the multiple function of these proteins. Elevated levels of HSP70 following diverse inciting causes have led researchers to conclude that HSP70 is involved in cellular protection in the normothermic environment [4, 17, 18]. A wide range of noxious stimuli, such as hypoxia, ischemia/reperfusion, hypoglycemia, endotoxemia, inflammation, and exposure to heavy toxic metals or reactive oxygen species (ROS), induce HSP70 expression in a large number of tissues. Since HSPs respond to environmental changes, expression in organs that are 'outside' the organism (for example, skin, lung, gastrointestinal epithelium) may occur in the absence of any apparent in-sult [17–24].

It has been demonstrated, both *in vivo* and *in vitro*, that exposure to a mild stress, such as heat pretreatment, induces high levels of HSP70. Increased HSP70 levels may confer protection from subsequent noxious stimuli and result in 'cytoprotection'. This should be of benefit against cellular injury caused by inflammation and infection [17–23]. Thus, altering HSP70 expression might be of importance in modulating highly lethal inflammatory diseases.

## Heat Shock Proteins as 'Disease Regulators': Sepsis and Acute Respiratory Distress Syndrome (Fig. 1)

Sepsis, as well as the related systemic inflammatory response syndrome (SIRS), and multiple organ dysfunction syndrome (MODS), are the leading causes of death in patients in surgical intensive care units (ICUs) [24, 25]. The lung is the organ most affected in MODS, with pulmonary dysfunction taking the form of the acute respiratory distress syndrome (ARDS), an often lethal inflammatory disorder of the lung [26]. Recent data from the USA indicate that the mortality rate associated with ARDS is greater than 35% [26].

ARDS is characterized by an increased inflammatory process in the lungs. In this disorder, alveolar epithelial cells are damaged and ultimately may be destroyed [27,28]. While some contributory pathophysiologic mechanisms have been identified, most remain obscure. Therefore, a better understanding of the fundamental biological changes leading to ARDS would be of scientific and therapeutic value.

Several papers have explored the role of HSP70 in a model of lipopolysaccharide (LPS)-induced lung injury. These investigators concluded that heat pre-treatment

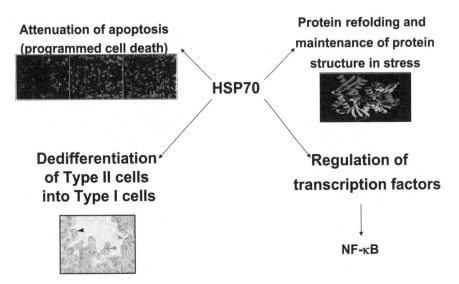

**Fig. 1.** Cytoprotective functions of heat shock protein (HSP)-70 of potential importance in lung injury and organ failure

induced HSP70 expression that protected the lungs against ventilator-induced lung injury (VILI) by decreasing cytokine transcription in the lung [29].

LPS stimulates the production and the release of many endogenous mediators of sepsis. These include tumor necrosis factor alpha (TNF-$\alpha$), interleukin (IL)-1 and IL-6 [29]. A distinct profile in the expression of genes encoding members of the HSP70 family was demonstrated in leukocytes obtained from different phases of the disease course in septic patients [30]. These findings strongly suggest that HSP70 may play a role in the outcome of septic shock patients [30]. Further, studies proved that in an animal model of ARDS, heat pretreatment prevented mortality [31].

Previous studies had revealed that sepsis induced by cecal ligation and double puncture (CLP) resulted in an ARDS-like state characterized by neutrophil accumulation and protein-rich interstitial edema formation [27, 31, 32-38]. Using this model, we found impaired hepatic expression of several essential liver-specific genes, including those encoding proteins that catalyze gluconeogenesis, $\beta$-oxidation of fatty acids, ureagenesis, and bile acid transport [39–41]. Further, we have demonstrated inappropriate downregulation of the expression of several key genes within the lung. These include surfactant proteins (SP)-A and (SP)-B and, most importantly, HSP70 [27, 42, 43]. We found that HSP70 mRNA increased after a sham operation but failed to increase after CLP [27]. HSP70 protein levels were unchanged after either CLP or sham operation. Therefore, HSP70 mRNA fails to increase after CLP despite significant damage to alveolar cells. This lack of increase in HSP70 implies profound pulmonary epithelial dysfunction, similar to our findings in the liver, and is supported by several other studies indicating that sepsis and endotoxemia impair HSP70 expression [23, 27, 32, 44]. These experiments led us to investigate in depth the role of HSP70 in ARDS and inflammation, by using an adenovirus (AdHSP) to enhance HSP70 expression [38].

We have demonstrated that intratracheal administration of AdHSP significantly attenuates lung injury in rats with sepsis-induced respiratory distress [38]. AdHSP, when compared to phosphate buffer saline (PBS) or a virus expressing a marker protein (AdGFP), attenuated CLP-induced neutrophil accumulation, septal thickening, interstitial fluid accumulation, and alveolar protein exudation [38]. More importantly, AdHSP treatment significantly decreased mortality in rats subjected to CLP [38]. In contrast to studies that provoked the entire heat shock response [31, 45, 46], our investigations present a unique approach to explore the effects of HSP70 on a single tissue, the lung [32]. We previously documented that AdHSP preferentially increases HSP70 expression in pulmonary epithelial cells [38]. An interesting finding was that 48 hours following CLP, virus uptake occurred primarily in pulmonary epithelial cells, especially type II pneumocytes [32].

## HSP70 Inhibits Pro-inflammatory Cell Signaling Pathways in ARDS

The heat shock response is known to modulate inflammation [2]. The mechanisms that have been investigated involve the attenuation of both cytokine-induced inflammatory mediator production and apoptosis [2,22,31,45]. Both processes are important in the pathogenesis of ARDS [48–50]. This involves cytokines such as TNF-$\alpha$ and IL-1$\beta$ [48–50,54].

HSP70 inhibits the apoptotic machinery including the apoptosome, the caspase activation complex, and apoptosis inducing factor [55–57]. HSP70 also participates in the proteasome-mediated degradation of apoptosis-regulatory proteins [58].

TNF-$\alpha$ and IL-1$\beta$ exert their effects in part via cell signaling pathways involving the nuclear transcription factor, nuclear factor-$\kappa$B (NF-$\kappa$B) [59–61]. This important acute inflammatory pathway is modulated by HSP70. NF-$\kappa$B is a dimeric protein, most often consisting of two subunits, p50 and p65 (Rel A). Normally, this dimer is retained in the cytoplasm by an inhibitory molecule, I$\kappa$B$\alpha$ [62]. An essential step in NF-$\kappa$B activation is I$\kappa$B$\alpha$ degradation. This permits the migration of NF-$\kappa$B into the nucleus where it can initiate transcription [61,62]. Degradation of I$\kappa$B$\alpha$ involves three sequential biochemical reactions. The first is phosphorylation of I$\kappa$B$\alpha$ by I$\kappa$B kinase (IKK). IKK is a complex molecule that contains two catalytic subunits, IKK$\alpha$ and IKK$\beta$, an essential regulatory subunit IKK$\gamma$also called NF-$\kappa$B essential modulator (or NEMO) [63], and a recently identified co-modulator, the 105 kDa protein, ELKS [64–66]. The dominant catalytic subunit in inflammation is IKK$\beta$ [61]. Phosphorylation of I$\kappa$B$\alpha$ is followed by poly-ubiquitination by SCF$^{\beta\text{-TrCP}}$ ubiquitin ligase and, finally, proteolysis by the 26S proteasome [67–70].

Several *in vitro* models have proven that heat shock or elevated levels of HSP70 suppresses NF-$\kappa$B activity and that this inhibition of NF-$\kappa$B results in a general reduction in the inflammatory response [44,46,71,73]. However, the exact molecular mechanism of the HSP70–NF-$\kappa$B interaction is still unknown. Ran et al. [74] demonstrated that HSP70 promotes rather than inhibits TNF-mediated cell death, by binding to IKK$\gamma$. This resulted in inhibition of IKK activity and consequently inhibited NF-$\kappa$B-dependent antiapoptotic gene induction [74]. Earlier, Yoo et al. demonstrated that HSP70 prevented phosphorylation of I$\kappa$B$\alpha$ by IKK$\beta$ [71].

Both activation and modulation of inflammation require coupling of extra-cellular signals with intra-cellular events, processes involving a number of specific biochemical pathways. We investigated the hypothesis that AdHSP limits sepsis-induced acute inflammation within alveolar epithelial cells in part by suppressing NF-$\kappa$B activation. In contrast to the observations of others [71,74], we found that HSP70 reduced, but did not abolish, IKK$\beta$ activity. More importantly, we have uncovered a novel mechanism of I$\kappa$B$\alpha$ stabilization that results from an association with HSP70 [75]. HSP70 binds to an incomplete protein degradative complex composed of phosphorylated-ubiquitinated I$\kappa$B$\alpha$sgF-$\kappa$B, and partial IKK complexes that contain ELKS, IKK$\beta$s and/or IKK$\gamma$g(NEMO). The association of HSP70 leads to stabilization of these intermediate complexes in a way that prevents proteasomal degradation of I$\kappa$B$\alpha$. Consequently, NF-$\kappa$B is retained in the cytoplasm and is unable to induce inflammatory responses.

## Conclusion

Hsps are important mediators of a number of key intracellular reactions. Of importance to the care of the critically ill are their involvement in protein repair and tertiary structure. HSP70 is known to modulate inflammation and apoptosis. In models of acute lung injury and ARDS, over-expression of HSP70 improves outcome, ameliorates lung injury and attenuates inflammation. The involvement of HSP70 in other aspects of lung injury and in other components of MODS is under investigation.

*Acknowledgement.* Supported in part by NIH Grant GM 059930.

## References

1. Davis TR (1974) Effects of heat on animals and man. Prog Biometeorol 1:228–238, 635–637
2. De Maio A (1999) Heat shock proteins: facts, thoughts and dreams. Shock 11:1–12
3. Snoeckx LH, Cornelussen RN, Van Nieuwenhoven FA, Reneman RS, Van Der Vusse GJ (2001) Heat shock proteins and cardiovascular pathophysiology. Physiol Rev 81:1461–1497
4. Feder ME, Hofmann GE (1999) Heat-shock proteins, molecular chaperones, and the stress response: evolutionary and ecological physiology. Annu Rev Physiol 61:243–282
5. Pilon M, Schekman R (1999) Protein translocation: how Hsp70 pulls it off. Cell 11:679–682
6. Kregel KC (2002) Heat shock proteins: modifying factors in physiological stress responses and acquired thermotolerance. J Appl Physiol 92:2177–2186
7. Frydman J (2001) Folding of newly translated proteins *in vivo*: the role of molecular chaperones. Annu Rev Biochem 70:603–647
8. Hartl FU, Hayer-Hartl M (2002) Molecular chaperones in the cytosol: from nascent chain to folded protein. Science 295:1852–1858
9. Yerbury JJ, Stewart EM, Wyatt AR, Wilson MR (2005) Quality control of protein folding in extracellular space. EMBO Rep 6:1131–1136
10. Rajan RS, Illing ME, Bence NF, Kopito RR (2001) Specificity in intracellular protein aggregation and inclusion body formation. Proc Natl Acad Sci USA 98:13060–13065
11. Hinault MP, Ben-Zvi A, Goloubinoff P (2006) Molecular chaperones: Cellular fold-controlling factors of toxic protein aggregates in neurodegenerative diseases. J Mol Neurosci (in press)
12. Hartl FU (1996) Molecular chaperones in cellular protein folding. Nature 381:571–579
13. Bukau B, Horwich AL (1998) The Hsp70 and Hsp60 chaperone machines. Cell 92:351–366
14. Whitesell L, Lindquist SL (2005) Hsp90 and the chaperoning of cancer. Nat Rev Cancer 5:761–772
15. Wegele H, Muller L, Buchner J (2004) Hsp70 and Hsp90-a relay team for protein folding. Rev Physiol Biochem Pharmacol 151:1–44
16. Westerheide SD, Morimoto RI (2005) Heat shock response modulators as therapeutic tools for diseases of protein conformation. J Biol Chem 280:33097–33100
17. Marber MS, Mestril R, Chi SH, Sayen MR, Yellon DM, Dillmann WH (1995) Overexpression of the rat inducible 70-kD heat stress protein in a transgenic mouse increases the resistance of the heart to ischemic injury. J Clin Invest 95:1446–1456
18. Kluck CJ, Patzelt H, Genevaux P, et al (2002) Structure-function analysis of HscC, the Escherichia coli member of a novel subfamily of specialized Hsp70 chaperones. J Biol Chem 277:41060–4169

19. Bellmann K, Wenz A, Radons J, Burkart V, Kleemann R, Kolb H (1995) Heat shock induces resistance in rat pancreatic islet cells against nitric oxide, oxygen radicals and streptozotocin toxicity in vitro. J Clin Invest 95:2840–2845
20. Klosterhalfen B, Hauptmann S, Tietze L, et al (1997) The influence of heat shock protein 70 induction on hemodynamic variables in a porcine model of recurrent endotoxemia. Shock 7:358–363
21. Tacchini L, Schiaffonati L, Pappalardo C, Gatti S, Bernelli-Zazzera A (1993) Expression of Hsp70, immediate-early response and heme oxygenase genes in ischemic-reperfused rat liver. Lab Invest 68:465–471
22. Wong HR, Wispe JR (1997) The stress response and the lung. Am J Physiol 273:L1–19
23. Schroeder S, Lindemann C, Hoeft A, et al (1999) Impaired inducibility of heat shock protein 70 in peripheral blood lymphocytes of patients with severe sepsis. Crit Care Med 27:1080–1084
24. Milberg JA, Davis DR, Steinberg KP, Hudson LD (1995) Improved survival of patients with acute respiratory distress syndrome (ARDS): 1983–1993. JAMA 273:306–309
25. Baue AE, Durham R, Faist E (1998) Systemic inflammatory response syndrome (SIRS), multiple organ dysfunction syndrome (MODS), multiple organ failure (MOF): are we winning the battle? Shock 10:79–89
26. Rubenfeld GD, Caldwell E, Peabody E, et al (2005) Incidence and outcomes of acute lung injury. N Engl J Med 353:1685–1693
27. Weiss YG, Bouwman A, Gehan B, Schears G, Raj N, Deutschman CS (2000) Cecal ligation and double puncture impairs heat shock protein 70 (Hsp70) expression in the lungs of rats. Shock 13:19–23
28. Smart SJ, Casale TB (1994) TNF-alpha-induced transendothelial neutrophil migration is IL-8 dependent. Am J Physiol 266:L238–L245
29. Vreugdenhil HA, Haitsma JJ, Jansen KJ, et al (2003) Ventilator-induced heat shock protein 70 and cytokine mRNA expression in a model of lipopolysaccharide-induced lung inflammation. Intensive Care Med 29:915–922
30. Durand P, Bachelet M, Brunet F, et al. (2000) Inducibility of the 70 kD heat shock protein in peripheral blood monocytes is decreased in human acute respiratory distress syndrome and recovers over time. Am J Respir Crit Care Med, 161:286–292
31. Villar J, Ribeiro SP, Mullen JB, Kuliszewski M, Post M, Slutsky AS (1994) Induction of the heat shock response reduces mortality rate and organ damage in a sepsis-induced acute lung injury model. Crit Care Med 22:914–921
32. Weiss YG, Tazelaar J, Gehan BA, et al (2001) Adenoviral vector transfection into the pulmonary epithelium after cecal ligation and puncture in rats. Anesthesiology 95:974–982
33. Rosenfeld MA, Yoshimura K, Trapnell BC, et al (1992) In vivo transfer of the human cystic fibrosis transmembrane conductance regulator gene to the airway epithelium. Cell 68:143–155
34. Dong JY, Wang D, Van Ginkel FW, Pascual DW, Frizzell RA (1996) Systematic analysis of repeated gene delivery into animal lungs with a recombinant adenovirus vector. Hum Gene Ther 7:319–331
35. Touqui L, Arbibe L (1999) A role for phospholipase A2 in ARDS pathogenesis. Mol Med Today 5:244–249
36. Weiss YG, Bellin L, Kim PK, et al (2001) Compensatory hepatic regeneration after mild, but not fulminant, intraperitoneal sepsis in rats. Am J Physiol Gastrointest Liver Physiol 280:G968–G973
37. Artigas A, Bernard GR, Carlet J, et al (1998) The American-European Consensus Conference on ARDS, part 2. Ventilatory, pharmacologic, supportive therapy, study design strategies and issues related to recovery and remodeling. Intensive Care Med 24:378–398
38. Weiss YG, Maloyan A, Tazelaar J, Raj N, Deutschman CS (2002) Adenoviral transfer of Hsp70 into pulmonary epithelium ameliorates experimental acute respiratory distress syndrome. J Clin Invest 110:801–806

39. Andrejko KM, Chen J, Deutschman CS (1998) Intrahepatic STAT-3 activation and acute phase gene expression predict outcome after CLP sepsis in the rat. Am J Physiol 275:G1423–G1429
40. Deutschman CS, De Maio A, Buchman TG, Clemens MG (1993) Sepsis-induced alterations in phosphoenolpyruvate carboxykinase expression: the role of insulin and glucagon. Circ Shock 40:295–302
41. Deutschman CS, Andrejko KM, Haber BA, et al (1997) Sepsis-induced depression of rat glucose-6-phosphatase gene expression and activity. Am J Physiol 273:R1709–R1718
42. Schears GJ, Costarino AT (1999) Complexity of inflammatory mediators in acute respiratory distress syndrome (ARDS). J Pediatr 135:144–146
43. Malloy J, McCaig L, Veldhuizen R, et al (1997) Alterations of the endogenous surfactant system in septic adult rats. Am J Respir Crit Care Med 156:617–623
44. Ofenstein JP, Heidemann S, Juett A, Sarnaik A (1998) Endotoxin inhibits heat induced Hsp70 in rats. Crit Care Med 26 (Suppl 1):A 138 (abst)
45. Mosser DD, Caron AW, Bourget L, et al (2000) The chaperone function of hsp70 is required for protection against stress-induced apoptosis. Mol Cell Biol 20:7146–7159
46. Guzhova IV, Darieva ZA, Melo AR, Margulis BA (1997) Major stress protein Hsp70 interacts with NF-κB regulatory complex in human T-lymphoma cells. Cell Stress Chaperones 2:132–139
47. Jaattela M, Wissing D, Bauer PA, Li GC (1992) Major heat shock protein hsp70 protects tumor cells from tumor necrosis factor cytotoxicity. EMBO J 11:3507–3512
48. Kitamura Y, Hashimoto S, Mizuta N, et al (2001) Fas/FasL-dependent apoptosis of alveolar cells after lipopolysaccharide-induced lung injury in mice. Am J Respir Crit Care Med 163:762–769
49. Serrao KL, Fortenberry JD, Owens ML, Harris FL, Brown LA (2001) Neutrophils induce apoptosis of lung epithelial cells via release of soluble Fas ligand. Am J Physiol Lung Cell Mol Physiol 280:L298–L305
50. Matute-Bello G, Liles WC, Steinberg KP, et al (1999) Soluble Fas ligand induces epithelial cell apoptosis in humans with acute lung injury (ARDS). J Immunol 163:2217–2225
51. Petrache I, Verin AD, Crow MT, Birukova A, Liu F, Garcia JG (2001) Differential effect of MLC kinase in TNF-alpha-induced endothelial cell apoptosis and barrier dysfunction. Am J Physiol Lung Cell Mol Physiol 280:L1168–L1178
52. Baud V, Karin M (2001) Signal transduction by tumor necrosis factor and its relatives. Trends Cell Biol 11:372–377
53. Akira S, Hoshino K, Kaisho T (2000) The role of Toll-like receptors and MyD88 in innate immune responses. J Endotoxin Res 6:383–387
54. Bromberg Z, Deutschman CS, Weiss YG (2005) Heat shock protein 70 and the acute respiratory distress syndrome. J Anesth 19:236–242
55. Beere HM, Wolf BB, Cain K, et al (2000) Heat-shock protein 70 inhibits apoptosis by preventing recruitment of procaspase-9 to the Apaf-1 apoptosome. Nat Cell Biol 2:469–475
56. Ravagnan L, Gurbuxani S, Susin SA, et al (2001) Heat-shock protein 70 antagonizes apoptosis-inducing factor. Nat Cell Biol 3:839–843
57. Saleh A, Srinivasula SM, Balkir L, Robbins PD, Alnemri ES (2000) Negative regulation of the Apaf-1 apoptosome by Hsp70. Nat Cell Biol 2:476–483
58. Garrido C, Schmitt E, Cande C, Vahsen N, Parcellier A, Kroemer G (2003) HSP27 and HSP70: potentially oncogenic apoptosis inhibitors. Review Cell Cycle 2:579–584
59. Christman JW, Sadikot RT, Blackwell TS (2000) The role of nuclear factor-κB in pulmonary diseases. Chest 117:1482–1487
60. Hoffmann A, Levchenko A, Scott ML, Baltimore D (2002) The IkappaB-NF-kappaB signaling module: temporal control and selective gene activation. Science 298:1241–1245
61. Chen LW, Egan L, Li ZW, Greten FR, Kagnoff MF, Karin M (2003) The two faces of IKK and NF-kappa B inhibition: prevention of systemic inflammation but increased local injury following intestinal ischemia-reperfusion. Nat Med 9:575–581

62. Ghosh S, May MJ, Kopp ER (1998) NF-κB and Rel proteins: Evolutionarily conserved mediators of immune responses. Annu Rev Immunol 16:225–260
63. Yamamoto Y, Kim DW, Kwak YT, Parjapati S, Verma U, Gaynor RB (2001) IKKγ/NEMO facilitates the recruitment of the IκB proteins into the IκB Kinase complex. J Biol C lem 276:36327–36336
64. Mercurio F, Zhu H, Murray BW, et al (1997) IKK1 and IKK2: Cytokine-activated IκB kinases essential for NF-κB activation. Science 278:860–866
65. Poyet JL, Srinivasula SM, Lin JH, et al (2000) Activation of the I kappa B kinases by RIP via IKKgamma /NEMO-mediated oligomerization. J Biol Chem 275:37966–37977
66. Ducut Sigala JL, Bottero V, Young DB, Shevchenko A, Mercurio F, Verma IM (2004) Activation of transcription factor NF-κB requires ELKS, an IκB kinase regulatory subunit. Science 304:1963–1967
67. Read MA, Brownell JE, Gladysheva TB, et al (2000) Nedd8 modification of cul-1 activates SCF(beta(TrCP)-dependent ubiquitination of I KappaB alpha. Mol Cell Biol 20:2326–2333
68. Ben-Neriah Y (2002) Regulatory functions of ubiquitination in the immune system. Nat Immunol 3:20–26
69. Ciechanover A, Orian A, Schwartz A (2000) Ubiquitin-mediated proteolysis: biological regulation via destruction. BioEssays 22:442–451
70. Adams J (2003) The proteasome: structure, function, and role in the cell. Cancer Treat Rev 29 (suppl 1):3–9
71. Yoo CG, Lee S, Lee CT, Kim YW, Han SK, Shim YS (2000) Anti-inflammatory effect of heat shock protein induction is related to stabilization of I kappa B alpha through preventing I kappa B kinase activation in respiratory epithelial cells. J Immunol 164:5416–5123
72. Curry HA, Clemens RA, Shah S, et al (1999) Heat shock inhibits radiation-induced activation of NF-kappaB via inhibition of I-kappaB kinase. J Biol Chem 274:23061–23067
73. Malhotra V, Kooy NW, Denenberg AG, Dunsmore KE, Wong HR (2002) Ablation of the heat shock factor-1 increases susceptibility to hyperoxia-mediated cellular injury. Exp Lung Res 28:609–622
74. Ran R, Lu A, Zhang L, et al (2004) Hsp70 promotes TNF-mediated apoptosis by binding IKK gamma and impairing NF-kappa B survival signaling. Genes Dev 18:1466–1481
75. Weiss YG, Bromberg Z, Goloubinoff P, Deutschman CS (2005) HSP-70 Expression in the lung attenuates ARDS by disrupting NF-κB. Intensive Care Med 31 (suppl 1):S45 (abst)

# Fibrosis in the Acute Respiratory Distress Syndrome

D.C.J. Howell, R.C. Chambers, and G.J. Laurent

## Introduction

Sepsis often leads to severe pulmonary dysfunction and a large proportion of patients will develop acute lung injury/acute respiratory distress syndrome (ALI/ARDS) [1]. Although sepsis is frequently an initiating factor in the development of ALI/ARDS, the etiology of ALI/ARDS is diverse and the disorders associated with the condition can broadly be divided into those which cause direct or indirect lung injury (Table 1). The current American/European definition of the condition has been designed to reflect the underlying severity of lung injury in ALI/ARDS (Table 2). Although not specifically part of the diagnostic criteria, it is well documented that a proportion of patients with ALI/ARDS develop aggressive pulmonary fibrosis that ultimately leads to their demise.

Table 1. Etiology of ALI/ARDS

| Direct Lung Injury | Indirect Lung Injury |
| --- | --- |
| Bronchopneumonia | Sepsis |
| Gastric aspiration | Multiple trauma with shock |
| Pulmonary contusion | Drug overdose |
| Inhalational injury | Acute pancreatitis |
| Near-drowning | Transfusion-associated acute |
| Reperfusion injury | lung injury (TRALI) |
| Fat emboli | Cardiopulmonary bypass |

## Pathogenesis of ALI/ARDS

ALI/ARDS is classically thought to exhibit three phases: i) exudative/inflammatory; ii) proliferative; and iii) fibrotic (reviewed in [2]). Briefly, the exudative phase is characterized histologically by diffuse alveolar damage as the microvascular endothelial and alveolar epithelium, which form the alveolar-capillary barrier, are disrupted. Intense neutrophil infiltration is also a major feature of this phase of

Table 2. Diagnostic criteria in ALI/ARDS

|  | Acute lung injury | Acute respiratory distress syndrome |
|---|---|---|
| Chest Xray | Bilateral infiltrates | Bilateral infiltrates |
| Clinical scenario | Acute onset | Acute onset |
| Pulmonary artery wedge pressure | < 18 mmHg | < 18 mmHg |
| Oxygenation | $PaO_2/FiO_2$ ratio < 300 mmHg | $PaO_2/FiO_2$ ratio < 200 mmHg |

ALI/ARDS. Once injured, the endothelial barrier becomes increasingly permeable resulting in highly proteinaceous, hemorrhagic pulmonary edema fluid flooding into alveoli, with resultant formation of fibrinous hyaline membranes. Epithelial integrity is also breached, as a result of damage to type I and II pneumocytes, which leads to exacerbation of alveolar edema as permeability of the epithelium increases and its resorptive function ceases. In addition, as type II cells are also injured, surfactant production is reduced. Lack of efficient endothelial and epithelial repair is thought to be critical in the progression of ALI/ARDS as the endothelium plays a vital role in remodeling of the alveolar capillary barrier [3], and an intact epithelial layer plays an important role in suppressing fibroblast proliferation and matrix production.

During the proliferative phase of ALI/ARDS, damage to the delicate capillary network of the lung is a major feature with intimal proliferation in small blood vessels. Following necrosis of type I pneumocytes, the epithelial basement membrane is exposed and type II cells proliferate in an attempt to repair the damaged epithelium. Fibroblasts/myofibroblasts emerge in the interstitial space and alveolar lumen. As fibrinous exudates become organized, they are replaced by collagen fibrils. The fibrotic phase is characterized by extensive alveolar septal and intra-alveolar fibrosis, as well as myointimal thickening and mural fibrosis of vessels, which contribute to the degree of pulmonary hypertension observed in this condition. There is a progressive increase in lung collagen with the duration of the condition, the severity of which correlates with increase in mortality.

A concept that has been challenged over recent years concerns the sequential relationship of the three phases of ALI/ARDS. Whereas it was once thought that these were distinct and develop as the condition progresses, there is now increasing evidence that there is much overlap between the three phases. In particular, a number of studies have shown that the fibrotic/fibroproliferative response occurs much earlier than previously thought. For example, N-terminal procollagen peptide III (N-PCP-III), which is a marker of collagen turnover, is elevated in bronchoalveolar lavage (BAL) fluid and tracheal aspirates from patients with ALI/ARDS within 24 hours of diagnosis [4–6]. In addition, fibroproliferation has been shown to occur early in ALI/ARDS and also predicts a poor outcome [7]. Another more recent study has further shown that extensive thin-section computed tomography (CT) changes, indicative of fibroproliferation, are independently predictive of a poor prognosis in patients with clinical early-stage ALI/ARDS [8].

## What Drives the Fibrotic Response in ALI/ARDS?

A number of factors, including genetic influences, oxidant stress, anti-apoptotic agents, and excessive mechanical ventilation, leading to shear-stress of alveoli, are likely to play critical roles in orchestrating the fibrotic response to lung injury in ALI/ARDS. In addition, pro-inflammatory and pro-fibrotic cytokines, chemokines, and growth factors are released from resident and recruited inflammatory cells that influence the progression of this condition. Although many potential fibrotic mediators have been proposed to play a role in chronic forms of pulmonary fibrosis, such as usual interstitial pneumonia [9, 10], less is currently known about specific factors that directly affect fibroproliferation and the resultant fibrotic response in ALI/ARDS. However, a number of candidates have been identified from human and animal studies. For example, levels of the potent pro-fibrotic mediators, transforming growth factor-$\alpha$ (TGF-$\alpha$) and platelet derived growth factor (PDGF), are increased in BAL fluid obtained from patients with ALI/ARDS [11, 12]. Furthermore, expression of a tumor necrosis factor-$\alpha$ (TNF-$\alpha$) transgene in murine lung leads to an alveolitis that steadily progresses to fibrosis, suggesting the possible importance of this cytokine in ALI/ARDS [13]. In addition, we have recently obtained evidence that angiotensin II, possibly generated locally within the lung, may play an important role in the fibrotic response to experimentally-induced lung injury, at least in part via the action of TGF-$\beta$ [14]. Th-2 cytokines, including IL-4 and IL-13, have also been implicated in the pathogenesis of fibroproliferative lung disorders [15]. More recently, BAL fluid from patients with ALI/ARDS was shown to contain active TGF-$\beta$1 which was capable of inducing procollagen I promoter activity in human lung fibroblasts *in vitro* [16]. Finally, there is increasing evidence that a prevailing procoagulant microenvironment with generation of coagulation proteinases such as thrombin and factor Xa, may also play a crucial role in regulating the fibrotic response in this condition.

## Evidence for the Role of the Coagulation Cascade in ALI/ARDS

Consistent with the concept that the coagulation cascade is activated in ALI/ARDS, extravascular and intra-alveolar accumulation of fibrin is a characteristic feature of this condition [17, 18]. The excessive procoagulant activity observed in the lung in ALI/ARDS is thought to arise from an imbalance between pro- and anti-coagulant factors. For example, BAL fluid from patients with ALI/ARDS has been shown to contain tissue factor/factor VII/VIIa complexes [18], which can activate factor X and trigger activation of the extrinsic pathway of coagulation.

The prevailing balance between the pro- and anti-coagulant state in the lung following injury is also affected by regulatory mechanisms, which control the clearance of deposited fibrin (fibrinolysis). This process, which occurs at all sites of wound healing, is initiated when plasminogen is converted to plasmin by the proteinases, urokinase-type plasminogen activator (u-PA) or tissue-type plasminogen activator (t-PA). Plasmin subsequently cleaves fibrin into a range of fibrin degradation products (FDPs). Fibrinolytic activity in the vasculature is largely under the control of t-PA; whereas extravascular fibrinolysis in the lung is controlled by u-PA. The conversion of plasminogen to plasmin by t-PA and u-PA is regulated by the endogenous inhibitor, plasminogen activator inhibitor-1 (PAI-1). PAI-1 activity is increased in ALI/ARDS, particularly in the alveolar compartment, thus favoring fibrin persistence [19]. The fibrinolytic system is also influenced by the plasma glycoprotein thrombin-activatable fibrinolysis inhibitor (TAFI). During fibrin degradation, plasmin exposes C-terminal lysine residues on the fibrin molecule to potentiate its clearance. TAFI cleaves these residues, which, therefore, favors fibrin persistence. Although it has not been shown in patients with ALI/ARDS, it is noteworthy that levels of TAFI are increased in BAL fluid from patients with interstitial lung disease [20].

In terms of a deficiency of anticoagulant factors, levels of antithrombin are reduced in patients with ALI/ARDS [21]. In addition, it has been shown that levels of protein C in the intra-alveolar compartment from patients with ALI/ARDS are reduced compared with plasma levels and correlate with a poor clinical outcome [22,23]. Levels of the major endogenous inhibitor of the extrinsic coagulation cascade, tissue factor pathway inhibitor (TFPI), are markedly increased following experimental lung injury [24]. However, studies by Gando and colleagues [25] suggest that systemic activation of the tissue factor-dependent pathway is not adequately balanced by TFPI in patients with ARDS.

A number of studies performed in experimental animal models have examined the effects of modulating the coagulation cascade in ALI/ARDS. For example, exogenous delivery of the highly specific direct thrombin inhibitor, hirudin, or of antithrombin, have been shown to be protective in animal models of ALI/ARDS [26–28]. In addition, administration of heparin, which inhibits coagulation proteinases by potentiating the formation of antithrombin/serine proteinase complexes, but also has anti-inflammatory properties, leads to improved gas exchange in an animal model of ALI/ARDS [29]. Heparin has also been shown to attenuate bleomycin-induced pulmonary fibrosis in mice [30], although in this study, it was uncertain whether heparin was delivered at an anticoagulant dose and whether the protective effects were due to its direct anti-proliferative effects, or due to blocking proteinase activity. The animal model of bleomycin-induced fibrosis, based on intratracheal delivery of this agent, is a well-established model of ALI/ARDS. Characteristic pathogenetic features of ALI/ARDS are observed in the lung following bleomycin instillation, including the rapid influx of inflammatory cells, an increase in microvascular permeability, and aggressive fibroproliferation, culminating in established interstitial fibrosis. Of note, intratracheal administration of activated protein C (APC) and intratracheal gene transfer of TFPI both attenuate bleomycin-induced fibrosis in rodent studies [31, 32]. BAL fluid levels of the coagulation proteinase, thrombin, are increased in this animal model of ALI/ARDS [33].

## Thrombin and Proteinase Activated Receptors (PARs)

In addition to its critical role in blood coagulation, thrombin exerts potent cellular responses via its ability to activate the family of proteinase activated receptors (PARs). A number of these cellular effects are likely to play important roles in inflammatory and tissue repair processes in ALI/ARDS and will, therefore, be discussed in greater detail.

The PARs belong to the family of seven transmembrane G-protein coupled receptors, which exhibit a unique mechanism of activation that involves the un-masking of a tethered ligand by limited proteolysis of specific amino acid sequences from the N-terminus of the receptor [34]. Following proteolytic cleavage, the newly generated tethered ligand binds intramolecularly to the second extracellular loop of the receptor, inducing a conformational shape change that allows it to interact with heterotrimeric G-proteins and initiate downstream signaling responses. To date, four PARs have been characterized, of which three, PAR-1, -3, and -4, are activated by thrombin. Synthetic peptides corresponding to the tethered ligands of PAR-1, -2 and -4 are capable of mimicking a number of cellular responses elicited by their respective endogenous activators. The first PAR to be cloned and char-acterized was PAR-1 [34], which has subsequently been shown to be the major receptor involved in mediating thrombin's cellular effects, in particular in terms of fibroblast responses [35–37]. PAR-1 has a wide tissue distribution and is present on a number of cell types including platelets, endothelial cells, epithelial cells, fibroblasts, smooth muscle cells, monocytes, lymphocytes, mast cells, and certain tumor cell lines (reviewed in [38]). PAR-2 and PAR-4 are similarly expressed on numerous cell types in the airways, blood, and cardiovascular system, whereas PAR-3 appears to have a more restricted expression pattern.

## PAR-Mediated Cellular Effects of Thrombin Pertinent to Fibrosis in ALI/ARDS

PAR-1 is the major high-affinity thrombin signaling receptor and is abundantly ex-pressed in the injured lung. PAR-1 mediated cellular responses elicited by thrombin that are likely to be important in the pathogenesis of ALI/ARDS include the ability of thrombin to promote platelet aggregation, influence vascular tone and perme-ability, stimulate angiogenesis and vascular repair, and promote inflammatory cell trafficking. Of particular importance to the fibrotic response in ALI/ARDS, throm-bin is a fibroblast mitogen and chemoattractant [39–41]. In addition, thrombin stimulates lung fibroblast differentiation to the myofibroblast phenotype [42, 43] and mesenchymal cell procollagen production and gene expression [36, 44]. These effects can be mimicked with PAR-1 agonists; whereas fibroblasts derived from PAR-1 deficient mice are unresponsive to thrombin in terms of MAP kinase signaling, proliferation [35], and procollagen α1(I) gene promoter activity [45]. Thrombin has bee nshown to be a major fibroblast mitoge nin BAL fluid from patie nts with pulmonary fibrosis associated with systemic sclerosis [46, 47]. To our knowledge, similar studies in patients with ARDS/ALI have not yet been reported.

There is good evidence that most of the cellular effects of thrombin are mediated via the induction and release of secondary mediators [38]. For example, PAR-1 activation by thrombin induces the production and release of PDGF, connective tissue growth factor (CTGF), TGF-β and pro-inflammatory mediators, such as IL-6, IL-8 and monocyte chemotactic protein-1 (MCP-1/CCL2). These mediators are, in turn, responsible for thrombin's mitogenic, pro-fibrotic, and pro-inflammatory effects via both autocrine and paracrine mechanisms.

We have specifically examined the procoagulant and downstream cellular effects of thrombin and PAR-1 activation in the bleomycin model of ALI *in vivo* using the direct thrombin inhibitor, UK-156406, in rats [48] and comparing responses in wild type and PAR-1 knockout (PAR-1 -/-) mice [49]. These studies revealed that thrombin and PAR-1 immunoreactivity in the lung were markedly increased following bleomycin instillation and were predominantly associated with fibroblasts and infiltrating macrophages. This is, to our knowledge, the first demonstration that expression of thrombin and PAR-1 is increased in a model of ALI/ARDS. In animals given bleomycin, lung collagen content characteristically doubled and was preceded by significant elevations in α1(I) procollagen and CTGF mRNA levels. However, in bleomycin-treated animals receiving an anticoagulant dose of UK-156046, lung collagen accumulation was significantly attenuated, a feature that was also preceded by a significant reduction in α1(I) procollagen and CTGF gene expression.

The protective effect of direct thrombin inhibition in this model may have been due to blocking thrombin's procoagulant (fibrin generation) or PAR-mediated cellular effects. In order to specifically dissect the potential contribution of PAR-1 activation in this model, we examined the response of PAR-1 -/- mice. Total lung collagen accumulation following bleomycin injury was dramatically reduced in PAR-1 -/- mice compared with that found in correspondingly injured wild type animals, as was BAL fluid inflammatory cell recruitment and microvascular permeability. This protection was associated with attenuation in lung levels of the potent PAR-1 inducible pro-inflammatory and pro-fibrotic growth factors, MCP-1, CTGF, and TGF-β [49]. Taken together, these data provide evidence that thrombin and PAR-1 play a critical role in inflammation, microvascular leak, and fibrotic responses in this model of ALI and may, therefore, also contribute to the pathogenesis of ALI/ARDS in humans.

## Emerging Concepts Regarding PARs and Fibrosis

A number of important studies have been published that have challenged conventional dogma on coagulation cascade proteinases and PAR activation (Fig. 1). It was previously thought that thrombin was the only major activator of PAR-1, -3 and -4 and that trypsin and mast cell tryptase activated PAR-2 [50]. However, it is now known that thrombin is not the only coagulation proteinase that is capable of exerting functional responses via proteolytic cleavage of PAR-1. Limited proteolysis of PAR-1 by factor Xa initiates downstream functional effects, such as fibroblast proliferation and procollagen production [45,51]. Furthermore, plasmin has been shown to activate PAR-1 to induce the expression of Cyr 61, a member of the CCN family of proteins which includes CTGF [52]. Riewald and Ruf have also shown that nascent factor Xa, in the procoagulant transient tissue factor-factor VIIa-factor Xa ternary complex generated following activation of the extrinsic coagulation cascade, signals via both PAR-1 and PAR-2 in endothelial cells [53]. This study raises the possibility that tissue factor dependent initiation of the coagulation cascade is mechanistically coupled to PAR-dependent cellular signaling.

There is good evidence that PAR-2 can be transactivated by cleaved PAR-1 [54] and that the tissue factor-factor VIIa complex can also signal via PAR-2 in endothelial cells [55]. Non-coagulation proteinases, such as trypsin, elastase, and the neutrophil proteinase, cathepsin G, have also been shown to cleave PAR-1. This was previously thought to occur at non-activating sites producing no functional effects [38, 56]. However, neutrophil elastase has recently been shown to induce apoptosis in human lung epithelial cells via a PAR-1 dependent mechanism. Since epithelial cell apoptosis is a central process in ALI/ARDS [57,58], this observation may be particularly relevant in the context of this condition.

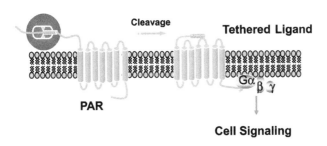

| Receptor | Activator |
|---|---|
| PAR-1 | Thrombin, factor Xa, tissue factor-FVIIa-FXa, neutrophil elastase, plasmin |
| PAR-2 | Factor Xa, TF-FVIIa-FXa |
| PAR-3 | Thrombin |
| PAR-4 | Thrombin, cathepsin G |

**Fig. 1.** Potential activators of proteinase activated receptors (PARs) in ALI/ARDS

Of particular pertinence to the pathogenesis of sepsis, the anticoagulant, APC, has recently also been shown to be capable of activating PAR-1 on endothelial cells, via a process that utilizes the endothelial protein C receptor (EPCR) as a co-receptor [59]. These studies suggest that rather than producing deleterious effects, activation of PAR-1 by APC on the endothelium is cytoprotective and anti-inflammatory. A model has been proposed based on the existence of different threshold concentrations of thrombin within the vasculature, exerting opposing effects. This model suggests that at low concentrations of thrombin, below the procoagulant threshold, thrombin binds to thrombomodulin. Formation of the resultant stoichiometric complex inhibits the enzymatic activity of thrombin and blocks direct PAR-1 activation. Thrombin bound to thrombomodulin can then favorably cleave zymogen protein C to its product, APC. Both substrate and product of this reaction bind to the EPCR. Endogenous production of APC by thrombin is dependent on EPCR binding. EPCR-bound APC subsequently cleaves PAR-1 and induces anti-inflammatory events. When thrombin is generated at higher concentrations that exceed the procoagulant threshold, PAR-1 is activated via the transient tissue factor-factor VIIa-factor Xa complex when coagulation is initiated and in the propagation phase of thrombin generation, which is required for the conversion of fibrinogen to fibrin. In terms of the relevance of these events to excessive intravascular coagulation, such as in sepsis, once the procoagulant threshold is exceeded, disease progression is rapid and this may negate the protective effects of EPCR-bound APC activation of PAR-1 [60]. This may be a plausible mechanism by which APC exerts the favorable effects observed in the PROWESS trial in humans [61]. However, this theory is not universally accepted and is currently at the center of a very interesting debate [62,63]. In contrast to a clear role for PAR-1 in the bleomycin model of ALI, two murine studies have shown that PAR-1 deficiency is not protective in models of endotoxemia [64,65]. However, the former study showed that a combination of PAR-2 deficiency and thrombin inhibition was associated with a favorable outcome [64], suggesting that blockade of all PAR-mediated cellular effects may be necessary for protection in endotoxemia. The contribution of PAR-1 (and other PARs) may, therefore, be dependent on both the nature and the initiating site of lung injury.

## Clinical Implications and Conclusion

Despite intense research efforts, there are still no pharmacological agents which have been shown to improve mortality rates in ALI/ARDS. The recent North American Late Steroid Rescue Study (LaSRS), conducted by the ARDSNet group, assessed the role of methylprednisolone based on previous favorable results in a smaller study [5]. Patients receiving steroids had early physiologic and clinical benefit, displaying improved oxygenation and lung compliance, and earlier withdrawal of mechanical ventilation. However, there was no difference in mortality at 60 and 180 days compared with the control group. Subgroup analysis showed that if BAL fluid procollagen III peptide levels were high at enrolment into the study, there was a survival benefit with steroid therapy, suggesting that identification of patients with an early fibrotic phenotype may be vital to aid the development of successful pharmacological strategies in the future (presented at the American Thoracic Society Conference, San Diego, 2005).

A number of fibrotic mediators have been identified in ALI/ARDS, including TGF-$\alpha$, TGF-$\beta$ and TNF-$\alpha$, which, if successfully targeted, may lead to a therapeutic breakthrough for the treatment of this condition. We further propose that modulation of the coagulation cascade, and more specifically, PAR-1 mediated cellular effects of coagulation proteinases, may also warrant further evaluation as potential therapeutic targets in this condition (Fig. 2). As described above, a number of anticoagulant agents, such as TFPI, site inactivated factor VIIa, heparin, and APC, have shown promise in animal models of ALI/ARDS, but successful clinical trials using these agents have yet to be described. Furthermore, the potential risk of bleeding complications observed in the recent PROWESS trial of APC in sepsis [61] suggests that the use of direct thrombin inhibitors or other anticoagulants in ALI/ARDS may prove problematic. PAR-1 antagonists and blocking antibodies have been developed as potential anti-thrombotic agents [66,67] and PAR-1 antagonist peptides have been shown to be anti-thrombotic and successful in preventing restenosis in an animal model of vascular thrombosis in non-human primates [68,69], suggesting that a suitable agent for use in humans is a realistic

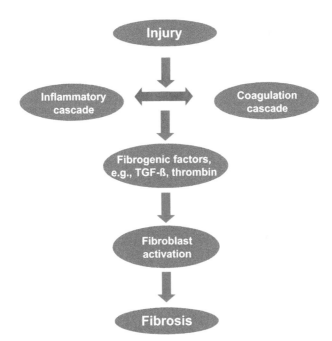

**Fig. 2.** Potential mechanism for the interaction of the coagulation cascade in the fibrotic pathway in ALI/ARDS. TGF: transforming growth factor

possibility. Strategies aimed at blocking PAR-1 may provide a unique opportunity for the treatment of ALI/ARDS by selectively interfering with the pro-fibrotic and pro-inflammatory effects of excessive proteinase signaling, whilst avoiding potential hemostatic complications associated with direct proteolytic inhibitors.

# References

1. Ware LB, Matthay MA (2000) The acute respiratory distress syndrome. N Engl J Med 342:1334–1349
2. Bellingan GJ (2002) The pulmonary physician in critical care * 6: The pathogenesis of ALI/ARDS. Thorax 57:540–546
3. Orfanos SE, Mavrommati I, Korovesi I, et al (2004) Pulmonary endothelium in acute lung injury: from basic science to the critically ill. Intensive Care Med 30:1702–1714
4. Clark JG, Milberg JA, Steinberg KP, et al (1995) Type III procollagen peptide in the adult respiratory distress syndrome. Association of increased peptide levels in bronchoalveolar lavage fluid with increased risk for death. Ann Intern Med 122:17–23
5. Meduri GU, Headley AS, Golden E, et al (1998) Effect of prolonged methylprednisolone therapy in unresolving acute respiratory distress syndrome: a randomized controlled trial. JAMA 280:159–165
6. Chesnutt AN, Matthay MA, Tibayan FA, et al (1997) Early detection of type III procollagen peptide in acute lung injury. Pathogenetic and prognostic significance. Am J Respir Crit Care Med 156:840–845
7. Marshall RP, Bellingan G, Webb S, et al (2000) Fibroproliferation occurs early in the acute respiratory distress syndrome and impacts on outcome. Am J Respir Crit Care Med 162:1783–1788
8. Ichikado K, Suga M, Muranaka H, et al (2006) Prediction of prognosis for acute respiratory distress syndrome with thin-section CT: validation in 44 cases. Radiology 238:321–329
9. McAnulty RJ, Laurent GJ (1995) Pathogenesis of lung fibrosis and potential new therapeutic strategies. Exp Nephrol 3:96–107
10. Chapman HA (2004) Disorders of lung matrix remodeling. J Clin Invest 113:148–157
11. Madtes DK, Rubenfeld G, Klima LD, et al (1998) Elevated transforming growth factor-alpha levels in bronchoalveolar lavage fluid of patients with acute respiratory distress syndrome. Am J Respir Crit Care Med 158:424–430
12. Snyder LS, Hertz MI, Peterson MS, et al (1991) Acute lung injury. Pathogenesis of intraalveolar fibrosis. J Clin Invest 88:663–673
13. Miyazaki Y, Araki K, Vesin C, et al (1995) Expression of a tumor necrosis factor-alpha transgene in murine lung causes lymphocytic and fibrosing alveolitis. A mouse model of progressive pulmonary fibrosis. J Clin Invest 96:250–259
14. Marshall RP, Gohlke P, Chambers RC, et al (2004) Angiotensin II and the fibroproliferative response to acute lung injury. Am J Physiol Lung Cell Mol Physiol 286:L156–L164
15. Jakubzick C, Choi ES, Joshi BH, et al (2003) Therapeutic attenuation of pulmonary fibrosis via targeting of IL-4- and IL-13-responsive cells. J Immunol 171:2684–2693
16. Budinger GR, Chandel NS, Donnelly HK, et al (2005) Active transforming growth factor-beta1 activates the procollagen I promoter in patients with acute lung injury. Intensive Care Med 31:121–128
17. Bachofen M, Weibel ER (1982) Structural alterations of lung parenchyma in the adult respiratory distress syndrome. Clin Chest Med 3:35–56
18. Idell S, Gonzalez K, Bradford H, et al (1987) Procoagulant activity in bronchoalveolar lavage in the adult respiratory distress syndrome. Contribution of tissue factor associated with factor VII. Am Rev Respir Dis 136:1466–1474

19. Prabhakaran P, Ware LB, White KE, Cross MT, Matthay MA, Ohnan MA (2003) Elevated levels of plasminogen activator inhibitor-1 in pulmonary edema fluid are associated with mortality in acute lung injury. Am J Physiol Lung Cell Mol Physiol 285:L20–L28

20. Fujimoto H, Gabazza EC, Hataji O, et al (2003) Thrombin-activatable fibrinolysis inhibitor and protein C inhibitor in interstitial lung disease. Am J Respir Crit Care Med 167:1687–1694

21. Kirschstein W, Heene DL (1985) Fibrinolysis inhibition in acute respiratory distress syndrome. Scand J Clin Lab Invest Suppl 178:87–94

22. Ware LB, Fang X, Matthay MA (2003) Protein C and thrombomodulin in human acute lung injury. Am J Physiol Lung Cell Mol Physiol 285:L514–L521

23. Matthay MA, Ware LB (2004) Plasma protein C levels in patients with acute lung injury: prognostic significance. Crit Care Med 32 (Suppl 5):S229–S232

24. Sabharwal AK, Bajaj SP, Ameri A, et al (1995) Tissue factor pathway inhibitor and von Willebrand factor antigen levels in adult respiratory distress syndrome and in a primate model of sepsis. Am J Respir Crit Care Med 151:758–767

25. Gando S, Kameue T, Matsuda N, et al (2003) Imbalances between the levels of tissue factor and tissue factor pathway inhibitor in ARDS patients. Thromb Res 109:119–124

26. Hoffmann H, Siebeck M, Spannagl M, et al (1990) Effect of recombinant hirudin, a specific inhibitor of thrombin, on endotoxin-induced intravascular coagulation and acute lung injury in pigs. Am Rev Respir Dis 142:782–788

27. Schmidt B, Davis P, La-Pointe H, et al (1996) Thrombin inhibitors reduce intrapulmonary accumulation of fibrinogen and procoagulant activity of bronchoalveolar lavage fluid during acute lung injury induced by pulmonary overdistention in newborn piglets. Pediatr Res 39:798–804

28. Uchiba M, Okajima K (1997) Antithrombin III (AT III) prevents LPS-induced pulmonary vascular injury: novel biological activity of AT III. Semin Thromb Hemost 23:583–590

29. Abubakar K, Schmidt B, Monkman S, et al (1998) Heparin improves gas exchange during experimental acute lung injury in newborn piglets. Am J Respir Crit Care Med 158:1620–1625

30. Piguet PF, Van GY, Guo J (1996) Heparin attenuates bleomycin but not silica-induced pulmonary fibrosis in mice: possible relationship with involvement of myofibroblasts in bleomycin, and fibroblasts in silica-induced fibrosis. Int J Exp Pathol 77:155–116

31. Yasui H, Gabazza EC, Tamaki S, et al (2001) Intratracheal administration of activated protein C inhibits bleomycin-induced lung fibrosis in the mouse. Am J Respir Crit Care Med 163:1660–1668

32. Kijiyama N, Ueno H, Sugimoto I, et al (2006) Intratracheal gene transfer of tissue factor pathway inhibitor attenuates pulmonary fibrosis. Biochem Biophys Res Commun 339:1113–1119

33. Tani K, Yasuoka S, Ogushi F, et al (1991) Thrombin enhances lung fibroblast proliferation in bleomycin-induced pulmonary fibrosis. Am J Respir Cell Mol Biol 5:34–40

34. Vu TK, Hung DT, Wheaton VI, Coughlin SR (1991) Molecular cloning of a functional thrombin receptor reveals a novel proteolytic mechanism of receptor activation. Cell 64:1057–1068

35. Trejo J, Connolly AJ, Coughlin SR (1996) The cloned thrombin receptor is necessary and sufficient for activation of mitogen-activated protein kinase and mitogenesis in mouse lung fibroblasts. Loss of responses in fibroblasts from receptor knockout mice. J Biol Chem 271: 21536–21541

36. Chambers RC, Dabbagh K, McAnulty RJ, Gray AJ, Blanc-Brude O, Laurent GJ (1998) Thrombin stimulates fibroblast pro-collagen production via proteolytic activation of protease-activated receptor 1. Biochem J 333:121–127

37. Chambers RC, Leoni P, Blanc-Brude O, Wembridge DE, Laurent GJ (2000) Thrombin is a potent inducer of connective tissue growth factor production via proteolytic activation of protease-activated receptor-1. J Biol Chem 275:35584–35591

38. Dery O, Corvera C, Steinhoff M, Bunnett NW (1998) Proteinase-activated receptors:novel mechanisms of signalling by serine proteases. Am J Physiol 274:C1429–C1452

39. Dawes KE, Gray AJ, Laurent GJ (1993) Thrombin stimulates fibroblast chemotaxis and replication. Eur J Cell Sci 61:126–130
40. Chen LB, Buchanan JM (1975) Mitogenic activity of blood components. I. Thrombin and prothrombin. Proc Natl Acad Sci USA 72:131–135
41. Carney DH, Cunningham DD (1978) Cell surface action of thrombin is sufficient to initiate division of chick cells. Cell 14:811–823
42. Bogatkevich GS, Tourkina E, Silver RM, et al (2001) Thrombin differentiates normal lung fibroblasts to a myofibroblast phenotype via the proteolytically activated receptor-1 and a protein kinase C-dependent pathway. J Biol Chem 276:45184–45192
43. Bogatkevich GS, Tourkina E, Abrams CS, et al (2003) Contractile activity and smooth muscle {alpha}-actin organization in thrombin-induced human lung myofibroblasts. Am J Physiol Lung Cell Mol Physiol 285:L334–L343
44. Dabbagh K, Laurent GJ, McAnulty RJ, et al (1998) Thrombin stimulates smooth muscle cell procollagen synthesis and mRNA levels via a PAR-1 mediated mechanism. Thromb Haemost 79:405–409
45. Blanc-Brude OP, Archer F, Leoni P, et al (2005) Factor Xa stimulates fibroblast procollagen production, proliferation, and calcium signaling via PAR1 activation. Exp Cell Res 304:16–27
46. Hernandez-Rodriguez NA, Cambrey AD, Harrison NK, et al (1995) Role of thrombin in pulmonary fibrosis. Lancet 346:1071–1073
47. Ohba T, McDonald JK, Silver RM (1994) Scleroderma bronchoalveolar lavage fluid contains thrombin, a mediator of human lung fibroblast proliferation via induction of platelet-derived growth factor alpha-receptor. Am J Respir Cell Mol Biol 10:405–412
48. Howell DC, Goldsack NR, Marshall RP, et al (2001) Direct thrombin inhibition reduces lung collagen, accumulation, and connective tissue growth factor mRNA levels in bleomycin-induced pulmonary fibrosis. Am J Pathol 159:1383–1395
49. Howell DC, Johns RH, Lasky JA, et al (2005) Absence of proteinase-activated receptor-1 signaling affords protection from bleomycin-induced lung inflammation and fibrosis. Am J Pathol 166:1353–1365
50. Macfarlane SR, Seatter MJ, Kanke T, et al (2001) Proteinase-activated receptors. Pharmacol Rev 53:245–282
51. Blanc-Brude OP, Chambers RC, Leoni P, Dik WA, Laurent GJ (2001) Factor Xa is a fibroblast mitogen via binding to effector-cell protease receptor-1 and autocrine release of PDGF. Am J Physiol Cell Physiol 281:C681–C689
52. Pendurthi UR, Ngyuen M, Andrade-Gordon P (2002) Plasmin induces Cyr61 gene expression in fibroblasts via protease-activated receptor-1 and p44/42 mitogen-activated protein kinase-dependent signalling pathway. Arterioscler Thromb Vasc Biol 22:1421–1426
53. Riewald M, Ruf W (2001) Mechanistic coupling of protease signalling and initiation of coagulation by tissue factor. Proc Natl Acad Sci USA 98:7742–7747
54. O'Brien PJ, Molino M, Kahn M, et al (2001) Protease activated receptors: theme and variations. Oncogene 20:1570–1581
55. Camerer E, Huang W, Coughlin SR (2000) Tissue factor- and factor X-dependent activation of protease-activated receptor 2 by factor VIIa. Proc Natl Acad Sci USA 97:5255–5260
56. Nakayama T, Hirano K, Shintani Y, et al (2003) Unproductive cleavage and the inactivation of protease-activated receptor-1 by trypsin in vascular endothelial cells. Br J Pharmacol 138:121–130
57. Suzuki T, Moraes TJ, Vachon E, et al (2005) Proteinase-activated receptor-1 mediates elastase-induced apoptosis of human lung epithelial cells. Am J Respir Cell Mol Biol 33:231–247
58. Laurent GJ (2005) No bit PARt for PAR-1. Am J Respir Cell Mol Biol 33:213–215
59. Riewald M, Petrovan RJ, Donner A, et al (2002) Activation of endothelial cell protease activated receptor 1 by the protein C pathway. Science 296:1880–1882
60. Ruf W, Riewald M (2003) Tissue factor-dependent coagulation protease signalling in acute lung injury. Crit Care Med 31 (Suppl 4): S231–S237

61. Bernard GR, Vincent JL, Laterre PF, et al (2001) Recombinant human protein C Worldwide Evaluation in Severe Sepsis (PROWESS) study group. Efficacy and safety of recombinant human activated protein C for severe sepsis. N Engl J Med 344:699–709

62. Ruf W (2005) Is APC activation of endothelial cell PAR1 important in severe sepsis?: Yes. J Thromb Haemost 3:1912–1914

63. Esmon CT (2005) Is APC activation of endothelial cell PAR1 important in severe sepsis?: No. J Thromb Haemost 3:1910–1911

64. Pawlinski R, Pedersen B, Schabbauer G, et al (2004) Role of tissue factor and protease-activated receptors in a mouse model of endotoxemia. Blood 103:1342–1347

65. Camerer E, Cornelissen I, Kataoka H, et al (2006) Roles of protease-activated receptors in a mouse model of endotoxemia. Blood 107:3912–3921

66. Brass LF (1997) Thrombin receptor antagonists: a work in progress. Coron Artery Dis 8:49–58

67. Bernatowicz MS, Klimas CE, Hartl KS, Peluso M, Allegretto NJ, Seiler SM (1996) Development of potent thrombin receptor antagonist peptides. J Med Chem 39:4879–4887

68. Andrade-Gordon P, Derian CK, Maryanoff BE, et al (2001) Administration of a potent antagonist of protease-activated receptor-1 (PAR-1) attenuates vascular restenosis following balloon angioplasty in rats. J Pharmacol Exp Ther 298:34–42

69. Derian CK, Damiano BP, Addo MF (2003) Blockade of the thrombin receptor protease-activated receptor-1 with a small-molecule antagonist prevents thrombus formation and vascular occlusion in nonhuman primates. J Pharmacol Exp Ther 304:855–861

# Resolution of Inflammation

G. Bellingan

## Introduction

Although sepsis is one of the leading causes of death world-wide, by far the most typical outcome is for the body to mount an effective inflammatory response overcoming the inciting challenge and for inflammation to then fully resolve. Until recently, inflammatory resolution had simply been assumed to occur passively by 'switching off' the influx signals, a response that ignored the need for many active processes to occur. A multitude of processes are now recognized as playing a part in both limiting the extent of inflammation and driving resolution. Despite this, research into the actual process of resolution, rather than simply those mediators known to limit the extent of the acute pro-inflammatory response, has until recently been very sparse. In addition to anti-inflammatory cytokines, new families of anti-inflammatory agents, such as the resolvins and lipoxins, are now coming to the fore. Likewise, for leukocyte clearance, the contribution of apoptosis and the importance of cellular emigration are being increasingly recognized as vital. Key changes in cellular programming and pro-resolution cell profiles are also being described.

## The Course of Inflammation

To understand resolution, we first need to outline some of the processes involved in the inflammatory process itself. Generally the body aims to keep inflammatory responses compartmentalized. However, loss of membrane and cellular integrity can allow inflammation to become systemic. Severe systemic inflammation has a high mortality, with death typically due to ongoing organ dysfunction and new nosocomial sepsis rather than inability to clear the initial pathogens. It is now accepted that an aggressive inflammatory responses is central to the development of multi-organ dysfunction syndrome (MODS) although the mechanisms whereby this occurs are not clear. The nosocomial sepsis that is so typical of the later course of such patients in the intensive care unit (ICU) can occur as a consequence of organ dysfunction prolonging their stay and increasing the risk of infection. We also recognize that such infections develop in the context of a failure of the body to mount an effective response to nosocomial infection due to temporary, though often prolonged, depression of the immune system; a condition termed

immunoparesis [1]. Not all patients with severe sepsis progress to immunoparesis or multi-organ dysfunction or fibrosis; indeed, the most common course for
inflammation is for it to successfully clear the inciting pathogen and to resolve.

## Normal Inflammatory Resolution

The most fundamental requirement for the successful resolution of either acute
innate or acute adaptive immunity is to neutralize and eliminate the initiating injurious agent. Failure to achieve this will lead to chronic inflammation with the nature
of the agent in question dictating the etiology of the developing chronic immune
response. Successfully dispensing with the inciting stimulus signals a cessation
of pro-inflammatory mediator synthesis (eicosanoids, chemokines, cytokines, cell
adhesion molecules, etc.) and leads to their catabolism, halting further leukocyte
recruitment and edema formation. These are probably the very earliest requirements for the resolution of acute inflammation, the outcome of which signals the
next stage, that of cell clearance. Inflammation is typified by neutrophil (PMN)
then mononuclear leukocyte influx and resolution requires the elimination of these
PMNs and subsequent clearance of the mononuclear cells. During these evolving
stages, there is a variable myofibroblast presence, depending on the inciting challenge, the persistence of the inflammatory response, and the cytokine milieu. The
cytokine profile evolves in parallel with the inflammatory response and this is, in
part, due to the presence of different effector cells and also to the phenotype of the
cells present.

This chapter reviews the process of resolution under three general headings.
First, those 'stop' signals – cytokines, chemokines and other mediators – that are
known to limit the pro-inflammatory response and may also contribute directly to
resolution. Second, the process of apoptosis, which, if induced either too early or
too extensively, is implicated in both persisting inflammation and immunoparesis.
Apoptosis is also central to the normal resolution of the inflammatory process once
the inciting stimuli have been eliminated. Finally, the process of cellular emigration
which is assuming increasing importance in leukocyte clearance and the return of
the tissue to normal structure and function.

## Endogenous Anti-inflammatory Processes

### Anti-inflammatory Cytokines

It is well recognized that the body attempts to balance inflammation by elaborat-
ing a range of endogenous compensatory anti-inflammatory peptides including
interleukin (IL) receptor antagonist (IL-1ra), IL-4, IL-10, and IL-13 [2]. These are
typically expressed later during the inflammatory response than the early tumor
necrosis factor-alpha (TNF-$\alpha$), IL-1, and IL-6 response. These anti-inflammatory

cytokines can act both to limit inflammation and to promote resolution. They have also been implicated in the process of immunoparesis, although the extent to which they are involved in, or essential for, these different roles is not clear.

IL-1ra is a naturally occurring inhibitor of IL-1, produced during inflammation and has a significantly greater avidity than IL-1 in binding to the IL-1 type I receptor. IL-1ra thus acts as a competitive antagonist of IL-1α and IL-1β, attenuating IL-1 activity *in vitro* and *in vivo*. A dynamic balance between IL-1 agonists and IL-1ra appears to exist [3]. Experimental models suggested a powerful anti-inflammatory effect from an infusion of IL-1ra that should be effective for Gram-positive, Gram-negative, and other pro-inflammatory states. A major clinical trail of IL-1ra, however, was unable to demonstrate any significant survival benefit for this agent in sepsis.

IL-4 and IL-10 are both T helper cell type 2 (Th2)-derived cytokines that are usually considered to be anti-inflammatory in nature. The role of IL-4 in sepsis is more complicated than initially believed. Hultgren et al. have shown that the outcome from sepsis and arthritis in IL-4 knockout mice depends on the genetic background of the mouse; IL-4 deficiency caused 70% lethality after staphylococcal challenge in 129SV mice compared to full survival in 129SV wild types while in C57BL/6, deficiency of IL-4 increased survival compared to the wild type [4]. Using murine malaria as the challenge, Saeftel et al. showed that 60 to 80% of IL-4 deficient mice survived whilst all BALB/c controls succumbed and the surviving knockout mice had increased natural killer (NK) cells and enhanced inducible nitric oxide synthase (iNOS) expression and were able to eliminate parasites. These findings suggested that interferon-gamma (IFN-γ) producing NK cells and NO are vital for clearance of parasite load [5].

IL-10, in particular, has been shown to inhibit a variety of innate and adaptive immune activities, including blocking synthesis of a number of pro-inflammatory mediators, including IFN-γ, IL-1, TNF, IL-12, and CXC and CC chemokines. IL-10 also acts at the post-translational level to increase endocytosis of monocyte human leukocyte antigen (HLA)-DR and this may augment other mechanisms of immunoparesis. Exogenous administration of IL-10 has been shown to protect from injury in response to lipopolysaccharide (LPS) and other challenges. Moreover, IL-10 has been shown to enhance resolution of pulmonary inflammation by promoting PMN apoptosis [6].

IL-10 can be detrimental to the host under conditions of microorganism invasion and this is a major concern [7]. Indeed, both protective and harmful effects have been demonstrated for IL-10, depending upon the time of intervention. It has been postulated that IL-10 functions as a temporal regulator of the transition from a reversible phase of sepsis to a later irreversible phase of shock. Using a cecal ligation and puncture (CLP) model, Latifi et al. demonstrated that the onset of lethality in IL-10 knockout mice occurred earlier than in wild-type mice and was associated with significant elevations in TNF-α and IL-6. Furthermore, refractory shock developed earlier in the IL-10 knockout animals and IL-10 administration could rescue this phenotype [8].

IL-13 is a 12 kDa cytokine that is a potent stimulator of eosinophil, lymphocyte, and macrophage-rich inflammation and is integral to tissue fibrosis and parenchymal proteolysis [9]. IL-13 dysregulation is thought to play an important role in the pathogenesis of a variety of diseases, including asthma, pulmonary and hepatic fibrosis, fungal pneumonitis, viral pneumonia, and chronic obstructive pulmonary disease (COPD). It can induce vascular cell adhesion molecule (VCAM)-1 expression and activate and inhibit the apoptosis of eosinophils; activation of signal transducer and activator of transcription-6 (STAT6) is believed to mediate these biological effects [10]. IL-13 levels are elevated in patients with the systemic inflammatory response syndrome (SIRS) and are also higher in those with infectious rather than non-infectious causes of SIRS. However, a low IL-13 level may be associated with a worse outcome in sepsis, certainly for children [11, 12]. IL-13 and IL-4 have overlapping effector profiles; this is at least partially due to the shared use of receptor components. However, IL-13 and IL-4 can be produced by different cells and are differentially regulated by mediators such as IFN-α. IL-13 acts via macrophages to stimulate the production of mRNA for wound repair proteins, such as matrix metalloproteases (MMPs), and is important for the production of collagen. Hence IL-13 is believed to have a key function in tissue repair and fibrosis.

Even pro-inflammatory cytokines can have anti-inflammatory effects and *vice versa*. For example, IL-12 is produced by macrophages and is a potent inducer of IFN-γ, which acts in a positive feedback fashion inducing further IL-12. IFN-γ does, however, also lead to inhibition of key chemokines, such as macrophage inflammatory protein (MIP)-1α. TNF-α exposure will inhibit IFN-γ driven IL-12 production through both IL-10 dependent and independent mechanisms. Experiments using TNF-α knockout mice suggest that this TNF-α response is important in limiting the extent of inflammation over time [13]. IL-18 is another IFN-γ inducing factor produced by macrophages. IL-18 can decrease IL-12 production, and is also important in pathogen elimination [14].

A newly emerging group of proteins, the suppressor of cytokine signaling (SOCS) family (discovered in 1997), is now understood to regulate innate immunity at the level of cytokine signaling. This family has been demonstrated to play a role in the negative regulation of interleukins, interferons, and TNF and it is conceivable that they also regulate the Toll-like receptor (TLR) ligands and, thus, innate immunity. SOCS-1 acts as a negative regulatory molecule of the JAK-STAT signal cascade and a critical negative regulating factor for LPS signal pathways. SOCS-1 expression is induced in macrophages stimulated with LPS and SOCS-1-deficient mice are highly sensitive to LPS-induced shock, producing increased levels of inflammatory cytokines [15].

## Cytokine Receptors and Anti-inflammatory Signals

### Decoy Receptors

The biology of many cytokines, as well as the interactions with their receptors, is complex. IL-1, for example, binds to both IL-1 type I receptor, through which signal transduction occurs, and to an IL-1 type II or 'decoy' receptor that does not signal [16]. The exact role of such receptors in regulating the immune response is not clear at present.

## Soluble Receptors

A number of cytokine receptors are found circulating in truncated forms. Typically, these remain able to bind their cytokine ligand, but are unable to transduce a signal because they lack a cytoplasmic tail [17]. They thus act to competitively inhibit the activity of the cytokine and, in this way, can limit the pro-inflammatory responses to the cytokines. Such soluble receptors can be produced in two ways. Differential mRNA splicing can lead to elaboration of soluble receptors lacking the membrane-spanning domains for cell-associated protein receptors, such as the TNF receptor 2 (p75 or TNF-R2), IL-4, granulocyte macrophage colony stimulating factor (GM-CSF), and IL-11. Proteolytic cleavage of the membrane-anchored receptors by metalloproteases from the cell surface is the second major route for generation of soluble receptors. This mechanism includes generation of soluble TNF receptor 1 (sTNF-R1), IL-1 type II receptor, CD62 ligand, transforming growth factor (TGF)-β receptor, and platelet-derived growth factor (PDGF) receptor. For TNF, for example, cellular activation by agents, such as LPS, induces rapid shedding of membrane TNFR. sTNFR are present constitutively in serum at concentrations that increase significantly in infectious diseases. Soluble TLR2 is another example; these are released constitutively from monocytes and are able to modulate cell activation and could provide a powerful mechanism for regulating cell activation [18, 19].

## Receptor-driven Apoptosis

Another mechanism whereby cytokine receptors can limit inflammation is through the induction of apoptosis, should this process occur at the appropriate time. The archetypal receptors for this include the TNF-R1, along with the Fas receptor [20]. These receptors contain a domain, known as the 'death domain', that is essential for the transduction of apoptotic signals (see later for detailed discussion of apoptosis).

## Balance of Pro- and Anti-inflammatory Mediators

The degree to which anti-inflammatory cytokines, soluble receptors, and decoy receptors balance the actions of pro-inflammatory cytokines and modulate inflammation are not clear. Investigators are increasingly reporting that the ratios of pro and anti-inflammatory counterparts correlate with outcomes in inflammatory states [21, 22]. What is not understood yet is whether anti-inflammatory cytokines simply balance the pro-inflammatory ones or is there a temporal relationship, with early pro-inflammatory elaboration being dampened down and later switched off by anti-inflammatory cytokines and if so what are the molecular mechanisms for this? Finally it is not clear if these mechanisms actually lead to cellular clearance and resolution or simply act as a 'stop' signal to the pro-inflammatory responses [23].

## Other Endogenous Immunomodulatory Agents

### Adenosine

Adenosine is a purine nucleoside that has been increasingly recognized as an important negative regulator in inflammation [24]. Inflammation causes tissue damage leading to adenosine release. Adenosine binds to G-protein coupled adenosine $A_{2A}$ receptors ($A_{2A}R$) and increases intracellular cyclic AMP, reducing the activity of nuclear factor-κB (NF-κB) and downregulating the inflammatory response. Stimulation of the adenosine receptor also decreases TLR-induced release of cytokines. Importantly, inflammation also acts to increase expression of the $A_{2A}R$. It has now been shown that inflammation is dramatically enhanced in $A_{2A}R$ deficient mice. Thiel et al. recently proposed that tissue inflammation induced local hypoxia and this could be important in augmenting the adenosine-driven protective response; in addition, they postulated that hyperoxia would abolish the protective hypoxic response and could enhance tissue damage [25]. Using an endotoxin challenge that significantly impaired gas exchange, this group showed that endotoxin-challenged mice breathing 10% oxygen (hypoxia) had a low mortality and, in the survivors, lung inflammation was less severe than in those breathing room air. Hypoxia also significantly reduced pulmonary PMN accumulation and improved gas exchange compared with normoxia, suggesting it acted to protect the lung from additional inflammatory damage. Hypoxia was also associated with elevated adenosine concentrations. In contrast, when mice were exposed to 100% oxygen, the toxicity of the challenge was dramatically increased compared to those challenged in normoxic conditions. Moreover, PMN expression of $A_{2A}R$ mRNA was reduced when exposed to high concentrations of oxygen.

### Lipoxins, Epilipoxins, and Resolvins

Lipoxins serve as anti-inflammatory signals that regulate key steps in leukocyte trafficking [26]. They are trihydroxytetraene-containing eicosanoids generated rapidly during cell-cell interactions in the blood stream or through leukocyte-epithelial cell interactions at the mucosa. The primed PMN is a key player in lipoxin biosynthesis which involves the insertion of molecular oxygen and then conversion into 15-hydroperoxyeicosatetraenoic acid (15-HPETE) which is rapidly converted to either lipoxin $A_4$, or lipoxin $B_4$. These agents are vasodilators and can inhibit leukocyte chemotaxis, block NK cell cytotoxicity, and can reduce the vascular permeability changes associated with sepsis [27]. *In vivo*, they have bee n shown to prevent leukocyte infiltration. There is some evidence that lipoxins may promote inflammatory cell resolution [28]. Linked with lipoxin synthesis is a decrease in leukotriene synthesis, providing a positive feedback to their anti-inflammatory effects. Aspirin also is implicated as it may acetylate cyclooxygenase (COX)-2, resulting in the conversion of arachidonic acid to 15R-HETE. 15R-HETE is released and transformed through transcellular routes to form 15-epilipoxin, which has similar anti-inflammatory actions. Lipoxins and aspirin-triggered epi-lipoxins also have been shown to regulate dendritic cell migration and IL-12 production. Despite pathogen clearance, absence of the lipoxin A4 biosynthetic pathways still results in uncontrolled inflammation and is lethal. There is a link to the SOCS family as lipoxins activate dendritic-cell triggered expression of SOCS-2. Absence of SOCS-2 leads to dendritic-cell hyper-responsiveness, refractory to inhibitory actions of lipoxin A4, although IL-10 can still provide downregulatory signals. SOCS-2 is also a crucial intracellular mediator of the anti-inflammatory actions of aspirin-induced lipoxins *in vivo* [29].

Other recently described local pro-resolution agents include the resolvins, docosatrienes, and neuroprotectins which all appear to have protective and pro-resolution actions [30]. Resolvins are derived from oxygenation of omega-3 polyunsaturated fatty acids (PUFAs), are capable of protective biological actions, and are present in exudates from resolving inflammation. Resolvin E1 is synthesized in the presence of aspirin, protects tissues from leukocyte-mediated injury, and may underlie any omega-3 protective actions [31].

## Galectin-3

Galectin-3 is a lectin with specificity for beta-galactosidase and is produced by inflammatory macrophages, endothelial, and epithelial cells [32]. Of interest to the field of resolution of inflammation, galectin-3 deficient mice show no difference in the number of leukocytes in the peritoneal cavity early after an inflammatory challenge [33]. However, after four days the galectin-3 deficient mice had significantly less recoverable PMN. Absence of galectin-3 did not induce more rapid cell death nor increased uptake by macrophages; this may indicate a specific role in the resolution phase of inflammation. These data indicate that galectins may play critical roles in the modulation of chronic inflammatory diseases. Galectin-3 has, however, also been shown to induce L-selectin shedding and IL-8 production in naive and primed PMN and can induce a respiratory burst [34], suggesting a role in the pathogenesis of inflammatory disease [35].

## Leptin

The adipocyte-derived hormone leptin, encoded by the *obese* (*ob*) gene, is an important regulator of energy expenditure and several endocrine and metabolic pathways. Plasma leptin levels rise in acute sepsis, whereas during chronic critical illness, leptin loses its diurnal variability and plasma levels fall [36, 37]. Leptin deficient *ob/ob* mice and fasted wild type mice are both hypersensitive to the lethal effects of endotoxin, an effect which is blunted by pre-treatment with exogenous leptin. Human congenital leptin deficiency is also associated with an increased predisposition to lethal infections and, in acute human sepsis, non-survivors had significantly lower circulating leptin levels compared to survivors [38]. These findings suggest that leptin is a key component of the host's immune/inflammatory response to sepsis and restoration of leptin may allow inflammatory resolution [39].

## Regulation of Inflammation by Local Inflammatory Cell Subpopulations

### T Helper Cells: Th1 and Th2 Cytokines and T Cell Switching

The local T cell population at the inflamed site plays a critical role in determining the cytokine milieu in that compartment. T cells recognize MHC bound antigen and are involved in cell mediated immunity. Following interaction with antigen, helper T cells undergo differentiation to effector cells [40–42]. Antigen-presenting cells, such as dendritic cells, facilitate this differentiation using the Notch pathway. Dendritic cells recognizing RNA, DNA, or LPS will promote Th1 differentiation, whereas dendritic cells recognizing more chronic infestations, such as nematodes, promote Th2 differentiation. Dendritic cells from specific tissues are also more likely to promote different T cell responses; with dendritic cells from bronchial and intestinal mucosa promoting development towards Th2 and splenic dendritic cells towards Th1. Notch is a receptor involved in decisions regarding cell fate. Mammals express 4 notch receptors, with five genes encoding ligands for Notch (Jagged1, Jagged2, Delta1, Delta3 and Delta4). Delta promotes Th1 responses while Jagged promotes Th2 responses. [43].

Th1 cells typically produce IFNγ and IL-2 while Th2 cells secrete IL-4, IL-5, and IL-13 (Table 1). Th1 responses are thought of as pro-inflammatory while Th2 responses are typically anti-inflammatory. Th2 is also an important regulator of extracellular matrix remodeling and is involved in activating collagen deposition while Th1 responses inhibit this process. The Th2 response should be thought of as an adaptive tissue healing mechanism rather than just an opposing mechanism to Th1. Th1 cells are involved in the defense against intracellular pathogens, such as bacteria, viruses, and parasites; these cells produce a delayed type hypersensitivity reaction, fight cancer cells, and are integral to the cell mediated immune response. A Th1 response usually involves complement fixing antibodies, activation of NK cells and further Th1 cytokine secretion. Th2 cells, meanwhile, produce an extra-cellular, humoral response that results in the upregulation of antibody production, particularly IgE. Th1 is responsible for organ specific autoimmune reactions such as diabetes and multiple sclerosis; Th2 is implicated in allergic responses [44, 45].

Sandler et al. used oligonucleotide microarray technology to look at the genes responsible for Th1 and Th2 cytokine profiles. They found that Th2-polarized mice upregulated genes associated with wound repair, arginase, MMPs and collagens while Th1-polarized mice upregulated genes associated with tissue damage [46].

Several factors are involved in determining whether a naive Th cell becomes a Th1 or Th2 cell, with the cytokines IL-12 and IL-4 being the most potent regula-

Table 1. Selected functions of some Th1 and Th2 cytokines

| Cytokine | Secreted by | Target cell/tissue to | Activity |
|---|---|---|---|
| IFNγ | Th1 cells,CD 8 cells,NK cells | Uninfected cells<br>Macrophages<br>Many cell types<br><br>Proliferating B cells<br><br><br>Th2 cells | → Inhibits viral replication<br>→ Enhances activity<br>→ Increases expression of class I and II MHC molecules<br>→ Induces class switch to IgG2a; blocks IL-4 induced class switch to IgE and IgG1<br>→ Inhibits proliferation |
| IL-2 | Th1 cells | Antigen-primed Th and CD8 cells<br>Antigen-specific T-cell clones<br>NK cells and CD8 cells | → Induces proliferation<br>→ Supports long term growth<br>→ Enhances activity |
| IL-4 | Th2 cells, mast cells, NK cells | Antigen-primed B cells<br>Activated B cells<br><br><br>Resting B cells<br>Thymocytes and T cells<br>Macrophages<br><br>Mast cells | → Co-stimulates activation<br>→ Stimulates proliferation and differentiation; induces class switch to IgG1 and IgE<br>→ Up-regulates class II MHC expression<br>→ Induces proliferation<br>→ Up-regulates class II MHC expression; increases phagocyte activity<br>→ Stimulates growth |
| IL-5 | Th2 cells, mast cells | Activated B cells<br><br>Eosinophils | → Stimulates proliferation and differentiation; induces class switch to IgA<br>→ Promotes growth and differentiation |
| IL-13 | Th2 cells | Macrophages | → Inhibits activation and release of inflammatory cytokines; important regulator of inflammatory response |

tors. Other factors involved include the antigen, co-stimulation, and the affinity of the T cell receptor [47].

Th2 maturation may also be influenced by IL-6, released by antigen presenting cells or other cells, such as fibroblasts and macrophages. Both Th1 and Th2 cytokines are able to upregulate proliferation of their own subset of T cells in a positive feedback loop and downregulate the opposite subset. Th1 and Th2 responses are not usually balanced; one will usually far outweigh the other. Some effector T cells can produce both IL-4 and IFNγ, suggesting that 'Th1' and 'Th2' cytokines can be produced by the same cell. This can lead to problems when assessing the cytokine response in plasma or brochoalveolar lavage (BAL) fluid and then referring to the response as Th1 or Th2 on the basis of cytokines. Commitment to Th1 or to Th2 is thought to be final; any switch in the levels of Th1 cells to Th2 cells, or vice versa in an immune response is thought to be due to new polarization of naive cells.

A Th2 cell response can be polarized to a Th1 cell response through the depletion of intracellular glutathione. A Th1 cell response can be polarized to a Th2 cell response by oxidized glutathione (GSH) [48]. High GSH in macrophages results in IL-12 secretion. GSH can be raised further by the interaction of these macrophages with IFNγ. IL-4 results in the reduction of GSH levels and therefore a polarization towards a Th2 response [49]. Hormones, such as melatonin, progesterone, or dehydroepiandrosterone, and nutrients, such as selenium or zinc, are also able to influence Th1/Th2 balance. For example, evidence suggests that progesterone promotes the production of IL-4 and IL-5 [50]. Some suggest that the overall control of these effects may occur via glucocorticoids and catecholamines. [51].

Th1 and Th2 cells express distinct patterns of death domain receptors following activation. The TNF-related apoptosis-inducing ligand (TRAIL) is seen only on Th2 cells, whereas CD95L is observed only in Th1 cells. Th2 cells are significantly more resistant to both TRAIL and CD95L induced apoptosis than Th1 cells. Hence, apoptosis may be important in determining the fate of T helper cells [52].

A third set of T cells has more recently been found to exist. These cells are known as T regulatory cells [53]. These CD4+CD25+ cells are the main producers of IL-10 and are thought to be involved in the regulation of fibrosis. T regulatory cells also produce TGF-β1. Gamma delta T cells also appear to be able to terminate host immune responses to infection and prevent chronic disease [54]. An interaction between peripheral gamma delta T cells and a population of pro-inflammatory macrophages occurs late in infection leading to the acquisition of cytotoxic activity by the T cells. Some data suggest that removal of macrophages either by emigration or local death is required to reduce inflammation [55]. Local apoptotic death of macrophages has also been demonstrated in the kidney in crescentic glomerulonephritis [56] and in the resolution of muscle inflammation [57], although, interestingly, only in one population of macrophages, those which were ED-1 positive, were numbers potentially controlled through apoptosis.

## Macrophage Switching

Macrophages are exposed to signals from the external milieu that alter their activation state. For example TGF-β generally acts in a pro-inflammatory fashion early in inflammation; it recruits monocytes, and activates them and leads to cytokine production. Later, however, TGF-β will act on macrophages to elicit more specific immunosuppressive actions [58]. This ability of macrophages to be programmed into specific phenotypes is called macrophage switching or alternative activation. Macrophages are involved in a variety of different functions in host defense and immunity despite being derived from a relatively homogeneous precursor population and specific stimuli, especially cytokines, lead to macrophages with different effector phenotypes [59,60].

The question arises: does inflammatory resolution need the presence of new macrophages destined to undertake new responses or can macrophages already present at the inflamed site switch to facilitate an anti-inflammatory and resolution role? CD163, a member of the scavenger receptor cysteine rich family, and CD206 are two surface markers which exhibit mutually exclusive induction patterns after stimulation by a panel of anti-inflammatory molecules. Porcheray et al. assessed the capacity of macrophages to switch from one activation state to another by determining the reversibility of CD163 and CD206 expression and of CCL18 production, indicating an intermediate or overlapping state [61]. These authors demonstrated that every activation state was rapidly and fully reversible, suggesting that a given cell may participate sequentially in both the induction and the resolution of inflammation.

## Apoptosis

### What Is Apoptosis?

Apoptosis progresses through distinct stages with cytoplasmic membrane ruffling and bleb formation which is accompanied by loss of cell volume. In the nucleus the chromatin condenses and the nucleus compacts [62–64]. Normally the next step is for apoptotic cells to be rapidly phagocytosed by tissue macrophages prior to any loss of cell membrane integrity. Haslett and Savill have shown that macrophages phagocytose only apoptotic PMNs and the phagocytosis of apoptotic cells at sites of inflammation has now been shown for the lung, gut, joint peritoneum, pleura, and kidney [65,66].

Apoptosis can be induced through a number of different mechanisms, including withdrawal of survival factors, the action of drugs, such as steroids and cytotoxics, irradiation, or free radicals. A number of genes specifically regulate apoptosis, including c-myc, p53, bak, bad and bcl-Xs, which induce apoptosis, and a number of suppressor genes, including bcl-2, bcl-Xl and mcl-1 [67,68]. Apoptotic death can also be signaled through one of a family of receptors known as death receptors. These are members of the TNF receptor super-family including CD120a (TNFR1),

Fas (Apo 1 or CD95), Fas ligand (FasL), and TRAIL or Apo2. [69, 70]. These receptors all contain a 60 amino acid intracellular death domain through which signals leading to the induction of programmed cell death are transduced.

Caspases are a family of 13 cysteine proteases that exist in inactive precursor form and can be placed into three major groups. The initiators (caspases 2, 8, 9, and 10) are activated in response to apoptotic signals and they in turn cleave the effector caspases (3, 6, and 7) into their active forms which drive the pro-apoptotic pathways (Fig. 1). There are a number of other caspases (1, 4, 5, 11, 12, and 13) which are involved in regulation of inflammatory rather than apoptotic pathways [71–75].

Apoptotic cells are specifically recognized through surface receptors including CD36, CD44 and phosphatidyl serine [76–78]. Many of the molecules involved in apoptotic cell uptake, including CD14, C-reactive protein (CRP) and complement, are components of the innate immune system [79]. A fundamental fact to recognize is that when macrophages phagocytose apoptotic cells they do not release pro-inflammatory mediators. This contrasts with their phagocytosis of pathogens or opsonized particles which elicits the release of pro-inflammatory mediators such as leukotrienes, and pro-inflammatory cytokines, like IL-8 and TNF-$\alpha$ [80,81]. The phagocytosis of apoptotic cells leads to the release of mediators such as TGF-$\beta$, IL-10, and PGE$_2$, which are all anti-inflammatory. Moreover, FasL is also released which induces further apoptosis in bystander cells [82–84].

The phagocytosis of apoptotic cells is extremely rapid and for this reason the accurate quantification of free apoptotic cells *in vivo* can be problematic.

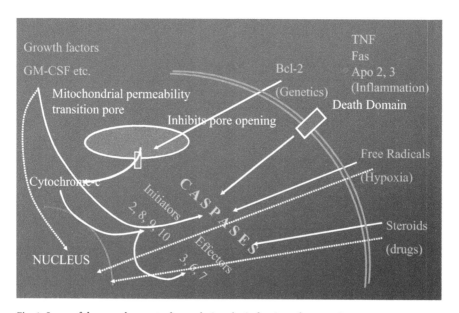

Fig. 1. Some of the complex controls regulating the induction of apoptosis

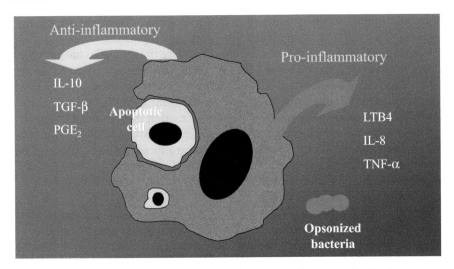

**Fig. 2.** Different effects of macrophage ingestion of apoptotic cells vs. opsonized pathogens

Macrophages are the main cells involved in clearance of apoptotic cells (Fig. 2), but are not the only cell populations capable of this. For example fibroblasts have also been shown to participate in the clearance response. Thus, apoptotic cell death and clearance by macrophages, as well as other cell populations, is a powerful anti-inflammatory mechanism and is uniquely suited to the resolution of inflammation.

## Apoptosis and Normal Inflammatory Resolution

PMNs have a life span of approximately 24 hours or less in the circulation before they undergo constitutive apoptosis. Thus, we should recognize that apoptosis is the normal fate of the PMN and what we are really considering in sepsis is the timing of this cell death. Similarly, eosinophils, like PMNs undergo constitutive apoptosis although over a more prolonged time span [85]. Apoptosis is also an essential part of normal lymphocyte maturation with up to 90% of immature T cells being deleted by apoptosis during positive and negative selection; a similar fate awaits B cell precursors that do not productively rearrange their immunoglobulin genes [86]. Monocytes also normally undergo constitutive apoptosis unless exposed to pro-inflammatory survival stimuli such as LPS, TNF-α, or M-CSF in which case they migrate into the site of inflammation to mature into macrophages [87]. Hence for the bulk of leukocytes, apoptosis is their normal fate and it is the understanding of when and how this silent and potentially powerful pro-resolution response should be activated that is important. Macrophages appear to be different; they can die by apoptosis, but this seems to require a significant noxious stimulus [88]. The normal fate of the inflammatory macrophage in successfully resolving acute inflammation is not to die at the inflamed site by apoptosis but instead to emigrate to the draining lymph nodes [89]. Finally, parenchymal cells probably undergo slow but steady apoptosis as part of normal repair and regeneration mechanisms.

Rather than excessive apoptosis, the usual response to sepsis is for the multiple pro-inflammatory signals (elevated TNF-$\alpha$, IFN-$\gamma$, or even decreased levels of IL-10) to prolong leukocyte survival. This has been well documented in conditions as diverse as sepsis, acute respiratory distress syndrome (ARDS), trauma, burns, bronchiectasis, and cystic fibrosis [90,91]. Drugs used in the treatment of sepsis, such as steroids, can also prolong PMN survival [92]. Delayed PMN apoptosis can ensure a vigorous inflammatory reaction and thus protect the host. However it is feasible that, through increased PMN numbers and persisting PMN activation, delayed PMN apoptosis is also responsible, at least in part, for some for the excessive tissue injury seen in severe sepsis.

Phagocytosis of apoptotic PMNs is part of the normal resolution response and this has been shown *in vivo* both in models of resolving inflammation and clinically in man. This feature is seen in many sites including in pulmonary inflammation, in the inflamed joint, the inflamed peritoneum, and in wound PMNs. For example, Meszaros et al. have shown that early in the inflammatory response, PMN in wounds have an increased resistance to apoptotic cell death; however, later in the inflammatory process they die by apoptosis and are phagocytosed locally by macrophages [93]. Similarly, Ishii et al. examined mechanisms controlling the elimination of PMNs during the resolution of acute pulmonary inflammation in rats [94], and again showed little evidence for any PMN apoptosis on day 0 but an increasing number of apoptotic PMN on day 1 to 3 as the lung inflammation subsided.

Macrophage ingestion of apoptotic cells can be modulated. This has been elegantly demonstrated by Godson and colleagues who showed that aspirin-triggered epilipoxins promote macrophage phagocytosis of apoptotic PMNs; steroids also increase the ability of macrophages to clear apoptotic cells [95,96].

## Emigration

Apoptosis and subsequent phagocytosis of PMNs still leaves the inflamed site populated by macrophages and lymphocytes. As noted earlier, macrophages can undergo apoptosis. However, in successfully resolving acute inflammation, they have been shown to be cleared not by apoptosis, but by emigration, passing into the lymphatics and draining specifically to the regional lymph nodes [89]. Only live macrophages can pass into the lymphatics, illustrating that this process is active and, more interestingly, resident macrophages are cleared at a very much slower rate than inflammatory macrophages. It has now been shown that part of the regulation of the rate of macrophage clearance resides in adhesion molecule expression on both the macrophages and the cells at the site of entry into the draining lymphatics [97]. For the peritoneum this site is the milky spot, a collection of mesothelial cells overlying the draining lymphatics and the site both for leukocyte entry into the peritoneum with the onset of inflammation and of exit with resolution. Unlike the studies by Hotchkiss et al. where the introduction of apoptotic cells prior to the induction of sepsis was harmful [98], it has recently been shown that the rate of inflammatory macrophage clearance from the inflamed site with resolution can be enhanced by phagocytosis of apoptotic cells [99]. Indeed, the instillation of apoptotic cells into the peritoneum drives a very rapid macrophage 'disappearance reaction' with rapid phagocytosis of all instilled apoptotic cells and localization of those macrophages that have phagocytosed these apoptotic cells to the milky spots of the greater omental lymphoid organ. Very late activating antigen (VLA)4 and VLA5, two beta$_1$ integrin adhesion molecules involved in cell transmigration, are important in regulating the adherence and subsequent lymphatic clearance of such macrophages. These adhesion molecules are also involved in the enhanced clearance of macrophages that have engulfed apoptotic cells. The beta$_2$ integrins also have a role in macrophage lymphatic emigration upon further activation of the macrophages [100]. Macrophage emigration into the draining lymphatics has not just been shown for the peritoneum but also with the resolution of kidney inflammation and with lung inflammation. Even Kupffer cells, long believed to be tissue fixed macrophages, have been shown to migrate using high resolution video microscopy [101].

Monocytes migrate into the inflamed site and adopt a pro-inflammatory phenotype where, along with the resident macrophages, they are vital in the phagocytosis and killing of pathogens and the orchestration of the pro-inflammatory response through their cytokine and chemokine elaboration [102–104]. With the waning of the inflammatory response, macrophages adopt different roles; they can undergo alternative activation, contribute to wound healing, and clear apoptotic cells, which then drives their emigration to the draining lymph nodes. Here they present antigen and thus further regulate the immune response. Of note, when macrophages are mixed into a co-culture of primed lymphocytes and antigen-laden dendritic cells, macrophages will downregulate the lymphocyte proliferation response. This suggests that the emigration of macrophages to the draining lymph nodes may have an anti-inflammatory action, dampening down non-compartmentalized activated adaptive immune response.

Macrophages are not the only cells in which emigration is important. Dendritic cells emigrate to regional lymph nodes very early during the inflammatory process, presenting antigen and initiating adaptive immune responses. Apoptotic cell ingestion can even modulate maturation of dendritic cells [105]. Similarly, lymphocytes, like macrophages, can be cleared by both apoptosis and emigration. Mature lymphocytes participate in a complex pattern of trafficking, passing from sites of inflammation into the lymph ducts to the regional lymph nodes. This T cell emigration is under specific chemokine control as CCR7 is required for T cell exit [106]. This same chemokine is induced on dendritic cells after interaction with apoptotic cells [107]. The presence of antigens can lead to expansion of specific cell populations. These cells can then cross back from the circulation into tissue or lymph nodes under the regulation of specific vascular and lymphocyte homing receptors as part of the pattern of lymphocyte recirculation [108].

The rate of lymph flow may also be important for inflammatory resolution. For example, it is known that NO is generated by lymphatic endothelial cells. This eNOS-generated NO regulates lymphatic fluid velocity. Hence, the possibility exists that NO may govern the rate of lymphatic leukocyte clearance.

## Fibrosis

Another consequence of dysregulated inflammation and inflammatory resolution is that of fibrosis and loss of tissue function. As with the rest of the inflammatory response, fibrosis is a vital part of normal healing, which, when excessive, can lead to severe consequences. This occurs in ARDS, but is also a feature of more chronic inflammation, such as cirrhosis and glomerulosclerosis. It is now apparent that the fibrotic response begins far earlier than previously recognized with profibrotic mediators apparent in lung lavage on the first day of ARDS [109]. Cytokines traditionally thought of for fibrosis include TGF-$\alpha$ and TGF-$\beta$, but more typical pro-inflammatory cytokines, such as TNF-$\alpha$, may also have important roles. ARDS is the only known lung fibrotic condition in which fibrosis can reverse. How this happens needs to be understood, harnessed, and developed as a therapy.

## Conclusion

Inflammation requires clearance of the inciting pathogen, then orchestrated removal of the burden of leukocytes and other cells influxed into the inflamed site along with dissipation of the pro (or anti) inflammatory mediator cascades. We now recognize that this resolution process is strictly controlled by a number of mediators and adhesion molecules. Apoptotic cell death, when timed appropriately, allows the non-phlogistic clearance of PMNs, monocytes and eosinophils. Macrophage engulfment of these apoptotic cells signals further anti-inflammatory processes, including additional programmed cell death, anti-inflammatory mediator release, and promotes active macrophage emigration which is the final route by which cell clearance is effected. Should these processes evolve successfully, then the tissue will return to its normal structure and function, but should this not proceed effectively then the body will limit further damage by evoking a fibrotic response to 'heal and seal' the damaged tissue.

## References

1. Marshall JC (2001) Inflammation, coagulopathy, and the pathogenesis of multiple organ dysfunction syndrome. Crit Care Med 29 (Suppl 7):S99–106

2. Pinsky MR (2001) Sepsis: a pro- and anti-inflammatory disequilibrium syndrome. Contrib Nephrol 132:354–366
3. Freeman BD, Buchman TG (2001) Interleukin-1 receptor antagonist as therapy for inflammatory disorders. Expert Opin Biol Ther 1:301–308
4. Hultgren O, Kopf M, Tarkowski A (1999) Outcome of Staphylococcus aureus-triggered sepsis and arthritis in IL-4-deficient mice depends on the genetic background of the host. Eur J Immunol 29:2400–2405
5. Saeftel M, Krueger A, Arriens S, et al (2004) Mice deficient in interleukin-4 (IL-4) or IL-4 receptor alpha have higher resistance to sporozoite infection with Plasmodium berghei (ANKA) than do naive wild-type mice. Infect Immun 72:322–331
6. Cox G (1996) IL-10 enhances resolution of pulmonary inflammation in vivo by promoting apoptosis of PMNs. Am J Physiol 271:L566–L571
7. Ayala A, Lehman DL, Herdon CD, et al (1994) Mechanism of enhanced susceptibility to sepsis following hemorrhage. Interleukin-10 suppression of T-cell response is mediated by eicosanoid-induced interleukin-4 release. Arch Surg 129:1172–1178
8. Latifi SQ, O'Riordan MA, Levine AD (2002) Interleukin-10 controls the onset of irreversible septic shock. Infect Immun 70:4441–4446
9. Lee PJ, Zhang X, Shan P, et al (2006) ERK1/2 mitogen-activated protein kinase selectively mediates IL-13-induced lung inflammation and remodeling in vivo. J Clin Invest 116:163–173
10. Zhou Zhu, Robert J. Homer, et al (1999) Elias Pulmonary expression of interleukin-13 causes inflammation, mucus hypersecretion, subepithelial fibrosis, physiologic abnormalities, and eotaxin production J Clin Invest 103:779–788
11. Socha LA, Gowardman J, Silva D, Correcha M, Petrosky N (2006) Elevation in interleukin 13 levels in patients diagnosed with systemic inflammatory response syndrome. Intensive Care Med 32:244–250
12. Blanco-Quiros A, Casado-Flores J, Garrote Adrados JA, Moro MN, Anton JA, Sanz EA (2005) Interleukin-13 is involved in the survival of children with sepsis. Acta Paediatr 94:1828–1831
13. Hodge-Dufour J, Marino MW, Horton MR, et al (1998) Inhibition of interferon gamma induced interleukin 12 production: a potential mechanism for the anti-inflammatory activities of tumor necrosis factor. Proc Natl Acad Sci USA 95:13806–13811
14. Bohn E, Sing A, Zumbihl R, et al (1998) IL-18 (IFN-gamma-inducing factor) regulates early cytokine production in, and promotes resolution of, bacterial infection in mice. J Immunol 160:299–307
15. Nakagawa R, Naka T, Tsutsui H, et al (2002) SOCS-1 participates in negative regulation of LPS responses. Immunity 17:677–687
16. Dinarello CA (1998) Interleukin-1 beta, interleukin-18, and the interleukin-1 beta converting enzyme. Ann NY Acad Sci 856:1–11
17. Fernandez-Botran R (1999) Soluble cytokine receptors: basic immunology and clinical applications. Crit Rev Clin Lab Sci 36:165–224
18. van der Poll T, van Deventer SJ (1999) Cytokines and anticytokines in the pathogenesis of sepsis. Infect Dis Clin North Am 13:413–426
19. Aderka D (1996) The potential biological and clinical significance of the soluble tumor necrosis factor receptors. Cytokine Growth Factor Rev 7:231–240
20. Fas SC, Fritzsching B, Suri-Payer E, Krammer PH (2006) Death receptor signaling and its function in the immune system. Curr Dir Autoimmun 9:1–17
21. Belli F, Capra A, Moraiti A, Rossi S, Rossi P (2000) Cytokines assay in peripheral blood and bronchoalveolar lavage in the diagnosis and staging of pulmonary granulomatous diseases. Int J Immunopathol Pharmacol 13:61–67
22. Whyte M, Hubbard R, Meliconi R, et al (2000) Increased risk of fibrosing alveolitis associated with interleukin-1 receptor antagonist and tumor necrosis factor-alpha gene polymorphisms. Am J Respir Crit Care Med 162:755–758

23. Goodman RB, Pugin J, Lee JS, Matthay MA (2003) Cytokine-mediated inflammation in acute lung injury. Cytokine Growth Factor Rev 14:523–535
24. Ohta A, Sitkovsky M (2001) Role of G-protein-coupled adenosine receptors in down regulation of inflammation and protection from tissue damage. Nature 414:916–920
25. Thiel M, Chouker A, Ohta A, et al (2005) Oxygenation inhibits the physiological tissue-protecting mechanism and thereby exacerbates acute inflammatory lung injury. PLoS Biol 3:e174
26. Serhan CN, Savill J (2005) Resolution of inflammation: the beginning programs the end. Nat Immunol 6:1191–1197
27. Filep JG, Khreiss T, Jozsef L (2005) Lipoxins and aspirin-triggered lipoxins in PMN adhesion and signal transduction. Prostaglandins Leukot Essent Fatty Acids 73:257–262
28. Maderna P, Godson C (2005) Taking insult from injury: lipoxins and lipoxin receptor agonists and phagocytosis of apoptotic cells. Prostaglandins Leukot Essent Fatty Acids. 73:179–187
29. Machado FS, Johndrow JE, Esper L, et al (2006) Anti-inflammatory actions of lipoxin A(4) and aspirin-triggered lipoxin are SOCS-2 dependent. Nat Med 12:330–334
30. Serhan CN (2004) A search for endogenous mechanisms of anti-inflammation uncovers novel chemical mediators: missing links to resolution. Histochem Cell Biol 122:305–321
31. Arita M, Clish CB, Serhan CN (2005) The contributions of aspirin and microbial oxygenase to the biosynthesis of anti-inflammatory resolvins: novel oxygenase products from omega-3 polyunsaturated fatty acids. Biochem Biophys Res Commun. 338:149–157
32. Ilarregui JM, Bianco GA, Toscano MA, Rabinovich GA (2005) The coming of age of galectins as immunomodulatory agents: impact of these carbohydrate binding proteins in T cell physiology and chronic inflammatory disorders. Ann Rheum Dis 64 (Suppl 4):iv96–103
33. Colnot C, Ripoche MA, Milon G, Montagutelli X, Crocker PR, Poirier F (1998) Maintenance of granulocyte numbers during acute peritonitis is defective in galectin-3-null mutant mice. Immunology 94:290–296
34. Nieminen J, St-Pierre C, Sato S (2005) Galectin-3 interacts with naive and primed PMNs, inducing innate immune responses. J Leukoc Biol 78:1127–1135
35. Zuberi RI, Hsu DK, Kalayci O, et al (2004) Critical role for galectin-3 in airway inflammation and bronchial hyperresponsiveness in a murine model of asthma. Am J Pathol 165:2045–2053
36. Waelput W, Brouckaert P, Broekaert D, Tavernier J (2002) A role for leptin in the systemic inflammatory response syndrome (SIRS) and in immune response. Curr Drug Targets Inflamm Allergy 1:277–289
37. Fiuza C, Suffredini AF (2001) Human models of innate immunity: local and systemic inflammatory responses. J Endotoxin Res 7:385–388
38. Bornstein SR, Licinio J, Tauchnitz R, et al (1998) Plasma leptin levels are increased in survivors of acute sepsis: associated loss of diurnal rhythm, in cortisol and leptin secretion. J Clin Endocrinol Metab 83:280–283
39. Matarese G, Moschos S, Mantzoros CS (2005) Leptin in immunology. J Immunol. 174:3137–3142
40. Liew FY (2001) Th1 and Th2 cells: a historical perspective. Nat Rev Immunol 2:55–60
41. Mosmann TR, Cherwinski H, Bond MW, Giedlin MA, Coffman RL (1986) Two types of murine helper T cell clone. Definition according to profiles of lymphokine activities and secreted proteins. J Immunol 136:2348–2357
42. Romagnani S (1991) Human Th1 and Th2 subsets: doubt no more. Immunol Today 12:256–257
43. Amsen D, Blander JM, Lee GR, Tanigaki K, Honjo T, Flavell RA (2004) Instruction of distinct CD4 T helper cell fates by different notch ligands on antigen-presenting cells. Cell 117:515–526
44. O'Garra A, Arai N (2000) The molecular basis of T helper 1 and T helper 2 cell differentiation. Trends Cell Biol 10:542–548

45. Gor D, Rose N, Greenspan N (2003) Th1-Th2: a procrustean paradigm. Nat Immunol 4:503–505
46. Sandler NG, Mentink-Kane MM, Cheever AW, Wynn TA (2003) Global gene expression profiles during acute pathogen-induced pulmonary inflammation reveal divergent roles for Th1 and Th2 responses in tissue repair. J Immunol 171:3655–3667
47. Murphy KM, Reiner SL (2002) The lineage decisions of helper T cells. Nat Rev Immunol 2:933–944
48. Peterson JD, Herzenberg LA, Vasquez K, Waltenbaugh C (1998) Glutathione levels in antigen-presenting cells modulate Th1 versus Th2 response patterns. Proc Natl Acad Sci USA 95:3071–3076
49. Kidd P (2003) Th1/Th2 balance: the hypothesis, its limitations, and implications for health and disease. Altern Med Rev 8:223–246
50. Piccinni MP, Scaletti C, Maggi E, Romagnani S (2000) Role of hormone controlled Th1 and Th2 type cytokines in successful pregnancy. J Neuroimmunol 109:30–33
51. Rook GA (1999) Glucocorticoids and immune function. Baill Clin Endocrinol Metab 13:567–581
52. Roberts AI, Devadas S, Zhang X, et al (2003) The role of activation-induced cell death in the differentiation of T-helper-cell subsets. Immunol Res 28:285–293
53. June CH, Blazar BR (2006) Clinical application of expanded CD4(+)25(+) cells. Semin Immunol 18:78–88
54. Carding SR, Egan PJ (2000) The importance of gamma delta T cells in the resolution of pathogen-induced inflammatory immune responses. Immunol Rev 173:98–108
55. Thepen T, van Vuuren AJ, Kiekens RC, Damen CA, Vooijs WC, van De Winkel JG (2000) Resolution of cutaneous inflammation after local elimination of macrophages. Nat Biotechnol 18:48–51
56. Lan HY, Mitsuhashi H, Ng YY, et al (1997) Macrophage apoptosis in rat crescentic glomerulonephritis. Am J Pathol 151: 531–538
57. Tidball JG, St Pierre BA (1996) Apoptosis of macrophages during the resolution of muscle inflammation. J Leukoc Biol 59:380–388
58. Ashcroft GS (1999) Bidirectional regulation of macrophage function by TGF-beta. Microbes Infect 1:1275–1282
59. Riches DW (1995) Signalling heterogeneity as a contributing factor in macrophage functional diversity. Semin Cell Biol 6:377–384
60. Lake FR, Noble PW, Henson PM, Riches DW (1994) Functional switching of macrophage responses to tumor necrosis factor-alpha (TNF alpha) by interferons. Implications for the pleiotropic activities of TNF alpha. J Clin Invest 93:1661–1669
61. Porcheray F, Viaud S, Rimaniol AC, et al (2005) Macrophage activation switching: an asset for the resolution of inflammation. Clin Exp Immunol 142:481–489
62. Cohen JJ, Kerr JF, Wyllie AH, Currie AR (1972) Apoptosis: a basic biological phenomenon with wide-ranging implications in tissue kinetics. Br J Cancer 26:239–257
63. Cohen JJ (1993) Programmed cell death and apoptosis in lymphocyte development and function. Chest 103:99S–101S
64. Mahidhara R, Billiar TR (2000) Apoptosis in sepsis. Crit Care Med 28:N105–N113
65. Haslett C (1999) Granulocyte apoptosis and its role in the resolution and control of lung inflammation. Am J Respir Crit Care Med 160:S5–11
66. Savill JS, Wyllie AH, Henson JE, Walport MJ, Henson PM, Haslett C (1989) Macrophage phagocytosis of aging PMNs in inflammation. Programmed cell death in the PMN leads to its recognition by macrophages. J Clin Invest 83:865–875
67. Hannah S, Cotter TG, Wyllie AH, Haslett C (1994) The role of oncogene products in PMN apoptosis. Biochem Soc Trans 22:253S
68. Camapana D, Cleveland JL (1996) Regulation of apoptosis in normal hemopoiesis and hematological disease. In: Brenner MK, Hoffbrand AV (eds) Recent Advances in Haematology. Churchill Livingstone, New York, pp 112–121

69. Lub-de Hooge MN, de Jong S, Vermot-Desroches C, Tulleken JE, de Vries EG, Zijlstra JG (2004) Endotoxin increases plasma soluble tumor necrosis factor-related apoptosis-inducing ligand level mediated by the p38 mitogen-activated protein kinase signaling pathway. Shock 22:186–188
70. De Freitas I, Fernandez-Somoza M, Essenfeld-Sekler E, Cardier JE (2004) Serum levels of the apoptosis-associated molecules, tumor necrosis factor-alpha/tumor necrosis factor type-I receptor and Fas/FasL, in sepsis. Chest 125:2238–2246
71. Wesche-Soldato DE, Lomas-Neira JL, Perl M, Jones L, Chung CS, Ayala A (2005) The role and regulation of apoptosis in sepsis. J Endotoxin Res 11:375–382
72. Ho PK, Hawkins CJ (2005) Mammalian initiator apoptotic caspases. FEBS J 272:5436–5453
73. Harwood SM, Yaqoob MM, Allen DA (2005) Caspase and calpain function in cell death: bridging the gap between apoptosis and necrosis. Ann Clin Biochem 42:415–431
74. Lavrik IN, Golks A, Krammer PH (2005) Caspases: pharmacological manipulation of cell death. J Clin Invest 115:2665–2672
75. Green DR (2005) Apoptotic pathways: ten minutes to dead. Cell 121:671–674
76. Savill J, Hogg N, Ren Y Haslett C (1992) Thrombospondin cooperates with CD36 and the vitronectin receptor in macrophage recognition of PMNs undergoing apoptosis. J Clin Invest 90:1513–1522
77. Fadok VA, Savill JS, Haslett C, et al. (1992) Different populations of macrophages use either the vitronectin receptor or the phosphatidylserine receptor to recognize and remove apoptotic cells. J Immunol 149:4029–4035
78. Hart SP, Dougherty GJ, Haslett C, Dransfield I (1997) CD44 regulates phagocytosis of apoptotic PMN granulocytes, but not apoptotic lymphocytes, by human macrophages. J Immunol 159:919–925
79. Devitt A, Moffatt OD, Raykundalia C, Capra JD, Simmons DL, Gregory CD (1998) Human CD14 mediates recognition and phagocytosis of apoptotic cells. Nature 392:505–509
80. Meagher LC, Savill JS, Baker A Fuller RW, Haslett C (1992) Phagocytosis of apoptotic PMNs does not induce macrophage release of thromboxane B2. J Leukoc Biol 52:269–273
81. Savill J, Dransfield I, Gregory C, Haslett C (2002) A blast from the past: clearance of apoptotic cells regulates immune responses. Nat Rev Immunol 2:965–975
82. Brown SB, Savill J (1999) Phagocytosis triggers macrophage release of Fas ligand and induces apoptosis of bystander leukocytes. J Immunol 162:480–485
83. Fadok VA Bratton DL, Konowal A, Freed PW, Westcott JY, Henson PM (1998) Macrophages that have ingested apoptotic cells in vitro inhibit pro-inflammatory cytokine production through autocrine/paracrine mechanisms involving TGFb, PGE2 and PAF. J Clin Invest 101:890–898
84. McDonald PP, Fadok VA, Bratton D, et al (1999) Transcriptional and translational regulation of inflammatory mediator production by endogenous TGF-beta in macrophages that have ingested apoptotic cells. J Immunol 163:6164–6172
85. Stern M, Savill J, Haslett C (1996) Human monocyte-derived macrophage phagocytosis of senescent eosinophils undergoing apoptosis. Mediation by alpha v beta 3/CD36/thrombospondin recognition mechanism and lack of phlogistic response. Am J Pathol 149:911–921
86. Van Parijs L, Abbas AK (1998) Homeostasis and self-tolerance in the immune system: turning lymphocytes off. Science 280:243–248
87. Mangan DF, Wahl SM (1991) Differential regulation of human monocyte programmed cell death (apoptosis) by chemotactic factors and pro-inflammatory cytokines. J Immunol 147:3408–3412
88. Zychlinsky A, Prevost MC, Sansonetti PJ (1992) Shigella flexneri induces apoptosis in infected macrophages. Nature 358:167–169
89. Bellingan GJ, Caldwell H, Howie SE, et al (1996) In vivo fate of the inflammatory macrophage during the resolution of inflammation: inflammatory macrophages do not die locally, but emigrate to the draining lymph nodes. J Immunol 157:2577–2585

90. Jimenez MF, Watson RW, Parodo J, et al (1997) Dysregulated expression of PMN apoptosis in the systemic inflammatory response syndrome. Arch Surg 132:1263–1269

91. Keel M, Ungethum U, Steckholzer U et al (1997) Interleukin-10 counterregulates proinflammatory cytokine-induced inhibition of PMN apoptosis during severe sepsis. Blood 90:3356–3363

92. Meagher LC, Cousin JM, Seckl JR, Haslett C (1996) Opposing effects of glucocorticoids on the rate of apoptosis in PMNic and eosinophilic granulocytes. J Immunol 156:4422–4428

93. Meszaros AJ, Reichner JS, Albina JE (1999) Macrophage phagocytosis of wound PMNs. J Leukoc Biol 65:35–42

94. Ishii Y, Hashimoto K, Nomura A, et al (1998) Elimination of PMNs by apoptosis during the resolution of acute pulmonary inflammation in rats. Lung 176:89–98

95. Reville K, Crean JK, Vivers S, Dransfield I, Godson C (2006) Lipoxin A4 redistributes myosin IIA and Cdc42 in macrophages: Implications for phagocytosis of apoptotic leukocytes. J Immunol 176:1878–1888

96. Liu Y, Cousin JM, Hughes J, et al (1999) Glucocorticoids promote nonphlogistic phagocytosis of apoptotic leukocytes. J Immunol 162:3639–3646

97. Bellingan GJ, Xu P, Cooksley H, et al (2002) Adhesion molecule-dependent mechanisms regulate the rate of macrophage clearance during the resolution of peritoneal inflammation. J Exp Med 196:1515–1521

98. Hotchkiss RS, Chang KC, Grayson MH, et al (2003) Adoptive transfer of apoptotic splenocytes worsens survival, whereas adoptive transfer of necrotic splenocytes improves survival in sepsis. Proc Natl Acad Sci USA 100:6724–6729

99. Bellingan G, Bottoms S, Xu P, Shock T, Laurent G (2004) Apoptotic Cells Promote Inflammatory Macrophage Clearance through a b1 Integrin Dependent Mechanism. Am J Respir Crit Care Med 171:A502 (abst)

100. Cao C, Lawrence DA, Strickland DK, Zhang L (2005) A specific role of integrin Mac-1 in accelerated macrophage efflux to the lymphatics. Blood 106:3234–3241

101. MacPhee PJ, Schmidt EE, Groom AC (1992) Evidence for Kuppfer cell migration along liver sinusoids from high resolution in vivo microscopy. Am J Physiol 263:G17–23

102. Geissmann F, Jung S, Littman DR (2003) Blood monocytes consist of two principle subsets with distinct migratory properties Immunity 19:71–82

103. Cailhier JF, Partolina M, Vuthoori S, et al (2005) Conditional macrophage ablation demonstrates that resident macrophages initiate acute peritoneal inflammation. J Immunol 174:2336–2342

104. Bellingan G (1999) Inflammatory cell activation in sepsis. Br Med Bull 55:12–29

105. Stuart LM, Lucas M, Simpson C, Lamb J, Savill J, Lacy-Hulbert A (2002) Inhibitory effects of apoptotic cell ingestion upon endotoxin-driven myeloid dendritic cell maturation. J Immunol 168:1627–1635

106. Debes GF, Bonhagen K, Wolff T, et al (2004) Chemokine receptor CCR7 required for T lymphocyte exit from peripheral tissues Nat Immunol 6:889–834

107. Hirao M, Onai N, Hiroishi K, et al (2000) CC chemokine receptor-7 on dendritic cells is induced after interaction with apoptotic tumor cells: critical role in migration from the tumor site to draining lymph nodes. Cancer Res 60:2209–2217

108. Tsokos GC, Liossis SN (1998) Lymphocytes, cytokines, inflammation, and immune trafficking. Curr Opin Rheumatol 10:417–425

109. Marshall RP, Bellingan G, Webb S, et al (2000) Fibroproliferation occurs early in the acute respiratory distress syndrome and impacts on outcome. Am J Respir Crit Care Med 162:1783–1788

# The Cellular Immune Respone

# Compartmentalized Activation of Immune Cells During Sepsis and Organ Dysfunction

J.-M. Cavaillon and M. Adib-Conquy

## Introduction

Bacterial sepsis is associated with the activation of immune cells by whole bacteria and by bacterial derived products resulting in a local and systemic inflammation. Very soon after the insult and the release of pro-inflammatory mediators, a regulatory anti-inflammatory response occurs. A subtle balance exists between pro- and anti-inflammatory mediators both locally and systemically. This balance, which evolves with time, is the reflection of a complex network of amplifying and down-regulating signals, and is modulated by specific surrounding cells that differ from one compartment to another. For example, the nature of mononuclear phagocytes differs greatly from one place to another, and circulating monocytes, resident macrophages in tissues, and adherent macrophages in cavities display specific properties. Accordingly, the inflammatory response varies from one compartment to another. The most striking differences exist between tissues and the blood compartment. In this chapter, we will focus on the activation of leukocytes during sepsis and systemic inflammatory response syndrome (SIRS), with the emphasis that leukocytes are present in most tissues and that their responsiveness and their contribution may differ from one compartment to another.

### Activating Stimuli

#### Immune Cell Activation by Bacteria

During infection, live bacteria and whole bacteria killed following the action of complement, defensins, anti-microbial peptides, or antibiotics interact with immune cells. Furthermore, bacterial-derived products, either actively secreted (exotoxins), released from the cell surface (e.g., lipopolysaccharide [LPS], peptidoglycan), or derived from inside cells (e.g., bacterial DNA, heat-shock proteins [HSP]) are also present within the cellular microenvironment. Whole bacteria and pathogen-associated microbial products (PAMPs) are potent activators of immune cells and following their interaction with specific sensors (e.g., Toll-like receptors [TLR], NOD1 and NOD2 molecules) induce the production of inflammatory cytokines. For example, in *in vitro* cultures of human mononuclear cells, the levels of tumor necrosis factor (TNF), one of the main inflammatory cytokines, induced by whole *Streptococcus pyogenes* are higher than those reached in response to streptococcal exotoxins; in contrast the levels of induced IL-8 are similar, and only exotoxins induce lymphotoxin-alpha [1]. Similarly, the levels of TNF induced by whole Gram-negative bacteria are far higher than those obtained in the presence of corresponding amounts of LPS [2]. However, while the intensity of the response may vary between whole bacteria and some isolated PAMPs, the spectrum of activity may be rather similar. This was the case when dendritic cells were studied by microarray technology after activation with *Escherichia coli* and LPS. Huang et al. [3] showed that LPS was able to mimic whole bacteria and accounted for almost the entire bacterial response. Indeed, among the different ligands of TLR, endotoxin (LPS) that specifically induces TLR4-dependent signaling, leads to the highest gene transcription in macrophages. The major role of endotoxin during Gram-negative infection can account for the differences observed between Gram-negative and Gram-positive infections. For example, the gene expression pattern of human blood leukocytes activated with either LPS or heat-killed *Staphylococcus aureus*, revealed that 155 identical genes were upregulated in response to LPS but downregulated after activation with *S. aureus*; in contrast 208 identical genes were downregulated in response to LPS but upregulated upon exposure to *S. aureus* [4]. Surprisingly, only 17 genes were differentially expressed in the liver of mice after Gram-negative or Gram-positive sepsis, while 166 common genes were upregulated and 130 downregulated [5].

## Role of Endotoxin and Other Pathogen-associated Microbial Products

As expected, circulating endotoxin is found in patients with Gram-negative sepsis, but it can also be detected in patients with Gram-positive and fungal infection [6]. Most importantly, similar to the likely situation with circulating cytokines [7], it is probable that detectable endotoxin within the blood stream of SIRS and sepsis patients may be underestimated. Indeed, in sepsis the presence of large amounts of endotoxin has been described linked to platelets, erythrocytes, and monocytes. Thus, it is possible that even in the absence of detectable circulating endotoxin, all patients deal with this powerful microbial agent. Thus, the presence of endotoxin in non-infectious SIRS patients may contribute to the generalized activation seen in tissues, similar to what has been described in models of sepsis and septic shock.

It is worth mentioning that many of the severe insults that require admission of patients to intensive care units (ICU) are associated with the presence of detectable amounts of endotoxin within the blood stream, independent of any infection. For example, plasma endotoxin has been found in 92% of patients after cardiac surgery with cardiopulmonary bypass [8], in 71% of patients undergoing abdominal aortic surgery after clamp release [9], in 61% of burn and trauma patients [10], in 57% of ICU patients [11], and in 46% of patients resuscitated after cardiac arrest [12]. The biological relevance of these levels of circulating endotoxin has been shown in different clinical settings. In patients resuscitated after cardiac arrest, the levels of circulating interleukin (IL)-6, IL-10, and IL-1 receptor antagonist (IL-1ra) were higher among patients with detectable circulating endotoxin [12]. In meningococcal disease, the plasma levels of LPS positively correlated with those of circulating chemokines [13].

In addition to translocated endotoxin, it is obvious, although poorly demonstrated, that other PAMPs can reach the blood stream. For example, bacterial peptidoglycan-associated lipoprotein can be detected in the blood of mice with peritonitis [14]. Bacterial peptidoglycan has been detected in the blood of rats after hemorrhagic shock [15], and it is most probable that fragmented bacterial DNA could also be found in the blood compartment.

Failure of the gut barrier remains central to the hypothesis that endotoxin reaches the systemic circulation *via* the portal route or *via* lymphatic vessels. Endotoxins escaping from the gut lumen contribute to activation of the host's inflammatory mechanisms, leading subsequently to tissue injury and multiple organ failure (MOF). In addition, local activation of the immune inflammatory system occurs, accompanied by a local production of cytokines and other immune inflammatory mediators [9]. These intestinal-derived mediators may result in a further exacerbation of the systemic inflammatory response. As stated by Swank and Deitch [16], "even if the immune inflammatory system, rather than the gut, is the "motor of" MOF, the gut remains one of the major pistons that turns the motor."

Within tissues, cells are exposed to more than one signal, and multiple stimuli act in synergy leading to an enhanced production of inflammatory cytokines. For example, synergy has been reported between endotoxin and other microbial TLR agonists or NOD ligands, Gram-positive-derived exotoxins, viral infection, hypoxia, glucose, anaphylatoxin C5a, or thrombin. In most cases, these synergies lead to more severe organ failure. Similarly, the addition of inflammatory cytokines (e.g., interferon [IFN]-γ, granulocyte-macrophage colony-stimulating factor [GM-CSF], TNF), further increases LPS-induced macrophage activity and LPS-induced lethality.

## Nature of Immune Cells Activated Within Tissues

### Macrophages

Within tissues, resident macrophages are undoubtedly an important source of inflammatory cytokines and mediators. However, very little information is available concerning these cell populations and most reports have addressed macrophages obtained from cavities.

In the case of hemorrhage, alveolar macrophages produce IL-1β and TNF-α (Table 1). Following injection of LPS in human volunteers [17] or in rats [18], the *ex vivo* production of IL-1 or TNF by alveolar macrophages was enhanced. This was not observed in mice [19], but it is most probable that the timing between the systemic delivery of LPS and the time when broncho-alveolar macrophages were collected and studied was responsible for this difference, rather than a difference

**Table 1.** Some examples of *in vivo* activation of immune cells within tissues during sepsis or SIRS as assessed by the production of mediators of inflammation

| Tissue compartmentalization of immune cells | Experimental model or clinical settings | Inflammatory mediators (technique) | References |
|---|---|---|---|
| **Liver** | | | |
| Mouse Kupffer cells | LPS i.p. injection | IL-1α, IL-1β, TNF (immunocytochemistry) | Chensue et al, Am J Pathol 1991; 138:395 |
| Mouse Kupffer cells | hemorrhage | TNF, IL-1β, TGFβ (mRNA) | Zhu et al. Cytokine 1995; 7:8 |
| Rat Kupffer cells | thermal injury | IL6 (mRNA) | Wu et al. Shock 1995; 3:268 |
| Mouse Kupffer cells | Cecal ligature & puncture | TNF, IL-6 (mRNA) | Wang et al. Arch Surg 1997; 132:364 |
| Mouse infiltrating leukocytes | live *S. aureus* i.v. | TNF, IL-1, IL-6 (immunocytochemistry) | Yao et al. Infect Immun 1997; 65:3889 |
| Rat Kupffer cells | LPS or live *E. coli* i.v. | IL-1α, IL-1 (immunocytochemistry) | Ge et al. J infect Dis 1997; 176:1313 |
| Macaque monkey infiltrating neutrophils | LPS i.v. injection | Tissue factor mRNA (in situ hybridization) | Todoroki et al. Surgery 2000; 127:209 |
| Human Kupffer cells | sepsis | HO-1 (immunocytochemistry) | Clark et al. Malar J 2003; 2:41 |
| **Spleen** | | | |
| Rat splenocytes | LPS i.v. injection | IL-1α, IL-1β, IL-1Ra (mRNA) | Ulich et al. Am J Pathol 1992; 141:61 |
| Mouse splenocytes | LPS i.p. injection | CAT reporter gene expression | Giroir et al. J Clin Invest 1992; 90:693 |
| Rat splenocytes | live *E. coli* i.v. | IL-1α, TNF, IL-6, IFNγ (mRNA) | Byerley et al. Am J Physiol 1992; 261:E728 |
| Rat adherent splenocytes | intestinal ischemial/reperfusion | TNF (bioassay) | Cohen et al. Lymphokine Cytokine Res 1992; 11:215 |
| Mouse splenocytes (other than MØ) | SEB i.p. injection | TNF, Ltα, IL-2, IFNγ (mRNA) | Bette et al. J Exp Med 1993; 178:1531 |
| Mouse splenocytes | LPS i.p. & CLP | TNF (bio-activity), IL-1β RIA) | Villa et al. Clin Diagn Lab Immunol 1995; 2:549 |
| Rat marginal zone macrophages | LPS or live *E. coli* i.v. | IL-1α, IL-1β (immunohistochemistry) | Ge et al. J infect Dis 1997; 176:1313 |
| Mouse splenocytes | LPS ± M-CSF i.p. injection | TNF, IL-6 (mRNA) | Chapoval et al. J Leukoc Biol 1998 ; 63:245 |
| Mouse splenocytes | hemorrhage | TNF (ELISA) | Molina et al. Life Sci 2000; 66:399 |

Table 1. (continued)

| Tissue compartmentalization of immune cells | Experimental model or clinical settings | Inflammatory mediators (technique) | References |
|---|---|---|---|
| **Lung** | | | |
| Rat alveolar neutrophils | LPS i.t. injection | IL-1βs IL-1Ra (mRNA) | Ulich et al. Am J Pathol 1992; 141: 61 |
| Human alveolar macrophages | ARDS | IL-1 (RIA) | Jacobs et al. Am Rev Respir Dis 1989; 140:1686 |
| Human alveolar macrophages | ARDS | TNF (mRNA) | Tran Van Nhieu et al. Am Rev Respir.Dis 1993; 147: 1585 |
| Human alveolar macrophages | ARDS | IL-8 (immunocytochemistry) | Donnelly et al. Lancet 1993; 341: 643 |
| Rat pulmonary macrophages | LPS i.v. injection | Leukotriene (immunocytochemistry) | Tanaka et al. Virchows Arch 1994; 424: 273 |
| Mouse alveolar macrophages | hemorrhage | IL-1β, TNF (mRNA) | Shenkar et al. Am J Respir Cell Mol Biol 1994; 10:290 |
| Mouse intraparenchymal mononuclear cells | hemorrhage | IL-1β, IFNγ, IL-10 (mRNA) | Shenkar et al. Am J Respir Cell Mol Biol 1994; 10:290 |
| Mouse intraparenchymal mononuclear cells | hemorrhage | IL-6, TNF (mRNA) | Abraham et al. J Exp Med 1995; 181: 569 |
| Mouse intraparenchymal mononuclear cells | hemorrhage | TGFβ (mRNA) | Le Tulzo et al J Clin Invest 1997; 99: 1516 |
| Sheep intravascular leukocytes | LPS infusion | TNF (immunocytochemistry) | Cirelli et al. J Leukoc Biol 1995; 57: 820 |
| Mouse infiltrating leukocytes | live S. aureus i.v. | TNF, IL-1, IL-6 (immunocytochemistry) | Yao et al. Infect Immun 1997; 65: 3889 |
| Human alveolar macrophages | cardiopulmonary bypass | TNF, IL-8 ex vivo release (ELISA) | Tsuchida et al. Am J Respir Crit.Care Med 1997; 156: 932 |
| Mouse intraparenchymal neutrophils | hemorrhage / LPS i.p. injection | IL-1β (immunocytochemistry) | Parsey et al. J Immunol 1998; 160: 1007 |
| Human alveolar macrophages | ARDS | membrane TNF (flow cytometry) | Armstrong et al. Am J Respir Cell Moll Biol 2000; 22: 68 |
| Human pulmonary macrophages | sepsis | HO-1 (immunocytochemistry) | Clark et al. Malar J 2003; 2: 41 |
| Mouse bronchoalveolar cells | LPS i.v. injection | TNF ex vivo release (ELISA) | Fitting et al. J Infect Dis 2004; 189: 129 |

**Table 1.** (continued)

| Tissue compartmentalization of immune cells | Experimental model or clinical settings | Inflammatory mediators (technique) | References |
|---|---|---|---|
| **Heart** | | | |
| Mouse infiltrating leukocytes | live *S. aureus* i.v. | TNF, IL-1, IL-6 (immunocytochemistry) | Yao et al. Infect Immun 1997; 65: 3889 |
| Canine mast cells & infiltrating mononuclear cells | ishemia reperfusion | TNF ((immunocytochemistry) | Frangogiannis et al. Circulation 1998; 98: 699 |
| | ishemia reperfusion | IL-6 (mRNA) | Frangogiannis et al. Circulation 1998; 98: 699 |
| Mouse infiltrating leukocytes | LPS i.p. injection | IL-6 (immunocytochemistry) | Kadokami et al. Am J Physiol 2001; 280: H2281 |
| **Gut** | | | |
| Rat intraepithelial lymphocytes | trauma / hemorrhage | IL-6 *ex vivo* release (bio-assay) | Wang et al. J Surg Res 1998; 79: 39 |
| Mouse intraepithelial lymphocytes | LPS injection | IFNγ (ELISA) | Nüssler et al. Shock 2001; 16: 454 |
| **Peritoneum** | | | |
| Mouse peritoneal macrophages | cecal ligature & puncture | TNF & IL-1β mRNA | McMasters et al. J Surg Res 1993; 54: 426 |
| Mouse peritoneal macrophages | hemorrhage | TNF, IL-1β, IL-6 mRNA | Zhu et al. Immunol 1994; 83: 378 |
| Mouse mast cells | cecal ligature & puncture | TNF (effect of anti-TNF) | Echtenacher et al. Nature 1996; 381: 75 |
| Rat peritoneal macrophages | LPS i.v. injection or hemorrhage | TNF & IL-6 mRNA | Tamion et al. Am J Physiol 1997; 273: G314 |
| Mouse peritoneal cells | LPS i.p. injection | IL-6 (ELISA, mRNA) & TNF mRNA | Chapoval et al. J Leukoc Biol 1998; 63: 245 |
| Rat peritoneal macrophages | hemorrhage | HO-1 mRNA | Tamion et al. Am J Respir Crit Care Med 2001; 164:1933 |
| Mouse peritoneal cells | LPS i.v. injection | TNF *ex vivo* release (ELISA) | Fitting et al. J Infect Dis 2004; 189: 129 |
| Human emigrated PMN | peritonitis | IL-8 (mRNA) | Holzer et al. Shock 2005; 23: 501 |
| **Brain** | | | |
| Rat microglial cells | LPS i.v. injection | IL-1β (mRNA) | Buttini et al. Neuroscience 1995, 65, 523 |
| Human cerebrospinal fluids cells | bacterial meningitis | TNF, Ltα, IL-1βmRNA | Rieckmann et al. Res. Exp. Med 1995; 195: 17 |
| Human cerebrospinal fluids cells | bacterial meningitis | TNF & TGFβ mRNA | Ossege et al. J Neurol Sci 1996; 144: 1 |
| Mouse microglia-like cells | LPS i.p. injection | IL-12p40 (mRNA) | Park et al. Biochem Biophys Res Commun 1996, 224: 391 |

**Table 1.** (continued)

| Tissue compartmentalization of immune cells | Experimental model or clinical settings | Inflammatory mediators (technique) | References |
|---|---|---|---|
| **Bone marrow** | | | |
| Mouse eosinophil, neutrophils, monocytes | LPS i.v. injection | TNF (immunomicroscopy) | Schmauder-Chock et al. Histochem J 1994; 26:142 |
| Mouse bone marrow cells | LPS i.v. injection | G-CSF, MIP-2 (mRNA) | Zhang et al. Shock 2005; 23: 3444 |
| **Blood** | | | |
| Human circulating leukocytes | sepsis | IL-8 (mRNA ) | Friedland et al. Infect Immun 1992; 60: 2402 |
| Human PBMC | trauma | IL-10 mRNA | Hauser et al. Shock 1995; 4: 247 |
| Human PBMC | ICU patients | IL-1β (flow cytometry) | Yentis et al. Clin. Exp. Immunol 1995; 100: 330 |
| Mouse PBMC | LPS injection | IL-10 mRNA | Barsig et al. Eur J Immunol 1995; 25: 2888 |
| Human circulating leukocytes | sepsis | cell-associated IL-8 (ELISA) | Marie et al. Infect Immun 1997; 65: 865 |
| Human lymphocytes & monocytes | fracture soft-tissue hematomas | membrane TNF (flow cytometry) | Hauser et al. J Trauma 1997; 42:895 |
| Human PBMC | sepsis | IL-18 (mRNA) | Mathiak et al. Shock 2001; 15: 176 |
| Mouse PBMC | LPS i.v. injection | *ex vivo* TNF release (ELISA) | Fitting et al.J Infect Dis 2004; 189: 129 |
| Human PBMC | sepsis | HO-1 mRNA | Reade et al. Br J Anaesth 2005; 94: 468 |

ARDS: acute respiratory distress syndrome; CAT: chloramphenicol acetyltransferase; G-CSF: granulocyte-colony stimulating factor; HO: heme oxygenase; IFN: interferon; IL: interleukin; i.p.: intraperitoneal; i.t.: intratracheal; i.v.: intravenous; LPS: lipopolysaccharide; MIP: macrophage inflammatory protein; PBMC: peripheral blood mononuclear cells; SEB: Staphylococcal enterotoxin B superantigen; TGF: transforming growth factor; TNF: tumor necrosis factor;

between species. When a non-infectious insult was localized to the lungs, as in the case of human acute respiratory distress syndrome (ARDS), or after lung irradiation in baboons [20], *ex vivo* cytokine production was also enhanced. In contrast, during local or remote infections, alveolar macrophage responsiveness was significantly reduced [21]. The activation of intracellular signaling pathways has been studied in *ex vivo* analysis. Schwartz et al. [22] observed an increased activation of nuclear factor-kappa B (NF-κB) in alveolar macrophages from patients with ARDS. Moine et al. [23] subsequently showed decreased cytoplasmic levels of p50, p65, and c-Rel in alveolar macrophages from patients with ARDS, consistent with an enhanced translocation of NF-κB dimers from the cytoplasm to the nucleus.

In humans, the study of peritoneal macrophages obtained from continuous ambulatory peritoneal dialysis patients revealed that LPS-activated cells released significantly more IL-1β during peritonitis as compared with the infection-free period [24]. In women with endometriosis, spontaneous and LPS-induced production of TNF-α, IL-6, IL-8, IL-10, IL-12, and nitric oxide (NO) by peritoneal macrophages was higher than in controls [25]. Following trauma/hemorrhage, LPS-induced production of TNF and IL-6 by liver Kupffer cells was enhanced [26]. This was also the case for IL-6 production in a burn model [27].

Macrophage reactivity has been mainly associated with the pro-inflammatory response, although these cells most probably also contribute to the release of anti-inflammatory mediators such as IL-1ra, IL-10, transforming growth factor-β (TGF-β), soluble TNF receptor (sTNFR), and heme oxygenase-1 (HO-1). HO-1 serves as a 'protective' molecule by virtue of its anti-inflammatory, anti-apoptotic, and anti-proliferative actions. HO-1 was expressed by peritoneal macrophages in a rat hemorrhagic shock model, and by Kupffer cells in human sepsis, HO-1 (Table 1).

## Neutrophils

In murine models of hemorrhage or of endotoxemia, activation of NF-κB, cAMP responsive element binding protein (CREB), mitogen extracellular signal-regulated kinase (MEK-1/2), and extracellular signal-regulated kinase (Erk2) was found in alveolar neutrophils but not in blood neutrophils [28, 29]. These reports further illustrate the profound differences that exist from one compartment to another for a similar cell population. Similarly, in human sepsis the production of both IL-12 isoforms after *ex vivo* stimulation was significantly higher with alveolar neutrophils than with autologous blood neutrophils [30]. Studying human blood and peritoneal neutrophils, Chollet-Martin's group [31] showed that TNF-α converting enzyme (TACE) was upregulated at the neutrophil surface during severe peritonitis. This finding could be related to a paracrine regulatory loop involving some TACE substrates such as TNF, L-selectin, and TNF receptors.

## Lymphocytes

In contrast to the hyporeactivity of the circulating lymphocytes observed in sepsis and SIRS (see below), it has bee nreported that lymphocytes de rived from inflamed tissues are activated, primed, and fully responsive to *ex vivo* stimulation. This has been particularly well illustrated in studies of intraepithelial lymphocytes from small intestinal mucosa after laparotomy and hemorrhage, or after endotoxemia (Table 1).

## Natural Killer Cells

Natural killer (NK) cells contribute to the pathogenesis of sepsis and SIRS [32,33]. NK cells are a major source of IFNγ, produced in response to different cytokines such as IL-12, IL-15, IL-18, and IL-21 or by high mobility group box protein (HMGB)-1. NK-derived IFNγ and NK cells contact prime macrophages that contribute to bacterial clearance and inflammatory cytokine production.

## Mast Cells

One of the striking parameters of inflammation is its rapid occurrence and the fast release of inflammatory cytokines and mediators. Numerous experimental approaches suggest that cells containing preformed TNF, such as mast cells, play a central role. The contribution of mast cells has been established in zymosan-induced peritoneal inflammation, and inflammation following myocardial ischemia-reperfusion (Table 1). Mast cell degranulation is a key event in the granulocyte infiltration and tissue dysfunction associated with intestinal ischemia-reperfusion [34]. It is noteworthy that TNF-producing mast cells are required to achieve an efficient innate immune response in peritonitis after cecal ligation and puncture (CLP), and after peritoneal or intranasal infection with *Klebsiella pneumoniae* [35,36]. Mast cells are directly activated by microbial derived compounds such as peptidoglycan and endotoxin and subsequently release a vast array of cytokines that govern innate immunity and inflammation.

## Differences between Compartments

In sepsis and SIRS, the response varies from one organ to another. The most convincing proof of this concept has been provided by Peter Ward's group [37] who examined the gene expression in different tissues in a CLP model of sepsis in rat. They reported that the sepsis response elicited gene expression profiles that were either organ-specific, common to more than one organ, or distinctly opposite in some organs. For example, in the latter case, the expression of about 15 genes was increased in the liver and decreased in the spleen. The nature of the specific chemokines expressed after insult differed from one tissue to another. For example, in the CLP murine model, macrophage-inflammatory protein-2 (MIP-2) was mainly expressed in the lung while keratinocyte-derived chemokine (KC) was found in the liver [38]. After injection of LPS in mice, regulated upon activation, normal T-cell expressed and secreted (RANTES) was far more abundant in the lung than in the liver [39]. Furthermore, the cascade of events may also vary from one compartment to another. For example, after injection of LPS, NF-κB activation in the liver was mediated through TNF- and IL-1 receptor-dependent pathways, but, in the lungs, LPS-induced NF-κB activation was largely independent of these receptors [40]. Most interestingly, neutralization of TNF, by pretreatment with an adenovirus-mediated TNF receptor fusion protein before injection of LPS in the mouse, reduced plasma levels of IL-6, MCP-1, and IL-12, whereas heart expression of these cytokines was unaffected [41].

In the lungs, alveolar macrophages behave differently as compared to macro-phages from other tissues. Although data are still missing in humans, mouse alveolar macrophages do not produce IL-10, do not express TLR9, and are thus insensitive to bacterial DNA, and fail to produce IFNβ in response to TLR4 or TLR3 agonists. Another specificity of the lungs may explain why this organ is often the first and the most common to fail in septic shock and SIRS. One of the characteristics of the lungs is the local presence of GM-CSF, a cytokine essential for normal pulmonary physiology and resistance to local infection. However, the critical role for GM-CSF in pulmonary homeostasis may well be a disadvantage in the case of endotoxin-induced lung inflammation. The synergy between GM-CSF- and LPS-induced signaling is well recognized, and, interestingly, neutralization of GM-CSF suppresses LPS-induced lung inflammation. Another striking observation is the absence of deactivation after a preliminary exposure to heat-killed Gram-negative bacteria or repeated exposure to LPS. In models where one would have expected an induction of endotoxin tolerance, a priming effect to live *E. coli*-induced lung injury or chronic pulmonary inflammation was induced. We suspect that there is a parallel between these observations and the capacity of GM-CSF to prevent or reverse the induction of endotoxin tolerance.

Another aspect of the cell reactivity within one given organ is its specific microenvironment. A fascinating observation was made years ago by Callery et al. [42]. These investigators reported that a high hepatic arginase activity occurs within the liver, resulting in negligible local arginine levels. Accordingly, they performed LPS-stimulated cultures of Kupffer cells in media with or without (-) L-arginine. In arginine (-) cultures, TNF production was significantly reduced, whereas prostaglandin-E2 (PGE2) production was amplified. Cyclooxygenase blockade upregulated the production of TNF. This influence of arginine on the production of TNF-α appeared unique to Kupffer cells because both TNF and PGE2 levels increased when peritoneal, pleural, and alveolar macrophages were stimulated by LPS in arginine (-) medium. The authors suggested that this response may reflect an evolutionary adaptation of Kupffer cells to their local hepatic environment; thus, despite continuous exposure to gut-derived endotoxin under normal conditions, Kupffer cells fail to generate detrimental cytokine responses.

## Local Detection of an On-going Process of Inflammation

During a localized and moderate infection, inflammatory mediators are released at the site of infection. In contrast, with systemic inflammation, most tissues contribute to the release of inflammatory mediators. As shown in Table 1, in sepsis and in sepsis-like experimental models, inflammatory mediators can be produced by immune cells present in most organs. Mediators were identified in tissues using mRNA levels, by immunochemistry, ELISA, or with bioactivity assays, and following their release in *ex vivo* culture.

### Lungs

There are numerous examples that illustrate the presence of enhanced levels of pro-inflammatory cytokines in bronchoalveolar lavages (BAL) following chest injury, ventilator-associated pneumonia, and in patients with ARDS or bacterial pneumonia. In the latter case, Dehoux et al. [21] elegantly demonstrated compartmentalized cytokine production. They showed higher levels of inflammatory cytokines in BAL fluid recovered from the involved lung of patients with unilateral pneumonia as compared to the contralateral, non-involved lung. Inflammatory cytokines were also found in pleural effusions of patients with pneumonia [43]. Thermal injury led to the expression of TNF mRNA in lung [44]. In MOF patients with ARDS, the presence of higher IL-1$\beta$ levels in pulmonary capillary blood than in peripheral vein blood strongly suggested the production of this cytokine within the tissue and its pouring out in the downstream vein [45].

Systemic injection of endotoxin induced gene expression of IL-1$\alpha$, IL-1$\beta$ and IL-1ra in lungs of rats, and of TNF in mice and sheep. In murine lungs, TNF was also produced after peritonitis, or after injection of *S. aureus* (Table 1). In contrast, intravenous administration of endotoxin in human volunteers did not lead to an enhanced expression of TNF, IL-1, IL-6 or IL-8 mRNA among bronchoalveolar cells [46]. An elegant *in vivo* imaging study performed in transgenic mice by Carlsen and coworkers [47] showed NF-$\kappa$B activation in numerous tissues following intravenous injection of LPS, particularly in lungs, skin, spleen, and small intestine. In contrast, liver, kidney, heart, muscle, and adipose tissues displayed less intense activities. Following LPS-injection in mice, we studied cells derived from different compartments and showed that tolerance to endotoxin, as monitored by *ex vivo* TNF production in response to LPS, was compartmentalized. Indeed, bronchoalveolar cells were less prone than splenocytes, peritoneal cells, and bone marrow cells to develop tolerance to endotoxin. Another interesting approach was reported by Molina et al. [48] who studied the levels of TNF after an LPS injection in rats that had previously undergone hemorrhagic-shock. When compared to sham animals, plasma levels of TNF were lower, whereas levels of TNF in BAL were far higher. From these observations, it appears that remote or systemic infection leads to an inflammatory response within the lungs.

The inflammatory process is also accompanied by the release of anti-inflammatory mediators. Soluble TNFR levels were increased in BAL fluid of patients who developed ARDS. Similarly, after chest trauma, sTNFRI and II and IL-1ra were present in plasma and in BAL fluid. Soluble TNFR was present in greater amounts in pleural effusion than in plasma of septic and non-septic ICU patients. Donnelly and colleagues [49] reported that low concentrations of the anti-inflammatory cytokines IL-10 and IL-1ra in BAL fluid obtained from patients with early ARDS were closely associated with poor prognosis. These results stand in apparent contrast to the relationship between high plasma levels of anti-inflammatory cytokines and poor outcome in SIRS patients.

## Liver

Douzinas et al. [45] showed in MOF patients with hepatic involvement that IL-6 levels were higher in hepatic sinusoidal blood than in peripheral vein blood. These results strongly suggest the production of the mentioned cytokine within the tissue and its pouring out in the downstream vein. Thermal injury led to the expression of TNF mRNA in liver. Similarly, injection of endotoxin induced gene expression of IL-1α, IL-1β and IL-1ra in rat liver, and TNF mRNA expression in mice. TNF was also induced in liver after *S. aureus* injection and in peritonitis models. Concomitantly, IL-10 mRNA expression was rapidly induced in murine liver (1 hour), and to a lesser extent in lungs and kidney. Kupffer cells contribute to the production of inflammatory cytokines and HO-1 (Table 1).

## Spleen

In the case of hemorrhage or thermal injury in mice, the spleen contributed to the production of TNF and IL-1β. In mice and rats, experimental peritonitis, and injection of LPS, *E. coli*, or Staphylococcal exotoxin led to TNF, IL-1α, IL-1β and IL-1ra expression in the spleen (Table 1), and to NF-κB activation [47]. However, IL-10 mRNA expression was also rapidly induced in spleen (1 hour).

In contrast, the *ex vivo* LPS-induced production of TNF by spleen cells was reduced in hemorrhage, trauma/hemorrhage, abdominal surgery, and sepsis models. This stands true also when IL-1 and IL-6 were investigated as well as for concanavalin A-induced IL-2 and IFNγ. In contrast, in most studies that addressed thermal injury, TNF, IL-1, and IL-6 production was increased upon LPS stimulation. A similar upregulation of the production of these three cytokines was also reported using a T-cell mitogen. This clear cut difference between various SIRS and burn models should encourage investigators to address whether putative circulating mediators could deactivate or prime spleen cells depending upon the nature of the insult.

## Gut

In the case of hemorrhage, elevated levels of IL-6 and TNF in the portal vein suggest a contribution from the gut to the inflammatory response [50]. High levels of portal vein TNF have been found during abdominal aortic surgery in man [9]. Both of these studies illustrate that hypoperfused gut can be a source of circulating TNF. Following intravenous injection of LPS in mice, NF-κB activation was observed in the small intestine [47]. In rats, TNF mRNA was expressed in the wall of the jejunum, and gene expression of IL-1α, IL-1β, and IL-1ra was found in the bowel.

## Peritoneum

Inflammatory cytokines were found in the ascites fluid of patients with pancreatitis, as well as in the peritoneal fluid of patients with appendicitis and peritonitis. Soluble TNF receptors I and II were also present in great excess as compared to TNF in ascites of patients with acute pancreatitis [51], illustrating the concomitant expression of both pro- and anti-inflammatory mediators.

## Brain

Pro-inflammatory cytokines and IL-1ra. were found in the cerebrospinal fluid (CSF) of patients with bacterial meningitis. TNF and TGFβ were found within leukocytes derived from the CSF of patients with meningitis (Table 1). In brains of patients who died from septic shock, immunohistochemical analysis revealed the expression of TNF in glial cells and of inducible NO synthase (iNOS) in vessel walls [52]. TNF mRNA was found in rat brain after intravenous injection of LPS. Low expression of IL-10 mRNA, but high TGFb mRNA expression was found in brain following *Haemophilus influenzae*-induced meningitis in infant rats [53].

## Heart

In the case of hemorrhage, the heart contributes to TNF and IL-1β production. Injection of LPS in mice led to the appearance of TNF in the heart as well as to the expression of HO-1. Immunochemistry analysis revealed that TNF production was mainly due to inflammatory and interstitial cells [54]. TNF expression was also observed in the heart after injection of *S. aureus* (Table 1).

## Bone Marrow

Endotoxin treatment resulted in the appearance of TNF in the secretory granules of all eosinophils, neutrophils, and monocytes in the bone marrow (Table 1).

## Muscle

Injection of LPS induced the expression of inflammatory cytokines in muscle, and led to NF-κB activation [47]. An increased expression of the inducible isoforms of cyclooxygenase (COX-2) was detected by Western-blot in muscle biopsies of septic patients, as compared to controls [55]. Furthermore, TNF was found in muscle biopsies of patients with septic cellulitis [56], and HO-1 was detected in the skeletal muscle of patients with septic myopathies [55]

## Other Tissues

In human septic shock caused by cellulitis, TNF, IL-1β and iNOS were found in skin, muscle fat, artery at the very site of infection, and in inflamed and putrescent areas [56]. LPS injection led to the appearance of TNF in mesangial cells of the kidney. Using the CAT reporter gene expression, Giroir et al. [57] also showed gene activation in kidney, in uterus, and in islet of Langherans. Finally, subcutaneous injection of LPS induced the expression of inflammatory cytokines in ocular tissues. Thus, almost all tissues can contribute to the production of inflammatory mediators during systemic inflammation. In numerous cases, the resident or infiltrating leukocytes are the main activated cells.

## The Blood Compartment

Proof of activation of circulating leukocytes is rare, as, probably, in most cases the analysis occurred once activated cells have marginated towards tissues. We showed in an *ex vivo* analysis that the spontaneous production of TNF by murine blood leukocytes was significantly enhanced 1 h after intravenous injection of LPS. At a later time (8 h), after intraperitoneal injection of LPS in mice, peripheral blood mononuclear cells (PBMC) also expressed IL-10 mRNA. In humans, IL-8 mRNA, but not IL-6 or TNF mRNA, was found in circulating leukocytes of patients with localized and septicemic *Pseudomonas pseudomallei* infection (Table 1).

Many events contribute to modify the nature of circulating leukocytes. During infection, a boost of hematopoiesis leads to a rise in new naive cells within the blood stream. Following an encounter with microbial products, circulating cells may be activated and marginate towards the tissues. Accordingly, numerous modifications in circulating leukocytes have been reported in sepsis and SIRS. This includes up- and down-regulation of many membrane markers. Decreased human leukocyte antigen D-related (HLA-DR) surface expression on monocytes is a well-known phenomenon, but the expression of other surface markers was found to be reduced (e.g., TNFR p75, CD14, CD71, CD86). In contrast, expression of TNFR p50, CD40, CD48, CD64, CD89, TLR4, triggering receptor expressed on myeloid cells (TREM)-1, and tissue factor was increased.

As a consequence of bathing within an immunosuppressive milieu, circulating blood leukocytes display a major alteration of their immune status [58]. Lymphocytes show a reduced capacity to proliferate in response to mitogen and to produce cytokines upon *ex vivo* activation. In response to bacterial stimuli, monocytes from septic patients exhibit an attenuated respiratory burst, and monocytes from critically ill patients synthesize less leukotriene C4 than healthy controls in response to calcium ionophore. The main feature of blood monocytes, lymphocytes, and neutrophils from septic patients is their reduced capacity to produce pro-inflammatory cytokines when further activated in *in vitro* cultures. In fact, the same observation has been found in all types of SIRS. Attempts to decipher the mechanisms underlying the altered responsiveness to LPS revealed an impaired activation of NF-κB that was reminiscent of the observation made in cells rendered tolerant to LPS [59, 60]. Furthermore, the expression of interleukin-1 receptor-associated kinase (IRAK)-M, a negative regulator of TLR-dependent signaling, was more rapidly upregulated following a second endotoxin challenge in monocytes isolated from septic patients than from healthy controls [61]. However, it is important to mention that the responsiveness to certain agonists is maintained and that the production of anti-inflammatory cytokines (e.g., IL-1ra, IL-10) is often enhanced. For example, leukocytes from trauma patients and from patients resuscitated after cardiac arrest produced similar amounts of TNF as did healthy controls when exposed to heat-killed *S. aureus*, while their response to LPS was dramatically reduced [12, 62]. More recently, we made a similar observation with monocytes from sepsis patients (Adib-Conquy et al., unpublished data). Accordingly, the reduced capacity of circulating leukocytes to produce cytokines upon activation is not a global defect, and the terms 'anergy', 'immunodepression', and 'immunoparalysis', often used to qualify the phenomenon, are excessive, and probably the term 'leukocyte reprogramming' best defines the exact nature of the phenomenon [63].

## Leukocyte Recruitment as a Key Factor of Local Inflammation

Following LPS injection, or in sepsis models (e.g., CLP), injury and altered functions of heart, lung, kidney, or liver have been regularly reported. These alterations are associated with an important influx of leukocytes. This recruitment within tissues implies the adhesion of circulating leukocytes to endothelium, a step involving numerous adhesion molecules. Targeting many of these molecules with specific antibodies resulted in an improvement in organ function, reduced local inflammation, and, in some models, improved survival. For example, beneficial effects of anti-intercellular adhesion molecule-1 (ICAM-1), anti-vascular cell adhesion molecule-1 (VCAM-1), anti-P-selectin, anti-L-selectin, anti-E-selectin, anti-lymphocyte function associated antigen (LFA1), anti-CD18, and anti-CD11b have been reported following LPS administration in rabbit, rat, or mouse. However, in some experimental models, these antibodies failed to induce any improvement. For example, in a baboon model of sepsis after infusion of live *E. coli*, anti-ICAM-1, anti-L selectin, and anti E-selectin did not protect against lung injury and did not improve survival. Similarly, anti-LFA-1 did not protect against a lethal injection of LPS in mice, and anti-CD18 worsened cardiovascular function in a canine model of septic shock. The involvement of different adhesion molecules may be specific to each compartment and probably also depends upon the experimental model used. This complexity is underscored by experiments in which antibody blockade or absence of ICAM-1 (gene knockout) abrogated LPS-induced cardiac dysfunction but did not reduce neutrophil accumulation. The deleterious effect of leukocyte recruitment within tissues is further illustrated by the beneficial effect of substances targeting alpha-chemokine receptors (CXCR), and more precisely CXCR1 and CXCR2.

Recruited neutrophils are undoubtedly key players in the perpetuation of the inflammatory process. Reduced apoptosis, priming, and enhanced activity are hallmark features of neutrophils in SIRS patients. For example, neutrophil depletion before burn injury prevented the early vascular leakage of albumin and ede ma in the ileum and je junum; although their depletion had less effect on the later stages of burn-induced microvascular injury in the intestine [64]. Neutrophils also contribute to the release of inflammatory cytokines. Data indicate that IL-1β-producing neutrophils rapidly traffic to the lungs in response to hemorrhage or endotoxemia, and may contribute to the development of lung injury after blood loss and sepsis [65]. Other mediators are specifically released by neutrophils. In a model of TNF-induced acute lung injury (ALI), neutrophil elastase inhibitor attenuated the inflammatory process by inhibiting the alveolar epithelial and vascular endothelial injury triggered by activated neutrophils. Peripheral blood neutrophils derived from animals 24 hours post-hemorrhage, exhibited an *ex vivo* decrease in apoptotic frequency and an increase in respiratory burst capacity. Interestingly, adoptive transfer of neutrophils from hemorrhaged, but not control animals, to neutropenic recipients reproduced ALI when subsequently challenged with sepsis, implying that this priming was mediated by neutrophils.

## The Cross-talk Between Compartments

### How Does the Inflammatory Response Spread from Organ to Organ?

The presence of circulating endotoxin may explain how so many tissues are activated in the setting of sepsis. As previously mentioned, the gut may be a source of systemic endotoxin in a variety of clinical settings. In some circumstances, the lungs may also be a source of endotoxin: in a rabbit model, it was shown that ventilator strategy can favor endotoxin translocation from the lungs after an endotracheal instillation of LPS [66]. Insulted organs can be a site for synthesis of inflammatory mediators and the associated increase in vascular and epithelial permeability favors the leakage of mediators from one compartment to another. For example, following lung injury or pneumonia, it was demonstrated that systemic TNF originated from a pulmonary source. Another example of cross-talk between compartments was illustrated by the significant correlation we found between levels of TGF-β in pleural effusion and BAL fluid [43]. However, it is worth mentioning that this may not always be the case since we failed to find any correlation between the levels of cytokines in pleural effusion and in plasma. Numerous experimental models have shown that limb, liver, intestinal, or renal ischemia-reperfusion induced-injury lead to acute inflammatory lung injury. It was reported that this phenomenon was induced by macrophage-derived products such as IL-1 and TNF. In contrast, neither TNF nor LPS were responsible for pulmonary inflammation following induction of peritonitis in mice. Other mediators, locally released and present in the blood stream, may contribute to the spreading of the inflammatory process, igniting local pathologies. Potential candidates are: C5a anaphylatoxin generated after complement activation as illustrated by the capacity of anti-C5 antibodies to reduce remote organ injury after intestinal ischemia/reperfusion; HMGB1 released by necrotic cells; IFNγ that contributes to endotoxin-induced death, and to lung inflammation after CLP; macrophage migration inhibitory factor (MIF), a circulating inflammatory cytokine in SIRS patients; leukotriene B4 (LTB4) as illustrated by the blunted lung injury following limb ischemia in sheep treated with lipoxygenase inhibitors; soluble MD2 that participates in the activation of TLR4-positive epithelial cells by endotoxin; and microbial products other than LPS, such as bacterial DNA, that possess a strong capacity to induce inflammatory mediators and induce septic shock. Activated circulating leukocytes can also propagate the inflammatory processes, as previously mentioned for neutrophils from hemorrhaged animals. Of course, one should not forget the well recognized deleterious effects of IL-1 and TNF either in the periphery or within the tissues. Systemic TNF has been shown to induce ARDS, while IL-1 has been suggested to be the main local inflammatory actor in ARDS.

A recent investigation demonstrated the cross-talk between liver and lungs during endotoxemia in piglets. When only lungs were perfused, endotoxin caused pulmonary hypertension and neutropenia, but oxygenation was maintained, TNF and IL-6 levels were minimally elevated, and there was no lung edema. In contrast, when both the liver and lungs were perfused with endotoxin, marked hypoxemia, a large increase in perfusate levels of TNF and IL-6, and severe lung edema were observed. NF-κB activation in lungs was also greatest when the liver was in the perfusion circuit.

## The Peripheral Nervous System as a Link Between Compartments

Besides the cross-talk between compartments that occurs by an exportation/importation of inflammatory mediators *via* the blood stream, another link exists, orchestrated by the brain via the pain fibers, the cholinergic neurons, and the sympathetic neurons. The release of pro-inflammatory neuromediators (e.g., substance P, norepinephrine) or anti-inflammatory neuromediators (e.g., acetylcholine, epinephrine) within the tissues, contributes to favor or limit the inflammatory response [67]. However, the effects of catecholamines on inflammation are complex. This is illustrated by the observation that epinephrine favors IL-8 production but represses that of NO, and decreases TNF production *in vitro via* $\beta_2$-adrenergic receptors. Tracey's group reported that vagal nerve stimulation attenuated hypotension and reduced levels of TNF in plasma and liver of LPS-treated rats [68]. These protective effects were mediated by acetylcholine and the α7 subunit of nicotinic receptors found on the surface of macrophages [69]. A similar receptor was also identified on endothelial cells, and in response to acetylcholine, the expression of adhesion molecules and chemokine production induced by TNF was reduced [70]. *In vivo*, cholinergic stimulation blocked recruitment of leukocytes. These findings identify the endothelium as a target of anti-inflammatory cholinergic mediators.

Studies that make use of chemical sympathectomy reveal an opposite effect of the sympathetic nervous system on the control of intraperitoneally delivered Gram-negative or Gram-positive bacteria [71]. Ablation of the sympathetic nervous system decreased the dissemination of Gram-negative bacteria through a mechanism of increased secretion of peritoneal TNF, improved phagocytic response of peritoneal cells, and increased influx of monocytes into the peritoneal cavity. In contrast, sympathectomy increased the Gram-positive bacterial tissue burden that was caused by a reduction in corticosteroid release, and was associated with a decrease in IL-4 secretion from peritoneal cells and in the influx of lymphocytes into the peritoneal cavity. In both models, the peritoneal wall was the critical border for systemic infection. These results show the dual role of the sympathetic nervous system in sepsis. It can be favorable or unfavorable, depending on the innate immune effector mechanisms necessary to overcome infection.

## Conclusion

Compartmentalization of the inflammatory response is a key feature of sepsis and SIRS. Tissue injury can be initiated far away from a distant insult. Blood borne elements are supposed to prevent initiation of deleterious inflammatory response within tissues. However, other circulating elements contribute to the ignition of inflammation at remote sites.

## References

**Note** For additional references, the reader is referred to the paper by Cavaillon JM and Annane D. Compartmentalization of the inamma tory response in sepsis and SIRS. J Endotoxin Res 12 151 70, 2006

1. Müller-Alouf H, Alouf J, Gerlach D, Ozegowski J, Fitting C, Cavaillon JM (1994) Comparative study of cytokine release by human peripheral blood mononuclear cells stimulated with Streptococcus pyogenes superantigen erythrogenic toxins, heat-killed streptococci and lipopolysaccharide. Infect Immun 62:4915–4921
2. Cavaillon JM (1994) Cytokines and macrophages. Biomed Pharmacother 48:445–453
3. Huang Q, Liu D, Majewski P, et al (2001) The plasticity of dendritic cell responses to pathogens and their components. Science 294:870–875
4. Feezor RJ, Oberholzer C, Baker HV, et al (2003) Molecular characterization of the acute inflammatory response to infections with gram-negative versus gram-positive bacteria. Infect Immun 71:5803–5813

5. Yu SL, Chen HW, Yang PC, et al (2004) Differential gene expression in gram-negative and gram-positive sepsis. Am J Respir Crit Care Med 169:1135–1143
6. Opal SM, Scannon PJ, Vincent JL, et al (1999) Relationship between plasma levels of lipopolysaccharide (LPS) and LPS-binding protein in patients with severe sepsis and septic shock. J Infect Dis 180:1584–1598
7. Cavaillon JM, Munoz C, Fitting C, Misset B, Carlet J (1992) Circulating cytokines: the tip of the iceberg ? Circ Shock 38:145–152
8. Suojaranta-Ylinen R, Ruokonen E, Pulkki K, Mertsola J, Takala J (1997) Preoperative glutamine loading does not prevent endotoxemia in cardiac surgery. Acta Anaesthesiol Scand 41, 385-91.
9. Cabie A, Farkas JC, Fitting C, et al (1993) High levels of portal TNFα during abdominal aortic surgery in man. Cytokine 5:448–453
10. Kelly JL, O'Sullivan C, O'Riordain M, et al (1997) Is circulating endotoxin the trigger for the systemic inflammatory response syndrome seen after injury ? Ann Surgery 225:530–543
11. Marshall JC, Foster D, Vincent JL, et al (2004) Diagnostic and prognostic implications of endotoxemia in critical illness: results of the MEDIC study. J Infect Dis 190:527–534
12. Adrie C, Adib-Conquy M, Laurent I, et al (2002) Successful cardiopulmonary resuscitation after cardiac arrest as a "sepsis like" syndrome. Circulation 106:562–568
13. Moller AS, Bjerre A, Brusletto B, Joo GB, Brandtzaeg P, Kierulf P (2005) Chemokine patterns in meningococcal disease. J Infect Dis 191:768–775
14. Hellman J, Roberts JDJ, Tehan MM, Allaire JE, Warren HS (2002) Bacterial peptidoglycan-associated lipoprotein is released into the bloodstream in gram-negative sepsis and causes inflammation and death in mice. J Biol Chem 277:14274–14280
15. Shimizu T, Tani T, Endo Y, Hanasawa K, Tsuchiya M, Kodama M (2002) Elevation of plasma peptidoglycan and peripheral blood neutrophil activation during hemorrhagic shock: plasma peptidoglycan reflects bacterial translocation and may affect neutrophil activation. Crit Care Med 30:77–82
16. Swank GM, Deitch EA (1996) Role of the gut in multiple organ failure: bacterial translocation and permeability changes. World J Surg 20:411–417
17. Smith PD, Suffredini AF, Allen JB, Wahl LM, Parrillo JE, Wahl SM (1994) Endotoxin administration to humans primes alveolar macrophages for increased production of inflammatory mediators. J Clin Immunol 14, 141–148
18. Christman JW, Petras SF, Hacker M, Absher PM, Davis GS (1988) Alveolar macrophage function is selectively altered after endotoxemia in rats. Infect Immun 56:1254–1259
19. Simpson SQ, Modi HN, Balk RA, Bone RC, Casey LC (1991) Reduced alveolar macrophage production of tumor necrosis factor during sepsis in mice and men. Crit Care Med 19:1060–1066
20. Cavaillon JM, Adib-Conquy M, Cloëz-Tayarani I, Fitting C (2001) Immunodepression in sepsis and SIRS assessed by ex vivo cytokine production is not a generalized phenomenon: a review. J Endotoxin Res 7:85–93
21. Dehoux MS, Boutten A, Ostinelli J, et al (1994) Compartmentalized cytokine production within the human lung in unilateral pneumonia. Am J Respir Crit Care Med 150:710–716
22. Schwartz MD, Moore E, Moore FA, et al (1996) Nuclear factor-kappa B is activated in alveolar macrophages from patients with acute respiratory distress syndrome. Crit Care Med 24:1285–1292
23. Moine P, McIntyre R, Schwartz MD, et al (2000) NF-κB regulatory mechanisms in alveolar macrophages from patients with acute respiratory distress syndrome. Shock 13:85–91
24. Fieren MWJA, Van Den Bemd GJ, Bonta IL (1990) Endotoxin-stimulated peritoneal macrophages obtained from continuous ambulatory peritoneal dialysis patients show an increased capacity to release interleukin-1b in vitro during infectious peritonitis. Eur J Clin Invest 20:453–457

25. Wu MY, Ho HN, Chen SU, Chao KH, Chen CD, Yang YS (1999) Increase in the production of IL-6, IL-10 and IL-12 by LPS stimulated peritoneal macrophages from women with endometriosis. Am J Reprod Immunol 41:106–111
26. Wichmann MW, Ayala A, Chaudry IH (1997) Male sex steroids are responsible for depressing macrophage immune function after trauma-hemorrhage. Am J Physiol 273:C1335-C1340.
27. Wu JZ, Ogle CK, Fisher JE, Warden GD, Ogle JD (1995) The mRNA expression and in vitro production of cytokines and other proteins by hepatocytes and Kupffer cells following thermal injury. Shock 3:268–273
28. Shenkar R, Abraham E (1999) Mechanisms of lung neutrophil activation after hemorrhage or endotoxemia: roles of reactive oxygen intermediates, NF-κB and cyclic AMP response element binding protein. J Immunol 163:954–962
29. Abraham E, Arcaroli J, Shenkar R (2001) Activation of extracellular signal-regulated kinases, NF-κB, and cyclic adenosine 5'-monophosphate response element binding protein in lung neutrophils occurs by differing mechanisms after hemorrhage or endotoxemia. J Immunol 166:522–530
30. Ethuin F, Delarche C, Gougerot-Pocidalo MA, Eurin B, Jacob L, Chollet-Martin S (2003) Regulation of interleukin 12 p40 and p70 production by blood and alveolar phagocytes during severe sepsis. Lab Invest 83:1353–1360
31. Kermarrec N, Selloum S, Plantefeve G, et al (2005) Regulation of peritoneal and systemic neutrophil-derived tumor necrosis factor-alpha release in patients with severe peritonitis: role of tumor necrosis factor-alpha converting enzyme cleavage. Crit Care Med 33:1359–1364
32. Badgwell B, Parihar R, Magro C, Dierksheide J, Russo T, Carson WE 3rd (2002) Natural killer cells contribute to the lethality of a murine model of Escherichia coli infection. Surgery 132:205–212
33. Goldmann O, Chhatwal GS, Medina E (2005) Contribution of natural killer cells to the pathogenesis of septic shock induced by Streptococcus pyogenes in mice. J Infect Dis 191:1280–1286
34. Kanwar S, Kubes P (1994) Mast cells contribute to ischemia-reperfusion-induced granulocyte infiltration and intestinal dysfunction. Am J Physiol 267:G316–G321
35. Echtenacher B, Männel D, Hültner L (1996) Critical protective role of mast cells in a model of acute septic peritonitis. Nature 381:75–77
36. Malavija R, Ikeda T, Ross E, Abraham S (1996) Mast cell modulation of neutrophil influx and bacterial clearance at sites of infection through TNFα. Nature 381:77–80
37. Chinnaiyan AM, Huber-Lang M, Kumar-Sinha C, et al (2001) Molecular signatures of sepsis: multiorgan gene expression profiles of systemic inflammation. Am J Pathol 159:1199–1209
38. Mercer-Jones MA, Shrotri MS, Peyton JC, Remick DG, Cheadle WG (1999) Neutrophil sequestration in liver and lung is differentially regulated by C-X-C chemokines during experimental peritonitis. Inflammation 23:305–319
39. VanOtteren GM, Strieter RM, Kunkel SL, et al (1995) Compartmentalized expression of RANTES in a murine model of endotoxemia. J Immunol 154:1900–1908
40. Koay MA, Christman JW, Wudel LJ, et al (2002) Modulation of endotoxin-induced NF-kappa B activation in lung and liver through TNF type 1 and IL-1 receptors. Am J Physiol Lung Cell Mol Physiol 283:L1247-L1254
41. Kadokami T, McTiernan CF, Kubota T, et al (2001) Effects of soluble TNF receptor treatment on lipopolysaccharide-induced myocardial cytokine expression. Am J Physiol 280: H2281-H2291
42. Callery MP, Mangino MJ, Flye MW (1991) A biologic basis for limited Kupffer cell reactivity to portal-derived endotoxin. Surgery 110:221–230
43. Marie C, Losser MR, Fitting C, Kermarrec N, Payen D, Cavaillon JM (1997) Cytokines and soluble cytokines receptors in pleural effusions from septic and nonseptic patients. Am J Respir Crit Care Med 156:1515–1522
44. Fang WH, Yao YM, Shi ZG, et al (2003) The mRNA expression patterns of tumor necrosis factor-alpha and TNFR-I in some vital organs after thermal injury. World J Gastroenterol 9: 1038–1044

45. Douzinas EE, Tsidemiadou PD, Pitaridis MT, et al (1997) The regional production of cytokines and lactate in sepsis-related multiple organ failure. Am Respir Crit Care Med 155:53–59
46. Boujoukos AJ, Martich GD, Supinski E, Suffredini AF (1993) Compartmentalization of the acute cytokine response in humans after intravenous endotoxin administration. J Appl Physiol 74:3027–3033
47. Carlsen H, Moskaug JO, Fromm SH, Blomhoff R (2002) In vivo imaging of NF-κB activity. J Immunol 168:1441–1446
48. Molina PE, Bagby GJ, Stahls P (2001) Hemorrhage alters neuroendocrine, hemodynamic, and compartment-specific TNF responses to LPS. Shock 16:459–465
49. Donnelly SC, Strieter RM, Reid PT, et al (1996) The association between mortality rates and decreased concentrations of interleukin-10 and interleukin-1 receptor antagonist in the lung fluids of patients with the adult respiratory distress syndrome. Ann Intern Med 125:191–196
50. Deitch EA, Xu D, Franko L, Ayala A, Chaudry IH (1994) Evidence favoring the role of the gut as a cytokine-generating organ in rats subjected to hemorrhagic shock. Shock 1:141–145
51. Dugernier TL, Laterre PF, Wittebole X, et al (2003) Compartmentalization of the inflammatory response during acute pancreatitis: correlation with local and systemic complications. Am J Respir Crit Care Med 168:148–157
52. Sharshar T, Gray F, Lorin de la Grandmaison G, et al (2003) Apoptosis of neurons in cardiovascular autonomic centres triggered by inducible nitric oxide synthase after death from septic shock. Lancet 362:1799–1805
53. Diab A, Zhu J, Lindquist L, Wretlind B, Link H, Bakhiet M (1997) Cytokine mRNA profiles during the course of experimental Haemophilus influenzae bacterial meningitis. Clin Immunol Immunopathol 85:236–245
54. Tanaka N, Kita T, Kasai K, Nagano T (1994) The immunocytochemical localization of tumor necrosis factor and leukotriene in the rat heart and lung during endotoxin shock. Virchows Arch 424:273–277
55. Rabuel C, Renaud E, Brealey D, et al (2004) Human septic myopathy: induction of cyclooxygenase, heme oxygenase and activation of the ubiquitin proteolytic pathway. Anesthesiology 101:583–590
56. Annane D, Sanquer S, Sebille V, et al (2000) Compartmentalised inducible nitric-oxide synthase activity in septic shock. Lancet 355:1143–1148
57. Giroir BP, Johnson JH, Brown T, Allen GL, Beutler B (1992) The tissue distribution of tumor necrosis factor biosynthesis during endotoxemia. J Clin Invest 90:693–698
58. Cavaillon JM, Fitting C, Adib-Conquy M (2004) Mechanisms of immunodysregulation in sepsis. Contrib Nephrol 144:76–93
59. Adib-Conquy M, Adrie C, Moine P, et al (2000) NF-κB expression in mononuclear cells of septic patients resembles that observed in LPS-tolerance. Am J Respir Crit Care Med 162:1877–1883
60. Adib-Conquy M, Asehnoune K, Moine P, Cavaillon JM (2001) Longterm impaired expression of nuclear factor-kB and IkBa in peripheral blood mononuclear cells of patients with major trauma. J Leukoc Biol 70:30–38
61. Escoll P, del Fresno C, Garcia L, et al (2003) Rapid up-regulation of IRAK-M expression following a second endotoxin challenge in human monocytes and in monocytes isolated from septic patients. Biochem Biophys Res Commun 311:465–472
62. Adib-Conquy M, Moine P, Asehnoune K, et al (2003) Toll-like receptor-mediated tumor necrosis factor and interleukin-10 production differ during systemic inflammation. Am J Respir Crit Care Med 168:158–164
63. Annane D, Bellissant E, Cavaillon JM (2005) Septic shock. Lancet 365:63–78
64. Sir O, Fazal N, Choudhry MA, Goris RJ, Gamelli RL, Sayeed MM (2000) Role of neutrophils in burn-induced microvascular injury in the intestine. Shock 14, 113–117
65. Parsey MV, Tuder RM, Abraham E (1998) Neutrophils are major contributors to intraparenchymal lung IL-1 beta expression after hemorrhage and endotoxemia. J Immunol 160:1007–1013

66. Murphy DB, Cregg N, Tremblay L, et al (2000) Adverse ventilatory strategy causes pulmonary-to-systemic translocation of endotoxin. Am J Respir Crit Care Med 162:27–33
67. Tracey KJ (2002) The inflammatory reflex. Nature 420:853–859
68. Borovikova LV, Ivanova S, Zhang M, et al (2000) Vagus nerve stimulation attenuates the systemic inflammatory response to endotoxin. Nature 405:458–462
69. Wang H, Yu M, Ochani M, et al (2003) Nicotinic acetylcholine receptor alpha7 subunit is an essential regulator of inflammation. Nature 421:384–388
70. Saeed RW, Varma S, Peng-Nemeroff T, et al (2005) Cholinergic stimulation blocks endothelial cell activation and leukocyte recruitment during inflammation. J Exp Med 201:1113–1123
71. Straub RH, Pongratz G, Weidler C, et al (2005) Ablation of the sympathetic nervous system decreases gram-negative and increases gram-positive bacterial dissemination: key roles for tumor necrosis factor/phagocytes and interleukin-4/lymphocytes. J Infect Dis 192:560–572

# The Neutrophil in the Pathogenesis of Multiple Organ Dysfunction Syndrome

Z. Malam and J.C. Marshall

## Introduction

Circulating neutrophils play a cardinal role in early host defenses against bacterial and viral pathogens. Originating from hematopoietic stem cells in the bone marrow, neutrophils – also known as polymorphonuclear neutrophils (PMNs) – mature to become terminally differentiated phagocytes that are incapable of cell division, and that synthesize only low levels of RNA and protein. They are recognized histologically by their multi-lobed nuclei and abundant cytoplasmic granules. The first description of neutrophils was by Elie Metchnikoff. Upon inserting rose thorns into the larvae of starfish, he observed that wandering mesodermal cells aggregated at the insertion site. These cells revealed phagocytic abilities, with the larger phagocytes termed macrophagocytes, more commonly known today as macrophages. The smaller phagocytic cells were termed microphagocytes, and subsequently granulocytes; neutrophils were the predominant cell type [1].

## Antimicrobial Defenses of the Neutrophil

### Neutrophil Localization at an Inflammatory Focus

The eradication of microbial pathogens is a complex and coordinated process. Initiation of neutrophil defense requires their recruitment from the circulation and from bone marrow reserves to the site of microbial invasion; this process is facilitated by a combination of host- and pathogen-derived chemotactic signals that include chemokines, cytokines, matrix metalloproteases, and products of the invading microbe [2]. Activated vascular endothelial cells and fibroblasts produce chemokines such as interleukin (IL)-8, which possess potent neutrophil chemotactic ability [3]. A concentration gradient at the site of inflammation induces neutrophils to migrate toward the source of chemokine release. Expression of surface chemokine receptors varies among neutrophils, and influences which neutrophil subsets are recruited. Host-derived and microbial factors such as lipopolysaccharide (LPS), tumor necrosis factor (TNF)-α, and platelet-activating factor (PAF) also enhance the response of neutrophils to subsequent stimuli [2]. For example, neutrophils primed with LPS produce significantly greater amounts of superoxide after exposure to the bacterial peptide, N-formyl-methionyl-leucyl-phenylalanine (fMLP) [4]. Furthermore, during inflammatory reactions, membrane receptor expression is augmented by selective exocytosis of cellular vesicles and granules enriched in membrane proteins mediating neutrophil recruitment and phagocytosis [5].

Recruitment of neutrophils to the microenvironment of microbial challenge is followed by their extravasation through the vascular endothelium, and accumulation in targeted tissue. Adhesion to activated endothelium results from the co-ordinated activities of selectins, selectin ligands, integrins, and members of the immunoglobulin superfamily [6]. Selectins are composed of three carbohydrate-recognizing members: E- and P-selectin expressed on activated endothelium, and L-selectin constitutively found on the surface of neutrophils [7]. Selectin ligands are characterized by intense glycosylation through N-linked carbohydrates and O-linked side chains [8]. Integrins are heterodimers that recognize extracellular matrix and cell surface glycoproteins, in addition to soluble molecules such as complement factor C3bi [6]. The $\beta 2$ integrins (CD11/CD18) are of particular importance in the neutrophil. Following stimulation, they undergo a conformational change that optimizes their interaction with members of the immunoglobulin superfamily, including intercellular adhesion molecule (ICAM)-1 and -2, vascular cell adhesion molecule (VCAM)-1, and platelet-endothelial cell adhesion molecule (PECAM)-1 [9].

Leukocyte-endothelial cell adhesion occurs in a coordinated and sequential fashion. The initial attachment between the neutrophil and the endothelial surface entails a loose tethering mediated by cell-surface L-selectin [10]. The primary ligand for selectins has been identified as the tetrasaccharide sialyl Lewis-X, although others include fucosylated and sulfated structures. During neutrophil activation, L-selectin is shed from the surface, facilitating extravascular passage: when shedding is blocked by a metalloprotease inhibitor, endothelial adherence and intravascular accumulation of neutrophils is increased [11]. Moreover, newly recruited neutrophils arriving at microvascular endothelium covered with leukocytes can attach to already adherent neutrophils via L-selectin-dependent mechanisms [12], perhaps through cell-surface P-selectin glycoprotein ligand-1 (PSGL-1) on neutrophils. Interestingly, L-selectin-deficient mice exhibited no defect in leukocyte adhesion and rolling following surgical tissue exteriorization [13], a process known to promote expression of P-selectin, suggesting that high P-selectin expression may provide an alternative to L-selectin-mediated adhesion.

Loosely attached neutrophils roll along the endothelial surface until firmer adhesion can take place. Endothelial P-selectin is necessary for early leukocyte rolling, since P-selectin antibodies can block constitutive [14] and trauma-induced [13] rolling. A P-selectin-independent rolling mechanism also exists; mice lacking P-selectin expression show no leukocyte rolling immediately following exteriorization of the mesentery, but do manifest rolling by 60-120 minutes following tissue trauma. The P-selectin ligand, PSGL-1, on neutrophils is necessary for P-selectin-dependent rolling; rolling was almost completely inhibited when neutrophils were pretreated with monoclonal blocking antibody to PSGL-1 [15]. E-selectin and

P-selectin demonstrate redundant roles in neutrophil rolling. Mice deficient in E-selectin and wild type mice pretreated with P-selectin antibody exhibited no deficiency in neutrophil recruitment into the peritoneal cavity during the first 6 hours following thioglycollate injection, but recruitment was blocked when E-selectin deficiency was combined with anti-P-selectin pretreatment [16].

Selectins mediate more than cell-cell adhesion. Ligation and cross-linking of L-selectin on neutrophils primes them for increased superoxide production and calcium influx following exposure to a chemoattractant [17]. L-selectin is also associated with increased adhesive properties of CD11a and CD11b and L-selectin clustering triggers p38 MAPK-mediated signal transduction to effect neutrophil shape change and release of secondary, tertiary, and secretory granules [18]. Similarly, P-selectin on endothelial cells supports superoxide production, neutrophil degranulation, and polarization in response to inflammatory mediators and bacterial peptides.

Firm adhesion of the neutrophil to the vascular endothelium is a prerequisite to extravascular migration into the tissues. Members of the β2-integrin family, particularly LFA-1 (CD11a/CD18) and Mac-1 (CD11b/CD18), mediate this state of firm adhesion. Patients with leukocyte adhesion deficiency I (LAD-I), characterized by the absence of CD18 integrins, show an inability to sustain neutrophil recruitment and experience recurrent life-threatening bacterial infections [19]. Severely compromised firm neutrophil adhesion and recruitment is also evident in mice with reduced CD18 expression [20]. Activated by mediators released from stimulated endothelium (for example IL-8 and PAF), the integrins bind to ICAM-1, their immunoglobulin ligand on the endothelial surface, although differing integrins bind different regions of the molecule. Circulating inflammatory mediators, such as IL-1, serve to upregulate ICAM-1 expression on activated endothelium. Neutrophil adhesion to ICAM-1 occurs sequentially, with LFA-1 binding first followed by Mac-1-mediated stabilization [21]. Confocal microscopy studies show that Mac-1 rapidly accumulates at the neutrophil-endothelium interface during initial contact and subsequently redistributes away from the site as the neutrophil spreads. During migration, this redistribution is directed to the leading edge with rapid formation and dissociation of Mac-1-dense macroaggregates [22].

Following firm adhesion, neutrophils traverse the endothelium paracellularly [23] or transcellularly [24]. PECAM-1 is essential for transendothelial migration, and is expressed at low levels on leukocytes but high levels (>106 molecules per cell) on the endothelium, localized in particular at endothelial intercellular junctions. Antibodies to PECAM-1 can block neutrophil transmigration through TNF-α-activated endothelial cell monolayers but exert no effect on adhesion. *In vivo* experiments demonstrate that PECAM-1 expression in mesenteric veins is critical for peritoneal neutrophil accumulation [25]. Recently, junctional adhesion molecule C (JAM-C) was identified as a novel receptor for Mac-1 on neutrophils. JAM-C localizes within interendothelial junctions and is co-distributed with the tight junction component, zonula occludens-1. Inhibiting JAM-C can significantly reduce transendothelial neutrophil migration; simultaneous blockade of PECAM-

1 almost completely abolishes this effect *in vitro*. In an *in vivo* murine model of acute thioglycollate-induced peritonitis, inhibition of JAM-C with soluble mouse JAM-C results in 50% reduced neutrophil transmigration [26].

## Pathogen Recognition and Uptake

Neutrophils recognize conserved molecules on the surface of invading microorganisms (for example, peptidoglycan on Gram-positive bacteria, and LPS on Gram-negative bacteria) through pattern recognition receptors that include CD14 and members of the Toll-like receptor (TLR) family [27]. Phagocytosis occurs through the extension of pseudopodia containing enzymes such as cathepsin G, myeloperoxidase, lactoferrin, gelatinase, and elastase [28]. Pathogen binding and uptake are facilitated by opsonization of the pathogen with host serum antibody and complement; opsonization of *Staphylococcus aureus* with human serum results in an eightfold increase in neutrophil phagocytosis within 10 minutes. Activation of the complement cascade promotes the deposition of serum complement proteins C3b, iC3b, and C1q on the pathogen surface. Neutrophils, in turn, possess receptors such as C1qR, CR1, and Mac-1 that recognize complement and FcεRI, FcεRII, FcαR, FcγRI, FcγRIIa, and FcγRIIIb that recognize the Fc-region of antibody [2]. Engagement of these receptors triggers individual signaling cascades that result in actin polymerization and localized membrane remodeling for particle ingestion. Together, they drive the formation of the phagosomal cup and its sealing following pathogen engulfment [29].

Phagosome maturation follows engulfment. The phagosome, through multiple and dynamic fusion events with potent secretory vesicles and granules, sequesters microbicidal peptides and proteolytic enzymes that facilitate microbial degradation. Neutrophil granules are classified into four categories: primary or azurophilic granules contain myeloperoxidase and membrane CD63; secondary or specific granules contain lactoferrin and membrane CD66b; tertiary granules contain gelatinase; and secretory vesicles contain albumin and express membrane alkaline phosphatase and CD35 (Table 1). For granular fusion with the phagosome to occur, changes in free cytosolic calcium must occur either by release from endoplasmic reticulum stores which in turn triggers an extracellular calcium influx [30] or by release from the phagosome itself [31]. Granules exhibit differential sensitivity to calcium, with secretory vesicles having the lowest threshold and azurophilic granules the highest. Calcium may exert its permissive effect on granule fusion through the rapid depolymerization of periphagosomal actin, which allows granules to access the phagosome [29]. Alternatively, calcium may catalyze coalescence of the apposed phagosome and granule membrane bilayer [32]. In addition to calcium, protein kinases such as protein kinase C isoforms [33] and members of the Src-family kinases [34] have been implicated in membrane fusion; however, their roles are still unclear.

Table 1. Neutrophil granule constituents

| Protein | Azurophil | Specific | Gelatinase | Secretory |
|---|:---:|:---:|:---:|:---:|
| **Membrane Proteins** | | | | |
| CD11b/CD18 | | • | • | • |
| CD16 | | | | • |
| CD45 | | | | • |
| CD63 | • | | | |
| CD66, CD67 | | • | | |
| CR1 | | | | • |
| Vacuolar H+-ATPase | • | | • | • |
| **Enzymes** | | | | |
| Collagenase | | • | | |
| Elastase | • | | | |
| Gelatinase | | • | • | |
| Heparanase | | • | | |
| Myeloperoxidase | • | | | |
| Proteinase-3 | • | | | |
| **Antimicrobial Peptides** | | | | |
| Bactericidal permeability-increasing protein | • | | | |
| Cathepsins | • | | | |
| Defensins | • | | | |
| hCAP-18 | | • | | |
| Lysozyme | • | • | • | |
| **Others** | | | | |
| α1-antitrypsin | • | | | |
| β2-microglobulin | | • | • | |
| Lactoferrin | | • | | |

## Pathogen Killing

Neutrophil cytotoxic mechanisms can be broadly characterized as oxygen-dependent and oxygen-independent. The former – effected through the generation of highly reactive oxygen species (ROS) – is termed the 'respiratory burst'. NADPH oxidase, a multi-unit membrane protein, assembles at the phagosome membrane following pathogen ingestion and neutrophil activation. Of the five glycoprotein subunits that make up NADPH oxidase, cytochrome b558 is the most abundant, and localizes in lipid rafts on the membrane. The remaining subunits translocate to lipid rafts in response to phagocytic stimulation, with the lipid rafts serving to anchor the NADPH oxidase subunits for optimal enzyme activation [35]. NADPH oxidase transfers electrons from cytoplasmic NADPH to oxygen, generating the superoxide anion ($O_2^-$) which subsequently can be converted to other ROS, including hydrogen peroxide ($H_2O_2$) and hypochlorous acid (HOCl) [29] (Fig. 1). HOCl oxidizes amino acids and nucleotides and exerts the strongest bactericidal effects. The importance of NADPH oxidase in antimicrobial activity is underlined by the observation that

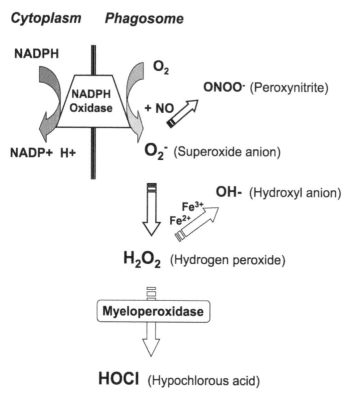

*Cytoplasm*    *Phagosome*

**Fig. 1.** Generation of reactive oxygen species by the neutrophil occurs following assembly of the multi-complex NADPH oxidase, that catalyzes the reduction of molecular oxygen through a series of intermediates to water. These intermediates are highly reactive oxidants, capable of inducing irreversible damage to proteins and lipids. From [111] with permission

patients with chronic granulomatous disease in which oxidase function is defective, are highly susceptible to recurrent bacterial infection [36].

Microbial killing also proceeds through oxygen-independent mechanisms involving anti-microbial peptides from azurophilic granules, proteolytic enzymes, and acidification of the pathogen-containing endosome [37]. Antimicrobial proteins and peptides such as defensins, permeability-increasing protein, and lysozyme increase bacterial permeability by disrupting anionic surfaces. Proteases such as neutrophil elastase and cathepsin G serve to breakdown bacterial proteins. Vacuolar ATPase is responsible for proton transport that leads to acidification, which then activates hydrolytic enzymes that function optimally under conditions of low pH (4.5-6.0) [37].

Pathogens are degraded and fragments are transported from early endosomes to late endosomes. Non-host peptides processed via the endosomal pathway become antigens that, in turn, are presented to T-cells. The antigen-presenting nature of macrophages and dendritic cells has been well characterized; however the role of the neutrophil as an antigen-presenting cell has traditionally been dismissed. Resting neutrophils harbor major histocompatibility complex (MHC) class I molecules on their surface and contain intracellular stores of both costimulatory and MHC class II molecules that bind to processed exogenous peptides, facilitating their trafficking to the cell surface, a key characteristic of a professional antigen-presenting cell [37]. Additional evidence for antigen-presenting function derives from the fact that neutrophils contain reserves of cathepsins B and D, lysosomal proteases necessary for antigen presentation [38]. Moreover antigen presentation during inflammation is facilitated by prolonged neutrophil survival resulting from the inhibition of apoptotic death by inflammatory cytokines that include IL-1, IL-6, TNF-$\alpha$, and interferon (IFN)-$\gamma$ [39,40]. Antigen presentation is rendered substantially more efficient when neutrophils travel to regional lymph nodes [37].

## Apoptosis and the Termination of Neutrophil-Mediated Inflammation

Clearance of neutrophils from an inflammatory focus occurs through apoptosis, or programmed cell death, of the neutrophil, followed by its uptake by fixed tissue macrophages [41]. Neutrophils are constitutively apoptotic cells, and the apoptotic program is activated within hours of their maturation and release from bone marrow stores [42].

### Cellular Mechanisms of Neutrophil Apoptosis

There are two major pathways of apoptosis or programmed cell death, termed the extrinsic and intrinsic pathways, and mediated through signals from the external environment, and endogenous cell stress, respectively. Cell death is effected through the activity of a family of intracellular enzymes known as caspases, a family of intracellular proteases that cleave their target proteins at conserved sites adjacent to the amino acid, aspartic acid.

Apoptosis, in response to stimuli in the external environment of the cell, is effected through the CD95 family of death receptors that includes the transmembrane proteins Fas and TNF receptor-1 having cysteine-rich extracellular domains and conserved cytoplasmic death domains [43]. Fas is activated by the binding of Fas ligand which initiates cross-linking of three receptor molecules and subsequent clustering of intracellular death domains [44]. Fas-associated death domain-containing protein (FADD) is recruited and binds to the cluster; this complex interacts with procaspase-8 through its death effector domain (DED). The resultant union of the three molecules forms the death-inducing signaling complex (DISC). Likewise, TNF-$\alpha$ binding to TNF receptor 1 results in receptor trimerization, bringing death domains nearer, and allowing TNF receptor-associated death domain-containing proteins (TRADDs) to bind to the receptor cluster via their death domains; this complex can then associate with FADD and procaspase-8 [43]. Binding of procaspase-8 via Fas or TNF receptor activation induces autocleavage and activation of caspase-8, which in turn, cleaves procaspase-3 to yield caspase-3. Caspase-3, in turn, cleaves a large number of substrates, from nuclear proteins to cytosolic structures and cytoskeletal elements, and also catalyzes the degradation of proteins crucial for neutrophil survival. Clustering of death receptors in ceramide-rich lipid rafts can also activate caspase-8 in the absence of ligand binding [45]. Intriguingly, TRADD proteins can bind TNF receptor-associated factor-2 (TRAF2) and receptor interacting protein (RIP) to activate the anti-apoptotic transcription factors, nuclear factor-kappa B (NF-κB) and activator protein (AP)-1 [43]. Since NF-κB and AP-1 commonly promote the expression of survival proteins, TNF-α has the ability to either promote or delay apoptosis [46].

Caspase-9 is the apical caspase of the intrinsic pathway, and its activation also results in activation of caspase-3 [47]. Caspase-9 is activated by stimuli that induce the release of cytochrome c from the mitochondrion, where it complexes in the cytoplasm with pro-caspase-9, and cytosolic apoptotic protease-activating factor (APAF), resulting in catalytic cleavage and activation of caspase-9 [48]; formation of this complex results in progression of apoptosis. Cytochrome c release from the mitochondrion is regulated by the levels and activities of pro-and anti-apoptotic members of the Bcl-2 family. For example, anti-apoptotic members Bcl-X and Mcl-1 are down-regulated during apoptosis [49], while pro-apoptotic members Bax, Bid, Bak, and Bad are constitutively expressed [50]. The pro-apoptotic function of these members results from their redistribution from the cytosol to the mitochondrion, resulting in disruption of mitochondrial membrane integrity and an increase in pore formation.

Constitutive neutrophil apoptosis is associated with increased mitochondrial inner membrane permeability, a reduction in mitochondrial transmembrane potential, and opening of mitochondrial permeability transition pores [51]. As a consequence, cytochrome c is released from the mitochondrion. Activation of the membrane-bound caspase, caspase-8, is also implicated in the induction of apoptosis [52].

## Inhibition of Neutrophil Apoptosis During Inflammation

Neutrophil survival is prolonged through the active inhibition of apoptosis during acute inflammation. A number of host-derived cytokines including TNF-α, IL-1β, IL-6, and granulocyte-macrophage colony-stimulating factor (GM-CSF) prolong neutrophil survival during acute inflammation (Table 2). Additionally, bacterial factors such as endotoxin, phenol-soluble modulins from S. epidermidis [53], lipotechoic acid from S. aureus [54], Escherichia coli verotoxin [55], Helicobacter pylori water-soluble surface proteins [56], and butyric acid and propionic acids from Gram-negative bacteria [57] all promote neutrophil survival. Furthermore, the process of endothelial transmigration can also signal delayed apoptosis. Endotoxin from the invading pathogen has been prominently implicated in different facets of delayed neutrophil apoptosis. TLR-1, -2, -4, -5, and -6 are present on neutrophils, and recognize a number of pathogen-specific molecular patterns [58]. TLR stimulation, in particular engagement of the LPS-receptor, TLR4 [59], delays neutrophil apoptosis. LPS induces expression of cellular inhibitor of apoptosis protein-2 (cIAP-2) resulting in accelerated degradation of caspase-3 [60]. Inhibition by LPS, or direct stimulation of TLR4, requires involvement of the PI3 kinase and Akt signaling pathways [61]; Erk and PI3 kinase/Akt signaling are necessary, but not sufficient for this delay. LPS and direct TLR4 stimulation also activate NF-κB [61]. Under normal conditions, this transcription factor is sequestered in the cytoplasm under control of its inhibitor, IκB. Stimuli that converge on the IκB kinase complex trigger phosphorylation and degradation of IκB, and expose the NF-κB nuclear localization sequence. This sequence promotes the translocation of activated NF-κB into the nucleus where it binds to consensus sites of responsive genes including genes encoding the Bcl-2 family of survival proteins, and members of the inhibitor of apoptosis proteins (IAP) family [62].

GM-CSF activates JAK-2/STAT-3 signaling pathways which upregulate cIAP-2 to delay programmed cell death in neutrophils [63], through signaling pathways involving PI3 kinase, Akt, and Erk [64]. An observed increase in levels of survival protein Mcl-1 may occur through one of two mechanisms: increased stability of the normally short-lived protein [64], or activation of the NF-κB transcription pathway [65]. GM-CSF may alternatively phosphorylate pro-apoptotic Bad at Ser-112

**Table 2.** Factors that delay neutrophil apoptosis

| |
|---|
| **Microbial Products** |
| Lipopolysaccharide (endotoxin) |
| Mannan |
| Lipoteichoic acid |
| Modulins from *S. epidermidis* |
| *E. coli* verotoxin |
| *H. pylori* surface proteins |
| Butyric acid |
| Propionic acid |
| |
| **Host-derived Mediators** |
| Interleukin-1β |
| Interleukin-2 |
| Interleukin-3 |
| Interleukin-4 |
| Interleukin-6 |
| Interleukin-8 |
| Tumor necrosis factor |
| Interferons |
| G-CSF |
| GM-CSF |
| Leptin |
| Pre-B cell colony-enhancing factor (PBEF) |
| |
| **Physiologic Processes** |
| Integrin engagement and transendothelial migration |

and Ser-136, inducing cytosolic translocation [66]. Phosphorylated Bad is unable to bind Bcl-2 and Bcl-X, with the result that apoptosis is inhibited [67]. Additionally granulocyte-colony stimulating factor (G-CSF) inhibits the translocation of pro-apoptotic Bax to mitochondria, with the result that cytochrome c release and caspase 3 activation are reduced [68]. An ROS-dependent mechanism of apoptotic delay caused by GM-CSF has also been proposed, but whether GM-CSF causes prolonged life by decreasing or increasing ROS generation is uncertain.

Other circulating factors from the inflammatory milieu that exert anti-apoptotic activity include type I and II IFNs. Both serve to upregulate cIAP-2, Mcl-1, and AP-1 via STAT-3 and JAK-2 signaling [63], and type I IFN-mediated delay occurs in a PI3 kinase-dependent manner necessitating PKC-δ and NF-κB activation [40]. Among the interleukins, IL-1β, IL-2, IL-3, IL-6, and IL-8 [69] show substantial capacity to inhibit apoptosis. A novel inflammatory cytokine, pre-B cell colony-enhancing factor (PBEF), has also been shown to play a late, but requisite, role in delayed neutrophil apoptosis, by reducing activity of caspases-3 and -8 [70]. Other pro-survival mediators associated with neutrophil longevity include C5a, fMLP, leukotriene B4 [71], and TNF-α [72], although studies of TNF-α have shown that it can both induce and inhibit apoptosis. Interestingly, downregulation of TNF-α receptors initiated during neutrophil transmigration is necessary for the delay. In fact, endothelial contact causes downregulation of all receptor-mediated apoptosis pathways, including Fas-activated cell death [73], implying that the neutrophil lifespan is determined as early as cell recruitment to the inflammatory site.

Finally, neutrophil proteins directly participating in apoptosis are differentially regulated during inflammation. Activated neutrophils display increased mitochondrial stability and diminished caspase-3 activity [74], and septic neutrophils maintain mitochondrial membrane integrity and the organelle further accumulates elevated levels of cytochrome c [75]. Caspase-3 transcription is downregulated, and caspase-9 transcription inhibited [75]. Since both mitochondria and caspases play pivotal roles in the control of cell fate, even minor perturbations of their abundance or activity in the cell can alter the expression of apoptosis.

## Activation of Neutrophil Apoptosis by Microbial Phagocytosis

In contrast to the inhibitory influences described above, bacterial phagocytosis activates neutrophil apoptosis, and reverses the cytokine-induced delay [76]. Cell death by apoptosis rather than necrosis limits local host tissue damage [50]. During apoptosis, the capacity of the neutrophil for chemotaxis, oxidative burst potential, and degranulation is lost, and cells manifest such hallmarks of apoptosis as cell shrinkage, chromatin compaction, and loss of the multilobed nuclear morphology [49].

Induction of apoptosis by bacterial ingestion appears to occur through two mechanisms: the engagement of surface death receptors [77], and the phagocytosis of opsonized pathogen targets [78]. Phagocytosis of E. coli results in the generation of ROS that have pro-apoptotic effects in neutrophils [79]. Apoptosis is also increased by immune complex or Fc-receptor-mediated phagocytosis, both of which generate ROS [79]. In fact, ROS production is crucial for both phagocytosis-induced cell death and the induction of apoptosis [80], and critical for normal clearance of neutrophils from inflammatory sites [81]. Further evidence supporting a role for ROS in inducing apoptosis lies in the upregulated expression of the pro-apoptotic Bax proteins following phagocytosis [82]; ROS can directly or indirectly modulate Bax expression [83]. However, the mechanism of the pro-apoptotic effects of ROS has yet to be defined, and a correlation between ROS production and apoptosis in phagocytosing neutrophils has not been found [84].

β2-integrins have also been implicated in phagocytosis-induced neutrophil death. Although β2-integrin engagement during endothelial transmigration delays apoptosis, β2-integrin-dependent phagocytosis promotes apoptosis by reducing activation of Akt. Patients with β2-integrin deficiency exhibit neutrophilia, suggesting that these receptors play a critical role in maintaining neutrophil homeostasis [85]. In murine peritonitis models, Mac-1 deficiency results in neutrophil accumulation and delayed neutrophil apoptosis; circulating neutrophil counts and their rates of apoptosis are normal, however, implying that Mac-1 regulation of neutrophil apoptosis is limited to inflamed tissue [80]. ROS have been associated with Mac-1-mediated phagocytosis as well, since this phagocytic pathway results in ROS production and a specific ROS threshold must be met for phagocytosis-induced apoptosis to occur [86]. Patients with chronic granulomatous disease (CGD) who lack functional NADPH oxidase show impaired phagocytosis-induced cell death [86]. Finally, caspases-8 and -3 are activated by Mac-1-dependent phagocytosis, and ROS are established requisites in caspase-8 cleavage and activation.

Neutrophil apoptosis following microbial phagocytosis is fundamental to the resolution of inflammation [2]. Oligonucleotide microarrays have identified transcriptional responses to the phagocytosis of microbes by neutrophils. Phagocytosis-induced apoptosis commences soon after pathogen ingestion [2]. Within 90 minutes of receptor-mediated phagocytosis, 256 genes undergo induction or repression; more than 30 of these genes encode proteins participating in three distinct pathways of apoptosis [87]. At 3 hours and 6 hours, gene expression analysis identified differential expression of 94 genes involved in cell fate, including upregulation of BAX, TLR2, and CASP-1 [87]; more than 20 pro-apoptotic molecules are upregulated, whereas genes encoding anti-apoptotic factors show either downregulation or no change in expression [87]. In contrast, genes encoding 133 important pro-inflammatory mediators or signal transduction molecules are downregulated during the induction of phagocytosis-induced neutrophil apoptosis, including IL-8, IL-10, C1q, and TLR-6 [2]. Thus, differential expression of genes that are central to the regulation of apoptosis plays a critical role in the resolution of inflammation, modulating both programmed cell death and pro-inflammatory capacity [2].

## The Role of the Neutrophil in Clinical Inflammation

A balance between neutrophil recruitment and removal at the site of injury or infection supports the divergent biologic imperatives of optimizing host defenses whilst minimizing host cytotoxicity. *In vivo*, disruption of apoptotic clearance contributes to sustained inflammation [88, 89], while deficiencies in apoptosis-promoting molecules such as NADPH oxidase and Mac-1 result in sustained neutrophil accumulation [80, 90, 91]. Neutrophils harvested from the systemic circulation [75] (Fig. 2), or lungs [92], of patients with sepsis show profound inhibition of apoptosis.

Neutrophils have been implicated in injury of the lung [93], liver [94] intestine [95], and kidney [96] following experimental infectious insult as well as in clinical sepsis, a state of prolonged systemic inflammation and the leading cause of death for patients in intensive care units (ICUs). Patients with sepsis exhibit widespread neutrophil infiltration of the lung [97] (Fig. 3) and distant organs [98]. Neutrophil apoptosis is profoundly inhibited in patients with sepsis [99, 100], multiple trauma and burn injury [101, 102], pancreatitis, and the acute respiratory distress syndrome (ARDS) [92]. The extent to which inappropriately prolonged neutrophil survival contributes to the expression of the multiple organ dysfunction

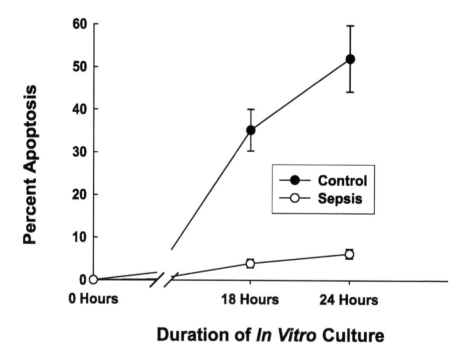

**Duration of *In Vitro* Culture**

**Fig. 2.** Neutrophils harvested from the systemic circulation of patients with sepsis show profound inhibition of the constitutive apoptotic program, with the result that survival after 24 hours of *in vitro* culture exceeds 90%. From [75] with permission

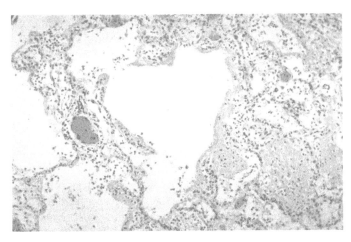

**Fig. 3.** Photomicrograph of the lung of a patient dying with acute respiratory distress syndrome (ARDS). Massive neutrophil infiltration is evident

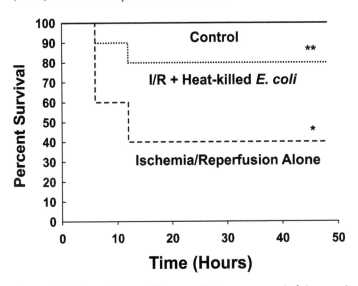

**Fig. 4.** Induction of neutrophil apoptosis improves survival in experimental intestinal ischemia/reperfusion (I/R) injury. Rats underwent laparotomy and intestinal I/R injury by occlusion of the superior mesenteric artery. Survival was 100% in sham-treated animals, but only 40% in those with intestinal I/R; pulmonary neutrophilia was prominent in these animals. Intratracheal instillation of heat-killed *E. coli* prior to intestinal I/R resulted in attenuation of neutrophilia, and a significant improvement in survival. * $p < 0.05$ vs sham-treated animals; ** $p < 0.05$ vs animals with I/R alone. From [103] with permission

syndrome is unknown. In animal models of intestinal ischemia/reperfusion injury, however, acceleration of apoptosis of neutrophils infiltrating the lung by the intra-tracheal instillation of heat-killed *E. coli* results in improved rates of survival [103] (Fig. 4).

## Conclusion

The neutrophil is a key contributor to the innate immune response. The anti-microbial activity of the neutrophil is non-selective, and so the resolution of neutrophil-mediated inflammation must be regulated to prevent tissue injury. The execution of a controlled cell death program after phagocytosis serves this dual role – resolving inflammation, and preventing damage to healthy host tissue [2]. While the process of neutrophil apoptosis is increasingly well understood, the molecular pathways involved remain incompletely characterized. A better under-standing of the processes underlying programmed cell death in neutrophils will aid in the development of therapies for treatment of neutrophil-mediated inflam-matory disease states.

A variety of therapeutic interventions have been proposed that target differing aspects of the neutrophil response to infection. Preventing neutrophil recruitment across the vascular endothelium may potentially involve the selectins, since P- and E-selectins are solely expressed on endothelial cells after induction by cy-tokines [104]. Small sized inhibitors of selectin-mediated capture and rolling are under development, and studies in a rat model show promising results with the inhibitor molecule, bimosiamose [105]. Downregulating the activation of neu-trophils through manipulation of intracellular signaling molecules, such as NF-κB or PI3 kinase, has also been proposed although, to date, no specific inhibitors have yielded efficacy in this regard [104]. Studies targeting the cytotoxic products of neutrophil activation suggest that the antioxidants vitamin C and E can reduce su-peroxide production by neutrophils in patients with anti-neutrophil cytoplasmic antibody-associated vasculitis, though further studies are necessary [106]. Finally, manipulating neutrophil apoptosis for safe disposal of neutrophils is paramount in resolving inflammation, and compounds that promote this have been identified including lipoxins [107], annexin 1 [108], and prostaglandin D2 [109]. Specifically, lipoxin B4 and 15-epi-lipoxin B4 can stimulate the removal of apoptotic neutrophils by macrophages [110].

## References

1. Segal AW (2005) How neutrophils kill microbes. Annu Rev Immunol 23:197–223
2. Kobayashi SD, Voyich JM, DeLeo FR (2003) Regulation of the neutrophil-mediated inflam-matory response to infection. Microbes Infect 5:1337–1344

3. Zlotnik A, Yoshie O (2000) Chemokines: a new classification system and their role in immunity. Immunity 12:121–127
4. DeLeo FR, Renee J, McCormick S, et al (1998) Neutrophils exposed to bacterial lipopolysaccharide upregulate NADPH oxidase assembly. J Clin Invest 101:455–463
5. Witko-Sarsat V, Rieu P, Scamps-Latscha B, Lesavre P, Halbwachs-Mecarelli L (2000) Neutrophils: molecules, functions and pathophysiological aspects. Lab Invest 80:617–653
6. Ley K (1996) Molecular mechanisms of leukocyte recruitment in the inflammatory process. Cardiovasc Res 32:733–742
7. McEver RP (1994) Selectins. Curr Opin Immunol 6:75–84
8. Varki A (1994) Selectin ligands. Proc Natl Acad Sci U S A 91:7390–7397
9. Hynes RO (1992) Integrins: versatility, modulation, and signaling in cell adhesion. Cell 69:11–25
10. Ley K, Tedder TF (1995) Leukocyte interactions with vascular endothelium. New insights into selectin-mediated attachment and rolling. J Immunol 155:525–528
11. Walcheck B, Kahn J, Fisher JM, et al (1996) Neutrophil rolling altered by inhibition of L-selectin shedding in vitro. Nature 380:720–723
12. Bargatze RF, Kurk S, Butcher EC, Jutila MA (1994) Neutrophils roll on adherent neutrophils bound to cytokine- induced endothelial cells via L-selectin on the rolling cells. J Exp Med 180:1785–1792
13. Ley K, Bullard DC, Arbones ML, et al (1995) Sequential contribution of L- and P-selectin to leukocyte rolling in vivo. J Exp Med 181:669–675
14. Nolte D, Schmid P, Jager U, et al (1994) Leukocyte rolling in venules of striated muscle and skin is mediated by P-selectin, not by L-selectin. Am J Physiol 267:H1637–H1642
15. Norman KE, Moore KL, McEver RP, Ley K (1995) Leukocyte rolling in vivo is mediated by P-selectin glycoprotein ligand-1. Blood 86:4417–4421
16. Labow MA, Norton CR, Rumberger JM, et al (1994) Characterization of E-selectin-deficient mice: demonstration of overlapping function of the endothelial selectins. Immunity 1:709–720
17. Waddell TK, Fialkow L, Chan CK, Kishimoto TK, Downey GP (1995) Signaling functions of L-selectin. Enhancement of tyrosine phosphorylation and activation of MAP kinase. J Biol Chem 270:15403–15411
18. Smolen JE, Petersen TK, Koch C, et al (2000) L- selectin signaling of neutrophil adhesion and degranulation involves p38 mitogen-activated protein kinase. J Biol Chem 275:15876–15884
19. Anderson DC, Springer TA (1987) Leukocyte adhesion deficiency: an inherited defect in the Mac-1, LFA-1, and p150,95 glycoproteins. Annu Rev Med 38:175–194
20. Wilson RW, Ballantyne CM, Smith CW, et al (1993) Gene targeting yields a CD18-mutant mouse for study of inflammation. J Immunol 151:1571–1578
21. Hentzen ER, Neelamegham S, Kansas GS, et al (2000) Sequential binding of CD11a/CD18 and CD11b/CD18 defines neutrophil capture and stable adhesion to intercellular adhesion molecule-1. Blood 95:911–920
22. Rochon YP, Kavanagh TJ, Harlan JM (2000) Analysis of integrin (CD11b/CD18) movement during neutrophil adhesion and migration on endothelial cells. J Microsc 197 ( Pt 1):15–24
23. Del MA, Zanetti A, Corada M, et al (1996) Polymorphonuclear leukocyte adhesion triggers the disorganization of endothelial cell-to-cell adherens junctions. J Cell Biol 135:497–510
24. Feng D, Nagy JA, Pyne K, Dvorak HF, Dvorak AM (1998) Neutrophils emigrate from venules by a transendothelial cell pathway in response to FMLP. J Exp Med 187:903–915
25. Chosay JG, Fisher MA, Farhood A, Ready KA, Dunn CJ, Jaeschke H (1998) Role of PECAM-1 (CD31) in neutrophil transmigration in murine models of liver and peritoneal inflammation. Am J Physiol 274:G776–G782
26. Chavakis T, Keiper T, Matz-Westphal R, et al (2004) The junctional adhesion molecule-C promotes neutrophil transendothelial migration in vitro and in vivo. J Biol Chem 279:55602–55608

27. Kurt-Jones EA, Mandell L, Whitney C, et al (2002) Role of toll-like receptor 2 (TLR2) in neutrophil activation: GM- CSF enhances TLR2 expression and TLR2-mediated interleukin 8 responses in neutrophils. Blood 100:1860–1868
28. Brinkmann V, Reichard U, Goosmann C, et al (2004) Neutrophil extracellular traps kill bacteria. Science 303:1532–1535
29. Lee WL, Harrison RE, Grinstein S (2003) Phagocytosis by neutrophils. Microbes Infect 5:1299–1306
30. Stendahl O, Krause KH, Krischer J, et al (1994) Redistribution of intracellular Ca2+ stores during phagocytosis in human neutrophils. Science 265:1439–1441
31. Lundqvist-Gustafsson H, Gustafsson M, Dahlgren C (2000) Dynamic ca(2+)changes in neutrophil phagosomes A source for intracellular ca(2+)during phagolysosome formation? Cell Calcium 27:353–362
32. Peters C, Mayer A (1998) Ca2+/calmodulin signals the completion of docking and triggers a late step of vacuole fusion. Nature 396:575–580
33. Korchak HM, Rossi MW, Kilpatrick LE (1998) Selective role for beta-protein kinase C in signaling for O-2 generation but not degranulation or adherence in differentiated HL60 cells. J Biol Chem 273:27292–27299
34. Mohn H, Le C, V, Fischer S, Maridonneau-Parini I (1995) The src-family protein-tyrosine kinase p59hck is located on the secretory granules in human neutrophils and translocates towards the phagosome during cell activation. Biochem J 309 ( Pt 2):657–665
35. Shao D, Segal AW, Dekker LV (2003) Lipid rafts determine efficiency of NADPH oxidase activation in neutrophils. FEBS Lett 550:101–106
36. Burg ND, Pillinger MH (2001) The neutrophil: function and regulation in innate and humoral immunity. Clin Immunol 99:7–17
37. Ishikawa F, Miyazaki S (2005) New biodefense strategies by neutrophils. Arch Immunol Ther Exp (Warsz ) 53:226–233
38. Kimura Y, Yokoi-Hayashi K (1996) Polymorphonuclear leukocyte lysosomal proteases, cathepsins B and D affect the fibrinolytic system in human umbilical vein endothelial cells. Biochim Biophys Acta 1310:1–4
39. Cowburn AS, Deighton J, Walmsley SR, Chilvers ER (2004) The survival effect of TNF-alpha in human neutrophils is mediated via NF-kappa B-dependent IL-8 release. Eur J Immunol 34:1733–1743
40. Wang K, Scheel-Toellner D, Wong SH, et al (2003) Inhibition of neutrophil apoptosis by type 1 IFN depends on cross-talk between phosphoinositol 3-kinase, protein kinase C-delta, and NF-kappa B signaling pathways. J Immunol 171:1035–1041
41. Fadeel B, Kagan VE (2003) Apoptosis and macrophage clearance of neutrophils: regulation by reactive oxygen species. Redox Rep 8:143–150
42. Haslett C (1992) Resolution of acute inflammation and the role of apoptosis in the tissue fate of granulocytes. Clin Sci (Lond) 83:639–648
43. Ashkenazi A, Dixit VM (1998) Death receptors: signaling and modulation. Science 281:1305–1308
44. Akgul C, Edwards SW (2003) Regulation of neutrophil apoptosis via death receptors. Cell Mol Life Sci 60:2402- 2408
45. Scheel-Toellner D, Wang K, Assi LK, et al (2004) Clustering of death receptors in lipid rafts initiates neutrophil spontaneous apoptosis. Biochem Soc Trans 32:679- 681
46. Ward C, Chilvers ER, Lawson MF, et al (1999) NF-kappaB activation is a critical regulator of human granulocyte apoptosis in vitro. J Biol Chem 274:4309–4318
47. Weinmann P, Gaehtgens P, Walzog B (1999) Bcl-Xl- and Bax-alpha-mediated regulation of apoptosis of human neutrophils via caspase-3. Blood 93:3106–3115
48. Li P, Nijhawan D, Budihardjo I, et al (1997) Cytochrome c and dATP-dependent formation of Apaf-1/caspase- 9 complex initiates an apoptotic protease cascade. Cell 91:479–489
49. Moulding DA, Quayle JA, Hart CA, Edwards SW (1998) Mcl- 1 expression in human neutrophils: regulation by cytokines and correlation with cell survival. Blood 92:2495–2502

50. Akgul C, Moulding DA, Edwards SW (2001) Molecular control of neutrophil apoptosis. FEBS Lett 487:318–322
51. Green DR, Reed JC (1998) Mitochondria and apoptosis. Science 281:1309–1312
52. Liles WC, Kiener PA, Ledbetter JA, Aruffo A, Klebanoff SJ (1996) Differential expression of Fas (CD95) and Fas ligand on normal human phagocytes: Implications for the regulation of apoptosis in neutrophils. J Exp Med 184:429- 440
53. Liles WC, Thomsen AR, O'Mahony DS, Klebanoff SJ (2001) Stimulation of human neutrophils and monocytes by staphylococcal phenol-soluble modulin. J Leukoc Biol 70:96-102
54. Lotz S, Aga E, Wilde I, et al (2004) Highly purified lipoteichoic acid activates neutrophil granulocytes and delays their spontaneous apoptosis via CD14 and TLR2. J Leukoc Biol 75:467–477
55. Liu J, Akahoshi T, Sasahana T, et al (1999) Inhibition of neutrophil apoptosis by verotoxin 2 derived from Escherichia coli O157:H7. Infect Immun 67:6203–6205
56. Kim JS, Kim JM, Jung HC, Song IS, Kim CY (2001) Inhibition of apoptosis in human neutrophils by Helicobacter pylori water-soluble surface proteins. Scand J Gastroenterol 36:589–600
57. Stehle HW, Leblebicioglu B, Walters JD (2001) Short- chain carboxylic acids produced by gram-negative anaerobic bacteria can accelerate or delay polymorphonuclear leukocyte apoptosis in vitro. J Periodontol 72:1059–1063
58. Takeda K, Akira S (2004) Microbial recognition by Toll- like receptors. J Dermatol Sci 34:73–82
59. Sabroe I, Prince LR, Jones EC, et al (2003) Selective roles for Toll-like receptor (TLR)2 and TLR4 in the regulation of neutrophil activation and life span. J Immunol 170:5268–5275
60. Mica L, Harter L, Trentz O, Keel M (2004) Endotoxin reduces CD95-induced neutrophil apoptosis by cIAP-2- mediated caspase-3 degradation. J Am Coll Surg 199:595–602
61. Francois S, El BJ, Dang PM, Pedruzzi E, Gougerot- Pocidalo MA, Elbim C (2005) Inhibition of neutrophil apoptosis by TLR agonists in whole blood: involvement of the phosphoinositide 3-kinase/Akt and NF-kappaB signaling pathways, leading to increased levels of Mcl-1, A1, and phosphorylated Bad. J Immunol 174:3633–3642
62. Ward C, Walker A, Dransfield I, Haslett C, Rossi AG (2004) Regulation of granulocyte apoptosis by NF-kappaB. Biochem Soc Trans 32:465–467
63. Sakamoto E, Hato F, Kato T, et al (2005) Type I and type II interferons delay human neutrophil apoptosis via activation of STAT3 and up-regulation of cellular inhibitor of apoptosis 2. J Leukoc Biol 78:301–309
64. Derouet M, Thomas L, Cross A, Moots RJ, Edwards SW (2004) Granulocyte macrophage colony-stimulating factor signaling and proteasome inhibition delay neutrophil apoptosis by increasing the stability of Mcl-1. J Biol Chem 279:26915–26921
65. Watson RW, Rotstein OD, Parodo J, Bitar R, Marshall JC (1998) The IL-1 beta-converting enzyme (caspase-1) inhibits apoptosis of inflammatory neutrophils through activation of IL-1 beta. J Immunol 161:957–962
66. Cowburn AS, Cadwallader KA, Reed BJ, Farahi N, Chilvers ER (2002) Role of PI3-kinase-dependent Bad phosphorylation and altered transcription in cytokine- mediated neutrophil survival. Blood 100:2607–2616
67. Downward J (1999) How BAD phosphorylation is good for survival. Nat Cell Biol 1:E33–E35
68. Maianski NA, Mul FP, van Buul JD, Roos D, Kuijpers TW (2002) Granulocyte colony-stimulating factor inhibits the mitochondria-dependent activation of caspase-3 in neutrophils. Blood 99:672–679
69. Hofman P (2004) Molecular regulation of neutrophil apoptosis and potential targets for therapeutic strategy against the inflammatory process. Curr Drug Targets Inflamm Allergy 3:1–9
70. Jia SH, Li Y, Parodo J, et al (2004) Pre-B cell colony- enhancing factor inhibits neutrophil apoptosis in experimental inflammation and clinical sepsis. J Clin Invest 113:1318–1327

71. Lee E, Lindo T, Jackson N, et al (1999) Reversal of human neutrophil survival by leukotriene B(4) receptor blockade and 5-lipoxygenase and 5-lipoxygenase activating protein inhibitors. Am J Respir Crit Care Med 160:2079–2085
72. van den Berg JM, Weyer S, Weening JJ, Roos D, Kuijpers TW (2001) Divergent effects of tumor necrosis factor alpha on apoptosis of human neutrophils. J Leukoc Biol 69:467–473
73. Tennenberg SD, Finkenauer R, Wang T (2002) Endothelium down-regulates Fas, TNF, and TRAIL-induced neutrophil apoptosis. Surg Infect (Larchmt ) 3:351–357
74. Watson RW, O'Neill A, Brannigen AE, et al (1999) Regulation of Fas antibody induced neutrophil apoptosis is both caspase and mitochondrial dependent. FEBS Lett 453:67- 71
75. Taneja R, Parodo J, Jia SH, Kapus A, Rotstein OD, Marshall JC (2004) Delayed neutrophil apoptosis in sepsis is associated with maintenance of mitochondrial transmembrane potential and reduced caspase-9 activity. Crit Care Med 32:1460–1469
76. Watson RW, Redmond HP, Wang JH, Bouchier-Hayes D (1996) Bacterial ingestion, tumor necrosis factor-alpha, and heat induce programmed cell death in activated neutrophils. Shock 5:47–51
77. Ward C, Dransfield I, Chilvers ER, Haslett C, Rossi AG (1999) Pharmacological manipulation of granulocyte apoptosis: potential therapeutic targets. Trends Pharmacol Sci 20:503–509
78. Watson RW, Redmond HP, Wang JH, Condron C, Bouchier-Hayes D (1996) Neutrophils undergo apoptosis following ingestion of Escherichia coli. J Immunol 156:3986–3992
79. Schettini J, Salamone G, Trevani A, et al (2002) Stimulation of neutrophil apoptosis by immobilized IgA. J Leukoc Biol 72:685–691
80. Coxon A, Rieu P, Barkalow FJ, et al (1996) A novel role for the beta 2 integrin CD11b/CD18 in neutrophil apoptosis: a homeostatic mechanism in inflammation. Immunity 5:653–666
81. Hampton MB, Vissers MC, Keenan JI, Winterbourn CC (2002) Oxidant-mediated phosphatidylserine exposure and macrophage uptake of activated neutrophils: possible impairment in chronic granulomatous disease. J Leukoc Biol 71:775–781
82. Kobayashi SD, Braughton KR, Whitney AR, et al (2003) Bacterial pathogens modulate an apoptosis differentiation program in human neutrophils. Proc Natl Acad Sci U S A 100:10948–10953
83. Kobayashi SD, Voyich JM, Braughton KR, et al (2004) Gene expression profiling provides insight into the pathophysiology of chronic granulomatous disease. J Immunol 172:636–643
84. Yamamoto A, Taniuchi S, Tsuji S, Hasui M, Kobayashi Y (2002) Role of reactive oxygen species in neutrophil apoptosis following ingestion of heat-killed Staphylococcus aureus. Clin Exp Immunol 129:479–484
85. Wehrle-Haller B, Imhof BA (2003) Integrin-dependent pathologies. J Pathol 200:481–487
86. Zhang B, Hirahashi J, Cullere X, Mayadas TN (2003) Elucidation of molecular events leading to neutrophil apoptosis following phagocytosis: cross-talk between caspase 8, reactive oxygen species, and MAPK/ERK activation. J Biol Chem 278:28443–28454
87. Kobayashi SD, Voyich JM, Buhl CL, Stahl RM, DeLeo FR (2002) Global changes in gene expression by human polymorphonuclear leukocytes during receptor-mediated phagocytosis: cell fate is regulated at the level of gene expression. Proc Natl Acad Sci U S A 99:6901–6906
88. Vandivier RW, Fadok VA, Hoffmann PR, et al (2002) Elastase-mediated phosphatidylserine receptor cleavage impairs apoptotic cell clearance in cystic fibrosis and bronchiectasis. J Clin Invest 109:661–670
89. Teder P, Vandivier RW, Jiang D, et al (2002) Resolution of lung inflammation by CD44. Science 296:155- 158
90. Rowe SJ, Allen L, Ridger VC, Hellewell PG, Whyte MK (2002) Caspase-1-deficient mice have delayed neutrophil apoptosis and a prolonged inflammatory response to lipopolysaccharide-induced acute lung injury. J Immunol 169:6401–6407
91. Segal BH, Kuhns DB, Ding L, Gallin JI, Holland SM (2002) Thioglycollate peritonitis in mice lacking C5, 5- lipoxygenase, or p47(phox): complement, leukotrienes, and reactive oxidants in acute inflammation. J Leukoc Biol 71:410–416
92. Matute-Bello G, Liles WC, Radella F, et al (1997) Neutrophil apoptosis in the acute respiratory distress syndrome. Am J Respir Crit Care Med 156:1969–1977

93. Abraham E (2003) Neutrophils and acute lung injury. Crit Care Med 31:S195–S199
94. Ho JS, Buchweitz JP, Roth RA, Ganey PE (1996) Identification of factors from rat neutrophils responsible for cytotoxicity to isolated hepatocytes. J Leukoc Biol 59:716–724
95. Kubes P, Hunter J, Granger DN (1992) Ischemia/reperfusion-induced feline intestinal dysfunction: importance of granulocyte recruitment. Gastroenterology 103:807–812
96. Lowell CA, Berton G (1998) Resistance to endotoxic shock and reduced neutrophil migration in mice deficient for the Src-family kinases Hck and Fgr. Proc Natl Acad Sci U S A 95:7580–7584
97. Steinberg KP, Milberg JA, Martin TR, Maunder RJ, Cockrill BA, Hudson LD (1994) Evolution of bronchoalveolar cell populations in the adult respiratory distress syndrome. Am J Respir Crit Care Med 150:113–122
98. Goris RJ, te Boekhorst TP, Nuytinck JK, Gimbrere JS (1985) Multiple-organ failure. Generalized autodestructive inflammation? Arch Surg 120:1109–1115
99. Jimenez MF, Watson RW, Parodo J, et al (1997) Dysregulated expression of neutrophil apoptosis in the systemic inflammatory response syndrome. Arch Surg 132:1263- 1269
100. Keel M, Ungethum U, Steckholzer U, et al (1997) Interleukin-10 counterregulates proinflammatory cytokine- induced inhibition of neutrophil apoptosis during severe sepsis. Blood 90:3356–3363
101. Chitnis D, Dickerson C, Munster AM, Winchurch RA (1996) Inhibition of apoptosis in polymorphonuclear neutrophils from burn patients. J Leukoc Biol 59:835–839
102. Ertel W, Keel M, Infanger M, Ungethum U, Steckholzer U, Trentz O (1998) Circulating mediators in serum of injured patients with septic complications inhibit neutrophil apoptosis through up-regulation of protein- tyrosine phosphorylation. J Trauma 44:767–775
103. Sookhai S, Wang JJ, McCourt M, Kirwan W, Bouchier-Hayes D, Redmond HP (2002) A novel therapeutic strategy for attenuating neutrophil-mediated lung injury in vivo. Ann Surg 235:285–291
104. Morgan MD, Harper L, Lu X, Nash G, Williams J, Savage CO (2005) Can neutrophils be manipulated in vivo? Rheumatology (Oxford) 44:597–601
105. Onai Y, Suzuki J, Nishiwaki Y, et al (2003) Blockade of cell adhesion by a small molecule selectin antagonist attenuates myocardial ischemia/reperfusion injury. Eur J Pharmacol 481:217–225
106. Harper L, Nuttall SL, Martin U, Savage CO (2002) Adjuvant treatment of patients with antineutrophil cytoplasmic antibody-associated vasculitis with vitamins E and C reduces superoxide production by neutrophils. Rheumatology (Oxford) 41:274–278
107. Goh J, Godson C, Brady HR, Macmathuna P (2003) Lipoxins: pro-resolution lipid mediators in intestinal inflammation. Gastroenterology 124:1043–1054
108. Perretti M, Flower RJ (2004) Annexin 1 and the biology of the neutrophil. J Leukoc Biol 76:25–29
109. Gilroy DW, Colville-Nash PR, McMaster S, Sawatzky DA, Willoughby DA, Lawrence T (2003) Inducible cyclooxygenase- derived 15-deoxy(Delta)12-14PGJ2 brings about acute inflammatory resolution in rat pleurisy by inducing neutrophil and macrophage apoptosis. FASEB J 17:2269–2271
110. Mitchell S, Thomas G, Harvey K, et al (2002) Lipoxins, aspirin-triggered epi-lipoxins, lipoxin stable analogues, and the resolution of inflammation: stimulation of macrophage phagocytosis of apoptotic neutrophils in vivo. J Am Soc Nephrol 13:2497–2507
111. Marshall JC (2005) Neutrophils in the pathogenesis of sepsis. Crit Care Med 33:S502–S505

# The Role of the Macrophage

J. Pugin

## Introduction

Ilia Metchnikoff made the first description of macrophages and their function in innate immunity at the end of the 19th century, and was awarded the Nobel Prize in 1908 for this discovery. Macrophages are phagocytic cells of myeloid lineage that originate from circulating monocytes and have transmigrated into tissues. They are present in virtually all tissues of the body where they carry out essential functions in maintaining normal homeostasis but also participate in pathological conditions [1]. Tissue macrophages are responsible for the non-inflammatory clearance of dying cells and debris [2]. Macrophages also sense their surrounding milieu for the presence of unusual stresses and/or the presence of non-self molecules and micro-organisms, recognized as dangerous to the body [3]. The engagement and activation of macrophages lead to responses that are typical of innate immunity, such as the rapid generation of an inflammatory response, and they also play a role as efficient effectors for the clearance of microorganisms [1]. Macrophages are also important in communicating with the adaptive arm of immunity, either as macrophages or as monocyte- or macrophage-derived dendritic cells [3]. They also participate in the presentation of non-self antigens to lymphocytes and secrete mediators, boosting adaptive immune responses. Finally, macrophages play a key role in wound healing and tissue repair, and possess natural tumoricidal activity.

## Origin of Tissue Macrophages

Circulating monocytes originate from myeloid bone marrow progenitors after a differentiation process under the control of cytokines and growth factors, particularly the stem cell factor, macrophage colony stimulating factor (M-CSF), and interleukin (IL)-3 [1]. Two different monocyte subpopulations are found in the circulation, recognizable by their expression of certain chemokine receptors and L-selectins [1]. The first population naturally migrates into tissue where they can settle for several months up to years, and acquire tissue specificity as resident peritoneal macrophages, alveolar macrophages, Kupffer cells, or microglial cells). Alternatively, under the control of cytokines and growth factors (essentially IL-4 and granulocyte-macrophage colony stimulating factor [GM-CSF]), monocytes can also transform into undifferentiated dendritic cells, such as Langerhans cells in the skin [3]. These cells will eventually migrate to lymphoid organs and become 'professional antigen-presenting cells' after adequate stimulation. Another phenotypically distinct monocyte sub-population can be recruited to tissues during inflammatory processes [1]. The recruitment process involves a series of precise mechanisms (specific chemokines of the CC family) and upregulation of leukocyte-endothelial adhesion molecules [4]. Such adhesion molecules are, at least in part, different under constitutive conditions compared to those involved in inflammation-induced trafficking of monocytes to tissues. The tissue microenvironment is key to the differentiation of the macrophage into a tissue-specific cell. The end-function of a hepatic Kupffer cell will be markedly different from that of a microglial cell or an alveolar macrophage, for example. The level of activation of these sentinel cells is also determined by the local balance between activator and de-activator cytokines (such as interferon [IFN]γ and IL-10, respectively). These mediators originate principally from epithelial cells and other cell populations of adaptive immunity in the surrounding tissue.

## Macrophages Express an Armada of Receptors

One of the major functions of the macrophage is to sense molecules and physical stresses in their microenvironment, in order to recognize the presence of foreign molecules [3]. Macrophages express a wide variety of receptors of innate immunity that recognize generally conserved microbial molecules. For example, they express high levels of CD14, a glycosyl-phosphatidylinositol glycoprotein, which binds several pathogen-associated molecular patterns (PAMPs), such as lipopolysaccharide (LPS), peptidoglycan, lipopeptides, mycobacterial lipoarabinomannan, and double-stranded RNA [5,6]. It is believed that CD14 'concentrates' microbial molecules at the macrophage surface allowing interactions with signaling receptors such as Toll-like receptors (TLRs). CD14 also enhances endocytosis of PAMPs and phagocytosis of osponized bacteria and yeasts [7]. The scavenger, complement, beta-glucan, mannose, and Fc receptors are among the receptors important for the clearance of microbial products. Importantly, although macrophages are capable of ingesting bacteria, this is performed more efficiently by another myeloid cell, the polymorphonuclear neutrophil, or PMN. Conversely, monocyte/macrophages are by far the best producers of inflammatory mediators in the body. Among the various monocyte/macrophage products are pro-inflammatory cytokines (tumor necrosis factor [TNF], IL-1, IL-6, macrophage migration inhibitory factor [MIF]), anti-inflammatory cytokines (IL-4, IL-10, IL-13, transforming growth factor [TGF]-β); chemokines (IL-8), growth factors (G-CSF), anti-microbial peptides (defensins, cathelicidins), lipid mediators (prostanoids, leukotrienes, platelet-activating factor [PAF]), oxygen and nitrogen radicals, and enzymes (lipases, proteases) [1].

## Role of Macrophages as Sentinel Cells

Although specific roles can be attributed to subclasses of macrophages depending on their location in various organs, a common feature of the macrophage is its sentinel role. They sense various noxious stimuli in their environment and elicit responses depending on the nature of the stimulus. In addition to microbial products, it has been shown that macrophages react to stimuli typical of tissue injury or stress, such as acidosis, extracellular ATP, tissue hypoxia, cell stretching, substance P, high mobility group box protein (HMGB)-1, uric acid, and proteolytic enzymes, including thrombin (Fig. 1). Compared with bacterial products, the magnitude of the macrophage activation is usually not as great with these latter stimuli. This introduces the important concept that these stimuli are sensed as 'danger signals' by macrophages. They may be considered as warning signs of tissue and cellular injury or dysfunction, and indicate that a foreign intruder, such as bacteria, might be dangerous [8,9]. The host should then be mounting an inflammatory reaction and an immune response. Synergistic responses between danger signals and bacterial molecules have been demonstrated both in animal and in *in vitro* studies. These effects could be the result of a synergism between transcription factors at the level of the promoter region of macrophage pro-inflammatory genes. It has also been demonstrated recently that danger signals induce the assembly of a cytoplasmic inflammasome, recruiting and activating caspase-1 [10–12]. This results in a massive increase in the production of the very potent local pro-inflammatory molecule, IL-1β.

The tissue macrophage is also believed to play a significant role in the pathogenesis of ventilator-induced lung injury (VILI), and possibly in the subsequent remote organ dysfunction [13,14]. The only perceptible effect of positive pressure mechanical ventilation, when applied to normal lungs with 'reasonable' volumes, is the recruitment of alveolar macrophages, dependent on the lung production of monocyte chemoattractant protein (MCP)-1 [15]. In these experiments, alveolar macrophages are primed by the mechanical stimulus to increase their cytoplasmic concentration of pro-inflammatory cytokine mRNAs, but do not secrete the proteins. It is only with a second hit, such as the presence of bacteria, for example, that they will respond with a rapid and massive local pro-inflammatory response, and a possible systemic spillover of mediators [16]. In many animal models, bacterial sepsis becomes lethal only when associated with burns, trauma, cerebral hemorrhage, aggressive mechanical ventilation, or hypovolemic shock. This leads to the concept of synergistic effects of noxious stimuli, and the necessity for two hits on the macrophage to observe a full-blown, clinically relevant inflammatory response plus end-organ dysfunction.

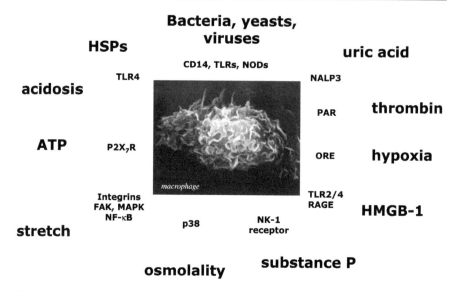

**Fig. 1.** Macrophages sense and are activated by molecules from the microbial world and by 'danger' signals from tissue injury. TLR: Toll-like receptor; NOD: nucleotide-binding oligomerization domain proteins; NALP: NACHT-, LRR- and pyrin domain (PYD)-containing proteins; PAR: protease-activated receptor; ORE: oxygen-responding element; RAGE: receptor for advanced glycation endproducts; NK-1: neurokinin-1; FAK: focal adhesion kinase; MAPK: mitogen activated protein kinase; NF-kB: nuclear factor-kappa B; P2X7R: purinergic P2X7 receptor; HSP: heat shock protein; HMGB-1: high-mobility group box-1 protein

## Macrophages Play a Central Role in the Pathogenesis of Sepsis

Because of their involvement in innate immunity, it is not a surprise that macrophages play a critical role in bacterial sepsis and in subsequent organ dysfunction. It is believed that excessive macrophage-induced inflammation is responsible for the loss of some organ functions, such as gas exchange in the lung [17]. Activated lung macrophages produce large amounts of pro-inflammatory cytokines, such as TNF and IL-1. In turn, these cytokines will stimulate pneumocytes and capillary endothelial cells to generate a strong chemokine gradient and recruit PMNs to the interstitium and the airspace [18]. In addition to its sentinel role, the macrophage plays a crucial role as an amplifier of the inflammatory and immune response. This inflammatory response is necessary for rapid and efficient clearance of a bacterial infection, but when such a response is excessive, it may become detrimental to lung integrity and function. Interestingly, neutrophilic infiltration in the lung (but also in some cases in the pleural space and the peritoneum) is not observed in other organs during severe sepsis and septic shock. Inflammatory cells are, for example, absent in the liver, the kidney, the central nervous system (CNS), or the gut despite evident dysfunction of these organs during bacterial sepsis [19]. Gut translocation of bacteria is not accompanied by massive hepatic (neutrophilic) inflammation, but drives an acute phase response, that is essentially dependent on macrophage IL-6 production [20]. In addition, Kupffer cells play an essential role in clearing bacteria and bacterial products from the portal circulation without generating a massive hepatic inflammatory reaction. This shows that the function of tissue macrophages depends on the organ involved, and that the Kupffer cell reaction to bacteria, for example, is markedly different from what is observed with alveolar macrophages.

Monocytes in the vascular compartment are also activated during bacterial sepsis. Interestingly, circulating monocytes are 'reprogrammed' and produce more anti-inflammatory mediators (IL-10, IL-1 receptor antagonist [IL-1ra], IL-4) than pro-inflammatory cytokines [21]. When stimulated *ex vivo*, monocytes from critically ill patients, and particularly from septic patients, have defective pro-inflammatory responses. The net inflammatory activity in septic plasma is in fact *anti-inflammatory* [17,22,23]. This systemic anti-inflammatory response may prevent excessive, non-specific, and deleterious systemic endothelial and leukocyte activation where it is unwanted, i.e., in the vascular compartment [22]. It may, therefore, help modulate effector leukocytes and focus inflammation at the infected site [22]. In addition, decreased surface expression of major histocompatibility complex (MHC) class II antigens, such as human leukocyte antigen (HLA)-DR, on the surface of circulating monocytes from patients with sepsis has been reported by several groups. This is mainly due to an IL-10-dependent sequestration of MHC class II molecules intracellularly [24], and is associated with poor outcome in patients with septic shock [25]. It remains unclear as to whether this phenotype persists in tissue macrophages after monocyte migration, and whether it is associated with impaired antigen presentation in monocyte-derived macrophages and dendritic cells.

Activation of coagulation and decreased fibrinolysis are important pathways in the pathogenesis of sepsis and related organ dysfunction [26,27]. This has recently been highlighted by the PROWESS trial showing that a recombinant form of activated protein C improved survival in patients with severe sepsis and septic shock [28]. During sepsis, coagulation is activated both in the vascular compartment (disseminated intravascular coagulation [DIC]) and in (some) organs, such as the alveolar compartment of the lung. The 'aberrant' expression of tissue factor is key to the initiation of DIC and in-organ coagulation [29]. Tissue factor is upregulated in monocytes and macrophages – but also in endothelial cells – after exposition to bacteria, bacterial products, and pro- inflammatory cytokines, and is responsible for the observed increased in "procoagulant activity" [29, 30]. Local and systemic inhibition of the fibrinolytic pathway, mainly dependent on the plasminogen-activation inhibitor (PAI)-1 protein may also participate in increased procoagulant activity during sepsis. PAI-1 is produced by activated monocyte/macrophages, among many other cell types [31]. Finally, monocytic cells express protease-activated receptors (PARs), which are receptors for serine proteases, such as thrombin. These receptors, at the interface of inflammation and coagulation pathways, can modulate the inflammatory response of monocytes and tissue macrophages [32–34].

It has recently been suggested that vagus nerve stimulation attenuates macrophage activation [35–37], as part of the newly discovered cholinergic anti-inflammatory pathway [38]. The acetylcholine α7-nicotinic receptor seems to be essential to modulate macrophage activation during sepsis [39].

Finally, although macrophages are involved in tissue remodeling and repair in various illnesses, this has been poorly studied in sepsis and related-organ dysfunction. Conceptually, macrophages are likely to play an important role in the resolution phase of sepsis and organ failure.

## Macrophage Products and Receptors: Therapeutic Targets?

Even though therapeutic strategies based on the systemic blockade of monocyte/macrophage-derived pro-inflammatory mediators have failed in the past, considerable interest still exists in developing modulators of macrophage function as potential therapies in sepsis and related organ dysfunction. TNF and IL-1 blockade in the lung has not been completely explored in sepsis-associated acute lung injury (ALI) or acute respiratory distress syndrome (ARDS), for example, despite ample demonstration that an intense pro-inflammatory reaction takes place in the lungs during sepsis. Blockade of late mediators associated with mortality in pre-clinical models of sepsis, such as HMGB-1, is also a valuable hypothesis to be tested [40, 41]. There may still be room in early septic shock for interventions that are directed to receptors recognizing bacterial products, but not interfering with bacterial clearance, such as TLRs [42]. Alternatively, therapies aimed at boosting the depressed immune functions of septic monocyte/macrophages, such as IFNγ and GM-CSF, have also been recently proposed and tested in small numbers of patients [43, 44]. Finally, therapeutic studies based on modulation of the macrophage α7 nicotinic receptor or triggering receptor expressed on myeloid cells (TREM)-1 are also underway [45].

## References

1. Cavaillon JM, Adib-Conquy M (2005) Monocytes/macrophages and sepsis. Crit Care Med 33 (12 Suppl):S506–509
2. Savill J (1998) Apoptosis. Phagocytic docking without shocking. Nature 392:442–443
3. Woodhead VE, Binks MH, Chain BM, Katz DR (1998) From sentinel to messenger: an extended phenotypic analysis of the monocyte to dendritic cell transition. Immunology 94:552–559
4. Muller WA, Randolph GJ (1999) Migration of leukocytes across endothelium and beyond: molecules involved in the transmigration and fate of monocytes. J Leukoc Biol 66:698–704
5. Pugin J, Heumann ID, Tomasz A, et al (1994) CD14 is a pattern recognition receptor. Immunity 1:509–516
6. Lee HK, Dunzendorfer S, Soldau K, Tobias PS (2006) Double- stranded RNA-mediated TLR3 activation is enhanced by CD14. Immunity 24:153–163

7. Poussin C, Foti M, Carpentier JL, Pugin J (1998) CD14- dependent endotoxin internalization via a macropinocytic pathway. J Biol Chem 273:20285–20291
8. Matzinger P (1994) Tolerance, danger, and the extended family. Annu Rev Immunol 12:991–1045
9. Matzinger P (2002)The danger model: a renewed sense of self. Science 296:301–305
10. Petrilli V, Papin S, Tschopp J (2005) The inflammasome. Curr Biol 15:R581
11. Martinon F, Petrilli V, Mayor A, Tardivel A, Tschopp J (2006) Gout-associated uric acid crystals activate the NALP3 inflammasome. Nature 440:237–241
12. Mariathasan S, Weiss DS, Newton K, et al (2006) Cryopyrin activates the inflammasome in response to toxins and ATP. Nature 440:228–232
13. Dunn I, Pugin J (1999) Mechanical ventilation of various human lung cells in vitro: identification of the macrophage as the main producer of inflammatory mediators. Chest 116 (Suppl 1):95S–97S
14. Pugin J, Dunn I, Jolliet P, et al (1998) Activation of human macrophages by mechanical ventilation in vitro. Am J Physiol 275:L1040–L1050
15. Bregeon F, Roch A, Delpierre S, et al (2002) Conventional mechanical ventilation of healthy lungs induced pro- inflammatory cytokine gene transcription. Respir Physiol Neurobiol 132:191–203
16. Bregeon F, Delpierre S, Chetaille B, et al (2005) Mechanical ventilation affects lung function and cytokine production in an experimental model of endotoxemia. Anesthesiology 102:331–339
17. Pugin J, Verghese G, Widmer MC, Matthay MA (1999) The alveolar space is the site of intense inflammatory and profibrotic reactions in the early phase of acute respiratory distress syndrome. Crit Care Med 27:304–312
18. Goodman RB, Pugin J, Lee JS, Matthay MA (2003) Cytokine- mediated inflammation in acute lung injury. Cytokine Growth Factor Rev 14:523–535
19. Hotchkiss RS, Swanson PE, Freeman BD, et al (1999) Apoptotic cell death in patients with sepsis, shock, and multiple organ dysfunction. Crit Care Med 27: 1230–1251
20. Koo DJ, Chaudry IH, Wang P (1999) Kupffer cells are responsible for producing inflammatory cytokines and hepatocellular dysfunction during early sepsis. J Surg Res 83:151–157.
21. Cavaillon JM, Adrie C, Fitting C, Adib-Conquy M (2005) Reprogramming of circulatory cells in sepsis and SIRS. J Endotoxin Res 11:311–320
22. Munford RS, Pugin J (2001) Normal responses to injury prevent systemic inflammation and can be immunosuppressive. Am J Respir Crit Care Med 163:316–321
23. Dugernier TL, Laterre PF, Wittebole X, et al (2003) Compartmentalization of the inflammatory response during acute pancreatitis: correlation with local and systemic complications. Am J Respir Crit Care Med 168:148–157
24. Fumeaux T, Pugin J (2002) Role of interleukin-10 in the intracellular sequestration of human leukocyte antigen-DR in monocytes during septic shock. Am J Respir Crit Care Med 166:1475–1482
25. Monneret G, Lepape A, Voirin N, et al (2006) Persisting low monocyte human leukocyte antigen-DR expression predicts mortality in septic shock. Intensive Care Med (in press)
26. Opal SM, Esmon CT (2003) Bench-to-bedside review: functional relationships between coagulation and the innate immune response and their respective roles in the pathogenesis of sepsis. Crit Care 7:23–38
27. Amaral A, Opal SM, Vincent JL (2004) Coagulation in sepsis. Intensive Care Med 30:1032–1040
28. Bernard GR, Vincent JL, Laterre PF, et al (2001) Efficacy and safety of recombinant human activated protein C for severe sepsis. N Engl J Med 344:699–709
29. Tilley R, Mackman N (2006) Tissue factor in hemostasis and thrombosis. Semin Thromb Hemost 32:5–10

30. Steinemann S, Ulevitch RJ, Mackman N (1994) Role of the lipopolysaccharide (LPS)-binding protein/CD14 pathway in LPS induction of tissue factor expression in monocytic cells. Arterioscler Thromb 14:1202–1209
31. Peiretti F, Bernot D, Lopez S, et al (2003) Modulation of PAI-1 and proMMP-9 syntheses by soluble TNFalpha and its receptors during differentiation of the human monocytic HL- 60 cell line. J Cell Physiol 196:346–353
32. Naldini A, Bernini C, Pucci A, Carraro F (2005) Thrombin- mediated IL-10 up-regulation involves protease-activated receptor (PAR)-1 expression in human mononuclear leukocytes. J Leukoc Biol 78:736–744
33. Roche N, Stirling RG, Lim S, et al (2003) Effect of acute and chronic inflammatory stimuli on expression of protease- activated receptors 1 and 2 in alveolar macrophages. J Allergy Clin Immunol 111:367–373
34. Colognato R, Slupsky JR, Jendrach M, Burysek L, Syrovets T, Simmet T (2003) Differential expression and regulation of protease-activated receptors in human peripheral monocytes and monocyte-derived antigen-presenting cells. Blood 102:2645–2652
35. de Jonge WJ, van der Zanden EP, The FO, et al (2005) Stimulation of the vagus nerve attenuates macrophage activation by activating the Jak2-STAT3 signaling pathway. Nat Immunol 6:844–851
36. Borovikova LV, Ivanova S, Zhang M, et al (2000) Vagus nerve stimulation attenuates the systemic inflammatory response to endotoxin. Nature 405:458–462
37. Borovikova LV, Ivanova S, Nardi D, et al (2000) Role of vagus nerve signaling in CNI-1493-mediated suppression of acute inflammation. Auton Neurosci 85:141–147
38. Pavlov VA, Wang H, Czura CJ, Friedman SG, Tracey KJ (2003) The cholinergic anti-inflammatory pathway: a missing link in neuroimmunomodulation. Mol Med 9:125–134
39. Wang H, Yu M, Ochani M, et al (2003) Nicotinic acetylcholine receptor alpha7 subunit is an essential regulator of inflammation. Nature 421:384–388
40. Yang H, Ochani M, Li J, et al (2004) Reversing established sepsis with antagonists of endogenous high-mobility group box 1. Proc Natl Acad Sci USA 101:296–301
41. Mantell LL, Parrish WR, Ulloa L (2006) Hmgb-1 as a therapeutic target for infectious and inflammatory disorders. Shock 25:4–11
42. Ulevitch RJ (2004) Therapeutics targeting the innate immune system. Nat Rev Immunol 4:512–520
43. Nierhaus A, Montag B, Timmler N, et al (2003) Reversal of immunoparalysis by recombinant human granulocyte-macrophage colony-stimulating factor in patients with severe sepsis. Intensive Care Med 29:646–651
44. Docke WD, Randow F, Syrbe U, et al (1997) Monocyte deactivation in septic patients: restoration by IFN-gamma treatment. Nat Med 3:678–681
45. Cohen J (2001) TREM-1 in sepsis. Lancet 358:776–778

# The Role of the Endothelium

W.C. Aird

## Introduction

The endothelium is a key modulator of systemic inflammation in critical illness. The goals of this chapter are to discuss how endothelial cells contribute to and are affected by the host response to infection and multiple organ dysfunction.

## A Primer in Endothelial Biology

When considering the role of the endothelium in health and disease, several important themes emerge:

### The Endothelium is a Spatially Distributed Organization

The endothelium, which lines blood vessels of the vascular tree, is a spatially distributed organ, extending to all recesses of the human body. The endothelium weighs 1 kg in an average-sized human and covers a surface area between 4,000–7,000 square meters. If arteries and veins are considered the conduits of the cardiovascular system, the capillaries are the 'business end' of the circulation, mediating the exchange of nutrients and gases between blood and underlying tissue. In keeping with Fick's law of diffusion, capillaries (and their endothelial lining) comprise the vast majority of the surface area of the circulation. Also in keeping with Ficks law of diffusion, capillaries are extraordinarily thin. They are basically three dimensional tubes of endothelium surrounded to a variable extent by occasional pericytes and extracellular matrix.

### The Endothelium is Derived from Lateral Plate Mesoderm

During embryogenesis, the endothelium is derived from lateral plate mesoderm. Hemangioblasts differentiate into angioblasts, which then migrate to the midline and coalesce to form the aorta and posterior cardinal vein to form the primary vascular plexus. This process, which is called vasculogenesis, is followed (and accompanied) by a highly coordinated series of steps that include angiogenesis, branching, establishment of arterial-venous identity, and stabilization and maturation of the vascular wall.

## The Endothelium Evolved in Concert with the Closed Circulation

In our need for oxygen, we are no different than the simplest organisms that inhabit the planet. For example, single cell aerobic organisms and tiny multicellular organisms (such as the flat worm) obtain their oxygen by simple diffusion. In larger multicellular organisms, the time-distance constraints of diffusion appear to mandate the existence of a pump (i. e., heart) that provides bulk flow delivery of oxygen to the various tissue of the body. In invertebrates, the cardiovascular system is said to be 'open' in the sense that the heart pumps blood ('hemolymph') into an open body cavity where it directly bathes all tissue cells. In vertebrates (fish, amphibians, reptiles, birds and mammals), blood is maintained within a closed vascular space. The open cardiovascular system of the invertebrate lacks an endothelial lining. In contrast, all vertebrates possess endothelium. Based on phylogenetic data, it appears that the closed circulation and the endothelium co-evolved approximately 550 million years ago. An interesting question is what were the selective pressures underlying the evolution of the endothelium? Did the high pressures associated with a closed circulation initially lead to the selection of a cell lining that limited leakage (by optimizing hydraulic conductivity and reflection co-efficient variables), prevented exsanguination (through the expression of procoagulants), and/or modulated regional flow (via release of nitric oxide [NO])?

## The Endothelium is a Multifunctional Organ

The endothelium is not an inert nucleated layer of cellophane, but rather participates in many physiological activities. The endothelium functions as a 'gatekeeper', regulating the transfer of cells and nutrients between blood and underlying tissue. The endothelium plays a key role in regulating hemostasis. Indeed, endothelial cells are mini-factories of hemostatic factors. On the procoagulant side, they express von Willebrand factor (vWF), plasminogen activator inhibitor (PAI)-1, and tissue factor. On the anticoagulant side, endothelial cells express thrombomodulin, endothelial protein C receptor (EPCR), heparan, tissue factor pathway inhibitor (TFPI), and tissue-type plasminogen activator (t-PA). The endothelium governs vasomotor tone, by releasing vasomotor molecules, most notably NO. Endothelial cells express pattern recognition receptors, including Toll-like receptor (TLR)-2 and TLR4, and thus participate in the earliest stages of innate immunity. In addition, endothelial cells are capable of releasing many inflammatory mediators.

## Endothelial Cell Heterogeneity

Endothelial cell phenotypes are differentially regulated in space and time, giving rise to the phenomenon of endothelial heterogeneity or vascular diversity (reviewed in [1, 2]). For example, from a functional standpoint, the endothelium displays remarkable division of labor. Endothelial cell-mediated regulation of white blood cell trafficking is primarily a property of postcapillary venules; endothelial-dependent vasomotor relaxation occurs in arterioles; barrier properties differ in different capillary beds across the body (e.g., compare the tight junctions of the blood brain barrier versus the loose, fenestrated, discontinuous endothelium of liver sinusoids); and each vascular bed employs unique formulas to balance local hemostasis [3]. For example, TFPI is expressed predominantly in capillary endothelial cells [4, 5], EPCR is preferentially expressed in venous and arterial endothelium [6], and thrombomodulin is expressed in blood vessels of all calibers in every organ, with the notable exception of the brain, where levels are virtually undetectable [7].

## Mechanisms of Endothelial Cell Heterogeneity

Each and every endothelial cell is analogous to a miniature adaptive input-output device. Input arises from the extracellular environment and may include biochemical and biomechanical forces. Output represents the cellular phenotype, and may include changes in cell shape, calcium flux, protein and/or mRNA expression, vasomotor tone, hemostatic balance, permeability, leukocyte trafficking, cell migration, proliferation, apoptosis, and/or release of inflammatory mediators. Input is coupled to output via non-linear signaling pathways that typically begin at the level of the cell surface and end at the level of transcriptional or post-transcriptional changes. Input differs across the vascular tree. For example, the blood brain barrier is exposed to paracrine mediators derived from surrounding astroglial cells, whereas endothelial cells lining capillaries of the heart are exposed to special regional forces and cardiomyocyte-derived paracrine factors. Since input varies across the vascular tree, so does output. In fact, if one could color code endothelial cell phenotypes according to the cell's proteome, transcriptome, and functional profile, the endothelium would display a rich color palette. If one were to then 'roll the film' the colors would fade in and fade out in concert with changes in the extracellular environment.

If the microenvironment were the sole cause of endothelial heterogeneity, then endothelial cells would be akin to a 'blank slate', blindly marching to the tune of the local tissue environment. Accordingly, if endothelial cells were removed from their native tissues and cultured *in vitro* under identical conditions, their phenotypes would drift towards one another, ultimately reaching identity. However, most data suggest that while cellular phenotypes do indeed drift towards each other, they never quite reach identity [8–10]. In other words, while some site-specific properties (i.e., those that 'wash out' in culture) are dependent on ongoing signals from the microenvironment, other vascular bed-specific properties are epigenetically fixed and mitotically heritable [10]. The relative contribution of microenvironment and epigenetic DNA modification in mediating endothelial cell heterogeneity may change with age or during disease.

## Endothelium in Disease

In traversing each and every organ/tissue in the body, the endothelium establishes a dialog that is unique to the underlying tissue. The endothelial-tissue interface is not only critical in homeostasis, but also plays a key role in mediating many focal vascular disease states. Based on our current knowledge, it may be argued that endothelial cells are involved in every disease state, either as a primary determinant of pathophysiology or as a victim of collateral damage (reviewed in [11]).

The two most common terms to describe endothelial cells in disease are endothelial cell activation and endothelial cell dysfunction. Endothelial cell activation is used to describe the phenotypic response of the endothelium to inflammatory stimuli. Endothelial cell activation is not an on-off switch. Rather, endothelial cells display a spectrum of response. That caveat notwithstanding, the activation phenotype usually consists of some combination of increased leukocyte adhesiveness, a procoagulant surface, and reduced barrier function. Importantly, the term activation does not address the cost of the phenotype to the host; the activation phenotype may be adaptive or non-adaptive.

For many physicians, the term endothelial cell dysfunction is synonymous with impaired endothelial-mediated vasomotor tone in atherosclerotic arteries. However, dysfunction is not limited in scope to one particular activity, disease, or vascular bed. Indeed, endothelial cell dysfunction may be defined as any endothelial phenotype – whether or not it meets the definition of activation – which represents a net liability to the host, as occurs, for example, locally in coronary artery disease or systemically in severe sepsis.

## Endothelial Diagnostics and Therapeutics

The endothelium has remarkable, yet largely untapped, diagnostic and therapeutic potential. From a diagnostic standpoint, few assays are currently available for monitoring endothelial cell health. The endothelium is not amenable to physical diagnostic maneuvers, such as inspection, palpation, percussion or auscultation. Unlike the kidney or liver, endothelial cell dysfunction is not associated with reliable changes in circulating biomarkers. Finally, the wide spatial distribution and thinness of the endothelium preclude conventional diagnostic imaging. An important, and urgent, goal is to develop a comprehensive diagnostic platform for dysfunctional endothelium.

The endothelium is an attractive therapeutic target. It is strategically situated between blood and underlying tissue, and thus is rapidly and preferentially exposed to systemically delivered agents. The endothelium is highly malleable and, therefore, responsive to therapeutic modalities. Finally, because the endothelium is tightly linked to the underlying tissue, it provides the pharmacotherapist with a direct 'line of communication' with each and every organ in the body.

## Endothelium in Critical Care

In keeping with the themes developed above, the following section will center on the endothelial cell as an input-output device, and in doing so will emphasize the critical role of the endothelium as a signal transducer in the host response to infection. An important caveat is that most of the evidence supporting a role for the endothelium in sepsis is derived from animal models. Although this represents an important and necessary starting point, the extent to which these data apply to the human condition remains to be determined.

### Input

Sepsis is associated with many changes in the extracellular environment that are sensed by endothelial cells. These include both biomechanical and biochemical forces.

#### Biomechanical

Under *in vivo* conditions, endothelium is normally exposed to protective levels and patterns of shear stress. Among the many benefits of laminar shear stress are the promotion of NO synthesis and release. In severe sepsis, a reduction in blood pressure may compromise levels of shear stress. Areas of no-flow are particularly vulnerable because the endothelial lining experiences both loss of shear stress and anoxia. An obligate feature of the cardiovascular system, as blood vessels branch and then merge, and as they twist and turn to conform to the closed-loop geometry of the circulation, is the existence of heterogeneous flow patterns across the vascular tree. For example, endothelial cells lining the straight segments of arteries are normally exposed to undisturbed laminar flow, whereas endothelial cells at bifurcations and curvatures experience disturbed laminar, and at times turbulent, flow [12, 13]. Atherosclerotic lesions preferentially form at these sites of disturbed flow. Endothelial cells in these regions have been shown to be primed for activation [12,14]. For example, they express increased levels of p65 nuclear factor-kappa B (NF-κB) in their cytoplasm [14]. Since NF-κB must translocate to the nucleus to exert its pro-inflammatory effects, these cells are analogous to a loaded gun. It has been argued that in atherosclerosis, systemic risk factors such as hypertension, hyperglycemia, and/or hyperlipidemia serve to 'pull the trigger', leading to nuclear translocation of NF-κB, upregulation of NF-κB-dependent genes, and plaque formation. An interesting question is whether an acute insult, such as sepsis, also has the capacity to push these cells over the edge. The answer appears to be yes. For example, endotoxin administration in mice resulted in significant nuclear translocation of NF-κB in regions of disturbed flow [14]. Interestingly, a recent study of septic baboons revealed selective induction of tissue factor at branch points of arteries [15]. The latter study is the first to convincingly demonstrate tissue factor expression in intact endothelium in response to sepsis, and suggests that flow-dependent hot spots of endothelial-derived tissue factor may contribute to activation of coagulation in sepsis.

Biochemical

Sepsis is associated with the release of many soluble mediators from non-endothelial cells and endothelial cells, which may then operate in paracrine and autocrine pathways, respectively, to activate the endothelium. In animal and human models of endotoxemia, the systemic administration of lipopolysaccharide (LPS) leads to a predictable and highly reproducible pattern of circulating inflammatory mediators, including, but certainly not limited to, cytokines and chemokines (for examples, see [16–20]). These are normally assayed by ELISA. In patients with severe sepsis, the pattern is less predictable. Of the various inflammatory biomarkers, interleukin (IL)-6 seems to be the most sensitive, being elevated in close to 100% of patients [21,22]. Similarly, the clotting cascade is activated in every patient with severe sepsis. Clotting is initiated by tissue factor (expressed by monocytes, and possibly endothelial cells), which activates factor VIIa, ultimately leading to increased thrombin generation, fibrin formation, and – at the extreme – clotting factor consumption. An elevated prothrombin time and partial thromboplastin time reflect consumption of clotting factors, and elevated D-dimers indicate increased production and degradation of fibrin. There are sensitive markers for thrombin generation, including thrombin-antithrombin complexes or F1+2. However, these assays remain investigational. It is important to recognize that the various serine proteases in the clotting cascade (most notably thrombin) are capable not only of activating their downstream substrate in the cascade, but also of binding to protease-activated receptors present on several cell types, including endothelial cells, resulting in a pro-inflammatory and procoagulant phenotype [23].

In large clinical studies, circulating levels of inflammatory and coagulation biomarkers have been correlated with severity of illness (for example, see [21]). However, at present, single markers do not exist for predicting outcome or tailoring therapy in individual patients. Such an eventuality will likely depend on two advances. One is the use of large scale ELISAs or proteomics to simultaneously survey dozens or hundreds of biomarkers in blood from patients with sepsis and then to apply state-of-the-art bioinformatics to interpret these data. Second is the need to leverage the wealth of information that is inherent in time series analyses, recognizing that the host response to infection is a highly dynamic process. For example, it is well established that temporal patterns of biomarker release vary on the order of hours (e. g., IL-6/IL-1 vs. tumor necrosis factor [TNF]-α) or days (e. g., high mobility group box protein [HMGB]-1 vs. IL-1/IL-6/TNF-α).

Like all multicellular organisms, the human body is a giant consortium of highly interactive cells, which creates all types of information highways and virtual organ systems. The endothelium is exposed on the luminal side to circulating cells, including leukocytes, red blood cells, and platelets. There is ample evidence supporting a role for cross-talk between the endothelium and each of these blood cell lineages. On the abluminal side, endothelial cells communicate with supporting cells (vascular smooth muscle cells and pericytes) and underlying parenchymal cells. Endothelial cells also communicate with each other at their lateral borders.

In sepsis, the communication lines break down and the dialog turns sour. As just one example, NADPH-mediated bursts of reactive oxygen species (ROS) from neutrophils have been shown to act in a juxtacrine manner to activate endothelial cells, resulting in phenotypic changes that include expression of TLR2 in endothelium [24].

There are other extracellular signals which do not fall neatly into the above categories and/or which interact with endothelial cells via receptor-independent mechanisms, yet are capable of activating the endothelium. These include hypoxia, high glucose, changes in osmolarity/pH, hypothermia/hyperthermia, and certain drugs.

### Role of Signal Input in Pathogenesis, Diagnostics, and Therapeutics

Sepsis is associated with many changes in the extracellular environment that may influence endothelial cell behavior. As mentioned above, no single marker or panel of markers is adequate for predicting clinical course in individual patients. Therapeutic strategies, aimed towards one or another mediator, have largely failed to improve survival in patients with severe sepsis. One interpretation of these disappointing results is that the inflammatory and coagulation cascades are sufficiently pleiotropic, redundant, and inter-dependent as to preclude single modality therapy. However, it is possible – indeed, likely – that many of the established therapies in sepsis exert their benefit at least partially through the endothelium (Table 1). For example, early intervention may promote rapid restoration of shear stress; low tidal volume ventilation may attenuate barotrauma to pulmonary endothelium; aggressive blood glucose control may be predicted to prevent deleterious effects of hyperglycemia on endothelial cells, and recombinant human activated protein C may reduce activation of inflammatory and coagulation pathways.

## Output

Inputs are pathogenic only insofar as they elicit a maladaptive response by the endothelium. Such phenotypes may be separated into two categories: structural and functional.

### Structural Changes

A number of studies have demonstrated that in response to sepsis, endothelial cells undergo morphological changes including contraction, swelling/blebbing, and frank denudation [15, 25]. The loss of endothelial surface may have several consequences. First, circulating blood is exposed to a procoagulant underlying extracellular matrix and tissue factor-expressing abluminal cells, leading to platelet adhesion and aggregation, and activation of the clotting cascade. Second, it is conceivable that dislodged endothelial cells contribute to the pool of circulating endothelial cells (normal circulating endothelial cell counts are 2–5 per ml of blood).

**Table 1.** Sepsis therapy targeted towards endothelial input-output

|  | Treatment | Comments | Ref |
|---|---|---|---|
| INPUT | | | |
| **Oxygen** | Supplemental oxygen to maintain oxygenation | Endothelial cells are highly sensitive to hypoxia | [56] |
| **pH** | Correction of acidosis | There is increasing evidence that endothelial cells are capable of sensing acidosis independent of hypoxia | [57, 58] |
| **Shear stress** | Fluid resuscitation and maintenance of blood pressure | Endothelial cells are highly sensitive to changes in shear stress; early goal-directed therapy may exert its benefit partly through promoting shear stress | [59, 60] |
| **Hyperthermia** | Body temperature control | Fever induces heat shock response | [61] |
| **Hyperglycemia** | Tight glucose control | Hyperglycemia may have deleterious effects on endothelial cells | [62–64] |
| **Cytokines** | | | |
| TNF-α | Anti-TNF-antibodies; receptor antagonists | TNF-α is a strong activator of endothelial cells; clinical trials have demonstrated inconsistent results | [65, 66] |
| IL-1, -6, -8 | Anti-IL-antibodies; receptor antagonists | Interleukins activate endothelial cells; clinical trials have failed | [67] |
| **Chemokines** | | | |
| PAF | PAF receptor antagonists; PAF acetylhydrolases | PAF is a potent phospholipid agonist that induces endothelial cell proliferation and permeability | [68–70] |
| MCP-1 | Anti-MCP antibodies; receptor antagonists | MCP binds to CCR2 on endothelial cells, inducing numerous pro-inflammatory signals | [71, 72] |
| **Serine proteases** | Anticoagulants | Thrombin binds to PAR on surface of endothelial cells, resulting in pro-inflammatory phenotype; selective anti-thrombin agents do not improve sepsis survival; rhAPC may exert its benefit partly through inhibition of thrombin-mediated signaling | [73, 74] |
| **Complement** | Anti-C5a-antibodies; receptor antagonists | C3a and C5a bind to receptors on endothelial cells | [75, 76] |
| **HMGB1** | Anti-C5a-antibodies; receptor antagonists | Late marker of sepsis; produced by and activates endothelial cells | [77–79] |
| **Bradykinin/HMWK** | Antagonists | Bradykinin and HMWK activate endothelial cells; clinical trials have failed | [80, 81] |
| **VEGF** | Anti-VEGF antibodies; receptor antagonists | VEGF binds to endothelial cell-specific receptors, and results in a pro-inflammatory phenotype | [82] |

Table 1. (continued)

| | Treatment | Comments | Ref |
|---|---|---|---|
| ROS | Antioxidants | Endothelial cells are highly sensitive to changes in redox state | [83, 84] |
| LPS | Anti-endotoxin antibodies | Clinical trials have failed | |
| **OUTPUT** | | | |
| **Leukocyte adhesion and transmigration** | Anti-adhesion molecule antibodies | ICAM-1, VCAM-1, P-selectin, E-selectin are expressed by activated endothelial cells and mediate increased adhesion of leukocytes to endothelium; PECAM-1 plays role in leukocyte transmigration | [85–87] |
| **Barrier dysfunction** | Sphingosine 1-phosphate administration; rhAPC; phosphodiesterase 2 inhibition | Sphingosine 1-phosphate appears to play a critical role in mediating barrier function; rhAPC may exert its benefit partly through sphingosine 1-phosphate-dependent reduction in endothelial cell permeability | [55, 88, 89] |
| **Vasomotor tone** | | | |
| NOS/NO | Nitric oxide donors/inhibitors | Recent evidence suggests that eNOS has a pro-inflammatory role in sepsis | [38, 81, 90, 92] |
| **Inflammatory mediators** | See above under input | Endothelial cells express TNF-$\alpha$, interleukins and many chemokines | |
| **Apoptosis** | Caspase inhibitors, rhAPC | Sepsis is associated with increased apoptosis of endothelial cells | [93, 94, 96] |
| **COUPLING** | | | |
| p38 MAPK | Chemical inhibitors | | [97–99] |
| NF-kB | Double-stranded oligodeoxynucleotides | rhAPC may exert its benefit partly through inhibition of NF-$\kappa$B activity | [100–102] |
| GSK3b | Chemical inhibitors | | [103] |

This table is not exhaustive but rather shows representative examples under each category. TNF, tumor necrosis factor; IL, interleukin; PAF, platelet activating factor; MCP, monocyte chemoattractant protein; PAR, protease-activated receptor; rhAPC, recombinant human activated protein C; HMGB1, high mobility group box 1; HMWK, high molecular weight kininogen; VEGF, vascular endothelial growth factor; ROS, reactive oxygen species; LPS, lipopolysaccharide; ICAM-1, intercellular adhesion molecule; VCAM, vascular cell adhesion molecule; NOS, nitric oxide synthase; NO, nitric oxide

Circulating endothelial cells may be identified using special stains for cell-specific markers, and they may be enumerated either manually or by fluorescence-activated cell sorter (FACS). Circulating endothelial cell levels have been shown to be increased in a number of pathological conditions associated with vascular injury, including sickle cell disease, thalassemia, cancer, pulmonary hypertension, vasculitides, and sepsis (reviewed in [26]). In one study, circulating endothelial cells – as measured by indirect immunofluorescence of the endothelial markers vWF and Fl-1 – were increased in patients with sepsis compared with normal volunteers and ICU patients who did not have sepsis [27]. Repair of denuded segments of the vasculature may occur by one of two mechanisms. First, neighboring endothelial cells may proliferate and migrate, thus sealing the hole. Second, circulating bone-marrow derived endothelial progenitor cells may become incorporated into the vascular wall. The latter mechanism has received much attention in the field of cardiology where studies show that the number of circulating endothelial progenitor cells correlates with positive outcomes and reflects the repair capacity of the host (reviewed in [28]). Few, if any such studies have been carried out in animal or human models of sepsis.

Another injury response is the release of microparticles. These tiny (0.5–3 M) submicroscopic membrane-bound particles are shed from multiple cell types, including endothelial cells. These microparticles may carry tissue factor, and therefore contribute to sepsis pathophysiology. Endothelial microparticles, which are assayed using FACS, have been shown to be increased in patients with severe sepsis [29].

## Functional Changes

The endothelium plays a central role in innate immunity and inflammation. For example, endothelial cells release vasomotor molecules, which result in increased blood flow to the site. Endothelial cells express increased levels of adhesion molecules on their cell surface, including E-selectin, P-selectin, vascular adhesion molecule (VCAM)-1, and intercellular adhesion molecule (ICAM)-1. These adhesion molecules bind to cognate ligands on the surface of leukocytes, and mediate their tethering, rolling, firm adhesion, and transendothelial migration (reviewed in [30, 31]). Normally, this process leads to the regulated transport of leukocytes into the extravascular space where they may engage pathogens, and contribute to tissue repair. An increase in endothelial permeability allows for the passage of plasma proteins into the interstitium, including complement proteins, immunoglobins, and clotting factors. Activated endothelial cells also express increased procoagulants and decreased anticoagulants. It is possible that the net shift in hemostatic balance towards the procoagulant side plays an essential role in 'walling off' the infection.

Sepsis represents an exaggerated/disseminated host response to infection. In preclinical models, there is a marked increase in the expression of cell adhesion molecules on the surface of the endothelium (for example, see [32]). The pattern of response differs between different vascular beds [33]. The induction of cell adhesion molecules correlates with increased trafficking of leukocytes. A biopsy is required to demonstrate induced levels of cell adhesion molecules on the surface of the endothelium. These are seldom carried out except for experimental purposes [34]. However, the various cell adhesion molecules may be released or cleaved at the cell surface by proteases such as neutrophil elastase. These soluble forms of the receptors circulate in the blood and may be measured using immunoassays (reviewed in [35]). However, levels of soluble receptors in the blood do not always correlate with *in situ* expression in the endothelium [33,34]. A limitation of these assays as surrogate markers for endothelial activation/dysfunction is that P-selectin, ICAM-1, and VCAM-1 are also expressed in non-endothelial cells. Only E-selectin is specific to the endothelial lineage. Of the various adhesion molecules, ICAM-1 has been shown to play a particularly important role in mediating leukocyte infiltration and sepsis mortality [33,36].

Two major isoforms contribute to the generation of NO in the vasculature: endothelial NO synthase (eNOS) and inducible NOS (iNOS). In animal models of sepsis, iNOS levels have been shown to be increased in many organs [37,38], whereas eNOS levels are generally downregulated [39,40]. Previous studies of arteries dissected from septic rodents have shown hyporesponsiveness of endothelial cells to acetylcholine [40]. In a rat model of cecal ligation and puncture, NOS inhibition reversed arteriolar hyporesponsiveness to catecholamines and endothelin in cremaster muscle [41]. eNOS and iNOS null mice are resistant to LPS-mediated shock, suggesting that NO plays a role in mediating hemodynamic instability in sepsis [38]. In addition, eNOS has been shown to promote pro-inflammatory effects of iNOS [38]. In contrast, iNOS contributes to impaired eNOS-mediated vasomotor reactivity [40]. Importantly, eNOS may protect against organ failure [42]. The benefit of eNOS-derived NO may be explained – at least in part – by its attenuating effect on platelet-endothelial and leukocyte-endothelial interactions [43–46].

Although every patient with severe sepsis has activation of their clotting cascade, it is not clear to what extent the endothelium contributes to the hemostatic imbalance. This gap in knowledge reflects the difficulty in assaying intact endothelium for hemostatic function. In mouse models, the systemic administration of LPS leads to vascular bed-specific changes in vWF expression in the endothelium [47]. Animal models of sepsis have also revealed widespread reduction in thrombomodulin expression. In patients with meningococcemia, skin biopsies revealed decreased expression of thrombomodulin and EPCR protein levels in dermal microvascular endothelium [48]. Like the cell adhesion molecules, thrombomodulin also circulates in soluble form. Previous studies have demonstrated that soluble thrombomodulin is elevated in ≈ 70% of patients with severe sepsis [21].

Of the various functions of the endothelium, the least understood – and possibly the most important in the context of sepsis – is the regulation of permeability. Bulk flow transfer of solutes and fluids occurs between (paracellular) or through (transcellular) endothelial cells. These routes are likely regulated by overlapping yet distinct molecular mechanisms. Platelet-endothelial cell adhesion molecule

(PECAM)-1 plays an important role in mediating inter-endothelial junctional integrity. Two recent studies have shown that deletion of PECAM-1 from mice results in increased permeability and sepsis mortality [49, 50].

### Role of Endothelial Output in Pathogenesis, Diagnostics, and Therapeutics

If sepsis is associated with significant denudation of endothelium, and if bone marrow-derived endothelial progenitor cells are capable of homing to these sites of injury, then perhaps therapies aimed towards promoting the mobilization and/or uptake of these progenitor cells will facilitate healing. From the standpoint of functional changes, it is not always clear which endothelial phenotypes are adaptive and which are maladaptive. In the case of NO, an argument may be made for inhibiting eNOS as a means of protecting against shock [51], while the counterargument – namely to increase eNOS levels – might be supported by the importance of minimizing microdomains of no-flow and/or to attenuate endothelial-blood cell interactions [52]. Despite evidence for a pathogenic role of cell adhesion molecules in animal models, there is little evidence supporting the use of anti-adhesion therapy in humans. Although it seems intuitive that clotting activation in sepsis is a maladaptive response (consider the patient with severe disseminated intravascular coagulation [DIC]), there are surprisingly few data to support this conclusion. Indeed, one interpretation of existing data is that activation of coagulation – provided that it is not excessive – is beneficial in sepsis [53, 54]. Recent evidence suggests that recombinant human activated protein C, a serine protease critically involved in the regulation of coagulation and inflammatory processes, prevents increased endothelial cell permeability and restores vascular integrity following inflammatory insult. These effects were shown to involve EPCR-mediated transactivation of the sphingosine 1-phosphate (S1P) receptor [55].

## Conclusion

In summary, the endothelium is a spatially distributed cell layer that displays significant heterogeneity in both structure and function. Endothelial heterogeneity reflects the capacity of the endothelium to meet the diverse needs of the underlying tissues. The endothelium plays an important role in mediating the host response to infection. Not only do endothelial cells express pattern recognition receptors, but they also govern local blood flow and vectorial transport of cells, solutes, and fluids across the vascular wall. The normal response to infection involves activation of endothelial cells without dysfunction. In sepsis, the endothelial response becomes excessive, sustained, and/or disseminated, at which point the activation phenotype poses a liability to the host and may be characterized as dysfunctional. Important goals for the future are to develop reliable diagnostic assays for monitoring the health of the endothelium and to elucidate those components of the endothelial response that are maladaptive and amenable to therapeutic targeting.

# References

1. Aird WC (2005) Spatial and temporal dynamics of the endothelium. J Thromb Haemost 3:1392–1406
2. Aird WC (2003) Endothelial cell heterogeneity. Crit Care Med 31 (Suppl 4):S221–S230.
3. Rosenberg RD, Aird WC (1999) Vascular-bed–specific hemostasis and hypercoagulable states. N Engl J Med 340:1555–1564
4. Broze GJ Jr (2003) The rediscovery and isolation of TFPI. J Thromb Haemost 1:1671–1675
5. Osterud B, Bajaj MS, Bajaj SP (1995) Sites of tissue factor pathway inhibitor (TFPI) and tissue factor expression under physiologic and pathologic conditions. Thromb Haemost 73:873–875
6. Laszik Z, Mitro A, Taylor FB Jr, Ferrell G, Esmon CT (1997) Human protein C receptor is present primarily on endothelium of large blood vessels: implications for the control of the protein C pathway. Circulation 96:3633–3640
7. Ishii H, Salem HH, Bell CE, Laposata EA, Majerus PW (1986) Thrombomodulin, an endothelial anticoagulant protein, is absent from the human brain. Blood 67:362–365
8. Lacorre DA, Baekkevold ES, Garrido I, et al (2004) Plasticity of endothelial cells: rapid dedifferentiation of freshly isolated high endothelial venule endothelial cells outside the lymphoid tissue microenvironment. Blood 103:4164–4172
9. Chi JT, Chang HY, Haraldsen G, et al (2003) Endothelial cell diversity revealed by global expression profiling. Proc Natl Acad Sci USA 100:10623–10628
10. Aird WC (2006) Mechanisms of endothelial cell heterogeneity in health and disease. Circ Res 98:159–162
11. Hwa C, Sebastian A, Aird WC (2005) Endothelial biomedicine: its status as an interdisciplinary field, its progress as a basic science, and its translational bench-to-bedside gap. Endothelium 12:139–151
12. Passerini AG, Polacek DC, Shi C, et al (2004) Coexisting proinflammatory and antioxidative endothelial transcription profiles in a disturbed flow region of the adult porcine aorta. Proc Natl Acad Sci USA 101:2482–2487
13. Dai G, Kaazempur-Mofrad MR, Natarajan S, et al (2004) Distinct endothelial phenotypes evoked by arterial waveforms derived from atherosclerosis-susceptible and -resistant regions of human vasculature. Proc Natl Acad Sci USA 101:14871–14876
14. Hajra L, Evans AI, Chen M, Hyduk SJ, Collins T, Cybulsky MI (2000) The NF-kappa B signal transduction pathway in aortic endothelial cells is primed for activation in regions predisposed to atherosclerotic lesion formation. Proc Natl Acad Sci USA 97:9052–9057
15. Lupu C, Westmuckett AD, Peer G, et al (2005) Tissue factor-dependent coagulation is preferentially up-regulated within arterial branching areas in a baboon model of Escherichia coli sepsis. Am J Pathol 167:1161–1172
16. Derhaschnig U, Reiter R, Knobl P, Baumgartner M, Keen P, Jilma B (2003) Recombinant human activated protein C (rhAPC; drotrecogin alfa [activated]) has minimal effect on markers of coagulation, fibrinolysis, and inflammation in acute human endotoxemia. Blood 102:2093–2098
17. Pajkrt D, van der Poll T, Levi M, et al (1997) Interleukin-10 inhibits activation of coagulation and fibrinolysis during human endotoxemia. Blood 89:2701–2705
18. de Jonge E, Dekkers PE, Creasey AA, et al (2000) Tissue factor pathway inhibitor dose-dependently inhibits coagulation activation without influencing the fibrinolytic and cytokine response during human endotoxemia. Blood 95:1124–1129
19. Derhaschnig U, Bergmair D, Marsik C, Schlifke I, Wijdenes J, Jilma B (2004) Effect of interleukin-6 blockade on tissue factor-induced coagulation in human endotoxemia. Crit Care Med 32:1136–1140
20. van der Poll T, Coyle SM, Levi M, et al (1997) Effect of a recombinant dimeric tumor necrosis factor receptor on inflammatory responses to intravenous endotoxin in normal humans. Blood 89:3727–3734

21. Kinasewitz GT, Yan SB, Basson B, et al (2004) Universal changes in biomarkers of co-agulation and inflammation occur in patients with severe sepsis, regardless of causative micro-organism. Crit Care 8:R82–R90
22. Bernard GR, Ely EW, Wright TJ, et al (2001) Safety and dose relationship of recombinant human activated protein C for coagulopathy in severe sepsis. Crit Care Med 29:2051–2059
23. Pawlinski R, Mackman N (2004) Tissue factor, coagulation proteases, and protease-activated receptors in endotoxemia and sepsis. Crit Care Med 32 (suppl 5):S293–S297
24. Fan J, Frey RS, Malik AB (2003) TLR4 signaling induces TLR2 expression in endothelial cells via neutrophil NADPH oxidase. J Clin Invest 112:1234–1243
25. Cybulsky MI, Chan MK, Movat HZ (1988) Acute inflammation and microthrombosis induced by endotoxin, interleukin-1, and tumor necrosis factor and their implication in gram-negative infection. Lab Invest 58:365–378
26. Khan SS, Solomon MA, McCoy JP Jr (2005) Detection of circulating endothelial cells and endothelial progenitor cells by flow cytometry. Cytometry B Clin Cytom 64:1–8
27. Mutunga M, Fulton B, Bullock R, et al (2001) Circulating endothelial cells in patients with septic shock. Am J Respir Crit Care Med 163:195–200
28. Liew A, Barry F, O'Brien T (2006) Endothelial progenitor cells: diagnostic and therapeutic considerations. Bioessays 28:261–270
29. Ogura H, Tanaka H, Koh T, et al (2004) Enhanced production of endothelial microparticles with increased binding to leukocytes in patients with severe systemic inflammatory response syndrome. J Trauma 56:823–830
30. Ley K (2003) The role of selectins in inflammation and disease. Trends Mol Med 9:263–268
31. Weber C (2003) Novel mechanistic concepts for the control of leukocyte transmigration: specialization of integrins, chemokines, and junctional molecules. J Mol Med 81:4–19
32. Lush CW, Cepinskas G, Sibbald WJ, Kvietys PR (2001) Endothelial E- and P-selectin expression in iNOS-deficient mice exposed to polymicrobial sepsis. Am J Physiol Gastrointest Liver Physiol 280:G291–297
33. Laudes IJ, Guo RF, Riedemann NC, et al (2004) Disturbed homeostasis of lung intercellular adhesion molecule-1 and vascular cell adhesion molecule-1 during sepsis. Am J Pathol 164:1435–1445
34. Leone M, Boutiere B, Camoin-Jau L, et al (2002) Systemic endothelial activation is greater in septic than in traumatic-hemorrhagic shock but does not correlate with endothelial activation in skin biopsies. Crit Care Med 30:808–814
35. Reinhart K, Bayer O, Brunkhorst F, Meisner M (2002) Markers of endothelial damage in organ dysfunction and sepsis. Crit Care Med 30 (Suppl 5):S302–S312
36. Xu H, Gonzalo JA, St Pierre Y, et al (1994) Leukocytosis and resistance to septic shock in intercellular adhesion molecule 1-deficient mice. J Exp Med 180:95–109
37. Cunha FQ, Assreuy J, Moss DW, et al (1994) Differential induction of nitric oxide synthase in various organs of the mouse during endotoxaemia: role of TNF-alpha and IL-1-beta. Immunology 81:211–215
38. Connelly L, Madhani M, Hobbs AJ (2005) Resistance to endotoxic shock in endothelial nitric-oxide synthase (eNOS) knock-out mice: a pro-inflammatory role for eNOS-derived no in vivo. J Biol Chem 280:10040–10046
39. Scott JA, Mehta S, Duggan M, Bihari A, McCormack DG (2002) Functional inhibition of constitutive nitric oxide synthase in a rat model of sepsis. Am J Respir Crit Care Med 165:1426–1432
40. Chauhan SD, Seggara G, Vo PA, Macallister RJ, Hobbs AJ, Ahluwalia A (2003) Protection against lipopolysaccharide-induced endothelial dysfunction in resistance and conduit vasculature of iNOS knockout mice. Faseb J 17:773–775
41. Hollenberg SM, Piotrowski MJ, Parrillo JE (1997) Nitric oxide synthase inhibition reverses arteriolar hyporesponsiveness to endothelin-1 in septic rats. Am J Physiol 272:R969–R974

42. Wang W, Mitra A, Poole B, et al (2004) Endothelial nitric oxide synthase-deficient mice exhibit increased susceptibility to endotoxin-induced acute renal failure. Am J Physiol Renal Physiol 287:F1044–1048
43. Radomski MW, Vallance P, Whitley G, Foxwell N, Moncada S (1993) Platelet adhesion to human vascular endothelium is modulated by constitutive and cytokine induced nitric oxide. Cardiovasc Res 27:1380–1382
44. Cerwinka WH, Cooper D, Krieglstein CF, Feelisch M, Granger DN (2002) Nitric oxide modulates endotoxin-induced platelet-endothelial cell adhesion in intestinal venules. Am J Physiol Heart Circ Physiol 282:H1111–H1117
45. Kubes P, Suzuki M, Granger DN (1991) Nitric oxide: an endogenous modulator of leukocyte adhesion. Proc Natl Acad Sci USA 88:4651–4655
46. Mitchell DJ, Yu J, Tyml K (1998) Local L-NAME decreases blood flow and increases leukocyte adhesion via CD18. Am J Physiol 274:H1264–H1268
47. Yamamoto K, de Waard V, Fearns C, Loskutoff DJ (1998) Tissue distribution and regulation of murine von Willebrand factor gene expression in vivo. Blood 92:2791–2801
48. Faust SN, Levin M, Harrison OB, et al (2001) Dysfunction of endothelial protein C activation in severe meningococcal sepsis. N Engl J Med 345:408–416
49. Carrithers M, Tandon S, Canosa S, Michaud M, Graesser D, Madri JA (2005) Enhanced susceptibility to endotoxic shock and impaired STAT3 signaling in CD31-deficient mice. Am J Pathol 166:185–196
50. Maas M, Stapleton M, Bergom C, Mattson DL, Newman DK, Newman PJ (2005) Endothelial cell PECAM-1 confers protection against endotoxic shock. Am J Physiol Heart Circ Physiol 288:H159–H164
51. Lopez A, Lorente JA, Steingrub J, et al (2004) Multiple-center, randomized, placebo-controlled, double-blind study of the nitric oxide synthase inhibitor 546C88: effect on survival in patients with septic shock. Crit Care Med 32:21–30
52. Buwalda M, Ince C (2002) Opening the microcirculation: can vasodilators be useful in sepsis? Intensive Care Med 28:1208–1217
53. Kerlin BA, Yan SB, Isermann BH, et al (2003) Survival advantage associated with heterozygous factor V Leiden mutation in patients with severe sepsis and in mouse endotoxemia. Blood 102:3085–3092
54. Aird WC (2003) Thrombin paradox redux. Blood 102:3077–3078
55. Finigan JH, Dudek SM, Singleton PA, et al (2005) Activated protein C mediates novel lung endothelial barrier enhancement: role of sphingosine 1-phosphate receptor transactivation. J Biol Chem 280:17286–17293
56. Ten VS, Pinsky DJ (2002) Endothelial response to hypoxia: physiologic adaptation and pathologic dysfunction. Curr Opin Crit Care 8:242–250
57. D'Arcangelo D, Facchiano F, Barlucchi LM, et al (2000) Acidosis inhibits endothelial cell apoptosis and function and induces basic fibroblast growth factor and vascular endothelial growth factor expression. Circ Res 86:312–318
58. Agullo L, Garcia-Dorado D, Escalona N, et al (2002) Hypoxia and acidosis impair cGMP synthesis in microvascular coronary endothelial cells. Am J Physiol Heart Circ Physiol 283:H917–H925
59. Barakat A, Lieu D (2003) Differential responsiveness of vascular endothelial cells to different types of fluid mechanical shear stress. Cell Biochem Biophys 38:323–343
60. Rivers E, Nguyen B, Havstad S, et al (2001) Early goal-directed therapy in the treatment of severe sepsis and septic shock. N Engl J Med 345:1368–1377
61. Hasday JD, Bannerman D, Sakarya S, et al (2001) Exposure to febrile temperature modifies endothelial cell response to tumor necrosis factor-alpha. J Appl Physiol 90:90–98
62. Wang L, Xing XP, Holmes A, et al (2005) Activation of the sphingosine kinase-signaling pathway by high glucose mediates the proinflammatory phenotype of endothelial cells. Circ Res 97:891–899

63. Han J, Mandal AK, Hiebert LM (2005) Endothelial cell injury by high glucose and heparanase is prevented by insulin, heparin and basic fibroblast growth factor. Cardiovasc Diabetol 4:12

64. van den Berghe G, Wouters P, Weekers F, et al (2001) Intensive insulin therapy in the critically ill patients. N Engl J Med 345:1359–1367

65. Panacek EA, Marshall JC, Albertson TE, et al (2004) Efficacy and safety of the monoclonal anti-tumor necrosis factor antibody F(ab')2 fragment afelimomab in patients with severe sepsis and elevated interleukin-6 levels. Crit Care Med 32:2173–2182

66. Pober JS (2002) Endothelial activation: intracellular signaling pathways. Arthritis Res 4 (suppl 3):S109–S116

67. Opal SM, Fisher CJ Jr, Dhainaut JF, et al (1997) Confirmatory interleukin-1 receptor antagonist trial in severe sepsis: a phase III, randomized, double-blind, placebo-controlled, multicenter trial. The Interleukin-1 Receptor Antagonist Sepsis Investigator Group. Crit Care Med 25:1115–1124

68. Opal S, Laterre PF, Abraham E, et al (2004) Recombinant human platelet-activating factor acetylhydrolase for treatment of severe sepsis: results of a phase III, multicenter, randomized, double-blind, placebo-controlled, clinical trial. Crit Care Med 32:332–341

69. Minneci PC, Deans KJ, Banks SM, Eichacker PQ, Natanson C (2004) Should we continue to target the platelet-activating factor pathway in septic patients? Crit Care Med 32:585–588

70. Hudry-Clergeon H, Stengel D, Ninio E, Vilgrain I (2005) Platelet-activating factor increases VE-cadherin tyrosine phosphorylation in mouse endothelial cells and its association with the PtdIns3'-kinase. Faseb J 19:512–520

71. Zisman DA, Kunkel SL, Strieter RM, et al (1997) MCP-1 protects mice in lethal endotoxemia. J Clin Invest 99:2832–2836

72. Hong KH, Ryu J, Han KH (2005) Monocyte chemoattractant protein-1-induced angiogenesis is mediated by vascular endothelial growth factor-A. Blood 105:1405–1407

73. Bernard GR, Vincent JL, Laterre PF, et al (2001) Efficacy and safety of recombinant human activated protein C for severe sepsis. N Engl J Med 344:699–709

74. Minami T, Sugiyama A, Wu SQ, Abid R, Kodama T, Aird WC (2004) Thrombin and phenotypic modulation of the endothelium. Arterioscler Thromb Vasc Biol 24:41–53

75. Buras JA, Rice L, Orlow D, et al (2004) Inhibition of C5 or absence of C6 protects from sepsis mortality. Immunobiology 209:629–635

76. Czermak BJ, Sarma V, Pierson CL, et al (1999) Protective effects of C5a blockade in sepsis. Nat Med 5:788–792

77. Kim JY, Park JS, Strassheim D, et al (2005) HMGB1 contributes to the development of acute lung injury after hemorrhage. Am J Physiol Lung Cell Mol Physiol 288:L958–965

78. Yang H, Ochani M, Li J, et al (2004) Reversing established sepsis with antagonists of endogenous high-mobility group box 1. Proc Natl Acad Sci USA 101:296–301

79. Andersson UG, Tracey KJ (2004) HMGB1, a pro-inflammatory cytokine of clinical interest: introduction. J Intern Med 255:318–319

80. Guo YL, Colman RW (2005) Two faces of high-molecular-weight kininogen (HK) in angiogenesis: bradykinin turns it on and cleaved HK (HKa) turns it off. J Thromb Haemost 3:670–676

81. Fein AM, Bernard GR, Criner GJ, et al (1997) Treatment of severe systemic inflammatory response syndrome and sepsis with a novel bradykinin antagonist, deltibant (CP-0127). Results of a randomized, double-blind, placebo-controlled trial. CP-0127 SIRS and Sepsis Study Group. JAMA 277:482–487

82. Nolan A, Weiden MD, Thurston G, Gold JA (2004) Vascular endothelial growth factor blockade reduces plasma cytokines in a murine model of polymicrobial sepsis. Inflammation 28:271–278

83. Armour J, Tyml K, Lidington D, Wilson JX (2001) Ascorbate prevents microvascular dysfunction in the skeletal muscle of the septic rat. J Appl Physiol 90:795–803

84. Heller AR, Groth G, Heller SC, et al (2001) N-acetylcysteine reduces respiratory burst but augments neutrophil phagocytosis in intensive care unit patients. Crit Care Med 29:272–276

85. Harlan JM, Winn RK (2002) Leukocyte-endothelial interactions: clinical trials of anti-adhesion therapy. Crit Care Med 30 (suppl 5):S214–S219
86. Bless NM, Tojo SJ, Kawarai H, et al (1998) Differing patterns of P-selectin expression in lung injury. Am J Pathol 153:1113–1122
87. Bogen S, Pak J, Garifallou M, Deng X, Muller WA (1994) Monoclonal antibody to murine PECAM-1 (CD31) blocks acute inflammation in vivo. J Exp Med 179:1059–1064
88. Peng X, Hassoun PM, Sammani S, et al (2004) Protective effects of sphingosine 1-phosphate in murine endotoxin-induced inflammatory lung injury. Am J Respir Crit Care Med 169:1245–1251
89. Seybold J, Thomas D, Witzenrath M, et al (2005) Tumor necrosis factor-alpha-dependent expression of phosphodiesterase 2: role in endothelial hyperpermeability. Blood 105:3569–3576
90. Szabo C, Southan GJ, Thiemermann C (1994) Beneficial effects and improved survival in rodent models of septic shock with S-methylisothiourea sulfate, a potent and selective inhibitor of inducible nitric oxide synthase. Proc Natl Acad Sci USA 91:12472–12476
91. Cobb JP, Natanson C, Hoffman WD, et al (1992) N omega-amino-L-arginine, an inhibitor of nitric oxide synthase, raises vascular resistance but increases mortality rates in awake canines challenged with endotoxin. J Exp Med 176:1175–1182
92. Laubach VE, Shesely EG, Smithies O, Sherman PA (1995) Mice lacking inducible nitric oxide synthase are not resistant to lipopolysaccharide-induced death. Proc Natl Acad Sci USA 92:10688–10692
93. Choi KB, Wong F, Harlan JM, Chaudhary PM, Hood L, Karsan A (1998) Lipopolysaccharide mediates endothelial apoptosis by a FADD-dependent pathway. J Biol Chem 273:20185–20188
94. Hotchkiss RS, Tinsley KW, Swanson PE, Karl IE (2002) Endothelial cell apoptosis in sepsis. Crit Care Med 30 (Suppl 5):S225–228
95. Kawasaki M, Kuwano K, Hagimoto N, et al (2000) Protection from lethal apoptosis in lipopolysaccharide-induced acute lung injury in mice by a caspase inhibitor. Am J Pathol 157:597–603
96. Cheng T, Liu D, Griffin JH, et al (2003) Activated protein C blocks p53-mediated apoptosis in ischemic human brain endothelium and is neuroprotective. Nat Med 9:338–342
97. Kan W, Zhao KS, Jiang Y, et al (2004) Lung, spleen, and kidney are the major places for inducible nitric oxide synthase expression in endotoxic shock: role of p38 mitogen-activated protein kinase in signal transduction of inducible nitric oxide synthase expression. Shock 21:281–287
98. Badger AM, Bradbeer JN, Votta B, Lee JC, Adams JL, Griswold DE (1996) Pharmacological profile of SB 203580, a selective inhibitor of cytokine suppressive binding protein/p38 kinase, in animal models of arthritis, bone resorption, endotoxin shock and immune function. J Pharmacol Exp Ther 279:1453–1461
99. Branger J, van den Blink B, Weijer S, et al (2002) Anti-inflammatory effects of a p38 mitogen-activated protein kinase inhibitor during human endotoxemia. J Immunol 168:4070–4077
100. Zingarelli B, Sheehan M, Wong HR (2003) Nuclear factor-kappaB as a therapeutic target in critical care medicine. Crit Care Med 31 (suppl 1):S105–S111
101. Matsuda N, Hattori Y, Jesmin S, Gando S (2005) Nuclear factor-kappaB decoy oligodeoxynucleotides prevent acute lung injury in mice with cecal ligation and puncture-induced sepsis. Mol Pharmacol 67:1018–1025
102. Gadjeva M, Tomczak MF, Zhang M, et al (2004) A role for NF-kappa B subunits p50 and p65 in the inhibition of lipopolysaccharide-induced shock. J Immunol 173:5786–5793
103. Dugo L, Collin M, Allen DA, et al (2005) GSK-3beta inhibitors attenuate the organ injury/dysfunction caused by endotoxemia in the rat. Crit Care Med 33:1903–1912

# Differential Effects of Pro-Inflammatory Mediators on Alveolar Epithelial Barrier Function

M.A. Matthay and J.-W. Lee

## Introduction

There has been considerable progress in understanding how the alveolar epithelium regulates fluid balance under normal and pathologic conditions [1]. There is a growing understanding of the important role of the alveolar epithelium in regulating inflammatory responses as well as in responding to several pathologic stimuli. Progress has been made possible because of the availability of excellent animal models for *in vivo* studies as well as several *in vitro* models including studies of cultured human alveolar epithelial type II cells. This chapter will focus on how four different inflammatory molecules (tumor necrosis factor [TNF]-$\alpha$, leukotriene $D_4$ (LTD$_4$), interleukin [IL]-1$\beta$, and transforming growth factor [TGF]-$\beta$) can exert differential effects on the barrier and fluid transport capacity of the alveolar epithelium with a particular focus on their relevance to acute lung injury (ALI).

## Normal Alveolar Epithelial Barrier

The normal alveolar epithelial barrier is very tight, resisting the passive movement of even small molecules and solutes such as electrolytes. Thus, the alveolar epithelium can be viewed as mostly impermeable to macromolecules such as proteins including albumin and immunoglobulins. Tight junctional proteins maintain this tight barrier between alveolar type I and type II epithelial cells [1].

In addition to these tight barrier properties, the alveolar epithelium has specialized functions that facilitate gas exchange. First, the alveolar epithelial type II cell is the source of surface active material, which is necessary for the maintenance of normal alveolar stability in the gas filled lung. Secondly, alveolar epithelial type II cells, as well as alveolar epithelial type I cells, have the capacity to remove excess alveolar fluid by vectorial ion transport. Sodium is taken up by apical ion channels and extruded actively by the basolateral Na/K-ATPase [1]. Chloride follows by unknown pathways under normal conditions and via the cystic fibrosis transmembrane conductance regulator (CFTR) under cAMP stimulated conditions [2,3]. Water follows the mini-osmotic gradient produced by vectorial transport of sodium and chloride into the interstitium and results in isomolar alveolar fluid clearance. Both catecholamine-dependent and catecholamine independent mechanisms can upregulate alveolar fluid clearance [2,4]. The best studied mechanisms are cAMP-dependent fluid clearance [1], which also has relevance at the time of birth when endogenous catecholamines upregulate alveolar fluid clearance [5]. Endogenous release of catecholamines has the capacity to upregulate alveolar fluid clearance under pathologic conditions of severe shock when there is a large increase in plasma catecholamine levels [6]. Delivery of a beta 2-adrenergic agonist to the distal airspaces of the lung markedly increases the rate of alveolar fluid clearance in several species, including the human lung [1].

## The Alveolar Epithelial Barrier to Pathologic Stimuli

Prior studies from our research group indicated that the alveolar epithelial barrier is remarkably resistant to injury. In these early studies, we instilled either autologus plasma or autologus serum into the distal airspaces of sheep. We found that large numbers of neutrophils and monocytes were chemoattracted to the alveoli, presumably secondary to release of chemotactic molecules from alveolar macrophages. The large numbers of inflammatory cells did not result in a change in alveolar epithelial permeability to protein [7]. Furthermore, fluid transport mechanisms were intact with a normal rate of alveolar fluid clearance.

A subsequent study in human volunteers was carried out to further assess the response of the alveolar epithelial to inflammatory stimuli [8]. Leukotriene $B_4$ (LTB$_4$) was instilled into the distal airspaces of human volunteers with a fiberoptic bronchoscope. The volunteers were lavaged subsequently at 4 and 24 hours in the LTB$_4$-instilled right middle lobe as well as in the contralateral control saline-instilled lingula. The results showed that large numbers of neutrophils were attracted to the alveoli, similar to the numbers of neutrophils lavaged from patients with acute respiratory distress syndrome (ARDS), but there was no increase in permeability to protein across the alveolar epithelium (Table 1). These results indicated that the epithelial barrier was resistant to injury and could permit the passage of inflammatory response cells, neutrophils and monocytes, to chemotactic stimuli in the airspaces without injuring the alveolar epithelium.

A subsequent experimental study in our laboratory demonstrated that instillation of *Escherichia coli* endotoxin into the distal airspaces of the sheep lung resulted in a large influx of neutrophils at both 4 hours and 24 hours in anesthetized as

**Table 1.** Bronchoalveolar lavage fluid cells and proteins after LTB$_4$ instillation in human lungs [8]

| Variable | NaCl | LTB$_4$ | P value |
|---|---|---|---|
| Total Cells ($10^6$) | $6.8 \pm 1.0$ | $26.4 \pm 5.0$ | 0.002 |
| Neutrophils (%) | $12.2 \pm 4.6$ | $55.7 \pm 6.0$ | 0.001 |
| Macrophages (%) | $82.7 \pm 5.9$ | $40.5 \pm 6.1$ | 0.001 |
| Total Protein (mg) | $15.4 \pm 4.8$ | $23.4 \pm 3.5$ | NS |

The data are the mean $\pm$ SE of data from 11 human subjects.

well as unanesthetized sheep. Again, similar to the studies with $LTB_4$, there was no change in alveolar epithelial permeability to protein in either the alveolar to the interstitial direction or from the vascular compartment to the airspaces. Also, the normal rate of alveolar fluid clearance was well preserved in these sheep studies over 24 hours [9].

When live bacteria were instilled into the airspaces, specifically *Pseudomonas aeruginosa*, there was evidence of a modest bidirectional increase in alveolar epithelial permeability. This finding was evident at both 4 and 24 hours in studies in sheep. Further, the rate of alveolar fluid clearance was diminished by the presence of bacteria and the alteration in epithelial barrier permeability. Nevertheless, there still was measurable net alveolar fluid clearance, although the rate of clearance was reduced [9]. Follow-up studies demonstrated that several products of *Pseudomonas* were responsible for the decrease in fluid clearance and the increase in lung epithelial permeability.

Several other studies in experimental animals using clinically relevant models of acute lung injury (ALI) demonstrated, as expected, that the alveolar epithelial barrier can be injured and that alveolar fluid clearance is reduced. For example, acid-induced lung injury, as a model of aspiration in humans, resulted in a reduction in alveolar fluid clearance proportionate to the degree of alveolar epithelial injury. In one study in rabbits, we found that an anti-IL-8 monoclonal antibody reduced acid-induced lung injury by reducing neutrophil mediated injury [10]. Also, in a more recent study, treatment with a beta-2 adrenergic agonist upregulated alveolar fluid clearance and decreased lung endothelial permeability in rats with acid-induced lung injury [11].

## Pro-inflammatory Molecules and Alveolar Epithelial Fluid Transport

We and other investigators have measured several pro-inflammatory mediators in the airspaces of patients with ALI as well as in animal models [12, 13]. The acute pro-inflammatory response is an important part of innate immunity that regulates neutrophil and monocyte influx designed to neutralize a variety of infectious agents and microbial products. The effects of some of these inflammatory molecules on alveolar epithelial function have resulted in several interesting effects.

For example, we discovered several years ago that TNF-α can markedly upregulate the rate of alveolar fluid clearance in rats with *Pseudomonas* pneumonia [14]. Another group of investigators confirmed this finding with a different model of ischemia-reperfusion and shock in rats [15]. Finally, additional studies by our group demonstrated that TNF-α has the capacity to upregulate sodium-dependent transport in both human type II cells as well as in the rat lung [16, 17]. There is also some evidence that prolonged exposure to TNF-α *in vitro* can have a depressant effect on gene expression and ion transport in the alveolar epithelium [18]. Thus, the presence of a pro-inflammatory molecule may upregulate alveolar fluid clearance, perhaps an adaptive response that is useful for the alveolar epithelium to minimize the quantity of excess fluid in the airspaces of the acutely injured and inflamed lung.

Another group of investigators discovered that $LTD_4$, a pro-inflammatory molecule, has the capacity to upregulate alveolar epithelial sodium and fluid transport [19]. Previous studies from our research group demonstrated that markedly elevated levels of $LTD_4$ are found in patients with ALI [20]. At that time we thought that the effects of $LTD_4$ were simply to increase vasoconstriction and broncoconstriction as part of the inflammatory response in the lung. However, this recent work indicates that $LTD_4$ can upregulate alveolar fluid clearance through increased activity and membrane localization of the Na/K-ATPase. The effect is mediated through the CysLT receptor 2, which was identified in both A549 cells and rat alveolar epithelial type II cells. Thus, both TNF-$\alpha$ and $LTD_4$ have the capacity to upregulate alveolar fluid clearance at the same time that they are enhancing the inflammatory responses in the airspaces of the lung.

There are other inflammatory molecules that we have studied that have the opposite effect on alveolar epithelial fluid transport. The best studied and perhaps the most relevant are IL-1$\beta$ and TGF-$\beta$1. Both of these cytokines are important in the pathogenesis of ALI and interestingly both of them appear to have deleterious effects on alveolar epithelial barrier function and the capacity of the epithelium to reabsorb edema fluid.

IL-1$\beta$ is one of the most biologically active cytokines in pulmonary edema and bronchoalveolar lavage (BAL) fluids of patients with ALI [21,22]. There is evidence that IL-1$\beta$ increases microvascular lung epithelial permeability based on both *in vitro* and *in vivo* models of ALI. IL-1$\beta$ also enhances alveolar epithelial repair by increasing cell spreading [23] and fibroblast proliferation [22]. In recent studies, we found that IL-1$\beta$ decreases expression of the epithelial sodium channel $\alpha$-subunit in alveolar epithelial cells via a p38 mitogen activated protein kinase (MAPK)-dependent signaling pathway. IL-1$\beta$ significantly reduced the amiloride-sensitive fraction of the transepithelial current and sodium transport across rat alveolar type II cell monolayers. IL-1$\beta$ also decreased both basal and dexamethasone-induced epithelial sodium channel $\alpha$-subunit ($\alpha$ENaC) mRMA levels and total and cell surface protein expression. The inhibitory effect of IL-1$\beta$ on $\alpha$ENaC expression was mediated by the activation of p38-MAPK in both rat and human alveolar type II cells [24]. These results provide evidence that IL-1$\beta$ may play an important role in reducing the resolution of alveolar edema in the acutely injured lung.

Another important cytokine with pro-inflammatory properties is TGF-$\beta$1. Recent work from our research group using mouse studies with both bleomycin and endotoxin-induced lung injury indicated that TGF-$\beta$1 is an important early mediator of lung injury by increasing permeability across the lung endothelium and epithelium [25]. In more recent studies, we determined that TGF-$\beta$1 significantly reduces the amiloride-sensitive fraction of sodium uptake and fluid transport across monolayers of both rat and human alveolar type II cells. TGF-$\beta$1 also significantly decreased $\alpha$ENaC mRNA and protein expression and inhibited expression of a luciferase reporter downstream of the $\alpha$ENaC promoter in lung epithelial cells.

The inhibitory effect was mediated by activation of the MAPK, ERK1/2 [26]. Also, TGF-β1 inhibited the amiloride-sensitive alveolar fluid transport in an *in vivo* rat model at a dose that was not associated with a change in epithelial protein permeability. These results, therefore, indicate that TGF-β1 can decrease the capacity of the alveolar epithelium to remove excess fluid from the distal airspace the lung.

## Gene Expression of Inflammatory and Transport Molecules in Human Alveolar Type II Cells

In order to explore the specific capacity of the alveolar epithelium to regulate the production of pro-inflammatory and ion transport genes, we have carried out a series of studies in cultured monolayers of human alveolar type II cells. Several experimental preparations have been used including the use of cytomix, a combination of IL-1β, TNF-α, and interferon (IFN)γ as well as authentic human pulmonary edema fluid from patients with ALI. In these studies, the cytomix preparation and the human edema fluid induce a marked increase in gene expression for several pro-inflammatory genes while at the same time inducing a marked decrease in gene expression for ion transport molecules as well as molecules that regulate epithelial cell permeability.

## Conclusions

In summary, there is convincing evidence that alveolar fluid clearance and the resolution of alveolar edema is driven by active vectorial ion transport (sodium and chloride) across the alveolar epithelium of the lung. Mortality in patients with ALI is significantly higher in the presence of impaired alveolar fluid clearance (Fig. 1) [27]. Several catecholamine dependent and independent mechanisms can markedly upregulate alveolar fluid clearance. Interestingly, evidence accumulated in the last 10 years indicates that several pro-inflammatory molecules that have a role in the pathogenesis of ALI by increasing lung vascular permeability can also play an important role in the capacity of the alveolar epithelium to modulate lung fluid balance. Specifically, TNF-α and LTD$_4$ can upregulate alveolar fluid clearance at the same time that they have pro-inflammatory effects in the nearby lung parenchyma. On the other hand, IL-1β and TGFβ have now been demonstrated to decrease alveolar epithelial fluid transport, thus probably contributing to the magnitude of ALI by diminishing the resolution of alveolar edema as well as enhancing the formation of lung edema. There is much to be learned about the differential effects of pro-inflammatory genes and their protein projects on lung fluid balance in the setting of ALI.

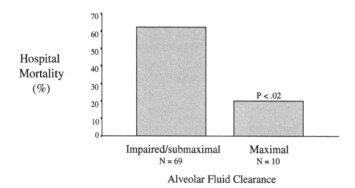

Fig. 1. These data demonstrates that submaximal or impaired alveolar fluid clearance in patients with acute lung injury is associated with a higher mortality when compared to patients with maximal alveolar fluid clearance. From [26] with permission

## References

1. Matthay MA, Folkesson HG, Clerici C (2002) Lung epithelial fluid transport and the resolution of pulmonary edema. Physiol Rev 82:569–600
2. Fang X, Fukuda N, Barbry P, Sartori C, Verkman AS, Matthay MA (2002) Novel role for CFTR in fluid absorption from the distal airspaces of the lung. J Gen Physiol 119:199–207
3. Fang X, Song Y, Hirsch J, et al (2006) Contribution of CFTR to Apical-basolateral Fluid Transport in Cultured Human Alveolar Epithelial Type II Cells. Am J Physiol Lung Cell Mol Physiol 290:L242–L249
4. Bertorello AM, Sznajder JI (2005) The dopamine Paradox in lung and kidney epitheliasharing the same target but operating different signaling networks. Am J Respir Cell Mol Biol 33:432–437
5. Walters DV, Olver RE (1978) The role of catecholamines in lung liquid absorption at birth. Pediatr Res 12:239–242
6. Pittet JF, Wiener-Kronish JP, McElroy MC, Folkesson HG, Matthay MA (1994) Stimulation of lung epithelial liquid clearance by endogenous release of catecholamines in septic shock in anesthetized rats. J Clin Invest 94:663–671
7. Matthay MA, Berthiaume Y, Staub NC (1985) Long-term clearance of liquid and protein from the lungs of unanesthetized sheep. J Appl Physiol 59:928–934
8. Martin TR, Pistorese BP, Chi EY, Goodman RB, Matthay MA (1989) Effects of leukotriene B4 in the human lung. Recruitment of neutrophils into the alveolar spaces without a change in protein permeability. J Clin Invest 84:1609–1619
9. Wiener-Kronish JP, Albertine KH, Matthay MA (1991) Differential responses of the endothelial and epithelial barriers of the lung in sheep to Escherichia coli endotoxin. J Clin Invest 88:864–875
10. Modelska K, Pittet JF, Folkesson HG, Courtney Broaddus V, Matthay MA (1999) Acid-induced lung injury. Protective effect of anti-interleukin-8 pretreatment on alveolar epithelial barrier function in rabbits. Am J Respir Crit Care Med 160:1450–1456
11. McAuley DF, Frank JA, Fang X, Matthay MA (2004) Clinically relevant concentrations of beta2-adrenergic agonists stimulate maximal cyclic adenosine monophosphate-dependent airspace fluid clearance and decrease pulmonary edema in experimental acid-induced lung injury. Crit Care Med 32:1470–1476

12. Pittet JF, Mackersie RC, Martin TR, Matthay MA (1997) Biological markers of acute lung injury: prognostic and pathogenetic significance. Am J Respir Crit Care Med 155:1187–1205
13. Pugin J, Verghese G, Widmer MC, Matthay MA (1999) The alveolar space is the site of intense inflammatory and profibrotic reactions in the early phase of acute respiratory distress syndrome. Crit Care Med 27:304–312
14. Rezaiguia S, Garat C, Delclaux C, et al (1997) Acute bacterial pneumonia in rats increases alveolar epithelial fluid clearance by a tumor necrosis factor-alpha-dependent mechanism. J Clin Invest 9:325–35
15. Borjesson A, Norlin A, Wang X, Andersson R, Folkesson HG (2000) TNF-alpha stimulates alveolar liquid clearance during intestinal ischemia-reperfusion in rats. Am J Physiol Lung Cell Mol Physiol 278:L3–L12
16. Fukuda N, Jayr C, Lazrak A, et al. (2001) Mechanisms of TNF-alpha stimulation of amiloride-sensitive sodium transport across alveolar epithelium. Am J Physiol Lung Cell Mol Physiol 280:L1258–L1265
17. Elia N, Tapponnier M, Matthay MA, et al (2003) Functional identification of the alveolar edema reabsorption activity of murine tumor necrosis factor-alpha. Am J Respir Crit Care Med 168:1043–1050
18. Dagenais A, Frechette R, Yamagata Y, et al (2004) Downregulation of αENaC activity and expression by TNF-alpha in alveolar epithelial cells. Am J Physiol Lung Cell Mol Physiol 286:L301–L311
19. Sloniewsky DE, Ridge KM, Adir Y, et al (2004) Leukotriene D4 activates alveolar epithelial Na,K-ATPase and increases alveolar fluid clearance. Am J Respir Crit Care Med 169:407–412
20. Matthay MA, Eschenbacher WL, Goetzl EJ (1984) Elevated concentrations of leukotriene D4 in pulmonary edema fluid of patients with the adult respiratory distress syndrome. J Clin Immunol 4:479–483
21. Pugin J, Verghese G, Widmer MC, Matthay MA (1999) The alveolar space is the site of intense inflammatory and profibrotic reactions in the early phase of acute respiratory distress syndrome. Crit Care Med 27:304–312
22. Olman MA, White KE, Ware LB, et al (2004) Pulmonary edema fluid from patients with early lung injury stimulates fibroblast proliferation through IL-1 beta-induced IL-6 expression. J Immunol 172:2668–2677
23. Geiser T, Atabai K, Jarreau PH, Ware LB, Pugin J, Matthay MA (2001) Pulmonary edema fluid from patients with acute lung injury augments in vitro alveolar epithelial repair by an IL-1beta-dependent mechanism. Am J Respir Crit Care Med 163:1384–1388
24. Roux J, Kawakatsu H, Gartland B, et al (2005) Interleukin-1beta decreases expression of the epithelial sodium channel alpha-subunit in alveolar epithelial cells via a p38 MAPK-dependent signaling pathway. J Biol Chem 280:18579–18589
25. Pittet JF, Griffiths MJ, Geiser T, et al (2001) TGF-beta is a critical mediator of acute lung injury. J Clin Invest 107:1537–1544
26. Frank J, Roux J, Kawakatsu H, et al (2003) Transforming growth factor-1 decreases expression of the epithelial sodium channel αENaC and alveolar epithelial vectorial sodium and fluid transport via an ERK1/2-dependent mechanism. J Biol Chem 278:43939–43950
27. Ware LB, Matthay MA (2001) Alveolar fluid clearance is impaired in the majority of patients with acute lung injury and the acute respiratory distress syndrome. Am J Respir Crit Care Med 163:1376–1383

# Mechanisms and Pathways of Dysfunction

# Macrocirculatory Disturbances

D. De Backer

## Introduction

Severe sepsis and septic shock are associated with a state of inadequate supply or inappropriate use of oxygen and nutrients by the cells, which may result in tissue hypoxia and lactic acidosis. Unless transient, this will lead to irreversible tissue damage and death. As tissue necrosis is uncommon in patients with septic shock [1], adaptations of organ metabolism are likely to occur in order to shut down some less essential metabolic pathways and to preserve vital functions. This will lead to the development of multiple organ failure (MOF), which can be reversed if the underlying sepsis can be cured. MOF is frequent in patients with severe sepsis, despite the restoration of whole-body hemodynamics. Early interventions aiming at normalizing some specific hemodynamic end-points improve outcome of patients in septic shock [2]. Nevertheless, many patients will still develop MOF and will ultimately die, suggesting that other factors were not corrected. Global hemodynamic alterations, blood flow redistribution, microvascular blood flow alterations, and direct cellular toxicity may play a crucial role in the development of MOF in these patients.

## Global Hemodynamic Alterations

Septic shock is a complex syndrome characterized by profound cardiovascular derangements, with alterations in cardiac function, blood flow redistribution between organs, and microcirculatory alterations (Table 1).

### Decreased Vascular Tone

Hypotension is a typical finding in sepsis. The endothelial dysfunction is responsible for a marked resistance to vasopressors. The contractile response of arteries and arterioles to norepinephrine or phenylephrine is decreased in sepsis [3], and this effect is mediated by circulating factors. Several factors have been implicated in this vasodilatory state. The role of nitric oxide (NO) has been clearly demonstrated [4, 5] but NO inhibitors have failed to improve survival in patients with septic shock even though these compounds increased arterial pressure. Vasopressin deficiency has also been reported [6, 7], but it is unlikely that vasopressin

**Table 1.** Principal hemodynamic alterations in septic shock

Systemic hemodynamic alterations:

    Decreased vascular tone
    Hypovolemia
        Absolute (increased permeability)
        Relative (blood pooling, especially in the splanchnic bed)
    Decreased venous compliance
    Myocardial dysfunction
        Systolic
        Diastolic

Regional blood flow alterations:

    Hepatosplanchnic area
    Kidneys
    Brain
Microvascular blood flow alterations

deficiency takes a prominent role in the early phases of sepsis as vasopressin levels are usually elevated at the onset of sepsis [7]. In addition to vasopressin deficiency, vasopressin resistance may also occur as there is desensitization of the vasopressin receptor, both in arteries and in venules [8, 9]. Inadequate cortisol levels or resistance to corticosteroids has also been suggested, especially in the late stages of sepsis, and hydrocortisone administration may help to restore the pressor response to norepinephrine in patients with septic shock [10]. Thus, it is likely that several mechanisms are implicated in the sepsis-induced vasodilatory state, but the contribution of each of these factors may vary over time.

## Decreased Venous Return

A decrease in venous return is always present in sepsis. Pinsky et al. [11] reported that endotoxin administration caused a marked decrease in venous tone within 5 min. At this time, endotoxin did not yet alter arterial vasomotor tone. The venous congestion is not equally distributed, with the splanchnic area more prone to develop venous pooling. By studying portal pressure/flow relationships, Ayuse et al. [12] reported that endotoxin increased the closing pressure without changes in the slope of the relationship. This leads to portal hypertension and venous pooling, which is further exacerbated since the veno-arterial response in the mesenteric artery is abolished.

    In addition, vascular permeability is increased in sepsis [13,14], and the combination of venous pooling and plasma losses results in severe hypovolemia. Finally, Stephan et al. [15] observed that the venous vascular compliance is decreased in septic patients, so that central venous pressure may underestimate the severity of hypovolemia.

The consequences of hypovolemia include low or inadequate cardiac output and redistribution of regional blood flows, especially at the expense of splanchnic and renal blood flows.

## Myocardial Depression

Septic shock is characterized by a high cardiac output and peripheral vasodilatation. However, various studies have demonstrated that myocardial contractility may be altered despite a normal or increased cardiac output. After administration of low doses of endotoxin to human healthy volunteers, Suffredini et al. [16] reported that the left ventricular ejection fraction was decreased although cardiac output increased. Myocardial depression is always observed in septic patients, whatever the method used to investigate cardiac function (e. g., echocardiography, isotopes), but its severity is variable and is related to outcome. Myocardial depression is related to the liberation of mediators of sepsis (e. g., cytokines, NO, etc), however the mechanisms responsible for myocardial depression are unclear. Myocardial contractility and relaxation are both affected. Histological changes are common and troponin can be released although coronary blood flow is increased and lactate is usually consumed by the heart. Nevertheless, myocardial depression resolves completely after resolution of sepsis.

## Altered Oxygen Extraction and $VO_2/DO_2$ Dependency

A large number of experimental studies have shown that oxygen extraction capabilities are impaired in sepsis and that this may lead to the development of dependence of oxygen consumption ($VO_2$) on oxygen delivery ($DO_2$), or $VO_2/DO_2$ dependency, even at normal values of $DO_2$ [17, 18]. Several factors may account for the altered extraction capabilities, including blood flow redistribution between the organs (due to the altered vascular tone), redistribution of blood flow within each organ (due to microvascular alterations), and altered use of oxygen by the cells (also called cytopathic hypoxia). The contribution of each of these factors is difficult to separate. As oxygen extraction is preserved in a perfused capillary [19], the role of decreased vascular tone and microcirculatory alterations seems to be prominent, at least in the early phases of sepsis. Due to methodological limitations, the reality of this phenomenon in humans has been difficult to demonstrate [20].

## Consequences of Global Hemodynamic Alterations

To what extent doe the hypotension induced by the decrease in vascular tone contribute to organ hypoperfusion and dysfunction in sepsis? In experimental studies, correction of hypotension by adrenergic agents has been shown to improve survival [21]. In patients, several studies have reported that the severity of hypotension is related to outcome [22]. In addition, the more severe the resistance to catecholamines, the greater the likelihood of developing organ failure and death [23, 24]. In a recent study, Varpula et al. [25] showed that a mean arterial pressure (MAP) level below 65 mmHg on arrival, during the first 6 hours, and the first 48 hours were independently associated with 30 day-mortality. Raising blood pressure above this level may not be associated with improved tissue perfusion [26, 27]. Accordingly, it may be considered that maintaining blood pressure above 65 mmHg is sufficient.

The combination of hypovolemia and myocardial dysfunction may be severe enough to impair cardiac output, leading to an inadequate $DO_2$ (whether $VO_2/DO_2$ dependency occurs or not). Many experimental studies have shown that cardiac output is initially low and that the hyperdynamic state can only be observed after fluid resuscitation [28, 29]. To what extent does impaired $DO_2$ play a role in the development of organ dysfunction? Several studies have reported that cardiac output and $DO_2$ are higher in survivors than in non-survivors [30–32]. In addition, it has been shown that early hemodynamic optimization is associated with a decreased risk of new onset organ failure and death [2]. What component of the decreased $DO_2$ is the most relevant? Early fluid administration prolongs survival time in animals [33], but its role in patients with septic shock, especially in prolonged shock, remains unclear. The role of inotropic agents is also controversial. Combining the findings of the studies by Rivers et al. [2] and Gattinoni et al. [34], it may be proposed that hemodynamic optimization using fluids, inotropic agents, and red blood cell transfusions may be beneficial in the early phases of sepsis. In the late stages of sepsis, maintaining $DO_2$ at high levels seems not to be beneficial, even though it seems reasonable to avoid tissue hypoperfusion. The lowest tolerable level of $DO_2$ has to be defined on an individual basis.

## Regional Blood Flow Alterations

In addition to systemic hemodynamic alterations, sepsis can induce profound alterations in blood flow distribution. These can lead to cerebral blood flow alterations, with possible loss of cerebral autoregulation, and alterations in renal and hepatosplanchnic blood flow.

### Hepatosplanchnic Hemodynamics

Important histological alterations can be observed in the gut [35] and the liver [36] during sepsis. Although a direct cytotoxic effect of NO or cytokines can be envisaged, an imbalance between oxygen supply and demand in the splanchnic area may participate in the development of organ failure [37].

#### Anatomic and Physiologic Considerations

The liver is supplied by a dual circulation. Hepatic artery and portal blood flow mix at the entry of the hepatic acinus, the functional liver unit, which is 2 mm wide. Before being drained by the hepatic vein, blood will provide oxygen and nutrients to the hepatocytes located in the sinusoids, but a wide $PO_2$ gradient can be observed between the periportal and the centrilobular zones, so that the latter is much more sensitive to decreases in oxygen supply. In normal circumstances, the hepatic vein saturation ($ShO_2$) is close to mixed venous oxygen saturation ($SvO_2$) so that the gradient between $ShO_2$ and $SvO_2$ is usually less than 10% [38].

The vascularization of the gut is also complex. In normal conditions, the distribution of blood flow to the different components is related to metabolic requirements. The amount of blood flow (by unit of weight) directed to the small intestine is twice the amount directed to the stomach or the colon, the mucosal and submucosal regions receiving 70% of total gut blood flow. Metabolism is also very high in this area since the gut mucosa accounts for 10–15% of total body protein production. In addition, the gut mucosa is particularly sensitive to alterations in blood flow due to the typical vascularization of the microvilli. The artery to the villus forms a right angle with the mesenteric artery so that plasma skewing occurs and hematocrit is lower in the mucosa than in the submucosa and serosa. Also, the artery is located in the center of the villus, surrounded by laces of veins in which the flows are in the opposite direction. This particular anatomical vascular network allows better absorption of the nutrients but also leads to countercurrent exchange of oxygen from the artery to the vein along their parallel course. Consequently, $PO_2$ decreases from the base of the villus to its tip, reaching values as low as 30 mmHg. In healthy humans, Temmesfeld-Wollbrück et al. [39] reported that oxygen saturation ranged from 50 to 100%.

### Effects of Sepsis on Hepatosplanchnic Blood Flow and Metabolism

The normal splanchnic $VO_2$ represents 20–35% of total $VO_2$ while splanchnic blood flow is equal to 25% of cardiac output. In sepsis, various studies [40,41] have reported a disproportionate increase in metabolic requirements in the splanchnic area (and especially in the liver with an increase in glucose output, lactate uptake, and protein synthesis). This increase in hepatosplanchnic metabolism exceeded the increase in splanchnic blood flow so that the gradient between $SvO_2$ and $ShO_2$ was increased, ranging between 20 and 40% [38,42]. We [43] reported that an increased gradient (higher than 10%) was associated with covariance of hepatosplanchnic $VO_2$ and $DO_2$ during dobutamine administration or application of positive end-expiratory pressure (PEEP) in septic patients.

The effects of sepsis on the gut are more difficult to investigate. In experimental studies on septic shock, mesenteric blood flow has been reported to be reduced, unchanged, or increased. Such differences may depend on the animal species, the technique used to investigate regional blood flow, and the amount of fluid administered. Even in experimental models in which mesenteric blood flow was increased, alterations in gut mucosal permeability, gut mucosal acidosis, and histological lesions can be observed [35]. Tugtekin et al. [44] reported that perfusion of the villi was markedly decreased and heterogeneous, and the authors ascribed the increase in gut mucosal $PCO_2$ to these alterations in mucosal blood flow. In addition, oxygen extraction capabilities are impaired by endotoxin, both in the liver and in the gut, and this could possibly be related to increased blood flow heterogeneity [45]. In septic patients, Temmesfeld-Wollbrück et al. [39] reported that gut oxygen saturation heterogeneity was increased and ranged from 0 to 70%.

In humans, liver dysfunction [46] and gut mucosal acidosis [47] are associated with a poor outcome.Even though therapeutic strategies using gastric mucosal pH as a goal yielded controversial results [48, 49], it seems reasonable to avoid interventions that could further impair hepatosplanchnic blood flow.

## Renal Perfusion

Renal failure frequently occurs in sepsis and several mechanisms have been implicated, including renal hypoperfusion [50]. The involvement of renal blood flow impairment in sepsis has been reviewed recently by Langenberg et al. [51]. These authors reported that renal blood flow was impaired in 62% of the 159 animal studies identified; in most of these studies renal blood flow impairment was associated with signs of under-resuscitation (hypodynamic shock). As the measurement of renal blood flow is difficult in critically ill patients, it remains uncertain whether renal blood flow alterations have a role in the development of acute renal failure in hyperdynamic sepsis. Indirect evidence suggests that afferent and efferent arterial tone in sepsis may be affected differently. Increasing MAP from 65 to 85 mmHg with norepinephrine, which acts primarily on the afferent arteriole, is not accompanied by any change in urine output or creatinine clearance [27], while partially replacing norepinephrine by vasopressin administration, which acts mostly on the efferent arteriole, increased both urine output and creatinine clearance [52].

## Cerebral Perfusion

The role of cerebral hypoperfusion in the development of septic encephalopathy is also controversial [53–55]. Although cerebral autoregulation theoretically protects the brain from whole body hemodynamic alterations [53], some authors have found that this regulatory mechanism may be lost in sepsis [56, 57]

## Conclusion

Sepsis induces profound metabolic and cardiovascular derangements. Although some indices indicate that cytopathic hypoxia may coexist, early correction of global hemodynamic alterations is essential. Regional blood flow alterations may persist after correction of systemic hemodynamics. Although a systematic increase in splanchnic blood flow may not be warranted, several arguments suggest that the maintenance of an adequate balance between oxygen supply and demand in the splanchnic area may be useful.

# References

1. Hotchkiss RS, Swanson PE, Freeman BD, et al. (1999) Apoptotic cell death in patients with sepsis, shock, and multiple organ dysfunction. Crit Care Med 27:1230–1251
2. Rivers E, Nguyen B, Havstadt S, et al. (2001) Early goal-directed therapy in the treatment of severe sepsis and septic shock. N Engl J Med 345:1368–1377
3. Hollenberg SM, Cunnion RE, Parrillo JE (1992) Effect of septic serum on vascular smooth muscle: In vitro studies using rat aortic rings. Crit Care Med 20, 993–998.
4. Landin L, Lorente JA, Renes E, Canas P, Jorge P, Liste D (1994) Inhibition of nitric oxide synthesis improves the vasoconstrictive effects of noradrenaline in sepsis. Chest 106:250–256
5. Pastor CM, Billiar TR (1995) Nitric oxide causes hyporeactivity to phenylephrine in isolated perfused livers from endotoxin-treated rats. Am J Physiol 268:G177–G182
6. Landry DW, Levin HR, Gallant EM, et al. (1997) Vasopressin deficiency contributes to the vasodilation of septic shock. Circulation 95:1122–1125
7. Sharshar T, Blanchard A, Paillard M, et al. (2003) Circulating vasopressin levels in septic shock. Crit Care Med 31:1752–1758
8. Roth BL, Spitzer JA (1987) Altered hepatic vasopressin and alpha 1-adrenergic receptors after chronic endotoxin infusion. Am J Physiol 252;E699–E702
9. Hollenberg SM, Tangora JJ, Piotrowski MJ, Easington C, Parrillo JE (1997) Impaired microvascular vasoconstrictive responses to vasopressin in septic rats. Crit Care Med 25:869–873
10. Annane D, Bellissant E, Sebille V, et al. (1998) Impaired pressor sensitivity to noradrenaline in septic shock patients with and without impaired adrenal function reserve. Br J Clin Pharmacol 46:589–597
11. Pinsky MR, Matuschak GM (1986) Cardiovascular determinants of the hemodynamic response to acute endotoxemia in the dog. J Crit Care 1:18–31
12. Ayuse T, Brienza N, Revelly JP, et al. (1995) Alterations in liver hemodynamics in an intact porcine model of endotoxin shock. Am J Physiol 268:H1106–H1114
13. O'Dwyer ST, Michie HR, Ziegler TR, Revhaug A, Smith RJ, Wilmore DW (1988) A single dose of endotoxin increases intestinal permeability in healthy humans. Arch Surg 123:1459-1464
14. Fink M P, Antonsson J B, Wang H, Rothschild HR (1991) Increased intestinal permeability in endotoxic pigs. Arch Surg 126:211–218
15. Stephan F, Novara A, Tournier B, et al. (1998) Determination of total effective vascular compliance in patients with sepsis syndrome. Am J Respir Crit Care Med 157:50–56
16. Suffredini AF, Fromm RE, Parker MM, et al. (1989) The cardiovascular response of normal humans to the administration of endotoxin. N Engl J Med 321:280–287
17. Nelson DP, Beyer C, Samsel RW, et al. (1987) Pathological supply dependence of O2 uptake during bacteremia in dogs. J Appl Physiol 63:1487–1492
18. Zhang H, Smail N, Cabral A, Cherkaoui S, Peny MO, Vincent JL (1999) Hepato-splanchnic blood flow and oxygen extraction capabilities during experimental tamponade: effects of endotoxin. J Surg Res 81:129–138
19. Ellis CG, Bateman RM, Sharpe MD, Sibbald WJ, Gill R (2002) Effect of a maldistribution of microvascular blood flow on capillary O(2) extraction in sepsis. Am J Physiol 282, H156–H164
20. Vincent JL, De Backer D (2004) Oxygen transport-the oxygen delivery controversy. Intensive Care Med 30:1990–1996
21. Sun Q, Tu Z, Lobo S, et al. (2003) Optimal Adrenergic Support in Septic Shock Due to Peritonitis. Anesthesiology 98:888–896
22. Bernardin G, Pradier C, Tiger F, et al. (1996) Blood pressure and arterial lactate level are early indicators of short-term survival in human septic shock. Intensive Care Med 22:17–25
23. Levy B, Dusang B, Annane D, et al. (2005) Cardiovascular response to dopamine and early prediction of outcome. A prospective multicenter study. Crit Care Med 33:2172–2177

24. Abid O, Akca S, Haji-Michael P, Vincent JL (2000) Strong vasopressor support may be futile in the intensive care unit patient with multiple organ failure. Crit Care Med 28:947–949
25. Varpula M, Tallgren M, Saukkonen K, Voipio-Pulkki LM, Pettila V (2005) Hemodynamic variables related to outcome in septic shock. Intensive Care Med 31:1066–1071
26. LeDoux D, Astiz M E, Carpati CM, Rackow EC (2000) Effects of perfusion pressure on tissue perfusion in septic shock. Crit Care Med 28:2729–2732
27. Bourgoin A, Leone M, Delmas A, Garnier F, Albanese J, Martin C (2005) Increasing mean arterial pressure in patients with septic shock: effects on oxygen variables and renal function. Crit Care Med 33:780–786
28. Cholley BP, Lang RM, Berger DS, Korcarz C, Payen D, Shroff SG (1995) Alterations in systemic arterial mechanical properties during septic shock: role of fluid resuscitation. Am J Physiol 269:H375–H384
29. De Backer D, Zhang H, Cherkhaoui S, Borgers M, Vincent JL (2001) Effects of dobutamine on hepato-splanchnic hemodynamics in an experimental model of hyperdynamic endotoxic shock. Shock 15:208–214
30. Shoemaker WC, Appel PL, Kram HB, Bishop MH, Abraham E (1993) Sequence of physiologic patterns in surgical septic shock. Crit Care Med 21:1876–1889
31. Shoemaker W C, Appel P L, Kram H B, Bishop MH, Abraham E (1993) Temporal hemodynamic and oxygen transport patterns in medical patients: septic shock. Chest 104:1529–1536
32. Tuchschmidt J, Fried J, Astiz M, Rackow E (1992) Elevation of cardiac output and oxygen delivery improves outcome in septic shock. Chest 102:216–220
33. Hollenberg S M, Dumasius A, Easington C, Collila SA, Neumann A, Parrillo JA (2001) Characterization of a hyperdynamic murine model of resuscitated sepsis using echocardiography. Am J Respir Crit Care Med 164:891–895
34. Gattinoni L, Brazzi L, Pelosi P, et al. (1995) A trial of goal-oriented hemodynamic therapy in critically ill patients. N Engl J Med 333:1025–1032
35. Sautner T, Wessely C, Riegler M, et al. (1998) Early effects of catecholamine therapy on mucosal integrity, intestinal blood flow, and oxygen metabolism in porcine endotoxin shock. Ann Surg 228:239–248
36. Tighe D, Moss R, Bennett D (1998) Porcine hepatic response to sepsis and its amplification by adrenergic receptor a1 agonist and a b2 antagonist. Clin Sci 95:467–478
37. Mythen MG, Webb AR (1994) The role of gut mucosal hypoperfusion in the pathogenesis of post-operative organ dysfunction. Intensive Care Med 20:203–209
38. Dahn MS, Lange MP, Jacobs LA (1988) Central mixed and splanchnic venous oxygen saturation monitoring. Intensive Care Med 14:373–378
39. Temmesfeld-Wollbrück B, Szalay A, Mayer K, Olschewski H, Seeger W, Grimminger F (1998) Abnormalities of gastric mucosal oxygenation in septic shock. Am J Respir Crit Care Med 157:1586–1592
40. Dahn MS, Mitchell RA, Lange MP, Smith S, Jacobs SA (1995) Hepatic metabolic response to injury and sepsis. Surgery 117:520–530
41. Dahn M S, Lange P, Lobdell K, Hans B, Jacobs LA, Mitchell RA (1987) Splanchnic and total body oxygen consumption differences in septic and injured patients. Surgery 101:69–80
42. Ruokonen E, Takala J, Uusaro A (1991) Effect of vasoactive treatment on the relationship between mixed venous and regional oxygen saturation. Crit Care Med 19:1365–1369
43. De Backer D, Creteur J, Noordally O, Smail N, Gulbis B, Vincent JL (1998) Does hepato-splanchnic $VO_2/DO_2$ dependency exist in critically ill septic patients? Am J Respir Crit Care Med 157:1219–1225
44. Tugtekin I, Radermacher P, Theisen M, et al. (2001) Increased ileal-mucosal-arterial $PCO_2$ gap is associated with impaired villus microcirculation in endotoxic pigs. Intensive Care Med 27:757–766
45. Madorin WS, Martin CM, Sibbald WJ (1999) Dopexamine attenuates flow motion in ileal mucosal arterioles in normotensive sepsis. Crit Care Med 27:394–400

46. Sakka SG, Reinhart K, Meier-Hellmann A (2002) Prognostic value of the indocyanine green plasma disappearance rate in critically ill patients. Chest 122:1715–1720
47. Levy B, Gawalkiewicz P, Vallet B, et al. (2003) Gastric capnometry with air-automated tonometry predicts outcome in critically ill patients. Crit Care Med 31:474–480
48. Gutierrez G, Palizas F, Doglio G, et al. (1992) Gastric intramucosal pH as a therapeutic index of tissue oxygenation in critically ill patients. Lancet 339:195–199
49. Gomersall CD, Joynt GM, Freebairn RC, Hung V, Buckley TA, Oh TE (2000) Resuscitation of critically ill patients based on the results of gastric tonometry: a prospective, randomized, controlled trial. Crit Care Med 28:607–614
50. Schrier RW, Wang W (2004) Acute renal failure and sepsis. N Engl J Med 351:159–169
51. Langenberg C, Bellomo R, May C, et al. (2005) Renal blood flow in sepsis. Crit Care 9:R363–R374
52. Patel BM, Chittock DR, Russell JA, Walley KR (2002) Beneficial effects of short-term vasopressin infusion during severe septic shock. Anesthesiology 96:576–582
53. Matta BF, Stow PJ (1996) Sepsis-induced vasoparalysis does not involve the cerebral vasculature: indirect evidence from autoregulation and carbon dioxide reactivity studies. Br J Anaesth 76:790–794
54. Pollard V, Prough DS, Deyo DJ, et al. (1997) Cerebral blood flow during experimental endotoxemia in volunteers. Crit Care Med 25:1700–1706
55. Bowton DL, Bertels NH, Prough DS, Stump DA (1989) Cerebral blood flow is reduced in patients with sepsis syndrome. Crit Care Med 17:399–403
56. Berre J, De Backer D, Moraine JJ, Vincent JL, Kahn RJ (1994) Effects of dobutamine and prostacyclin on cerebral blood flow velocity in septic patients. J Crit Care 9:1–6
57. Berre J, De Backer D, Moraine JJ, Melot C, Kahn RJ, Vincent JL (1997) Dobutamine increases cerebral blood flow velocity and jugular bulb hemoglobin saturation. Crit Care Med 25:392–398

# The Microcirculation Is a Vulnerable Organ in Sepsis

P.W.G. Elbers and C. Ince

## Introduction: The Microcirculation as a Key Organ in Septic Shock

There is now increasing evidence that the microcirculation is one of the key organs in the pathophysiology of sepsis and septic shock [1, 2]. However, its importance does not seem to be reflected in current clinical practice. In addition, the surviving sepsis campaign, a world wide effort to decrease sepsis related mortality, focuses only minimally on the importance of the microcirculatory organ [3]. By definition, sepsis is initiated by an infectious agent and the ultimate therapeutic strategy will therefore be its removal from the body. However, the systemic hostile inflammatory response that ensues from sepsis is the real culprit of this disease. The microcirculation is severely affected by this inflammatory response. At the same time, it is responsible for maintaining or even fueling the devastating disease process of sepsis and septic shock. Even in the face of stable systemic hemodynamics, the microcirculation may be at risk giving rise to regional dysoxia, causing multiple organ failure (MOF) and ultimately death.

Monitoring the microcirculation provides sensitive information on the severity of disease and the effect of therapies [4]. In addition, if sepsis is a disease of the microcirculation [5], resuscitating this organ may become as important as antibiotic therapy.

## The Microcirculation as a Functional System

The microcirculation is one of the largest organs in the body and by definition comprises vessels with a diameter roughly smaller than 100 micrometers, i.e., arterioles, capillaries, and venules, and the blood flowing in them. The entire length of the organ is lined with endothelial cells, which are surrounded by smooth muscle cells mainly in arterioles. Red blood cells (RBCs) and the various types of white blood cell (WBC) complete the cellular picture. However, the microcirculation also embraces a large number of other components including platelets, coagulation factors, and a plethora of cytokines and chemokines [6].

Among the many different microcirculatory functions, the delivery of oxygen to tissue is paramount. This is part of the microcirculation's larger function as an exchanger of nutrients and waste products and chemical or cellular signals. Pertaining to sepsis, however, it is also important to realize the pathogenic interplay

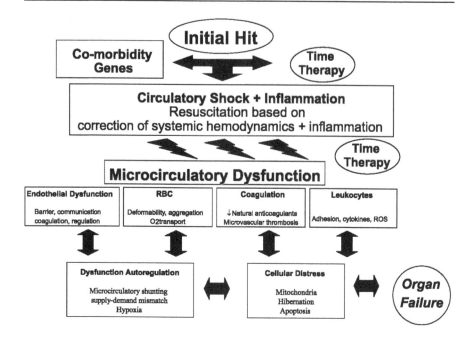

Fig. 1. Microcirculatory and mitochondrial distress syndrome is the condition whereby distributive alterations of microcirculatory control result in shunting and regional mis-match of oxygen supply and demand leading to cellular distress and organ failure. Circulatory failure as a result of sepsis can be initiated by various insults such as trauma, infection, and shock. The treatment of circulatory failure is initially based on correction of systemic variables. In distributive shock, however, systemic variables may be normal and regional hypoxia can persist due to microcirculatory shunting and dysfunction. Here, time and therapy contribute to the definition and nature of microcirculatory and mitochondrial distress syndrome. Left uncorrected, the different cellular and inflammatory components of the distressed microcirculation interact and increase in severity, fueling the respiratory distress of the parenchymal cells and ultimately leading to organ failure (adapted from [2] with permission)

of WBCs, RBCs, endothelium, and messenger molecules in inflammation and coagulation in the microcirculation [6].

It is, therefore, not surprising that this organ is a highly regulated one. Central to coordinating microcirculatory perfusion, and hence oxygen delivery ($DO_2$), is the endothelium. In order to meet the oxygen requirements of the cells, the endothelium will ultimately control arteriolar smooth muscle cell tone, both directly and via neurohumoral mechanisms, resulting in altered microcirculatory perfusion. This is achieved by mechanisms such as stress and strain sensing as well as detection of oxygen and metabolic waste products [7]. Endothelium produced nitric oxide (NO) deserves special attention in this context. Apart from its role as a mediator of the inflammatory cascade, the vasodilating properties of NO are important in regulating the distribution of perfusion.

The endothelium, helped by WBCs, platelets, and messenger molecules, is also involved in the regulation of inflammation and coagulation [8]. Interestingly, RBCs are nowadays considered to regulate perfusion by releasing vasodilators, such as NO [9] and ATP [10], when encountering oxygen deprived environments. In addition it has been shown that deoxyhemoglobin can convert nitrite to NO, causing arteriolar dilatation [11]. Thus, apart from transporting oxygen, RBCs effectively redirect flow and oxygen where it is needed.

## Scientific Importance of the Microcirculation

Realization of the importance of the microcirculation is growing, although the concept of microcirculatory disturbances in sepsis is not new. For several decades now, microcirculatory alterations have been recognized as important in pathophysiology [12, 13], and given attention as potential therapeutic targets [14].

One reason why the microcirculation has become an organ of increasing interest in critical care medicine is the validation [15] and clinical introduction [16] of orthogonal polarization spectral (OPS) imaging, which has allowed direct visualization of the human microcirculation in solid organs and mucous membranes for the first time. OPS imaging has revealed the important role of microcirculatory abnormalities in patients with sepsis, confirming results from animal models [17–19]. In addition, we recently validated a scoring system for quantification of microcirculatory abnormalities in sepsis [20] and introduced side stream dark field (SDF) imaging [2, 21] as a successor to OPS imaging.

## The Septic Microcirculation

In their hallmark clinical study of 50 patients with severe sepsis, De Backer and colleagues showed that functional vessel density and the proportion of perfused vessels smaller than 20 micrometer were significantly lower than in healthy controls, non-septic patients, and post-cardiac surgery patients [17]. In addition, microvascular deterioration was more severe in non-survivors. A later study by the same group showed that septic patients who did not survive their disease showed no improvement in microvascular perfusion whereas survivors did [18]. Our group reported comparable observations of sluggish microcirculatory perfusion in a small group of septic patients. These observations also independently showed sustained flow in larger vessels confirming that shunting of the capillaries of the microcirculation is a key feature of sepsis [2, 19, 22].

These findings are important because they show that there is indeed a microvascular problem in human sepsis, which is associated with organ dysfunction and death. It also shows the importance of looking at the actual vessels. There has been some confusion in the past, where plethysmography [23], xenon dilution [24], and laser Doppler flux [25] have been used as surrogate markers for microcirculatory perfusion. While observations using these techniques have brought useful data, it should be remembered that they cannot account for any degree of microcirculatory heterogeneity, a characteristic property of sepsis. For this reasons, these techniques should be considered as indicators of regional rather than microcirculatory perfusion.

Of particular note is that the clinical picture of a disturbed microcirculation in sepsis is paralleled by the abnormalities found in various animal models using intravital microscopy and carbon injection. Observations in mice, rats, and dogs invariably show a reduction in perfused capillary density, and stopped flow next to areas of hyperdynamic blood flow, resulting in increased heterogeneity in skeletal and intestinal microvascular beds, despite normotensive conditions [26–29]. It has also been shown experimentally that hemorrhagic shock does not affect microvascular perfusion as much as endotoxic shock for the same degree of hypotension [27].

An increased heterogeneity of the microcirculation was shown to provoke areas of hypoxia and generally impaired oxygen extraction, both mathematically and in a porcine model of septic shock [30]. This means that while some parts of the microcirculation may do relatively well after an insult, there may be other more vulnerable areas that are underperfused; we called these areas, microcirculatory weak units [22].

## Dysfunction of Individual Microcirculatory Components

To understand the causes of microcirculatory abnormalities in sepsis, the impact of sepsis on the different components of the microcirculation needs to be considered. A common finding has been the decreased reactivity of smooth muscle cells to vasostimulating drugs in experimental sepsis. This applies to both vasoconstrictors [31, 32] and vasodilators [33]. However, observations in humans show that the response to nitroglycerin and acetylcholine is still preserved, at least partially [17, 19]. Vasoconstrictor activity can be improved by inhibiting the formation of NO [34]. This is in agreement with observations of a severely deregulated state of the endothelium in sepsis, in which there is massive overexpression of inducible NO synthase (iNOS). As this expression is not homogeneous within tissues, the resulting heterogeneous vasodilatation may partly explain the variation in microcirculatory perfusion observed clinically [35–37].

Apart from its central role in sepsis, the endothelium also serves a passive role lining the vessel wall. In sepsis, this barrier becomes swollen and leaky allowing fluids to extravasate passively [38]. This leads to pooling of blood, which is lost from the macrocirculation, and edema formation, which is aggravated by a possible impairment in the glycocalyx [39] and a reduction in the anionic charge on endothelial cells [40, 41], allowing charged proteins to pass.

There are numerous interactions of WBCs and the endothelium during sepsis, representing the crossroads between inflammation and coagulation. Essentially a complex defense system against infectious agents, this interaction is responsible for the inflammatory response. Many mediators are released, including tumor necrosis factor (TNF)-$\alpha$, interleukin (IL)-1$\beta$, IL-8, E-selectin, P-selectin, and the intercellular adhesion molecules (ICAMs) [6,42]. All are responsible for activating neutrophils, while the latter three, produced both in endothelium and monocytes, are also associated with the initiation of a procoagulant state [43]. While leukocytes themselves become less deformable [44], and have a prolonged capillary transit time [45], potentially blocking microcirculatory flow, the procoagulant state can give rise to a coagulopathy of consumption, disseminated intravascular coagulation (DIC). This coagulopathy gives rise to microthrombi in the smallest of vessels, again disrupting flow, in addition to the induced risk of bleeding as a result of diminished levels of platelets and clotting factors, both in the micro- and macrocirculation [46].

The RBC is an underappreciated cell. By virtue of its hemoglobin content, it is responsible for the bulk transport of oxygen. RBCs have to pass through capillaries smaller than the cell itself, meaning that they have to deform to be able to pass in single file through the smallest vessels, where there is an effective capillary hemodilution, with hematocrits far lower than that in arterial blood [47]. In addition, a consistent finding both clinically and experimentally is that RBC deformability is decreased in sepsis. This decrease may be caused by direct binding of endotoxin to the RBC, complement coating of RBCs, membrane alterations associated with intracellular ATP changes or the formation of schistocytes in DIC [48–50]. Of specific interest is that the reduction in RBC deformability has been shown to be NO dependent [51], suggesting that the excessive NO production in sepsis may contribute to RBC dysfunction.

## Dysoxia and the Oxygen Extraction Paradox

The factors discussed above lead to a disturbed microcirculation which, if not corrected adequately, is associated with a very poor prognosis [18]. From this perspective, the microcirculation may be considered as the motor of sepsis [2]. The model that fits this viewpoint is that a disturbed microcirculation in sepsis will lead to an uneven distribution of tissue oxygenation leading to regional dysoxia in microcirculatory weak units, loss of cell viability, organ failure and death. It may, therefore, be meaningful to see if there is evidence linking microcirculatory abnormalities and dysoxia.

In terms of clinical practice, it is perhaps surprising that regional monitoring is not more routinely applied. Usually, clinicians rely on global parameters such as $DO_2$, oxygen uptake ($VO_2$), cardiac output, and arterial and central venous blood pressure. Urinary output, lactate levels and skin color or temperature are only nonspecific markers of regional perfusion. Circumstantial evidence of abnormal regional perfusion and dysoxia comes from the fact that patients can be dying even in the light of normal or even improving global parameters.

It is a common finding in clinical sepsis that there is a deficit in oxygen extraction rate. This is illustrated by a normal or high mixed venous oxygen saturation ($SvO_2$). However, trials aimed at maximizing tissue $DO_2$ did not improve outcome [52, 53]. This means that either the oxygen is not reaching the microcirculation or that cells and their mitochondria are simply not using it. Indeed mitochondrial dysfunction has been found to be associated with the severity and outcome of clinical sepsis [54]. This type of mitochondrial malfunction in the presence of normal to high amounts of tissue oxygenation has been termed cytopathic hypoxia [55]. Postulated mechanisms include reverse cytochrome inhibition by NO and peroxynitrite. One important study supporting the existence of cytopathic hypoxia examined pigs in which oxygen availability, as assessed by Clark electrodes, remained high while metabolic distress persisted as evidenced by a high intragastric $CO_2$ [56]. While cytopathic hypoxia may be one of the causes of metabolic dysfunction, evidence is gathering that microcirculatory blood flow is the main determinant of metabolic disturbance. Microcirculatory $PO_2$, assessed by palladium porphyrin phosphorescence, revealed that tissue $PO_2$ was less than venous $PO_2$ in a similar pig model [22]. These findings were direct evidence of shunting of oxygen transport from the microcirculation. Further evidence for this theory comes from a recent study by Creteur et al. in which they showed, amongst other findings, that increasing microcirculatory blood flow, as assessed by OPS imaging, with dobutamine, led to an increase in tissue $CO_2$ levels, confirming that capillary blood flow was an important factor in the metabolic challenge in this setting [57].

## Microcirculatory and Mitochondrial Distress Syndrome (MMDS)

The pathophysiology of severe sepsis unresponsive to treatment is determined at the level of the microcirculation and probably at the mitochondrial level. The time factor and the nature of treatment being applied are also important elements. We have termed these deleterious changes, the microcirculatory and mitochondrial distress syndrome (MMDS), in which time and therapy are considered as important modulating co-factors [2]. It is important to realize that MMDS is caused by the initial septic hit but then acts to maintain the septic process. Keeping in mind the pathophysiological mechanisms described previously, the microcirculation may be considered a motor of sepsis, effectively shutting down oxygen, nutrient, and medication supply to regions of tissue.

In addition, it should be remembered that the intricate process of microcirculatory organ function is very much dependent on the stage of the disease and the therapy given [2]. An intensive care unit (ICU) physician treating many septic patients will only rarely see one in whom at least some form of therapy has not been started, e.g., fluids, vasoactive agents, antibiotics, or steroids. This will also apply to the microcirculation in sepsis, where it would be more correct to take into account time and therapy when defining microcirculatory disorders. Since the microcirculatory organ can now be visualized in humans more readily, it is possible to directly observe the microscopic consequences of sepsis in man.

## Monitoring the Microcirculation

The hallmark of global hemodynamics in septic shock is that of a hyperdynamic circulation. This means an increased cardiac output, low arterial blood pressure, and decreased total peripheral resistance. However, this increased flow does not necessarily result in adequate tissue oxygenation in weak microcirculatory beds in vulnerable organs or their compartments. This paradox can only be explained by extreme heterogeneity of the microcirculation or massive arteriovenous shunting of blood flow, effectively bypassing at least some microcirculatory areas.

As has been pointed out above, it is very easy to miss regional perfusion and oxygenation deficits if solely relying on monitoring global parameters. Important studies by LeDoux et al. [58] and Bourgoin et al. [59] emphasize this idea, showing that resuscitating septic patients to a higher mean arterial pressure (MAP) using norepinephrine actually reduced urinary excretion, increased gastric $PCO_2$, and worsened capillary blood flow.

There is already a myriad of techniques to monitor the microcirculation or at least some form of regional tissue perfusion or oxygenation. Although a detailed overview is not within the scope of this chapter, some methods should be mentioned. The easiest available today is probably $SvO_2$ [60]. Although classically considered a global parameter, low $SvO_2$ values are indicative of tissue at risk of anaerobic metabolism. In the absence of a pulmonary artery catheter the clinician may use the central venous or right atrial oxygen saturation, $ScvO_2$ or $SraO_2$. Interpretation of these values should, however, be made with caution, as they do not correlate with individual $SvO_2$ values. However, following their trend may be useful in clinical practice [61]. Also of interest is the ateriovenous $PCO_2$ difference, essentially monitoring whether cells are actually doing their job and receiving the energy to do so, especially when combined with the arteriovenous $O_2$ content difference [62].

Monitoring regional oxygenation can be done by gastric pH or gastric, sublingual, buccal, esophageal, or tissue $PCO_2$ measurement, informing us about the splanchnic vascular bed [36,58,64,65]. For measurement of tissue oxygenation the clinician may use methods based on different forms of spectroscopy to measure microcirculatory hemoglobin saturation [36]. For the moment, the best available monitors of the human microcirculation are SDF and OPS imaging. The SDF imaging technique [21] seems promising as it completely avoids tissue reflectance by illuminating tissue from the side, rendering sharp images of the microcirculation, especially capillaries. An important point to remember, however, is that even though microcirculatory distress, especially measured sublingually, is a serious clinical observation which is associated with a bad prognosis, the microcirculation of other organs may remain unresponsive to therapy and need different recruitment procedures to return to normal function.

It should be noted that images of the septic microcirculation show considerable variation. Again, time and therapy play a very important role here. For example, we observed stagnant capillaries in pressure guided resuscitation in sepsis. In contrast, capillaries with continuous or even hyperdynamic flow may be observed next to capilliaries with stopped flow in ongoing fluid resuscitated sepsis. We are currently trying to classify these flow abnormalities in distributive shock based on actual moving pictures. This may be helpful in identifying the causes of these microcirculatory disturbances and perhaps in fine tuning our therapies.

## Resuscitating the Microcirculation

Knowledge of the pathophysiology of microcirculatory disturbances in sepsis can be used to resuscitate this organ. Loss of barrier function resulting in edema and the heterogeneity of the microcirculation will cause an effective loss of fluids to the global circulation. In addition, there is a flow redistribution at a regional level, predominantly away from vulnerable organs such as those of the splanch-nic region [65]. In order to recruit microcirculatory units that are not adequately perfused, it is important to administer fluids and inotropic agents as a first step in microcirculatory resuscitation. Fluids have been shown to increase tissue oxy-genation in an animal model [66]. In addition, dobutamine has been shown to increase microcirculatory perfusion and oxygenation in humans [57,67]. How-ever, this may not hold later on in sepsis underscoring the importance of time in MMDS. In addition, fluids are not effective in consolidating pathological shunting and cause redistribution of blood flow due to both hemorheological effects and altered regulatory properties of the vasculature [36].

While normalizing the systemic hemodynamic profile can be considered the first step in rescuing the microcirculation in shock, apparently adequate resuscita-tion based on systemic variables is not always affective in recruiting the microcir-culation. That is why direct monitoring of the microcirculation may be so crucial. Under such conditions other microcirculatory recruitment maneuvers may be considered.

The role of NO in sepsis is complex and incompletely understood [35]. However, it is now generally accepted that nonselective inhibition of NOS is not a good thing as it led to increased mortality in human sepsis as shown by the early termination of a phase III trial [68]. This is perhaps also the basis of ambiguous results of administering steroids, which non-selectively inhibit NOS in sepsis. However, as mentioned before, from a microcirculatory point of view, selective iNOS inhibition could be favorable in redistributing blood flow away from where it is not needed towards dysoxic regions. In fact, in a porcine model of septic shock, selective iNOS inhibition led to improved intestinal tissue oxygenation and normalization of the gastric $PCO_2$ gap [36]. Still, the need for a more robust understanding of iNOS inhibition, including issues such as the best timing and the degree of blockade, calls for cautiousness in clinical use of this strategy.

As far as the microcirculation is concerned, one should probably be careful with vasopressor therapy in sepsis. Although it is obvious from Ohm's law that at least some perfusion pressure is necessary for blood flow to different organs, resuscitating septic patients to fixed blood pressure endpoints using vasopressor agents may actually jeopardize microcirculatory flow. This was shown by Boerma et al. who administered a relatively high dose of vasopressin to a septic shock patient [69]. While urine output and blood pressure improved, sublingual microcirculation came to a halt and the patient died. When using vasopressors it may be advisable to monitor the microcirculation in some way. This has been done by Dubois et al. who showed that vasopressin at lower doses did not affect the sublingual microcirculation [70].

Vasodilators could resuscitate the microcirculation by improving flow and by raising capillary hematocrit [71]. As previously mentioned, it has been shown that the septic microcirculation is still responsive to acetylcholine [17]. Experimentally, we have shown that the NO donor, SIN-1, improved gastric $PCO_2$ in a porcine model of fluid resuscitated shock [36]. Commonly used NO donors in intensive care medicine are nitroglycerin and nitroprusside. In septic patients, marked improvement of microcirculatory flow was indeed observed after nitroglycerin infusion [19].

It may be counterintuitive that NO donating vasodilators and iNOS inhibiting agents can both be beneficial for the microcirculation, although theoretically, they can be combined. This problem can be circumvented, however, by using other vasodilators such as ketanserin, a 5-hydroxytryptamine antagonist. We used this agent in hypertension after cardiopulmonary bypass and preliminary results show a marked improvement in microvascular perfusion suggesting this approach may prove useful in sepsis. Another potentially useful agent in this respect is prostacyclin, which has been shown to improve oxygen consumption and delivery as well as improve gastric intramucosal pH (pHi) in human studies [72,73].

The vasodilator, pentoxifylline, is a phosphodiesterase inhibitor and has multiple modes of actions that could resuscitate the microcirculation. Pentoxifylline has experimentally been shown to improve cardiac output, RBC and WBC deformability and to interfere with leukocyte endothelial interaction, causing less WBC stasis [74–78]. In addition, recent research shows that pentoxifylline may act as an iNOS inhibitor thus possibly correcting microcirculatory perfusion maldistribution in sepsis [79]. Indeed, pentoxifylline improved oxygen extraction in an animal model [80], and in septic neonates it was even shown to induce a survival benefit. However, a large clinical trial, in adults or children, has not been conducted so far [81].

Interest in activated protein C (APC) started because of its anticoagulant activity, inactivating factors Va and VIIIa and increasing fibrinolysis [42]. As such it could counteract DIC and may help resuscitate the microcirculation. APC is currently the only drug that has shown a survival benefit in human sepsis; trials with other anticoagulant drugs have failed to do so [82]. This finding may be explained by the fact that APC also has anti-inflammatory properties. From a microcirculatory perspective, this is beneficial as APC has been shown to reduce endotoxin-induced leukocyte rolling and adhesion as well as improving small vessel blood flow [83]. In addition, APC is also known to block iNOS, which may be another explanation for the observed microcirculatory improvements [84].

## Conclusion

The microcirculation is a vulnerable organ in sepsis. At the same time, the diseased microcirculation fuels sepsis, leading to organ failure. Direct monitoring of the microcirculation itself or at least some indicator of regional perfusion may, therefore, be useful in assessing the course of disease.

However, it should be noted that the effectiveness of many microcirculatory recruitment maneuvers has not yet been confirmed in appropriate clinical trials. Similarly, although there is strong evidence that an improving microcirculation is associated with a better outcome, this is not necessarily a cause and effect relationship and resuscitation of the microcirculation has not been the subject of clinical investigation at the present time. Nevertheless, it is important to remember that normal or improving global hemodynamics or oxygen-derived parameters do not preclude microcirculatory dysfunction, multiple organ failure, and fatal outcome. The microcirculation may be the much-needed end-point of resuscitation of clinical sepsis and septic shock. In addition to accepted therapies, such as fluid resuscitation and inotropic support, promising microcirculatory resuscitating maneuvers including vasodilatation, iNOS inhibition, and multi-action drugs, such as APC, could complement the armamentarium of tomorrow's ICUs.

## References

1. Vincent JL, De Backer D (2005) Microvascular dysfunction as a cause of organ dysfunction in severe sepsis. Crit Care 9 (Suppl 4):S9–12
2. Ince C (2005) The microcirculation is the motor of sepsis. Crit Care 9 (Suppl 4):S13–19
3. Dellinger RP, Carlet JM, et al (2004) Surviving Sepsis Campaign guidelines for management of severe sepsis and septic shock. Intensive Care Med 30:536–555
4. Trzeciak S, Rivers EP (2005) Clinical manifestations of disordered microcirculatory perfusion in severe sepsis. Crit Care 9 (Suppl 4):S20–26
5. Spronk PE, Zandstra DF, Ince C (2004) Bench-to-bedside review: sepsis is a disease of the microcirculation. Crit Care 8:462–468
6. Lehr HA, Bittinger F, Kirkpatrick CJ (2000) Microcirculatory dysfunction in sepsis: a pathogenetic basis for therapy? J Pathol 190:373–386
7. Segal SS (2005) Regulation of blood flow in the microcirculation. Microcirculation 12:33–45
8. Vallet B (2002) Endothelial cell dysfunction and abnormal tissue perfusion. Crit Care Med 30 (Suppl 5):S229–234
9. Stamler JS, Jia L, Eu JP, et al (1997) Blood flow regulation by S-nitrosohemoglobin in the physiological oxygen gradient. Science 276:2034–2037
10. Gonzalez-Alonso J, Olsen DB, Saltin B (2002) Erythrocyte and the regulation of human skeletal muscle blood flow and oxygen delivery: role of circulating ATP. Circ Res 91:1046–1055
11. Cosby K, Partovi KS, Crawford JH, et al (2003) Nitrite reduction to nitric oxide by deoxyhemoglobin vasodilates the human circulation. Nat Med 9:1498–1505
12. Bains JW, Bond TP, Lewis SR (1965) Microcirculation in endotoxin shock. Surg Forum 16:484–485
13. Rudowski W (1967) [Disturbance of microcirculation in oligovolemic shock]. Pol Arch Med Wewn 38:261–266

14. Stehr K (1976) [Pathogenesis and therapy of shock in children (author's transl)]. Klin Padiatr 188:479–488
15. Mathura KR, Vollebregt KC, et al (2001) Comparison of OPS imaging and conventional capillary microscopy to study the human microcirculation. J Appl Physiol 2001, 91(1):74–78.
16. Groner W, Winkelman JW, Harris AG, et al (1999) Orthogonal polarization spectral imaging: a new method for study of the microcirculation. Nat Med 5:1209–1212
17. De Backer D, Creteur J, Preiser JC, Dubois MJ, Vincent JL (2002) Microvascular blood flow is altered in patients with sepsis. Am J Respir Crit Care Med 166:98–104
18. Sakr Y, Dubois MJ, De Backer D, Creteur J, Vincent JL (2004) Persistent microcirculatory alterations are associated with organ failure and death in patients with septic shock. Crit Care Med 32:1825–1831
19. Spronk PE, Ince C, Gardien MJ, Mathura KR, Oudemans-van Straaten HM, Zandstra DF (2002) Nitroglycerin in septic shock after intravascular volume resuscitation. Lancet 360:1395–1396
20. Boerma EC, Mathura KR, van der Voort PH, Spronk PE, Ince C (2005) Quantifying bedside-derived imaging of microcirculatory abnormalities in septic patients: a prospective validation study. Crit Care 9:R601–606
21. Ince C (2005) Sidestream dark field (SDF) imaging: an improved technique to observe sublingual microcirculation. Crit Care 2005 8 (Suppl 1):P72 (abst)
22. Ince C, Sinaasappel M (1999) Microcirculatory oxygenation and shunting in sepsis and shock. Crit Care Med 27:1369–1377
23. Astiz ME, DeGent GE, Lin RY, Rackow EC (1995) Microvascular function and rheologic changes in hyperdynamic sepsis. Crit Care Med 23:265–271
24. Finley RJ, Holliday RL, Lefcoe M, Duff JH (1975) Pulmonary edema in patients with sepsis. Surg Gynecol Obstet 140:851–857
25. Sair M, Etherington PJ, Peter Winlove C, Evans TW (2001) Tissue oxygenation and perfusion in patients with systemic sepsis. Crit Care Med 29:1343–1349
26. Lam C, Tyml K, Martin C, Sibbald W (1994) Microvascular perfusion is impaired in a rat model of normotensive sepsis. J Clin Invest 94:2077–2083
27. Nakajima Y, Baudry N, Duranteau J, Vicaut E (2001) Microcirculation in intestinal villi: a comparison between hemorrhagic and endotoxin shock. Am J Respir Crit Care Med 164:1526–1530
28. Drazenovic R, Samsel RW, Wylam ME, Doerschuk CM, Schumacker PT (1992) Regulation of perfused capillary density in canine intestinal mucosa during endotoxemia. J Appl Physiol 72:259–265
29. Ellis CG, Bateman RM, Sharpe MD, Sibbald WJ, Gill R (2002) Effect of a maldistribution of microvascular blood flow on capillary O(2) extraction in sepsis. Am J Physiol Heart Circ Physiol 282:H156–164
30. Humer MF, Phang PT, Friesen BP, Allard MF, Goddard CM, Walley KR (1996) Heterogeneity of gut capillary transit times and impaired gut oxygen extraction in endotoxemic pigs. J Appl Physiol 81:895–904
31. Baker CH, Sutton ET, Dietz JR (1992) Endotoxin alteration of muscle microvascular renin-angiotensin responses. Circ Shock 36:224–230
32. Baker CH, Sutton ET, Zhou Z, Dietz JR (1990) Microvascular vasopressin effects during endotoxin shock in the rat. Circ Shock 30:81–95
33. Tyml K, Yu J, McCormack DG (1998) Capillary and arteriolar responses to local vasodilators are impaired in a rat model of sepsis. J Appl Physiol 84:837–844
34. Hollenberg SM, Broussard M, Osman J, Parrillo JE (2000) Increased microvascular reactivity and improved mortality in septic mice lacking inducible nitric oxide synthase. Circ Res 86:774–778
35. Hauser B, Bracht H, Matejovic M, Radermacher P, Venkatesh B (2005) Nitric oxide synthase inhibition in sepsis? Lessons learned from large-animal studies. Anesth Analg 101:488–498

36. Siegemund M, van Bommel J, Schwarte LA, et al (2005) Inducible nitric oxide synthase inhibition improves intestinal microcirculatory oxygenation and $CO_2$ balance during endotoxemia in pigs. Intensive Care Med 31:985–992
37. Tugtekin IF, Radermacher P, Theisen M, et al (2001) Increased ileal-mucosal-arterial $PCO_2$ gap is associated with impaired villus microcirculation in endotoxic pigs. Intensive Care Med 27:757–766
38. Solomon LA, Hinshaw LB (1968) Effect of endotoxin on isogravimetric capillary pressure in the forelimb. Am J Physiol 214:443–447
39. van den Berg BM, Vink H, Spaan JA (2003) The endothelial glycocalyx protects against myocardial edema. Circ Res 92:592–594
40. Gotloib L, Shustak A, Jaichenko J, Galdi P (1988) Decreased density distribution of mesenteric and diaphragmatic microvascular anionic charges during murine abdominal sepsis. Resuscitation 16:179–192
41. Gotloib L, Shostak A, Galdi P, Jaichenko J, Fudin R (1992) Loss of microvascular negative charges accompanied by interstitial edema in septic rats' heart. Circ Shock 36:45–56
42. Hoffmann JN, Vollmar B, Laschke MW, Fertmann JM, Jauch KW, Menger MD (2005) Microcirculatory alterations in ischemia-reperfusion injury and sepsis: effects of activated protein C and thrombin inhibition. Crit Care 9 (Suppl 4):S33–37
43. McCuskey RS, Urbaschek R, Urbaschek B (1996) The microcirculation during endotoxemia. Cardiovasc Res 32:752–763
44. Poschl JM, Ruef P, Linderkamp O (2005) Deformability of passive and activated neutrophils in children with Gram-negative septicemia. Scand J Clin Lab Invest 65:333–339
45. Goddard CM, Allard MF, Hogg JC, Herbertson MJ, Walley KR (1995) Prolonged leukocyte transit time in coronary microcirculation of endotoxemic pigs. Am J Physiol 269:H1389–1397
46. Vincent JL, De Backer D (2005) Does disseminated intravascular coagulation lead to multiple organ failure? Crit Care Clin 21:469–477
47. Desjardins C, Duling BR(1987) Microvessel hematocrit: measurement and implications for capillary oxygen transport. Am J Physiol 252:H494–503
48. Poschl JM, Leray C, Ruef P, Cazenave JP, Linderkamp O (2003) Endotoxin binding to erythrocyte membrane and erythrocyte deformability in human sepsis and in vitro. Crit Care Med 31:924–928
49. Weed RI (1970) The importance of erythrocyte deformability. Am J Med 49:147–150
50. Hurd TC, Dasmahapatra KS, Rush BF Jr, Machiedo GW (1988) Red blood cell deformability in human and experimental sepsis. Arch Surg 123:217–220
51. Bateman RM, Jagger JE, Sharpe MD, Ellsworth ML, Mehta S, Ellis CG (2001) Erythrocyte deformability is a nitric oxide-mediated factor in decreased capillary density during sepsis. Am J Physiol Heart Circ Physiol 280:H2848–2856
52. Alia I, Esteban A, Gordo F, et al (1999) A randomized and controlled trial of the effect of treatment aimed at maximizing oxygen delivery in patients with severe sepsis or septic shock. Chest 115:453–461
53. Gattinoni L, Brazzi L, Pelosi P, et al (1995) A trial of goal-oriented hemodynamic therapy in critically ill patients. SvO2 Collaborative Group. N Engl J Med 333:1025–1032
54. Brealey D, Brand M, Hargreaves I, et al (2002) Association between mitochondrial dysfunction and severity and outcome of septic shock. Lancet 360:219–223
55. Fink MP (2002) Bench-to-bedside review: Cytopathic hypoxia. Crit Care 6:491–499
56. VanderMeer TJ, Wang H, Fink MP (1995) Endotoxemia causes ileal mucosal acidosis in the absence of mucosal hypoxia in a normodynamic porcine model of septic shock. Crit Care Med 23:1217–1226
57. Creteur J, De Backer D, Sakr Y, Koch M, Vincent J (2006) Sublingual capnometry tracks microcirculatory changes in septic patients. Intensive Care Med 32:516–523
58. LeDoux D, Astiz ME, Carpati CM, Rackow EC (2000) Effects of perfusion pressure on tissue perfusion in septic shock. Crit Care Med 28:2729–2732

59. Bourgoin A, Leone M, Delmas A, Garnier F, Albanese J, Martin C (2005) Increasing mean arterial pressure in patients with septic shock: effects on oxygen variables and renal function. Crit Care Med 33:780–786
60. Rivers EP, Ander DS, Powell D (2001) Central venous oxygen saturation monitoring in the critically ill patient. Curr Opin Crit Care 7:204–211
61. Dueck MH, Klimek M, Appenrodt S, Weigand C, Boerner U (2005) Trends but not individual values of central venous oxygen saturation agree with mixed venous oxygen saturation during varying hemodynamic conditions. Anesthesiology 103:249–257
62. Mekontso-Dessap A, Castelain V, Anguel N, et al (2002) Combination of venoarterial $PCO_2$ difference with arteriovenous $O_2$ content difference to detect anaerobic metabolism in patients. Intensive Care Med 28:272–277
63. Guzman JA, Dikin MS, Kruse JA (2005) Lingual, splanchnic, and systemic hemodynamic and carbon dioxide tension changes during endotoxic shock and resuscitation. J Appl Physiol 98:108–113
64. Weil MH, Nakagawa Y, Tang W, et al (1999) Sublingual capnometry: a new noninvasive measurement for diagnosis and quantitation of severity of circulatory shock. Crit Care Med 27:1225–1229
65. Duranteau J, Sitbon P, Teboul JL, et al (1999) Effects of epinephrine, norepinephrine, or the combination of norepinephrine and dobutamine on gastric mucosa in septic shock. Crit Care Med 27:893–900
66. Anning PB, Sair M, Winlove CP, Evans TW (1999) Abnormal tissue oxygenation and cardiovascular changes in endotoxemia. Am J Respir Crit Care Med 159:1710–1715
67. De Backer D, Creteur J, Preiser J, et al (2006) The effects of dobutamine on microcirculatory alterations in patients with septic shock are independent of its systemic effects. Crit Care Med 34:403–408
68. Llinares Tello F, Hernandez Prats C, Burgos San Jose A, et al (2004) [Replacement therapy with protein C for meningococcal sepsis and fulminant purpura in pediatric patients]. Farm Hosp 28:130–136
69. Boerma EC, van der Voort PH, Ince C (2005) Sublingual microcirculatory flow is impaired by the vasopressin-analogue terlipressin in a patient with catecholamine-resistant septic shock. Acta Anaesthesiol Scand 49:1387–1390
70. Dubois MJ, De Backer D, Creteur J, Anane S, Vincent JL (2003) Effect of vasopressin on sublingual microcirculation in a patient with distributive shock. Intensive Care Med 29:1020–1023
71. Buwalda M, Ince C (2002) Opening the microcirculation: can vasodilators be useful in sepsis? Intensive Care Med 28:1208–1217
72. Bihari D, Smithies M, Gimson A, Tinker J (1987) The effects of vasodilation with prostacyclin on oxygen delivery and uptake in critically ill patients. N Engl J Med 317:397–403
73. Radermacher P, Buhl R, Santak B, et al (1995) The effects of prostacyclin on gastric intramucosal pH in patients with septic shock. Intensive Care Med 21:414–421
74. Wang P, Ba ZF, Zhou M, Tait SM, Chaudry IH (1993) Pentoxifylline restores cardiac output and tissue perfusion after trauma-hemorrhage and decreases susceptibility to sepsis. Surgery 114:352–358
75. Mollitt DL, Poulos ND (1991) The role of pentoxifylline in endotoxin-induced alterations of red cell deformability and whole blood viscosity in the neonate. J Pediatr Surg 26:572–574
76. Tighe D, Moss R, Heath MF, Hynd J, Bennett ED (1989) Pentoxifylline reduces pulmonary leucostasis and improves capillary patency in a rabbit peritonitis model. Circ Shock 28:159–164
77. Schonharting MM, Schade UF (1989) The effect of pentoxifylline in septic shock–new pharmacologic aspects of an established drug. J Med 20:97–105
78. Puranapanda V, Hinshaw LB, O'Rear EA, Chang AC, Whitsett TL (1987) Erythrocyte deformability in canine septic shock and the efficacy of pentoxifylline and a leukotriene antagonist. Proc Soc Exp Biol Med 185:206–210

79. Trajkovic V (2001) Modulation of inducible nitric oxide synthase activation by immunosuppressive drugs. Curr Drug Metab 2:315–329
80. Fan J, Gong XQ, Wu J, Zhang YF, Xu RB (1994) Effect of glucocorticoid receptor (GR) blockade on endotoxemia in rats. Circ Shock 42:76–82
81. Haque K, Mohan P (2003) Pentoxifylline for neonatal sepsis. Cochrane Database Syst Rev CD004205
82. Macias WL, Yan SB, Williams MD, et al (2005) New insights into the protein C pathway: potential implications for the biological activities of drotrecogin alfa (activated). Crit Care 9 (Suppl 4):S38–45
83. Hoffmann JN, Vollmar B, Laschke MW, et al (2004) Microhemodynamic and cellular mechanisms of activated protein C action during endotoxemia. Crit Care Med 32:1011–1017
84. Isobe H, Okajima K, Uchiba M, et al (2001) Activated protein C prevents endotoxin-induced hypotension in rats by inhibiting excessive production of nitric oxide. Circulation 104:1171–1175

# The Cholinergic Anti-inflammatory Pathway: Connecting the Mind and Body

C.J. Czura, S.G. Friedman, and K.J. Tracey

> When the parts of the body and its humors are not in harmony, then the
> mind is unbalanced and melancholy ensues, but on the other hand, a quiet
> and happy mind makes the whole body healthy.

Papai Pariz Ferenc, 1680

## Introduction

The recent discovery of the 'cholinergic anti-inflammatory pathway' – the efferent
arm of an inflammatory reflex through which the central nervous system (CNS)
can monitor and regulate peripheral inflammation – has identified several possible
therapeutic approaches for inflammatory diseases. Acetylcholine, the primary neurotransmitter of the vagus nerve, interacts with nicotinic acetylcholine receptors
expressed on macrophages to prevent cytokine release, thereby attenuating the host
response to inflammatory stimuli [1–3]. This neurotransmitter receptor system on
cells of the innate immune system may explain, at least in part, the therapeutic
effects of several cholinergic agonists, including nicotine, which have proven effi-
cacious in inflammatory bowel disease [4]. Animals devoid of cholinergic-immune
system communication, either by surgical vagotomy or genetic disruption of the
α7 subunit of the acetylcholine receptor, are exquisitely sensitive to inflammatory
stimuli [2, 3]. These observations suggest that the vagus nerve, via acetylcholine,
regulates inflammatory responses to maintain immunological homeostasis.

Studies in animal models of systemic inflammation suggest that the cholinergic anti-inflammatory pathway can be harnessed therapeutically, because direct
electrical stimulation of the cervical vagus nerve attenuates pro-inflammatory
cytokine release and hypotension during endotoxemia or ischemia/reperfusion
injury [2, 3, 5]. The cholinergic anti-inflammatory pathway has enabled development of at least two therapeutic approaches to treat inflammatory diseases. Vagus
nerve stimulators are safe, clinically approved implantable devices used to treat
epilepsy that is refractory to medical therapy [6, 7]. Direct electrical stimulation
of the cervical vagus nerve in animals inhibits the release of pro-inflammatory
cytokines such as tumor necrosis factor (TNF) and interleukin (IL)-1β in endotoxemia, ischemia/reperfusion injury, and hemorrhagic shock, suggesting that
devices similar to those already in clinical use may be useful for inflammatory

disease. It is plausible to consider that modulation of vagus nerve activity through biofeedback may provide a method to rationally suppress inflammation. Biofeedback can be used to effectively modulate vagus nerve activity, as evidenced by alteration of heart rate, skin temperature, and the galvanic skin response. This raises the theoretical possibility that biofeedback may be used to modulate vagus nerve activity, which in turn controls the immune response in inflammatory disease.

## Identification of the Cholinergic Anti-inflammatory Pathway

Evolution has conferred redundant mechanisms to inhibit inflammation and prevent excessive release of TNF and other cytokines [8]. These anti-inflammatory mechanisms provide a critical level of control that restrains inflammation at the site of activation. An optimal inflammatory response leads locally to host defense against infection, stimulation of tissue remodeling and wound healing, and recovery. These beneficial inflammatory responses are mediated in part by TNF and other cytokines produced by inflammatory cells. Failure of the anti-inflammatory mechanisms to control the cytokine response during local inflammation can lead to systemic cytokine release, which induces wide-spread organ dysfunction, diffuse coagulation, hypotension, and death. Thus, uncontrolled systemic inflammatory responses can become more deleterious to the host than the initial insult.

TNF has been validated as a clinically important therapeutic target, because anti-TNF antibodies have significantly improved the lives of many patients with rheumatoid arthritis [9] and Crohn's disease [10]. Recent studies revealed that acetylcholine, the principle neurotransmitter of the vagus nerve, significantly attenuates the release of TNF and other pro-inflammatory cytokines (IL-1$\beta$, IL-6, IL-18, and high mobility group box protein 1 [HMGB1]) from human macrophages [2,3,11]. Direct electrical stimulation of the peripheral vagus nerve *in vivo*, during lethal endotoxemia in rodents, inhibits organ TNF synthesis, attenuates peak serum TNF levels, and prevents the development of shock [2,3]. Electrical vagus nerve stimulation and cholinergic agonists protect against inflammatory responses, at least in part, by inhibiting endothelial cell activation and leukocyte migration into local sites of inflammation [12]. The molecular interaction of acetylcholine with macrophages has been localized to the $\alpha7$ subunit of the nicotinic acetylcholine receptor, and subsequent downstream signaling inhibits the activity of the transcriptional activators, nuclear factor kappa B (NF-$\kappa$B), JAK2, and signal transducers and activators of transcription 3 (STAT3) [3,11–13]. Mice rendered genetically deficient in the $\alpha7$ subunit produce significantly more endotoxin-induced TNF as compared to wild-type mice, and vagus nerve stimulation fails to attenuate TNF release. These studies suggest that the CNS regulates peripheral inflammation via the cholinergic anti-inflammatory pathway in real time to maintain immunological homeostasis, and that this activity is critically dependent upon the $\alpha7$ subunit of the acetylcholine receptor.

## Functional Anatomy of the Vagus Nerve

The vagus nerve is well positioned at the interface of the immune and central nervous systems because it innervates the liver, spleen, lungs, kidneys, digestive tract, and other visceral organs that act as routes of entry or filters for pathogens and their products. The vagus nerve has motor functions in the larynx, diaphragm, stomach, and heart; and sensory functions in the ears, tongue, and visceral organs, including the liver. Inflammatory signals in peripheral tissues activate afferent signals in the vagus nerve that are relayed to the hypothalamus and stimulate the release of ACTH [14]. Afferent vagus nerve signaling has been implicated in the development of fever after administration of endotoxin [15]. It now appears that the vagus nerve is an integral component of a reflex loop that can detect and regulate inflammatory responses in real-time. Inflammation activates an ascending signal that can be relayed to the hypothalamus to activate humoral anti-inflammatory mechanisms; efferent vagus nerve signals can rapidly and specifically inhibit macrophages in tissues [1]. This new knowledge of the cholinergic anti-inflammatory pathway suggests that it may be possible to target peripheral cholingeric macrophage receptors.

## Clinically Approved Vagus Nerve Stimulators

The recent discovery that electrical stimulation of the vagus nerve protects against the lethal sequelae of endotoxemia suggests that this modality may be used to treat other inflammatory diseases [1–3, 5]. Application of either 1V or 5V to the cervical vagus nerve in endotoxemic rats prevents the development of significant hypotension, without suppressing heart rate. This vagus nerve stimulation protocol significantly inhibits TNF synthesis in the liver, heart, and other organs, and reduces serum cytokine levels in murine models of endotoxemia, sepsis, and peritonitis [2, 3, 16]. Vagus nerve stimulation is also effective in animal models of inflammation that are independent of endotoxin, including transient aortic occlusion with reperfusion injury [5], myocardial ischemia/reperfusion injury [17], carrageenan-induced hindlimb edema [18], and hypovolemic shock [19, 20].

Vagus nerve stimulation has been approved for clinical use by the Food and Drug Administration (FDA) for patients who suffer from complex partial seizures or generalized seizures where consciousness is lost, and do not respond to anticonvulsant medication, as well as for patients who are ineligible for brain surgery. It is also used as a treatment for photosensitive epilepsy and epilepsy resulting from head injury. Vagus nerve stimulation showed early promise in an open, acute phase pilot study of adults in a treatment-resistant major depressive episode [7, 21]. Clinical experience with vagus nerve stimulators in over 30,000 patients worldwide indicates that the modality is safe, and can reduce seizure rates by up to 45%; complications of immunosuppression or secondary infection have not been reported [22, 23].

## Vagus Nerve Stimulators as Anti-inflammatory Devices

The identification of the cholinergic anti-inflammatory pathway as an endogenous inflammatory control mechanism suggests that it may be possible to manipulate cytokine activity to therapeutic advantage. Preclinical studies using vagus nerve stimulation have shown that augmentation of efferent vagus nerve signaling attenuates cytokine release in several rodent models of inflammation [2,3,5,16–20]. Because inflammatory responses are an important component of many diverse diseases, and products of the innate immune system are being pursued as new therapeutic targets [24], it is intriguing to consider the use of vagus nerve stimulators as anti-inflammatory devices.

Presently available vagus nerve stimulation devices are implanted subcutaneously in the left chest wall, and a lead tunneled to the left vagus nerve. The generator is about the size of a small tape measure; three small leads are attached to the nerve in a procedure that takes 1 to 2 hours. For a few days following the procedure, the generator is programmed to stimulate the vagus nerve at regular intervals (e. g., for 30 seconds every 5 minutes) at a frequency established by the physician using a computer. If a seizure begins between intervals, the patient activates the stimulator by swiping a magnet over the chest where the device is implanted. Complications of the stimulator are restricted to tingling in the neck, hoarseness, and a slight cough during nerve stimulation, in addition to those associated with the surgery itself, such as injury to the vagus nerve, carotid artery, and internal jugular vein. It is now interesting to consider whether a modified device could be used in the future to treat inflammation.

### Inflammatory Bowel Disease

Several studies have demonstrated a reduced risk of developing ulcerative colitis in cigarette smokers as compared to nonsmokers [25, 26]. Nicotine, a cholinergic agonist, controls inflammation in ulcerative colitis by inhibiting pro-inflammatory cytokines (IL-2, IL-8, and IL-10) and by stimulating increased mucus production in the colon [27]. Ex-smokers with ulcerative colitis experience improvement in symptoms with nicotine gum, and transdermal nicotine patches combined with mesalamine or steroids result in clinical improvement in other patients [28].

Therapeutic targeting of cytokine activity has recently been validated as a treatment of Crohn's disease. Hommes et al. investigated inhibition of mitogen activated protein kinases (MAPKs), which are critical effectors mediating cytokine release, with the experimental therapeutic agent CNI-1493 in patients with Crohn's disease [29]. Twelve patients with severe Crohn's disease were randomly assigned to receive eithe r 8or 25 mg/m$^2$ CNI-1493 daily for 12 days. Clinical endpoints included safety, Crohn's Disease Activity Index, Inflammatory Bowel Disease Questionnaire, and the Crohn's Disease Endoscopic Index of Severity. Colonic biopsies prior to enrollment displayed enhanced JNK and p38 MAPK activation as compared with non-Crohn's disease samples. Treatment with CNI-1493 resulted in diminished JNK phosphorylation and TNF production, as well as significant clinical benefit and rapid endoscopic ulcer healing, with clinical responses observed in 67% of patients at four weeks, and 58% at eight weeks. Endoscopic improvement occurred in all but one patient. Fistula healing occurred in 80% of patients and steroids were tapered in 89% of patients. These observations suggest that inhibition of cytokine activity can improve the clinical course of patients suffering from Crohn's disease [29].

In subsequent experiments in rodent models of inflammation, CNI-1493 was observed to cross the blood-brain barrier and act as a pharmacological vagus nerve stimulator [30]. Parasympathetic efferent neurons derived from the vagus nerve provide major modulatory input to the gastrointestinal tract, and information from the gut reaches the CNS via the vagus nerve. Thus, pharmacologic vagus nerve stimulation, as well as electrical vagus nerve stimulation, may alter the clinical course of inflammatory bowel disease.

## Rheumatoid Arthritis

Recent studies have demonstrated that the microenvironment of rheumatoid synovial fluid is a pro-inflammatory milieu that contains high levels of TNF. TNF occupies a major pathogenic role in the development of rheumatoid arthritis joint destruction [31, 32]. Autonomic neuropathy occurs with increased frequency in patients with rheumatoid arthritis [33]. Toussirot et al. found a significant difference between the R-R interval variation during the Valsalva maneuver when rheumatoid arthritis patients were compared with control patients [34]. Tan et al. used sympathetic skin response (SSR) and tests of R-R interval variation to assess dysautonomia in patients with rheumatoid arthritis and frequent abnormalities were noted, regardless of whether or not there were clinical symptoms of autonomic dysfunction [35]. Our new understanding of the regulatory influence of vagus nerve activity on inflammation suggests that insufficient vagus nerve activity may underlie excessive TNF production in the joints of patients with rheumatoid arthritis. Patients may eventually be taught to control SSR and R-R interval variation through biofeedback, and they may reap the benefit of self-inhibition of TNF.

## Diabetes

TNF has been implicated in the development of autoimmune diabetes in studies of mice that are genetically susceptible to develop diabetes, and in clinical studies [36]. TNF also plays an important role in gestational diabetes, and is associated with dyslipidemia and hypertension in type 1 diabetes [37, 38]. Early activation of the inflammatory immune response may be a critical factor in juvenile type 1 diabetes [39, 40]. A recent study revealed that administration of nicotine to diabetes-prone mice prevents hyperglycemia, a finding that is consistent with a role for cholinergic regulation of this complication of inflammation [41]. Other complications of diabetes may be dependent upon excessive cytokine responses.

For example, Ohara et al. have shown that IL-6 and vascular endothelial growth factor (VEGF) are produced within the intraocular area, and contribute to the hyperpermeability of retinal vessels in preproliferative diabetic retinopathy [42]. High vitreous levels of soluble TNF receptors relate to retinopathy severity, and may be reactive products of inflammation [43]. Doganay et al. compared cytokine levels with grades of diabetic retinopathy and concluded that these molecules (TNF, NO, IL-1β, sIL-2R, IL-6, and IL-8) act together during the course of diabetic retinopathy, and may serve as therapeutic targets for this disease [44]. As with rheumatoid arthritis, autonomic dysfunction is also associated with diabetes. The potential contribution of diabetic neuropathy to reduced vagal regulation of inflammation during diabetes is unknown.

## Atherosclerosis

Excessive cytokine responses have been implicated in the pathogenesis of atherosclerosis [45]. Macrophages represent a significant cellular component of the atherosclerotic plaque, and synthesis of pro-inflammatory cytokines is necessary for fatty streak development. Elevated TNF receptor levels are associated with carotid atherosclerosis in patients less than 70 years old, suggesting that chronic subclinical inflammation could account for this association, and modification of these inflammatory pathways could be used to prevent atherosclerosis-associated stroke [46]. Atherogenesis is the consequence of a variety of effector mechanisms rather than the result of a single functional molecule or cell type; however, inflammation is pivotal to plaque formation. It will be interesting to determine if cholinergic modulation can retard this process and prevent or delay the complications of atherosclerosis.

## Biofeedback and Inflammation

For centuries patients and physicians have believed in the vague notion that an individual's 'state of mind' can influence somatic health. Folklore, art, and literature are replete with the themes that grief and depression are associated with increased disease susceptibility, and positive beliefs and expectations augur wellness. A familiar example is the death of a devoted spouse shortly after he or she buries their loved one. To students and some philosophical individuals, the fundamental relationship between a sense of well-being and health is indisputable.

The vagus nerve is a mixed nerve composed of approximately 80% sensory fibers relaying information between the brain from the head, neck, thorax and abdomen. The sensory afferent cell bodies of the vagus nerve reside in the nodose ganglion and transmit information to the area postrema and nucleus tractus solitarius (NTS), two regions that are active during peripheral inflammation. Ascending vagus nerve signals excite second-order neurons within the NTS via glutamate activity [47]. The NTS forms the apex of a vagus feedback loop that modulates visceral activity through two mechanisms: NTS neurons inhibit a subset of neurons within the dorsal motor nucleus of the vagus (DMV), which provide cholinergic excitatory signals to the viscera and the digestive tract; the NTS also suppresses visceral activity by activating other inhibitory DMV efferent neurons through nonadrenergic, noncholinergic pathways [37]. The NTS and DMV both contain blood vessels that lack a functional blood brain barrier, making these important circumventricular organs. This may allow these brain regions to receive sensory input from diffusible circulating factors such as lipopolysaccharide (LPS), TNF, or IL-1, in addition to afferent vagus nerve signals [48].

From the NTS, information is relayed to the rest of the brain via an autonomic feedback loop, direct projections to the medullary reticular formations, and through the parabrachial nucleus and the locus ceruleus. From the latter, connections emanate to the hypothalamus, the amygdala (mood regulation), and the entire forebrain (for a review see [49]). Recognition of common molecules and receptors in the immune, endocrine, and nervous systems validates the timeless supposition that the mind and body are connected. The cholinergic anti-inflammatory pathway may provide the neural substrate that links higher cortical function (mind) and immune responses (body). Some recent insight into central mechanisms that regulate efferent vagus nerve activity has been gained from pharmacological studies of the cholinergic anti-inflammatory pathway, which indicate that although nicotinic receptors are essential for neural regulation of inflammation in the periphery, muscarinic receptors within the brain can activate efferent vagus nerve signaling and inhibit cytokine release [50].

One implication of the anti-inflammatory activity of the efferent vagus nerve is that subjects may be trained to rationally augment vagus nerve activity; it may one day be possible to use this approach to modulate peripheral inflammatory and immune responses. This approach has been used in the treatment of headache [51], temporomandibular joint disorders [52], Raynaud's disease [53], hypertension [54], diabetes [55], urinary [56] and fecal incontinence [57], asthma [58], and intermittent claudication [59] with varying success. Electronic sensors and graphic displays monitor physiologic parameters such as heart rate, skin temperature, and muscle tension. Subjects learn to associate visual and auditory signals from a computer interface with changes in involuntary functions, and to recognize mental and physical states that induce desired physiologic changes regulated by the parasympathetic (vagus) nervous system (e.g., blood pressure reduction, warming of extremities, slowing of heart rate).

Classical teaching indicates that the parasympathetic nervous system rarely works in isolation; in most instances, the sympathetic nervous system, via epinephrine and norepinephrine, interacts with parasympathic acitivity, and the two systems working together finely tune homeostasis. Similarly, sympathetic and parasympathetic activities collaborate to maintain immunological homeostasis [1]. The sympathetic nervous system can increase circulating levels of catecholamines, which stimulate the release of the anti-inflammatory cytokine IL-10 via $\beta$-adrenergic receptors. The activities of the sympathetic nervous system are diverse; although the two branches of the autonomic nervous system act synergistically to control inflammation via catecholamine-induced IL-10 release, in different contexts epinephrine and norepinephrine can stimulate the release of pro-inflammatory cytokines and counteract the predominantly anti-inflammatory activity of the parasympathetic nervous system [60].

## Conclusion

As reviewed above, there is abundant evidence implicating autonomic dysfunction or cytokine excess in diseases with inflammatory pathology such as sepsis, Crohn's disease, and rheumatoid arthritis. The identification of a vagus nerve mechanism that regulates cytokine activity and immune cell activation now suggests that some neurological or nervous system disorders may in fact manifest as inflammatory conditions, and thus alter the optimal treatment. The ability to rationally modulate vagus nerve activity through biofeedback techniques now makes it plausible to consider how to study the regulation of cytokine synthesis in volunteer subjects and patients under varying states of vagus nerve activity.

## References

1. Tracey KJ (2002) The inflammatory reflex. Nature 420:853–859
2. Borovikova LV, Ivanova S, Zhang M, et al (2000) Vagus nerve stimulation attenuates the systemic inflammatory response to endotoxin. Nature 405:458–462
3. Wang H, Yu M, Ochani M, et al (2003) Nicotinic acetylcholine receptor alpha7 subunit is an essential regulator of inflammation. Nature 421:384–388
4. Pullan RD, Rhodes J, Ganesh S, et al (1994) Transdermal nicotine for active ulcerative colitis. N Engl J Med 330:811–815
5. Bernik TR, Friedman SG, Ochani M, et al (2002) Cholinergic anti-inflammatory pathway inhibition of tumor necrosis factor during ischemia reperfusion. J Vasc Surg 36:1231–1236
6. Labar D, Dean A (2002) Neurostimulation therapy for epilepsy. Curr Neurol Neurosci Rep 2:357–364
7. Nahas Z, Marangell LB, Husain MM, et al (2005) Two-year outcome of vagus nerve stimulation (VNS) for treatment of major depressive episodes. J Clin Psychiatry 66:1097–104
8. Tracey KJ (2005) Fatal Sequence: The Killer Within. Dana Press, Washington
9. Jobanputra P, Barton P, Bryan S, Burls A (2002) The effectiveness of infliximab and etanercept for the treatment of rheumatoid arthritis: a systematic review and economic evaluation. Health Technol Assess 621:1–110
10. Vermeire S, Louis E, Carbonez A, et al (2002) Demographic and clinical parameters influencing the short-term outcome of anti-tumor necrosis factor (infliximab) treatment in Crohn's disease. Am J Gastroenterol 979:2357–2363
11. Wang H, Liao H, Ochani M, et al (2004) Cholinergic agonists inhibit HMGB1 release and improve survival in experimental sepsis. Nat Med 10:1216–1221
12. Saeed RW, Varma S, Peng-Nemeroff T, et al (2005) Cholinergic stimulation blocks endothelial cell activation and leukocyte recruitment during inflammation. J Exp Med 201:1113–1123
13. de Jonge WJ, van der Zanden EP, The FO, et al (2005) Stimulation of the vagus nerve attenuates macrophage activation by activating the Jak2-STAT3 signaling pathway. Nat Immunol 6:844–851

14. Maier SF, Goehler LE, Fleshner M, Watkins LR (1998) The role of the vagus nerve in cytokine-to-brain communication. Ann N Y Acad Sci 840:289–300
15. Dantzer R (2001) Cytokine-induced sickness behavior: mechanisms and implications. Ann N Y Acad Sci 933:222–234
16. van Westerloo DJ, Giebelen IA, Florquin S, et al (2005) The cholinergic anti-inflammatory pathway regulates the host response during septic peritonitis. J Infect Dis 191:2138–2148
17. Mioni C, Bazzani C, Giuliani D, et al (2005) Activation of an efferent cholinergic pathway produces strong protection against myocardial ischemia/reperfusion injury in rats. Crit Care Med 33:2621–2628
18. Borovikova LV, Ivanova S, Nardi D, et al (2000) Role of vagus nerve signaling in CNI-1493-mediated suppression of acute inflammation. Auton Neurosci 85:141–147
19. Guarini S, Altavilla D, Cainazzo MM, et al (2003) Efferent vagal fibre stimulation blunts nuclear factor-kappaB activation and protects against hypovolemic hemorrhagic shock. Circulation 107:1189–1194
20. Guarini S, Cainazzo MM, Giuliani D, et al (2004) Adrenocorticotropin reverses hemorrhagic shock in anesthetized rats through the rapid activation of a vagal anti-inflammatory pathway. Cardiovasc Res 63:357–365
21. Marangell LB, Rush AJ, George MS, et al (2002) Vagus nerve stimulation (VNS) for major depressive episodes: one year outcomes. Biol Psychiatry 51:280–287
22. Binnie CD (2000) Vagus nerve stimulation for epilepsy: a review. Seizure 9:161–169
23. Labar D, Dean A (2002) Neurostimulation therapy for epilepsy. Curr Neurol Neurosci Rep 2:357–364
24. Riedemann NC, Guo RF, Ward PA (2003) The enigma of sepsis. J Clin Invest 112:460–467
25. Wolf JM, Lashner BA (2002) Inflammatory bowel disease: sorting out the treatment options. Cleve Clin J Med 69:621–626
26. Jani N, Regueiro MD (2002) Medical therapy for ulcerative colitis. Gastroenterol Clin North Am 31:147–166
27. Eliakim R, Fan QX, Babyatsky MW (2002) Chronic nicotine administration differentially alters jejunal and colonic inflammation in interleukin-10 deficient mice. Eur J Gastroenterol Hepatol 14:607–614
28. Lang KA, Peppercorn MA (1999) Promising new agents for the treatment of inflammatory bowel disorders. Drugs R D 1:237–244
29. Hommes D, van den Blink B, Plasse T, et al (2002) Inhibition of stress-activated MAP kinases induces clinical improvement in moderate to severe Crohn's disease. Gastroenterology 122:7–14
30. Bernik TR, Friedman SG, Ochani M, et al (2002) Pharmacological stimulation of the cholinergic anti-inflammatory pathway. J Exp Med 195:781–788
31. Burger D, Dayer JM (2002) The role of human T-lymphocyte-monocyte contact in inflammation and tissue destruction. Arthritis Res 4:S169–176
32. Ji H, Pettit A, Ohmura K, et al (2002) Critical roles for interleukin 1 and tumor necrosis factor alpha in antibody-induced arthritis. J Exp Med 196:77–85
33. Barendregt PJ, van der Heijde GL, Breedveld FC, et al (1996) Parasympathetic dysfunction in rheumatoid arthritis patients with ocular dryness. Ann Rheum Dis 55:612–615
34. Toussirot E, Serratrice G, Valentin P (1993) Autonomic nervous system involvement in rheumatoid arthritis. 50 cases. J Rheumatol 20:1508–1514
35. Tan J, Akin S, Beyazova M, Sepici V, Tan E (1993) Sympathetic skin response and R-R interval variation in rheumatoid arthritis. Two simple tests for the assessment of autonomic function. Am J Phys Med Rehabil 72:196–203
36. Plesner A, Greenbaum CJ, Gaur LK, et al (2002) Macrophages from high-risk HLADQB1*0201/*0302 type 1 diabetes mellitus patients are hypersensitive to lipopolysaccharide stimulation. Scand J Immunol 56:522–529
37. Kirwan JP, Hauguel-De Mouzon S, Lepercq J, et al (2002) TNF-alpha is a predictor of insulin resistance in human pregnancy. Diabetes 51:2207–2213

38. Idzior-Walus B, Mattock MB, Solnica B, et al (2001) Factors associated with plasma lipids and lipoproteins in type 1 diabetes mellitus: the EURODIAB IDDM Complications Study. Diabet Med 18:786–796
39. Erbagci AB, Tarakcioglu M, Coskun Y, et al (2001) Mediators of inflammation in children with type I diabetes mellitus: cytokines in type I diabetic children. Clin Biochem 34:645–650
40. Romano M, Pomilio M, Vigneri S, et al (2001) Endothelial perturbation in children and adolescents with type 1 diabetes: association with markers of the inflammatory reaction. Diabetes Care 24:1674–1678
41. Mabley JG, Pacher P, Southan GJ, et al (2002) Nicotine reduces the incidence of type I diabetes in mice. J Pharmacol Exp Ther 300:876–881
42. Ohara K, Funatsu H, Kitano S, Hori S, Yamashita H (2001) The role of cytokines in the pathogenesis of diabetic retinopathy. Nippon Ganka Gakkai Zasshi 105:213–217
43. Limb GA, Hollifield RD, Webster L, Charteris DG, Chignell AH (2001) Soluble TNF receptors in vitreoretinal proliferative disease. Invest Ophthalmol Vis Sci 42:1586–1591
44. Doganay S, Evereklioglu C, Er H, et al (2002) Comparison of serum NO, TNF-alpha, IL-1beta, sIL-2R, IL-6 and IL-8 levels with grades of retinopathy in patients with diabetes mellitus. Eye 16:163–170
45. Hansson GK (2001) Regulation of immune mechanisms in atherosclerosis. Ann N Y Acad Sci 947:157–165
46. Elkind MS, Cheng J, Boden-Albala B, et al (2002) Tumor necrosis factor receptor levels are associated with carotid atherosclerosis. Stroke 33:31–37
47. Rogers RC, McTigue DM, Hermann GE (1996) Vagal control of digestion: modulation by central neural and peripheral endocrine factors. Neurosci Biobehav Rev 20:57–66
48. Smith BN, Dou P, Barber WD, Dudek FE (1998) Vagally evoked synaptic currents in the immature rat nucleus tractus solitarii in an intact in vitro preparation. J Physiol 512:149–162
49. Pavlov VA, Wang H, Czura CJ, Friedman SG, Tracey KJ (2003) The cholinergic anti-inflammatory pathway: a missing link in neuroimmunomodulation. Mol Med 9:125–134
50. Pavlov VA, Ochani M, Gallowitsch-Puerta M, et al (2006) Central muscarinic cholinergic regulation of the systemic inflammatory response during endotoxemia. Proc Natl Acad Sci USA 103:5219–5223
51. Hermann C, Blanchard EB (2002) Biofeedback in the treatment of headache and other childhood pain. Appl Psychophysiol Biofeedback 27:143–162
52. Crider AB, Glaros AG (1999) A meta-analysis of EMG biofeedback treatment of temporomandibular disorders. J Orofac Pain 13:29–37
53. Middaugh SJ, Haythornthwaite JA, Thompson B, et al (2001) The Raynaud's Treatment Study: biofeedback protocols and acquisition of temperature biofeedback skills. Appl Psychophysiol Biofeedback 26:251–278
54. Yucha CB, Clark L, Smith M, et al (2001) The effect of biofeedback in hypertension. Appl Nurs Res 14:29–35
55. McGrady A, Horner J (1999) Role of mood in outcome of biofeedback assisted relaxation therapy in insulin dependent diabetes mellitus. Appl Psychophysiol Biofeedback 24:79–88
56. Gormley EA (2002) Biofeedback and behavioral therapy for the management of female urinary incontinence. Urol Clin North Am 29:551–557
57. Pager CK, Solomon MJ, Rex J, et al (2002) Long-term outcomes of pelvic floor exercise and biofeedback treatment for patients with fecal incontinence. Dis Colon Rectum 45:997–1003
58. Lehrer P, Smetankin A, Potapova T (2000) Respiratory sinus arrhythmia biofeedback therapy for asthma: a report of 20 unmedicated pediatric cases using the Smetankin method. Appl Psychophysiol Biofeedback 25:193–200
59. Aikens JE (1999) Thermal biofeedback for claudication in diabetes: a literature review and case study. Altern Med Rev 4:104–110
60. Bergmann M, Sautner T (2002) Immunomodulatory effects of vasoactive catecholamines. Wien Klin Wochenschr 114:752–761

# Coagulation in Sepsis

W.J. Wiersinga, M. Levi, and T. van der Poll

## Introduction

Activation of inflammatory and coagulation pathways is an important event in the pathogenesis of sepsis. In sepsis, which can be defined as the disadvantageous systemic host response to infection, the blood coagulation system is triggered. Activation of coagulation and deposition of fibrin as a consequence of inflammation can be considered instrumental in containing inflammatory activity to the site of infection. However, inflammation-induced coagulation may be detrimental in those circumstances when the triggered blood coagulation system is insufficiently controlled, which can lead to the clinical syndrome of disseminated intravascular coagulation (DIC) and microvascular thrombosis. In recent years, the vital roles of several elements of the hemostatic mechanism have, in part, been unraveled, including those of tissue factor, thrombin, protease-activated cell receptors (PARs), and activated protein C (APC). Clinical trials of recombinant anticoagulants for sepsis have been conducted, of which only recombinant human APC reduced the 28-day mortality of sepsis patients.

## Coagulation and Tissue Factor

Tissue factor is regarded as one of the primary initiators of the inflammation-induced coagulation cascade [1, 2]. Tissue factor is constitutively expressed by different cell types in the extravascular compartment, including pericytes, cardiomyocytes, smooth muscle cells, and keratinocytes. As a consequence of a disruption in the vascular integrity, tissue factor-expressing cells located in the underlying cell layers come into contact with bloodstream. In addition, during severe inflammation, cells present in or lining the circulation, in particular monocytes and endothelial cells, will also start expressing tissue factor. Interaction of tissue factor with factor VIIa, which circulates at low levels in the bloodstream, results in the activation of factor X either directly, or indirectly through the activation of factor IX. Activated factor X converts prothrombin (factor II) to thrombin, which finally induces the conversion of fibrin to fibrinogen, thereby inducing the formation of a blood clot. Amplification is required for adequate clot formation, which in particular takes place on phospholipid surfaces presented by activated platelets. Besides this more traditional role for cell-associated tissue factor, more recent evidence points to a role for blood-borne tissue factor in blood clotting. Indeed, microparticles bearing tissue factor and the P-selectin glycoprotein ligand-1 (PSGL-1, a protein expressed by leukocytes) have been found to be essential for the formation of thrombi at sites of injury (Fig. 1). Such microparticles, which can be released by monocytes upon activation by bacterial agonists or cytokines, readily bind to activated platelets through an interaction between PSGL-1 within the particle and its natural counter receptor, P-selectin, expressed by platelets. As a consequence, at sites of injury, activated platelets and tissue factor rich microparticles assemble, allowing for a potent and concentrated procoagulant response. Hence, activation of platelets may accelerate fibrin formation in several ways: by providing a phospholipid surface at which amplification of coagulation is facilitated and by concentrating tissue factor rich microparticles.

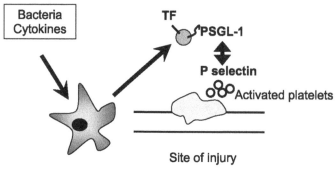

**Fig. 1.** Role of monocytes, platelets, and tissue factor rich microparticles in coagulation. Upon activation of monocytes by bacteria, endotoxin or cytokines, tissue factor (TF) expression is increased and microparticles containing tissue factor and the adhesion molecule P selectin glycoprotein ligand 1 (PSGL-1) are released. Tissue factor rich microparticles bind to activated platelets via an interaction between PSGL-1 and P selectin

The pivotal role of tissue factor in the activation of coagulation during a systemic inflammatory response syndrome, such as produced by endotoxemia or severe sepsis, has been established by many different experiments. Generation of thrombin in humans injected intravenously with a low dose of endotoxin, documented by a rise in the plasma concentrations of the prothrombin fragment F1+2 and of thrombin-antithrombin (TAT) complexes, was preceded by an increase in tissue factor mRNA levels in circulating blood cells, enhanced expression of tissue factor on circulating monocytes and the release of tissue factor-containing microparticles [3,4]. In line with this observation, baboons infused with a lethal dose of *Escherichia coli* demonstrated a sustained activation of coagulation, which was associated with enhanced expression of tissue factor on circulating monocytes, and patients with severe bacterial infection have been reported to express tissue factor activity on the surface of peripheral blood mononuclear cells [5]. More importantly, a number of different strategies that prevent the activation of the VIIa-tissue factor pathway in endotoxemic humans and chimpanzees, and in bacteremic baboons abrogate the activation of the common pathway of coagulation. In healthy humans injected with endotoxin, intravenous infusion of recombinant tissue factor pathway inhibitor (TFPI) at two different doses caused a dose-dependent inhibition of coagulation activation [6]. Strategies that potently inhibited coagulation activation in endotoxemic or bacteremic primates include antibodies directed against tissue factor or factor VII/VIIa, active site inhibited factor VIIa (Dansyl-Glu-Gly-Arg chloromethylketone or DEGR-VIIa), and TFPI [7–10].

## Anticoagulant Mechanisms

Blood clotting is controlled by three major anticoagulant proteins: TFPI, antithrombin, and APC [1, 2]. TFPI is an endothelial cell derived protease inhibitor that inactivates factor VIIa bound to tissue factor. Antithrombin inhibits factor Xa, thrombin, and factor IXa, as well as factor VIIa bound to tissue factor; these anticoagulant activities of antithrombin are accelerated by vascular heparin-like proteoglycans. The protein C system provides important control of coagulation by virtue of the capacity of APC to proteolytically inactivate factors Va and VIIa, thereby preventing the procoagulant activities of factors Xa and IXa. In the protein C system, thrombin functions as an anticoagulant: this pathway is triggered when thrombin binds to thrombomodulin on the vascular endothelium (Fig. 2) [11, 12]. Thrombomodulin-bound thrombin mediates the activation of protein C, an e ve nt that is augme nted by the e ndothelial protein C receptor (EPCR). Thrombin bound to thrombomodulin is efficiently inhibited by antithrombin and protein C inhibitor. Hence, thrombomodulin inhibits coagulation in various ways: by conversion of thrombin into an activator of protein C and by accelerating the inhibition of thrombin. Moreover, the thrombin-thrombomodulin complex can activate thrombin-activatable fibrinolysis inhibitor (TAFI), an endogenous fibrinolysis inhibitor that removes C-terminal lysine residues from fibrin thereby rendering fibrin less sensitive to the action of plasmin. Protein S serves as an essential cofactor for APC. Hemostasis is further controlled by the fibrinolytic system. Plasmin is the key enzyme of this system, which degrades fibrin clots. Plasmin is generated from plasminogen by a series of proteases, most notably tissue-type plasminogen activator (t-PA) and urokinase-type plasminogen activator (u-PA). The main inhibitor of plasminogen activator is plasminogen activator inhibitor-1 (PAI-1), which binds to t-PA and u-PA.

Several preclinical studies have supported the anticoagulant potencies of TFPI, antithrombin, and the protein C system *in vivo*. As discussed above, exogenous TFPI attenuated consumptive coagulopathy in septic primates [8]. Similarly, antithrombin treatment inhibited the procoagulant response during severe sepsis in baboons [13]. Infusion of APC into septic baboons prevented hypercoagulability and death, while inhibition of activation of endogenous protein C by a monoclonal antibody exacerbated the response to a lethal *E. coli* infusion, and converted

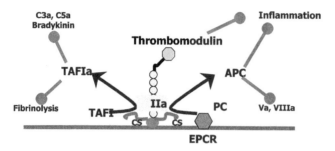

**Fig. 2.** Multiple functions of the thrombomodulin-thrombin complex. Thrombomodulin is essential for thrombin (IIa)-mediated activation of protein C (PC), a step that is further amplified by the endothelial cell protein C receptor (EPCR). Activated protein C (APC) inactivates coagulation cofactors Va and VIIIa, thereby reducing thrombin generation, and also directly impacts on inflammation (see text). Thrombomodulin also more directly suppresses inflammation. In addition, thrombomodulin is a cofactor for thrombin-mediated activation of thrombin-activatable fibrinolysis inhibitor (TAFI). Activated TAFI (TAFIa) cleaves basic C-terminal amino acid residues of its substrates, including fibrin, and thereby impairs efficient transformation of plasminogen to plasmin. TAFIa also inactivates the pro-inflammatory factors C3a, C5a, and bradykinin. Lines ending with an arrow indicate activation/generation. Lines ending with a bullet indicate inhibition

a sublethal model produced by a $LD_10$ dose of *E. coli* into a severe shock response associated with DIC and death [14]. Furthermore, treatment of baboons with an anti-EPCR monoclonal antibody, thereby reducing the efficiency by which protein C can be activated by the thrombin-thrombomodulin complex, was also associated with exacerbation of a sublethal *E. coli* infection into lethal sepsis with DIC [15]. Furthermore, interference with the bioavailability of protein S by administration of C4b binding protein, causing a decrease in free protein S levels, resulted in similar changes [16].

Severe sepsis is characterized by activation of tissue factor-dependent coagulation with concurrent inhibition of anticoagulant mechanisms: while tissue factor procoagulant activity is markedly enhanced, the activities of TFPI, antithrombin, the protein C-APC system and fibrinolysis are all impaired, resulting in a shift toward a net procoagulant state [17]. During a severe systemic inflammatory response syndrome, antithrombin levels are markedly decreased due to impaired synthesis (as a result of a negative acute phase response), degradation by elastase from activated neutrophils, and – quantitatively most importantly – consumption as a consequence of ongoing thrombin generation [1]. Pro-inflammatory cytokines can also cause reduced synthesis of glycosaminoglycans on the endothelial surface, which will also contribute to reduced antithrombin function, since these glycosaminoglycans can act as physiological heparin-like cofactors of antithrombin. The impairment of the protein C system during sepsis is the result of increased consumption of protein S and protein C, and decreased activation of protein C by downregulation of thrombomodulin on endothelial cells. Furthermore, protein S can be bound by the acute phase response protein, C4b-binding protein, thereby reducing the biological availability of this important cofactor for protein C. In

patients with severe meningococcal sepsis this downregulation of thrombomod-
ulin and consequent impaired activation of protein C was confirmed *in vivo* [18].
Finally, fibrinolysis is impaired in sepsis, primarily due to exaggerated release of
PAI-1 [1,17].

## Interaction Between Coagulation and Inflammation

It is now generally accepted that bidirectional interactions exists between coagulation and inflammation [1,2]. Cytokines are crucial soluble mediators of inflammation. Several pro-inflammatory cytokines can activate the coagulation system
*in vivo*, including tumor necrosis factor (TNF)-α, interleukin (IL)-1, IL-6 and
IL-12 [19–22]. Importantly, although anti-TNF-α treatment is highly protective
against mortality in experimental sepsis induced by intravenous administration
of live bacteria [23], elimination of TNF-α does not influence activation of coagulation in models of endotoxemia and sepsis [24, 25]. These data indicate that
mortality and activation of coagulation are not necessarily linked phenomena. Endogenous IL-6 may be involved in coagulation activation; in chimpanzees injected
with low dose endotoxin, treatment with an anti-IL-6 antibody prevented coagulation activation [26], although this IL-6 mediated procoagulant effect could not be
confirmed in healthy humans challenged with endotoxin using another anti-IL-6
antibody [27].

Interestingly, inhibition of coagulation by some, but not all, interventions also
influences the inflammatory response during experimental bacteremia. Interventions inhibiting the tissue factor pathway in lethal *E. coli* sepsis in baboons not
only prevented DIC, but also resulted in an increased survival [7, 8, 10]. These
findings contrast with interventions that block the coagulation system further
downstream: administration of factor Xa blocked in its active center by DEGR
failed to influence the outcome of bacteremic baboons, although completely inhibiting the development of DIC [28]. Moreover, administration of exogenous
APC or interference with the bioavailability of endogenous APC also impacts on
survival in this model [14–16]. In agreement with these finding, heterozygous protein C deficient mice demonstrated higher levels of pro-inflammatory cytokines
and increased neutrophil invasion in their lungs after intraperitoneal injection of
endotoxin [29]. These observations have led to the hypothesis that inhibition of
the VIIa-tissue factor pathway and exogenous or endogenous APC protect against
death not merely by an effect on the coagulation system, but (at least in part)
through effects on inflammatory responses different to the procoagulant response.

Proteases of the coagulation system, as well as anticoagulant proteins, can directly influence inflammatory processes. In this respect, PARs seem to play a pivotal
role in linking coagulation and inflammation [30, 31]. A typical feature of PARs
is that they serve as their own ligand. Proteolytic cleavage by an activated coagulation factor, including thrombin, factors VIIa and Xa, and APC (Table 1), leads
to exposure of a neo-amino terminus, which activates the same receptor, initiating transmembrane signaling (Fig. 3). Conversely, cathepsin G from granulocytes

**Table 1.** Proteases that activate the different protease-activated receptors (PARs)

| | |
|---|---|
| PAR-1 | thrombin, factor Xa, APC, granzyme A, trypsin |
| PAR-2 | trypsin, tryptase, factor VIIa, factor Xa, proteinase 3, Der P3 D9, acrosien |
| PAR-3 | thrombin |
| PAR-4 | thrombin, trypsin, cathepsin G |

cleaves PAR-1 at a different site from thrombin to generate a disabled receptor that cannot respond to thrombin.

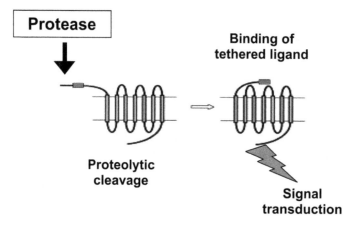

**Fig. 3.** Activation of protease-activated receptors (PARs). The general mechanism by which proteases cleave and activate PARs is the same: proteases cleave at specific sites within the extracellular amino terminus of the receptors; this cleavage exposes a new amino terminus that serves as a tethered ligand domain, which binds to conserved regions in the second extracellular loop of the cleaved receptor, resulting in the initiation of signal transduction

The PAR family consists of four members, PAR-1 to PAR-4, that are localized in the vasculature on endothelial cells, mononuclear cells, platelets, fibroblasts, and smooth muscle cells [30]. Low concentrations of thrombin activate PAR-1, whereas high concentrations are required to activate PAR-3 and PAR-4. In humans, thrombin activates platelets by cleavage of PAR-1 and PAR-4, whereas thrombin activates mouse platelets by cleavage of a PAR-3–PAR-4 complex. In primary endothelial cells, APC signaling is mediated through PAR-1, whereas tissue factor-factor VIIa-factor Xa can signal when PAR-1 is blocked, indicating that this signaling occurs through PAR-2. PAR-1 dependent APC signaling induces a number of genes that are known to downregulate pro-inflammatory signaling pathways and that inhibit apoptosis [32]. Thrombin activation of PAR-1 has been shown to induce the expression of pro-inflammatory cytokines and chemokines *in vitro*. In addition, endotoxin and TNF-α induction of IL-6 expression by cultured endothelial cells is enhanced by the activation of PAR-1 and PAR-2. Endotoxin and inflammatory cytokines also induce PAR-2 and PAR-4 expression in cultured endothelial cells. The activation of multiple PARs by coagulation proteases most probably enhances inflammation during sepsis. This is further underscored by a recent study in a mouse model of endotoxemia that showed that genetically modified mice expressing low levels of tissue factor exhibited reduced IL-6 expression and increased survival compared with control mice [33]. In contrast, hirudin inhibition of thrombin or a deficiency in either PAR-1 or PAR-2 did not affect IL-6 expression or mortality in this model. However, combining hirudin treatment to inhibit thrombin signaling through PAR-1 and PAR-4 with PAR-2 deficiency reduced endotoxin-induced IL-6 expression and increased survival [33]. Taken together, these studies suggest that activation of multiple PARs by coagulation proteases may contribute to inflammation in endotoxemia and sepsis. In vivo evidence for a role of coagulation-protease stimulation of inflammation comes from recent experiments showing that the administration of recombinant factor VIIa to healthy human subjects causes a small but significant 3 to 4-fold rise in plasma levels of IL-6 and IL-8 [34].

Antithrombin has also been found to impact on inflammation [2]. For example, antithrombin can diminish the expression of β2 integrins on leukocytes and, by binding to syndecan 4 (a proteoglycan on neutrophils), can inhibit chemokine-induced neutrophil migration. In addition, antithrombin can enhance prostacyclin formation and inhibit nuclear factor-κB (NF-kB) signaling in endothelial cells and can decrease tissue factor expression and IL-6 production by monocytes and endothelium. Much effort has been put into elucidating the mechanisms by which APC exerts its anti-inflammatory properties. APC inhibits inflammation indirectly through reducing thrombin generation and, thereby, thrombin-induced inflammation via PARs. However, APC also directly attenuates inflammation by inhibiting monocyte expression of tissue factor and TNF-α, NF-κB translocation, cytokine signaling, TNF-α induced upregulation of cell surface leukocyte adhesion molecules, and leukocyte-endothelial cell interactions [2, 12]. Thrombomodulin exerts anti-inflammatory effects at multiple levels (Fig. 2). First, thrombomodulin is essential for the activation of protein C to APC; as such, thrombomodulin is key to the anti-inflammatory properties of APC. Second, the activation of TAFI requires the thrombomodulin-thrombin complex, and activated TAFI has been demonstrated to suppress bradykinin activity and complement activation [35]. Furthermore, the lectin domain of thrombomodulin likely plays a direct role in the orchestration of inflammatory reactions. Indeed, genetically modified mice that lack the N-terminal lectin-like domain of thrombomodulin displayed a reduced survival after systemic endotoxin administration, showed increased neutrophil recruitment to the lungs, and responded with larger infarcts after myocardial ischemia/reperfusion injury [36]. Importantly, deletion of the lectin-like domain of thrombomodulin did not influence the capacity of thrombomodulin to activate protein C, indicating that the anti-inflammatory effects of this part of thrombomodulin are not mediated by APC. Finally, multiple interactions exist between inflammation and mediators of the fibrinolytic system [1, 37]. Fibrinolytic activators and inhibitors may modulate the inflammatory response by their effect on inflammatory cell recruitment and migration. For instance, uPAR (the receptor for u-PA) mediates leukocyte adhesion to the vascular wall or extracellular matrix components and its expression on leukocytes is strongly associated with their migratory and tissue-invasive potential. This is illustrated in a mouse model of bacterial pneumonia where uPAR deficient mice displayed a profoundly reduced neutrophil influx in the pulmonary compartment [38]. The plasma concentrations of PAI-1 are elevated in patients with sepsis, and such elevated circulating PAI-1 levels are highly predictive of an unfavorable outcome in sepsis patients [39]. It remains to be established whether the elevated PAI-1 levels are merely indicative of a strong inflammatory response of the host, rather than having any pathophysiological significance. Recent findings that a sequence variation in the gene encoding PAI-1 influences the development of septic shock in patients and in relatives of patients with meningococcal infection has provided circumstantial evidence that PAI-1 might play a functional role in the host response to bacterial infection [40]. Figure 4 presents a global overview of the bimodal interactions between coagulation and inflammation in sepsis.

## Coagulation Activation and Organ Failure

Patients with sepsis almost invariably show evidence of activation of the coagulation system. Although the majority of these patients do not have clinical signs of DIC, patients with a laboratory diagnosis of this syndrome are known to have a worse outcome than patients with normal coagulation parameters. A number of small clinical studies have suggested that sepsis-related DIC is associated with not only a high mortality but also with organ dysfunction and that attenuation of coagulation may ameliorate organ failure in this condition. In the placebo group of the PROWESS study (which addressed the efficacy of recombinant human APC in severe sepsis), patients with DIC displayed a mortality rate of 43% versus 27% in patients without DIC [41]. Similarly, in the KyberSept trial (addressing the efficacy of antithrombin in severe sepsis), 28-day mortality among placebo-treated patients with DIC was 40%, versus 22% in patients without this syndrome [42]. Data obtained from a large clinical study in 840 patients with severe sepsis have further suggested a direct relationship between coagulopathy and organ failure and death [43]. In this cohort, both baseline coagulation abnormalities (on admission) and first-day changes in the coagulation biomarkers, antithrombin, prothrombin time, and D-dimer, correlated with 28-day mortality. In addition, shifts in these coagulation markers during the first day of severe sepsis correlated with new organ dysfunctions, progression from single to multiple organ failure, and delayed resolution of existing organ dysfunction [43]. Thrombocytopenia is a common feature of DIC and in sepsis the extent of thrombocytopenia is correlated with an adverse outcome [44]. These findings have led to the hypothesis that systemic activation of coagulation can contribute to organ failure by inducing tissue hypoxia. However, the causal link between DIC and organ failure is still a matter of debate, one argument being that if micovascular thrombosis contributes to organ dysfunction

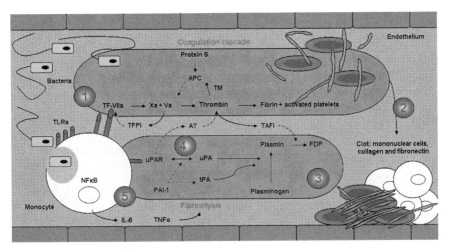

**Fig. 4.** Proposed bidirectional relation between inflammation and coagulation in sepsis. (1) Invading pathogens are recognized by the immune system through the Toll-like receptors (TLRs). After recognition, the coagulation cascade is activated by inducing tissue factor (TF) expression on monocytes and granulocytes. In sepsis decreased levels of free protein S and activated protein C (APC) are seen, ultimately leading to enhanced thrombin formation. (2) A fibrin clot with activated mononuclear cells is formed. In severe cases this may lead to disseminated intravascular coagulation. (3) The activated counteracting plasmin-mediated fibrinolysis leads to the formation of fibrin degradation products (FDP). (4) Furthermore, after binding to urokinase-type plasminogen activator (u-PA) the upregulated protease-activated receptors for u-PA (uPAR) on monocytes and granulocytes will enhance the fibrinolytic pathway. Plasminogen activator inhibitor-1 (PAI-1), which is strongly upregulated in sepsis, inhibits these fibrinolytic events. (5) Binding of, among others, tissue factor and thrombin to specific PARs on inflammatory cells may affect inflammation by inducing release of pro-inflammatory cytokines, which will further modulate coagulation and fibrinolysis. Straight and dashed arrows indicate stimulatory and inhibitory effects, respectively

in sepsis, anticoagulants would reduce organ failure and improve outcome [45]; as already alluded to above, down stream intervention in the coagulation cascade by DEGR-Xa did not influence lethality of bacteremic baboons, while completely inhibiting coagulation activation [28].

## Clinical Trials with Anticoagulants in Sepsis

After promising results from animal studies and small Phase II trials, three specific anticoagulant proteins were evaluated in large multinational clinical trials to test their efficacy in the treatment of severe sepsis: recombinant human APC, antithrombin, and TFPI [46–48]. As discussed above, during inflammation-induced activation of coagulation, such as seen in severe sepsis, the function of all of these endogenous anticoagulant pathways is impaired, which provides a clear rationale for exogenous administration of these agents.

Recombinant human APC, also known as drotrecogin alfa (activated), possesses anti-inflammatory, antithrombotic, and profibrinolytic properties. In the PROWESS study, in which 1690 patients with severe sepsis were randomized to receive APC or placebo, APC significantly reduced morbidity and mortality [46]. Patients treated with APC had a statistically and clinically significant reduction in 28-day mortality (24.7% in the treatment group and 30.8% in the placebo group; relative risk reduction, 19.4% [95% CI, 6.6%–30.5%]), this study, therefore, being the first published trial in sepsis to show a clear survival benefit. Importantly, APC is not effective in reducing mortality in patients with severe sepsis and a low risk of death (defined by an Acute Physiology and Chronic Health Evaluation [APACHE II] score < 25 or single-organ failure) [49].

Antithrombin was studied in a large phase III clinical trial involving 2,314 patients (the KyberSept study) [47]. Despite encouraging results obtained in earlier smaller trials [50], the phase III study failed to demonstrate a benefit of the use of exogenous antithrombin concentrate in patients with severe sepsis. After completion of this trial questions were raised about the dose of antithrombin used, which was lower than used in preclinical animal studies and may have influenced the possible anti-inflammatory effects of antithrombin. In addition, the concurrent use of heparin may have affected the trial results: there was a trend toward a survival benefit in patients who received antithrombin without heparin [47]. A recent posthoc analysis of this trial has indicated that antithrombin may improve outcome in patients with DIC not receiving heparin. In these patients, antithrombin reduced 28-day mortality by 14.6% when compared with placebo [42]. These findings await confirmation in a prospectively designed clinical trial.

TFPI (recombinant human TFPI, tifacogin) is the third anticoagulant that has been tested in a large, multicenter, phase III trial in patients with severe sepsis (the OPTIMIST trial) [48]. In spite of promising phase II data [51], treatment with TFPI failed to affect all-cause 28-day mortality. Remarkably, TFPI appeared to be relatively effective in the first half of the trial, but ineffective in the second half. Several post-hoc exploratory analyses were unable to explain this changing mortality pattern.

Heparin had a clear beneficial impact on the outcome in all the three phase III trials described. However, a firm conclusion cannot be drawn from these data since the administration of heparin was a post-randomization event. However, the use of heparin in sepsis remains an appealing (and cheap) treatment option. In a murine model of DIC, it was recently shown that low molecular weight heparin could attenuate LPS-induced multiple organ failure (MOF) [52]. Therefore, a well-conducted randomized, placebo-controlled trial of heparin administration in severe sepsis is warranted.

# Conclusion

Severe sepsis triggers clotting, diminishes the activity of natural anticoagulant mechanisms, and impairs the fibrinolytic system. Augmented interactions between inflammation and coagulation can give rise to a vicious cycle, eventually leading to dramatic events such as manifested in severe sepsis and DIC. Unraveling the role of coagulation and inflammation in sepsis will pave the way for new treatment targets in sepsis that can modify the excessive activation of these systems. At present it remains unclear whether anticoagulant therapy improves survival in severe sepsis; in addition, it remains uncertain whether the beneficial effect of recombinant human APC derives from its anticoagulant properties. These issues will be clarified as our understanding of the interplay between coagulation and inflammation during sepsis improves further in the very near future.

# References

1. Levi M, van der Poll T (2005) Two-way interactions between inflammation and coagulation. Trends Cardiovasc Med 15:254–259
2. Esmon CT (2005) The interactions between inflammation and coagulation. Br J Haematol 131:417–430
3. Franco RF, de Jonge E, Dekkers PE, et al (2000) The *in vivo* kinetics of tissue factor messenger RNA expression during human endotoxemia: relationship with activation of coagulation. Blood 96:554–559
4. Aras O, Shet A, Bach RR, et al (2004) Induction of microparticle- and cell-associated intravascular tissue factor in human endotoxemia. Blood 103:4545–4553
5. Osterud B, Flaegstad T (1983) Increased tissue thromboplastin activity in monocytes of patients with meningococcal infection: related to an unfavourable prognosis. Thromb Haemost 49:5–7
6. de Jonge E, Dekkers PE, Creasey AA, et al (2000) Tissue factor pathway inhibitor dose-dependently inhibits coagulation activation without influencing the fibrinolytic and cytokine response during human endotoxemia. Blood 95:1124–1129
7. Taylor FB, Jr., Chang A, Ruf W, et al (1991) Lethal *E. coli* septic shock is prevented by blocking tissue factor with monoclonal antibody. Circ Shock 33:127–134
8. Creasey AA, Chang AC, Feigen L, Wun TC, Taylor FB Jr, Hinshaw LB (1993) Tissue factor pathway inhibitor reduces mortality from Escherichia coli septic shock. J Clin Invest 91:2850–2856
9. Levi M, ten Cate H, Bauer KA, et al (1994) Inhibition of endotoxin-induced activation of coagulation and fibrinolysis by pentoxifylline or by a monoclonal anti-tissue factor antibody in chimpanzees. J Clin Invest 93:114–120
10. Taylor FB, Chang AC, Peer G, Li A, Ezban M, Hedner U (1998) Active site inhibited factor VIIa (DEGR VIIa) attenuates the coagulant and interleukin-6 and -8, but not tumor necrosis factor, responses of the baboon to LD100 Escherichia coli. Blood 91:1609–1615
11. Esmon CT (2003) The protein C pathway. Chest 124:26S-32S
12. Van de Wouwer M, Collen D, Conway EM (2004) Thrombomodulin-protein C-EPCR system: integrated to regulate coagulation and inflammation. Arterioscler Thromb Vasc Biol 24:1374–1383
13. Taylor FB Jr, Emerson TE Jr, Jordan R, Chang AK, Blick KE (1988) Antithrombin-III prevents the lethal effects of Escherichia coli infusion in baboons. Circ Shock 26:227–235

14. Taylor FB Jr, Chang A, Esmon CT, D'Angelo A, Vigano-D'Angelo S, Blick KE (1987) Protein C prevents the coagulopathic and lethal effects of Escherichia coli infusion in the baboon. J Clin Invest 79:918–925
15. Taylor FB Jr, Stearns-Kurosawa DJ, Kurosawa S, et al (2000) The endothelial cell protein C receptor aids in host defense against Escherichia coli sepsis. Blood 95:1680–1686
16. Taylor F, Chang A, Ferrell G, et al (1991) C4b-binding protein exacerbates the host response to Escherichia coli. Blood 78:357–363
17. Levi M, Ten Cate H (1999) Disseminated intravascular coagulation. N Engl J Med 341:586–592
18. Faust SN, Levin M, Harrison OB, et al (2001) Dysfunction of endothelial protein C activation in severe meningococcal sepsis. N Engl J Med 345:408–416
19. van der Poll T, Buller HR, ten Cate H, et al (1990) Activation of coagulation after administration of tumor necrosis factor to normal subjects. N Engl J Med 322:1622–1627
20. Jansen PM, Boermeester MA, Fischer E, et al (1995) Contribution of interleukin-1 to activation of coagulation and fibrinolysis, neutrophil degranulation, and the release of secretory-type phospholipase A2 in sepsis: studies in nonhuman primates after interleukin-1 alpha administration and during lethal bacteremia. Blood 86:1027–1034
21. Stouthard JM, Levi M, Hack CE, et al (1996) Interleukin-6 stimulates coagulation, not fibrinolysis, in humans. Thromb Haemost 76:738–742
22. Lauw FN, Dekkers PE, te Velde AA, et al (1999) Interleukin-12 induces sustained activation of multiple host inflammatory mediator systems in chimpanzees. J Infect Dis 179:646–652
23. Lorente JA, Marshall JC (2005) Neutralization of Tumor Necrosis Factor in Preclinical Models of Sepsis. Shock 24 (Suppl 1):107–119
24. Hinshaw LB, Tekamp-Olson P, Chang AC, et al (1990) Survival of primates in LD100 septic shock following therapy with antibody to tumor necrosis factor (TNF alpha). Circ Shock 30:279–292
25. van der Poll T, Coyle SM, Levi M, et al (1997) Effect of a recombinant dimeric tumor necrosis factor receptor on inflammatory responses to intravenous endotoxin in normal humans. Blood 89:3727–3734
26. van der Poll T, Levi M, Hack CE, et al (1994) Elimination of interleukin 6 attenuates coagulation activation in experimental endotoxemia in chimpanzees. J Exp Med 179:1253–1259
27. Derhaschnig U, Bergmair D, Marsik C, Schlifke I, Wijdenes J, Jilma B (2004) Effect of interleukin-6 blockade on tissue factor-induced coagulation in human endotoxemia. Crit Care Med 32:1136–1140
28. Taylor FB Jr, Chang AC, Peer GT, et al (1991) DEGR-factor Xa blocks disseminated intravascular coagulation initiated by Escherichia coli without preventing shock or organ damage. Blood 78:364–368
29. Levi M, Dorffler-Melly J, Reitsma PH, et al (2003) Aggravation of endotoxin-induced disseminated intravascular coagulation and cytokine activation in heterozygous protein C-deficient mice. Blood 101:4823–4827
30. Coughlin SR (2000) Thrombin signalling and protease-activated receptors. Nature 407:258–264
31. Ossovskaya VS, Bunnett NW (2004) Protease-activated receptors: contribution to physiology and disease. Physiol Rev 84:579–621
32. Riewald M, Petrovan RJ, Donner A, Mueller BM, Ruf W (2002) Activation of endothelial cell protease activated receptor 1 by the protein C pathway. Science 296:1880–1882
33. Pawlinski R, Pedersen B, Schabbauer G, et al (2004) Role of tissue factor and protease-activated receptors in a mouse model of endotoxemia. Blood 103:1342–1347
34. de Jonge E, Friederich PW, Vlasuk GP, et al (2003) Activation of coagulation by administration of recombinant factor VIIa elicits interleukin 6 (IL-6) and IL-8 release in healthy human subjects. Clin Diagn Lab Immunol 10:495–497
35. Myles T, Nishimura T, Yun TH, et al (2003) Thrombin activatable fibrinolysis inhibitor, a potential regulator of vascular inflammation. J Biol Chem 278:51059–51067

36. Conway EM, Van de Wouwer M, Pollefeyt S, et al (2002) The lectin-like domain of thrombomodulin confers protection from neutrophil-mediated tissue damage by suppressing adhesion molecule expression via nuclear factor kappaB and mitogen-activated protein kinase pathways. J Exp Med 196:565–577

37. Blasi F, Carmeliet P (2002) uPAR: a versatile signalling orchestrator. Nat Rev Mol Cell Biol 3:932–943

38. Rijneveld AW, Levi M, Florquin S, Speelman P, Carmeliet P, van Der Poll T (2002) Urokinase receptor is necessary for adequate host defense against pneumococcal pneumonia. J Immunol 168:3507–3511

39. Raaphorst J, Johan Groeneveld AB, Bossink AW, Erik Hack C (2001) Early inhibition of activated fibrinolysis predicts microbial infection, shock and mortality in febrile medical patients. Thromb Haemost 86:543–549

40. Hermans PW, Hazelzet JA (2005) Plasminogen activator inhibitor type 1 gene polymorphism and sepsis. Clin Infect Dis 41 (Suppl 7):S453–458

41. Dhainaut JF, Yan SB, Joyce DE, et al (2004) Treatment effects of drotrecogin alfa (activated) in patients with severe sepsis with or without overt disseminated intravascular coagulation. J Thromb Haemost 2:1924–1933

42. Kienast J, Juers M, Wiedermann CJ, et al (2006) Treatment effects of high-dose antithrombin without concomitant heparin in patients with severe sepsis with or without disseminated intravascular coagulation. J Thromb Haemost 4:90–97

43. Dhainaut JF, Shorr AF, Macias WL, et al (2005) Dynamic evolution of coagulopathy in the first day of severe sepsis: relationship with mortality and organ failure. Crit Care Med 33:341–348

44. Vanderschueren S, De Weerdt A, Malbrain M, et al (2000) Thrombocytopenia and prognosis in intensive care. Crit Care Med 28:1871–1876

45. Vincent JL, De Backer D (2005) Does disseminated intravascular coagulation lead to multiple organ failure? Crit Care Clin 21:469–477

46. Bernard GR, Vincent JL, Laterre PF, et al (2001) Efficacy and safety of recombinant human activated protein C for severe sepsis. N Engl J Med 344:699–709

47. Warren BL, Eid A, Singer P, et al (2001) Caring for the critically ill patient. High-dose antithrombin III in severe sepsis: a randomized controlled trial. JAMA 286:1869–1878

48. Abraham E, Reinhart K, Opal S, et al (2003) Efficacy and safety of tifacogin (recombinant tissue factor pathway inhibitor) in severe sepsis: a randomized controlled trial. JAMA 290:238–247

49. Abraham E, Laterre PF, Garg R, et al (2005) Drotrecogin alfa (activated) for adults with severe sepsis and a low risk of death. N Engl J Med 353:1332–1341

50. Eisele B, Lamy M, Thijs LG, et al (1998) Antithrombin III in patients with severe sepsis. A randomized, placebo-controlled, double-blind multicenter trial plus a meta-analysis on all randomized, placebo-controlled, double-blind trials with antithrombin III in severe sepsis. Intensive Care Med 24:663–672

51. Abraham E, Reinhart K, Svoboda P, et al (2001) Assessment of the safety of recombinant tissue factor pathway inhibitor in patients with severe sepsis: a multicenter, randomized, placebo-controlled, single-blind, dose escalation study. Crit Care Med 29:2081–2089

52. Slofstra SH, van 't Veer C, Buurman WA, Reitsma PH, ten Cate H, Spek CA (2005) Low molecular weight heparin attenuates multiple organ failure in a murine model of disseminated intravascular coagulation. Crit Care Med 33:1365–1370

# The Role of Insulin and Blood Glucose Control

L. Langouche, I. Vanhorebeek, and G. Van den Berghe

## Introduction

Patients who are critically ill, either as a results of a septic complication after extensive surgery or trauma, or those who present with organ failure often due to primary sepsis, have a high risk of death and suffer from substantial morbidity. The hypermetabolic stress response that usually follows any type of major trauma or acute illness is associated with hyperglycemia and insulin resistance, often referred to as 'stress diabetes' or 'diabetes of injury' [1, 2]. In critically ill patients, even in those who were not previously diagnosed with diabetes, glucose uptake is reduced in peripheral insulin sensitive tissues, whereas endogenous glucose production is increased, resulting in hyperglycemia. It has long been generally accepted that a moderate hyperglycemia in critically ill patients is beneficial to ensure the supply of glucose as a source of energy to organs that do not require insulin for glucose uptake, such as the brain and the immune system. However, an increasing body of evidence associates the upon-admission degree of hyperglycemia, as well as the duration of hyperglycemia during critical illness, with adverse outcome. The first evidence against the concept of tolerating hyperglycemia during critical illness came from two large, randomized, controlled trials, one in a group of surgical intensive care patients [3] and another in strictly medical intensive care patients [4]. The studies demonstrated that tight blood glucose control with insulin therapy significantly improves morbidity and mortality. Both blood glucose control and glucose-independent actions of insulin appear to contribute to the beneficial effects of the therapy [5].

## Hyperglycemia and Outcome in Critical Illness

The development of stress-induced hyperglycemia is associated with several clinically important problems in a wide array of patients with severe illness or injury. An increasing number of reports associate the upon-admission degree of hyperglycemia, as well as the duration of hyperglycemia during critical illness, with adverse outcome. In patients with severe brain injury, hyperglycemia was associated with longer duration of hospital stay, a worse neurological status, pupil reactivity, higher intracranial pressures, and reduced survival [6, 7]. In severely burned children, the incidence of bacteremia and fungemia, the number of skin grafting procedures, and the risk of death were higher in hyperglycemic than in normoglycemic patients [8]. In trauma patients, elevated glucose levels early after injury have been associated with infectious morbidity, a lengthier ICU and hospital stay, and increased mortality [9, 10]. Furthermore, this effect appeared to be independent of the associated shock or the severity of injury [10]. Trauma patients with persistent hyperglycemia had a significantly greater degree of morbidity and mortality [11]. A meta-analysis of studies on myocardial infarction revealed an association between hyperglycemia and increased risk of congestive heart failure or cardiogenic shock and in-hospital mortality [12]. Higher blood glucose levels predicted a higher risk of death after stroke and a poor functional recovery in those patients who survived [13]. A retrospective review of a heterogeneous group of critically ill patients indicated that even a modest degree of hyperglycemia occurring after admission to the intensive care unit (ICU) was associated with a substantial increase in hospital mortality [14]. A retrospective study on non-diabetic pediatric critically ill patients revealed a correlation of hyperglycemia with a greater in-hospital mortality rate and longer length of stay [15].

## Blood Glucose Control with Intensive Insulin Therapy

The landmark prospective, randomized, controlled clinical trial of intensive insulin therapy in a large group of patients admitted to the ICU after extensive or complicated surgery or trauma revealed major clinical benefits on morbidity and mortality [3]. In the conventional management of hyperglycemia, insulin was only administered when blood glucose levels exceeded 220 mg/dl, with the aim of keeping concentrations between 180 and 200 mg/dl, resulting in mean blood glucose levels of 150–160 mg/dl (hyperglycemia). In the intensive insulin therapy group, insulin was administered to patients by insulin infusion titrated to maintain blood glucose levels between 80 and 110 mg/dl which resulted in mean blood glucose levels of 90–100 mg/dl (normoglycemia). This intervention appeared safe as no hypoglycemia-induced adverse events were reported. Maintaining normoglycemia with insulin strikingly lowered ICU mortality by 43% (from 8.0% to 4.6%), the benefit being most pronounced in the group of patients who required intensive care for more than 5 days, with a mortality reduction from 20.2% to 10.6% (Fig. 1). Also, in-hospital mortality was lowered from 10.9% to 7.2% in the total group and from 26.3% to 16.8% in the group of long-stayers. Besides saving lives, insulin therapy largely prevented several critical illness-associated complications. The development of blood stream infections was reduced by 46%, of acute renal failure requiring dialysis or hemofiltration by 41%, of bacteremia by 46%, the incidence of critical illness polyneuropathy was reduced by 44%, the number of red blood cell (RBC) transfusions by 50%. Patients were also less dependent on prolonged mechanical ventilation and needed fewer days in intensive care. Although a large number of patients included in this study recovered from complicated cardiac surgery, the clinical benefits of this therapy were equally present in most other

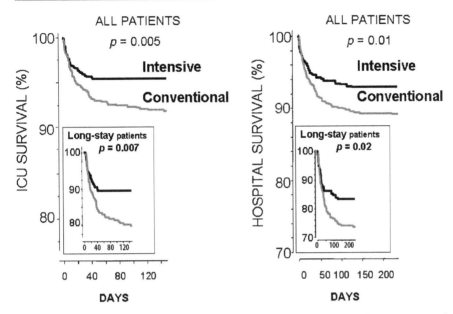

Fig. 1. Effects of intensive insulin therapy in the intensive care unit (ICU). Kaplan-Meier survival plots of patients from the Leuven study who received intensive insulin treatment (blood glucose maintained below 110 mg/dl; black) or conventional treatment (insulin administration only when blood glucose exceeded 220 mg/dl; gray) in the ICU. The upper panels display results from all patients; the lower panels display results for long-stay (> 5 days) ICU patients only. P values were determined with the use of the Mantel-Cox log-rank test. Adapted from [35] with permission

diagnostic subgroups. In the patients with isolated brain injury tight glycemic control protected the central and peripheral nervous system from secondary insults and improved long-term rehabilitation [16]. An important confirmation of the clinical benefits of intensive insulin therapy was recently obtained with the demonstration, by a large randomized controlled trial, that the Leuven protocol of glycemic control with insulin in adult surgical critically ill patients [3] was similarly effective in a strictly medical adult ICU patient population [4]. In this exclusively medical ICU population, in which sepsis is the most common trigger for ICU admission, intensive insulin therapy during ICU stay reduced morbidity among all intention-to-treat medical ICU patients and in those patients who were treated at least for a few days, it improved morbidity and reduced mortality. Morbidity benefits included prevention of kidney injury, reduced duration of mechanical ventilation, shorter ICU stay and shorter hospital stay, but not prevention of blood-stream infections. Among the long-stay patients, in-hospital mortality was reduced from 52.5% to 43.0%. These data indicate that the preventive effect on severe infections, observed in the surgical study, is not the most important pathway by which mortality is reduced with intensive insulin therapy.

In 'real-life' intensive care medicine, Jamie Krinsley evaluated the impact of implementing strict blood glucose control in a heterogeneous medical/surgical

ICU population [17]. A less strict blood glucose control was aimed for, a regimen chosen primarily to avoid inadvertent hypoglycemia; in this setting insulin therapy lowered mean blood glucose levels of 152 mg/dl in the baseline period to 131 mg/dl in the protocol period. Comparison with patient data before the implementation of the protocol showed a 29.3% reduction in hospital mortality, and a 10.8% decrease in length of ICU stay. Development of new renal insufficiency was 75% lower, and 18.7% fewer patients required RBC transfusion. Again, the number of patients acquiring infections did not change significantly, but the incidence was already low at baseline in this patient group [17]. Another small, prospective, randomized, controlled trial by Grey and Perdizet conducted in a predominantly surgical ICU, confirmed the beneficial effect of tight blood glucose control on the number of serious infections [18]. In this study, insulin therapy was targeted to glucose levels between 80 and 120 mg/dl, which resulted in a mean daily glucose levels of 125 mg/dl versus 179 mg/dl in the standard glycemic control group. A significant reduction in the incidence of total nosocomial infections, including intravascular device, bloodstream, intravascular device-related bloodstream, and surgical site infections was observed in the insulin group compared to the conventional approach [18].

## Insulin Resistance and Hyperglycemia

The stress imposed by any type of acute illness or injury leads to the development of insulin resistance, glucose intolerance, and hyperglycemia. Hepatic glucose production is upregulated in the acute phase of critical illness, despite high blood glucose levels and abundantly released insulin. Elevated levels of cytokines, growth hormone, glucagon, and cortisol might play a role in the increased gluconeogenesis [19–23]. Several effects of these hormones oppose the normal action of insulin, resulting in increased lipolysis and proteolysis which provide substrates for gluconeogenesis. Catecholamines, which are released in response to acute injury, enhance hepatic glycogenolysis and inhibit glycogenesis [24]. Apart from the upregulated glucose production, glucose uptake mechanisms are also affected during critical illness and contribute to the development of hyperglycemia. Due to immobilization of the critically ill patient, exercise-stimulated glucose uptake in skeletal muscle is supposedly absent [25, 26]. Furthermore, due to impaired insulin-stimulated glucose uptake by the glucose transporter 4 (GLUT-4) and due to impaired glycogen synthase activity, glucose uptake in heart, skeletal muscle, and adipose tissue is compromised [27–30]. However, total body glucose uptake is massively increased, but is accounted for by tissues that are not dependent on insulin for glucose uptake, such as brain and blood cells [1, 31]. The higher levels of insulin, impaired peripheral glucose uptake, and elevated hepatic glucose production reflect the development of insulin resistance during critical illness.

The mechanism by which insulin therapy lowers blood glucose in critically ill patients is not completely clear. These patients are thought to suffer from both hepatic and skeletal muscle insulin resistance, but data from liver and skeletal muscle biopsies harvested from non-survivors in the Leuven study, suggest that glucose levels are lowered mainly via stimulation of skeletal muscle glucose uptake. Indeed, insulin therapy did increase mRNA levels of GLUT-4, which controls insulin-stimulated glucose uptake in muscle, and of hexokinase-II, the rate-limiting enzyme in intracellular insulin-stimulated glucose metabolism [32]. On the other hand, hepatic insulin resistance in these patients is not overcome by insulin therapy. The hepatic expression of phospoenolpyruvate carboxykinase, the rate-limiting enzyme in gluconeogenesis, and of glucokinase, the rate-limiting enzyme for insulin-mediated glucose uptake and glycogen synthesis, was unaffected by insulin therapy [32, 33]. Moreover, circulating levels of insulin-like growth factor binding protein-1, normally under the inhibitory control of insulin, were also refractory to the therapy in the total population of both survivors and non-survivors [32].

## Preventing Glucose Toxicity with Intensive Insulin Therapy

It is striking that during the relatively short period that patients need intensive care, avoiding even a moderate level of hyperglycemia with insulin improves the most feared complications of critical illness. In critically ill patients, hyperglycemia thus appears much more acutely toxic than in healthy individuals whose cells can protect themselves by downregulation of glucose transporters [34]. This acute toxicity of high levels of glucose in critical illness might be explained by an accelerated cellular glucose overload and more pronounced toxic side effects of glycolysis and oxidative phosphorylation [35].

Hepatocytes, gastro-intestinal mucosal cells, pancreatic beta cells, renal tubular cells, endothelial cells, immune cells, and neurons are insulin-independent for glucose uptake, which is mediated mainly by the glucose transporters GLUT-1, GLUT-2, or GLUT-3 [1]. Cytokines, angiotensin II, endothelin-1, vascular endothelial growth factor (VEGF), transforming growth factor (TGF)-$\beta$ and hypoxia, all induced in critical illness, have been shown to upregulate the expression and membrane localization of GLUT-1 and GLUT-3 in different cell types [36–40]. This upregulation might overrule the normal downregulatory protective response against hyperglycemia. Moreover, GLUT-2 and GLUT-3 allow glucose to enter cells directly in equilibrium with the elevated extracellular glucose level which is present in critical illness [41]. Therefore, one would expect increased glucose toxicity in tissues where glucose uptake is mediated by non-insulin-dependent transport. Hyperglycemia has been linked to the development of increased oxidative stress in diabetes, in part due to enhanced mitochondrial superoxide production [42–44]. Superoxide interacts with nitric oxide (NO) to form peroxynitrite, a reactive species able to induce tyrosine nitration of proteins which affects their normal function [45]. During critical illness, cytokine-induced activation of NO synthase (NOS) increases NO levels, and hypoxia-reperfusion aggravates superoxide production, resulting in more peroxynitrite being generated [45]. When cells in critically ill patients are overloaded with glucose, high levels of peroxynitrite and superoxide are to be expected, resulting in inhibition of the glycolytic enzyme GAPDH, and mitochondrial complexes I and IV [42].

We recently demonstrated that prevention of hyperglycemia with insulin therapy protected both the ultrastructure and function of the hepatocytic mitochondrial compartment of critically ill patients, but no obvious morphological or pronounced functional abnormalities were detected in skeletal muscle of critically ill patients [46]. Mitochondrial dysfunction with disturbed energy metabolism is a likely cause of organ failure, the most common cause of death in the ICU. Prevention of hyperglycemia-induced mitochondrial dysfunction in other tissues that allow glucose to enter passively might explain some of the protective effects of intensive insulin therapy in critical illness.

## Metabolic and Non-Metabolic Effects of Blood Glucose Control with Intensive Insulin Therapy

Similar to the serum lipid profile of diabetic patients [47], lipid metabolism in critically ill patients is strongly deranged. Most characteristic are elevated triglycerides together with very low levels of high-density lipoprotein (HDL) and low-density lipoprotein (LDL) cholesterol [48–50]. Insulin therapy almost completely reversed this hypertriglyceridemia and substantially elevated HDL and LDL and the level of cholesterol associated with these lipoproteins [32]. Insulin treatment also decreased serum triglycerides and free fatty acids in burned children [51]. Multivariate logistic regression analysis revealed that improvement of the dyslipidemia with insulin therapy explained a significant part of the reduced mortality and organ failure in critically ill patients [32]. Given the important role of lipoproteins in transportation of lipid components (cholesterol, triglycerides, phospholipids, lipid-soluble vitamins) and endotoxin scavenging [52–54], a contribution to improved outcome might indeed be expected.

Critically ill patients become severely catabolic, with loss of lean body mass, despite adequate enteral or parenteral nutrition. Intensive insulin therapy might attenuate this catabolic syndrome of prolonged critical illness, as insulin exerts anabolic actions [55–58]. Intensive insulin treatment indeed resulted in higher total protein content in skeletal muscle of critically ill patients [46] and prevented weight loss in a rabbit model of prolonged critical illness [59].

Intensive insulin therapy prevented excessive inflammation, illustrated by decreased C-reactive protein (CRP) and mannose-binding lectin levels [60], independent of its preventive effect on infections [3]. Insulin therapy also attenuated the CRP response in an experimental animal model of prolonged critical illness induced by third degree burn injury [59]. Moreover, critically ill rabbits showed an increased capacity of monocytes to phagocytose and an increase in their ability to generate an oxidative burst when blood glucose levels were kept normal [59]. In burned children, administration of insulin resulted in lower pro-inflammatory cytokines and proteins, whereas the anti-inflammatory cascade was stimulated, although these effects were largely seen only late after the traumatic stimulus [51]. Insulin treatment attenuated the inflammatory response in thermally injured rats and endotoxemic rats and pigs [61–63]. Next to these anti-inflammatory effects of insulin, prevention of hyperglycemia may be crucial as well. Hyperglycemia inactivates immunoglobulins by glycosylation and, therefore, contributes to the risk of infection [64]. High glucose levels also negatively affected polymorphonuclear neutrophil (PMN) function and intracellular bactericidal and opsonic activity [65–68].

Critical illness also resembles diabetes mellitus in its hypercoagulation state [69, 70]. In diabetes mellitus, vascular endothelium dysfunction, elevated platelet activation, increased clotting factors, and inhibition of the fibrinolytic system all might contribute to this hypercoagulation state [71–75]. Insulin therapy indeed protected the myocardium and improved myocardial function after acute myocardial infarction, during open heart surgery, and in congestive heart failure [76]. Prevention of endothelial dysfunction also contributed to the protective effects of insulin therapy in critical illness in part via inhibition of excessive iNOS-induced NO release [77] and via reduction of circulating levels of asymmetric dimethylarginine, which inhibits the constitutive enzyme, endothelial NOS (eNOS), and hence the production of endothelial NO [78].

## Glucose Control or Insulin?

Multivariate logistic regression analysis of the results of the Leuven study [3] indicated that blood glucose control and not the insulin dose administered statistically explains most of the beneficial effects of insulin therapy on outcome of critical illness [5]. It appeared crucial to reduce blood glucose levels below 110 mg/dl for the prevention of morbidity events such as bacteremia, anemia, and acute renal failure. The level of hyperglycemia was also an independent risk factor for the development of critical illness polyneuropathy [5]. Finney et al. confirmed the independent association between hyperglycemia and adverse outcome in surgical ICU patients [79]. Our recent experiments in an animal model of critical illness, in which we independently manipulated the level of blood glucose and insulin [80], confirm the superior role of strict blood glucose control over the glycemia-independent effects of insulin, in obtaining the survival benefit as well as most of the morbidity benefits.

## Conclusion

Hyperglycemia in critically ill patients is a result of an altered glucose metabolism. Apart from the upregulated glucose production (both gluconeogenesis and glycogenolysis), glucose uptake mechanisms are also affected during critical illness and contribute to the development of hyperglycemia. The higher levels of insulin, impaired peripheral glucose uptake and elevated hepatic glucose production reflect the development of insulin resistance during critical illness.

Hyperglycemia in critically ill patients has been associated with increased mortality. Simply maintaining normoglycemia with insulin therapy improves survival and reduces morbidity in surgical and medical ICU patients, as shown by two large, randomized controlled studies. These results obtained from clinical studies were also confirmed in 'real-life' intensive care of a heterogeneous patient population admitted to a mixed medical/surgical ICU.

Prevention of glucose toxicity by strict glycemic control appears to be crucial, although other metabolic and non-metabolic effects of insulin, independent of glycemic control, may contribute to the clinical benefits.

## References

1. McCowen KC, Malhotra A, Bistrian BR (2001) Stress-induced hyperglycemia. Crit Care Clin 17:107–124
2. Thorell A, Nygren J, Ljungqvist O (1999) Insulin resistance: a marker of surgical stress. Curr Opin Clin Nutr Metab Care 2:69–78
3. Van den Berghe G, Wouters P, Weekers F, et al (2001) Intensive insulin therapy in critically ill patients. N Engl J Med 345:1359–1367
4. Van den Berghe G, Wilmer A, Hermans G, et al (2006) Intensive insulin therapy in medical intensive care patients. N Engl J Med 354:449–461
5. Van den Berghe G, Wouters PJ, Bouillon R, et al (2003) Outcome benefit of intensive insulin therapy in the critically ill: Insulin dose versus glycemic control. Crit Care Med 31:359–366
6. Rovlias A, Kotsou S (2000) The influence of hyperglycemia on neurological outcome in patients with severe head injury. Neurosurgery 46:335–342
7. Jeremitsky E, Omert LA, Dunham CM, Wilberger J, Rodriguez A (2005) The impact of hyperglycemia on patients with severe brain injury. J Trauma 58:47–50
8. Gore DC, Chinkes D, Heggers J, Herndon DN, Wolf SE, Desai M (2001) Association of hyperglycemia with increased mortality after severe burn injury. J Trauma 51:540–544
9. Yendamuri S, Fulda GJ, Tinkoff GH (2003) Admission hyperglycemia as a prognostic indicator in trauma. J Trauma 55:33–38
10. Laird AM, Miller PR, Kilgo PD, Meredith JW, Chang MC (2004) Relationship of early hyperglycemia to mortality in trauma patients. J Trauma 56:1058–1062
11. Bochicchio GV, Sung J, Joshi M, et al (2005) Persistent hyperglycemia is predictive of outcome in critically ill trauma patients. J Trauma 58:921–924
12. Capes SE, Hunt D, Malmberg K, Gerstein HC (2000) Stress hyperglycaemia and increased risk of death after myocardial infarction in patients with and without diabetes: a systematic overview. Lancet 355:773–778
13. Capes SE, Hunt D, Malmberg K, Pathak P, Gerstein HC (2001) Stress hyperglycemia and prognosis of stroke in nondiabetic and diabetic patients: a systematic overview. Stroke 32:2426–2432
14. Krinsley JS (2003) Association between hyperglycemia and increased hospital mortality in a heterogeneous population of critically ill patients. Mayo Clin Proc 78:1471–1478
15. Faustino EV, Apkon M (2005) Persistent hyperglycemia in critically ill children. J Pediatr 146:30–34
16. Van den Berghe G, Schoonheydt K, Becx P, Bruyninckx F, Wouters PJ (2005) Insulin therapy protects the central and peripheral nervous system of intensive care patients. Neurology 64:1348–1353

17. Krinsley JS (2004) Effect of an intensive glucose management protocol on the mortality of critically ill adult patients. Mayo Clin Proc 79:992–1000
18. Grey NJ, Perdrizet GA (2004) Reduction of nosocomial infections in the surgical intensive-care unit by strict glycemic control. Endocr Pract 10 (Suppl 2):46–52
19. Hill M, McCallum R (1991) Altered transcriptional regulation of phosphoenolpyruvate carboxykinase in rats following endotoxin treatment. J Clin Invest 88:811–816
20. Flores EA, Istfan N, Pomposelli JJ, Blackburn GL, Bistrian BR (1990) Effect of interleukin-1 and tumor necrosis factor/cachectin on glucose turnover in the rat. Metabolism 39:738–743
21. Lang CH, Dobrescu C, Bagby GJ (1992) Tumor necrosis factor impairs insulin action on peripheral glucose disposal and hepatic glucose output. Endocrinology 130:43–52
22. Sakurai Y, Zhang XJ, Wolfe RR (1996) TNF directly stimulates glucose uptake and leucine oxidation and inhibits FFA flux in conscious dogs. Am J Physiol 270:E864–E872
23. Khani S, Tayek JA (2001) Cortisol increases gluconeogenesis in humans: its role in the metabolic syndrome. Clin Sci (Lond) 101:739–747
24. Watt MJ, Howlett KF, Febbraio MA, Spriet LL, Hargreaves M (2001) Adrenaline increases skeletal muscle glycogenolysis, pyruvate dehydrogenase activation and carbohydrate oxidation during moderate exercise in humans. J Physiol 534:269–278
25. Richter EA, Ruderman NB, Gavras H, Belur ER, Galbo H (1982) Muscle glycogenolysis during exercise: dual control by epinephrine and contractions. Am J Physiol 242:E25–E32
26. Rodnick KJ, Piper RC, Slot JW, James DE (1992) Interaction of insulin and exercise on glucose transport in muscle. Diabetes Care 15:1679–1689
27. Wolfe RR, Durkot MJ, Allsop JR, Burke JF (1979) Glucose metabolism in severely burned patients. Metabolism 28:1031–1039
28. Wolfe RR, Herndon DN, Jahoor F, Miyoshi H, Wolfe M (1987) Effect of severe burn injury on substrate cycling by glucose and fatty acids. N Engl J Med 317:403–408
29. Stephens JM, Bagby GJ, Pekala PH, Shepherd RE, Spitzer JJ, Lang CH (1992) Differential regulation of glucose transporter gene expression in adipose tissue or septic rats. Biochem Biophys Res Commun 183:417–422
30. Virkamaki A, Yki-Jarvinen H (1994) Mechanisms of insulin resistance during acute endotoxemia. Endocrinology 134:2072–2078
31. Meszaros K, Lang CH, Bagby GJ, Spitzer JJ (1987) Contribution of different organs to increased glucose consumption after endotoxin administration. J Biol Chem 262:10965–10970
32. Mesotten D, Swinnen JV, Vanderhoydonc F, Wouters PJ, Van den Berghe G (2004) Contribution of circulating lipids to the improved outcome of critical illness by glycemic control with intensive insulin therapy. J Clin Endocrinol Metab 89:219–226
33. Mesotten D, Delhanty PJ, Vanderhoydonc F, et al (2002) Regulation of insulin-like growth factor binding protein-1 during protracted critical illness. J Clin Endocrinol Metab 87:5516–5523
34. Klip A, Tsakiridis T, Marette A, Ortiz PA (1994) Regulation of expression of glucose transporters by glucose: a review of studies in vivo and in cell cultures. FASEB J 8:43–53
35. Van den Berghe G (2004) How does blood glucose control with insulin save lives in intensive care? J Clin Invest 114:1187–1195
36. Pekala P, Marlow M, Heuvelman D, Connolly D (1990) Regulation of hexose transport in aortic endothelial cells by vascular permeability factor and tumor necrosis factor-alpha, but not by insulin. J Biol Chem 265:18051–18054
37. Shikhman AR, Brinson DC, Valbracht J, Lotz MK (2001) Cytokine regulation of facilitated glucose transport in human articular chondrocytes. J Immunol 167:7001–7008
38. Quinn LA, McCumbee WD (1998) Regulation of glucose transport by angiotensin II and glucose in cultured vascular smooth muscle cells. J Cell Physiol 177:94–102
39. Clerici C, Matthay MA (2000) Hypoxia regulates gene expression of alveolar epithelial transport proteins. J Appl Physiol 88:1890–1896

40. Sanchez-Alvarez R, Tabernero A, Medina JM (2004) Endothelin-1 stimulates the translocation and upregulation of both glucose transporter and hexokinase in astrocytes: relationship with gap junctional communication. J Neurochem 89:703–714
41. Tirone TA, Brunicardi FC (2001) Overview of glucose regulation. World J Surg 25:461–467
42. Brownlee M (2001) Biochemistry and molecular cell biology of diabetic complications. Nature 414:813–820
43. Giugliano D, Ceriello A, Paolisso G (1996) Oxidative stress and diabetic vascular complications. Diabetes Care 19:257–267
44. West IC (2000) Radicals and oxidative stress in diabetes. Diabet Med 17:171–180
45. Aulak KS, Koeck T, Crabb JW, Stuehr DJ (2004) Dynamics of protein nitration in cells and mitochondria. Am J Physiol Heart Circ Physiol 286:H30–H38
46. Vanhorebeek I, De Vos R, Mesotten D, Wouters PJ, Wolf-Peeters C, Van den Berghe G (2005) Protection of hepatocyte mitochondrial ultrastructure and function by strict blood glucose control with insulin in critically ill patients. Lancet 365:53–59
47. Taskinen MR (2001) Pathogenesis of dyslipidemia in type 2 diabetes. Exp Clin Endocrinol Diabetes 109 (Suppl 2):S180–S188
48. Lanza-Jacoby S, Wong SH, Tabares A, Baer D, Schneider T (1992) Disturbances in the composition of plasma lipoproteins during gram-negative sepsis in the rat. Biochim Biophys Acta 1124:233–240
49. Khovidhunkit W, Memon RA, Feingold KR, Grunfeld C (2000) Infection and inflammation-induced proatherogenic changes of lipoproteins. J Infect Dis 181 (Suppl 3):S462–S472
50. Carpentier YA, Scruel O (2002) Changes in the concentration and composition of plasma lipoproteins during the acute phase response. Curr Opin Clin Nutr Metab Care 5:153–158
51. Jeschke MG, Klein D, Herndon DN (2004) Insulin treatment improves the systemic inflammatory reaction to severe trauma. Ann Surg 239:553–560
52. Tulenko TN, Sumner AE (2002) The physiology of lipoproteins. J Nucl Cardiol 9:638–649
53. Harris HW, Grunfeld C, Feingold KR, Rapp JH (1990) Human very low density lipoproteins and chylomicrons can protect against endotoxin-induced death in mice. J Clin Invest 86:696–702
54. Harris HW, Grunfeld C, Feingold KR, et al (1993) Chylomicrons alter the fate of endotoxin, decreasing tumor necrosis factor release and preventing death. J Clin Invest 91:1028–1034
55. Zhang XJ, Chinkes DL, Irtun O, Wolfe RR (2002) Anabolic action of insulin on skin wound protein is augmented by exogenous amino acids. Am J Physiol Endocrinol Metab 282:E1308–E1315
56. Gore DC, Wolf SE, Sanford AP, Herndon DN, Wolfe RR (2004) Extremity hyperinsulinemia stimulates muscle protein synthesis in severely injured patients. Am J Physiol Endocrinol Metab 286:E529–E534
57. Agus MS, Javid PJ, Ryan DP, Jaksic T (2004) Intravenous insulin decreases protein breakdown in infants on extracorporeal membrane oxygenation. J Pediatr Surg 39:839–844
58. Hillier TA, Fryburg DA, Jahn LA, Barrett EJ (1998) Extreme hyperinsulinemia unmasks insulin's effect to stimulate protein synthesis in the human forearm. Am J Physiol 274:E1067–E1074
59. Weekers F, Giulietti AP, Michalaki M, et al (2003) Metabolic, endocrine, and immune effects of stress hyperglycemia in a rabbit model of prolonged critical illness. Endocrinology 144:5329–5338
60. Hansen TK, Thiel S, Wouters PJ, Christiansen JS, Van den Berghe G (2003) Intensive insulin therapy exerts antiinflammatory effects in critically ill patients and counteracts the adverse effect of low mannose-binding lectin levels. J Clin Endocrinol Metab 88:1082–1088
61. Jeschke MG, Klein D, Bolder U, Einspanier R (2004) Insulin attenuates the systemic inflammatory response in endotoxemic rats. Endocrinology 145:4084–4093
62. Klein D, Schubert T, Horch RE, Jauch KW, Jeschke MG (2004) Insulin treatment improves hepatic morphology and function through modulation of hepatic signals after severe trauma. Ann Surg 240:340–349

63. Brix-Christensen V, Andersen SK, Andersen R, et al (2004) Acute hyperinsulinemia restrains endotoxin-induced systemic inflammatory response: an experimental study in a porcine model. Anesthesiology 100:861–870
64. Black CT, Hennessey PJ, Andrassy RJ (1990) Short-term hyperglycemia depresses immunity through nonenzymatic glycosylation of circulating immunoglobulin. J Trauma 30:830–832
65. Nielson CP, Hindson DA (1989) Inhibition of polymorphonuclear leukocyte respiratory burst by elevated glucose concentrations in vitro. Diabetes 38:1031–1035
66. Perner A, Nielsen SE, Rask-Madsen J (2003) High glucose impairs superoxide production from isolated blood neutrophils. Intensive Care Med 29:642–645
67. Rassias AJ, Marrin CA, Arruda J, Whalen PK, Beach M, Yeager MP (1999) Insulin infusion improves neutrophil function in diabetic cardiac surgery patients. Anesth Analg 88:1011–1016
68. Rayfield EJ, Ault MJ, Keusch GT, Brothers MJ, Nechemias C, Smith H (1982) Infection and diabetes: the case for glucose control. Am J Med 72:439–450
69. Carr ME (2001) Diabetes mellitus: a hypercoagulable state. J Diabetes Complications 15:44–54
70. Calles-Escandon J, Garcia-Rubi E, Mirza S, Mortensen A (1999) Type 2 diabetes: one disease, multiple cardiovascular risk factors. Coron Artery Dis 10:23–30
71. Williams E, Timperley WR, Ward JD, Duckworth T (1980) Electron microscopical studies of vessels in diabetic peripheral neuropathy. J Clin Pathol 33:462–470
72. Patrassi GM, Vettor R, Padovan D, Girolami A (1982) Contact phase of blood coagulation in diabetes mellitus. Eur J Clin Invest 12:307–311
73. Carmassi F, Morale M, Puccetti R, et al (1992) Coagulation and fibrinolytic system impairment in insulin dependent diabetes mellitus. Thromb Res 67:643–654
74. Hughes A, McVerry BA, Wilkinson L, Goldstone AH, Lewis D, Bloom A (1983) Diabetes, a hypercoagulable state? Hemostatic variables in newly diagnosed type 2 diabetic patients. Acta Haematol 69:254–259
75. Garcia Frade LJ, de la Calle H, Alava I, Navarro JL, Creighton LJ, Gaffney PJ (1987) Diabetes mellitus as a hypercoagulable state: its relationship with fibrin fragments and vascular damage. Thromb Res 47:533–540
76. Das UN (2003) Insulin: an endogenous cardioprotector. Curr Opin Crit Care 9:375–383
77. Langouche L, Vanhorebeek I, Vlasselaers D, et al (2005) Intensive insulin therapy protects the endothelium of critically ill patients. J Clin Invest 115:2277–2286
78. Siroen MP, van Leeuwen PA, Nijveldt RJ, Teerlink T, Wouters PJ, Van den Berghe G (2005) Modulation of asymmetric dimethylarginine in critically ill patients receiving intensive insulin treatment: a possible explanation of reduced morbidity and mortality? Crit Care Med 33:504–510
79. Finney SJ, Zekveld C, Elia A, Evans TW (2003) Glucose control and mortality in critically ill patients. JAMA 290:2041–2047
80. Ellger B, Debaveye Y, Vanhorebeek I, et al (2006) Survival benefits of intensive insulin therapy in critical illness: impact of maintaining normoglycemia versus glycemia-independent actions of insulin. Diabetes 55:1096–1105

# Dysfunction of the Bioenergetic Pathway

M. Singer

## Introduction

Sepsis represents a whole-body inflammatory response to infection that often progresses to multiple organ failure (MOF). In this condition, organ function is altered in an acutely ill patient such that homeostasis cannot be maintained without interventions, including pharmacological and mechanical support, in the hope that recovery will eventually ensue once the severe inflammatory insult has subsided.

Despite three decades of intensive research and billions of pharmaceutical company dollars searching for immunotherapeutic magic bullets, mortality rates for sepsis-induced MOF have not changed dramatically. The incidence of sepsis is rising [1], and predicted to increase still further as elderly and immunosuppressed populations grow.

The syndrome of sepsis presents numerous paradoxes and many questions that remain unanswered. Why are some people more susceptible than others to a septic insult? How does excessive inflammation actually cause the organs to fail? Why do these failed organs look remarkably normal with minimal evidence of cell death [2]? Unlike many other conditions that cause single organ failure, why is there, in general, (near-) total recovery of organ function should the patient survive? Why is this recovery seen even in organs with poor regenerative capacity [3]?

This chapter will attempt to address at least some of these points, adopting the stance that mitochondrial dysfunction lies at the core of organ dysfunction (Fig. 1.). Recovery is thus contingent on the restoration of an adequately functioning bioenergetic pathway. I will suggest that this assumed 'failure' may actually represent an adaptive, last-ditch, protective response to enable eventual survival of the patient should they be 'fit' enough to endure the prolonged inflammatory insult.

## How Does Inflammation Lead to Organ Failure?

Genetic, immune, and exogenous factors (e.g., more pathogenic bacteria) are responsible for triggering an excessive degree of inflammation, yet precise mechanisms and interactions remain poorly understood. There is an increasing apprecia-

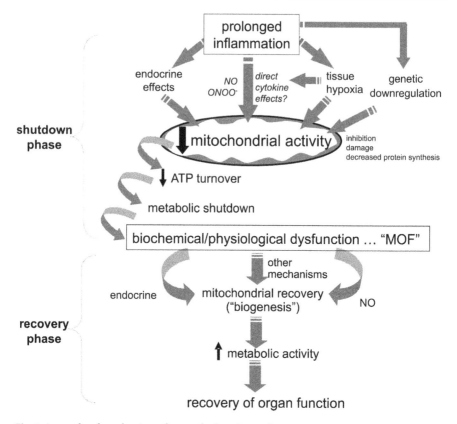

Fig. 1. A postulated mechanism of organ dysfunction and recovery

tion of the importance of other systems, such as the hormonal, immune, metabolic, and bioenergetic pathways in inducing organ dysfunction. The degree of perturbation of each of these systems has been independently associated with increased mortality. Furthermore, many of the conventional paradigms that have attempted to explain the underlying pathophysiology of organ failure have been successfully challenged in recent years. For example, the traditional belief held that organ failure was directly related to inflammatory mediator-induced release of vasoactive agents, activation and aggregation of neutrophils and platelets, and a disseminated intravascular coagulation (DIC) that would result in an abnormal microvasculature with consequent tissue hypoxia, cell death, and organ dysfunction. However, this dogma has been undermined by the findings of normal histology in the majority of affected organs [2], and a paradoxical rise in oxygen tension in tissues as varied as gut epithelium, bladder, and skeletal muscle [4–6]. As the tissue oxygen tension represents the local balance between supply and demand, this infers that oxygen is actually freely available but is not being utilized. Thus, the major problem in sepsis may lie at a cellular level. As cytochrome oxidase is by far the predominant consumer of molecular oxygen (> 90% of total body utilization), a mitochondrial pathology is, therefore, implicated in the pathophysiology of sepsis-induced MOF.

## Mitochondria in Health

The mitochondrion is the powerhouse of the body, being responsible for > 95% of ATP in most cell types. A number of other roles are increasingly appreciated, such as initiation of cell death pathways (apoptosis and necrosis), intracellular calcium regulation, oxygen sensing, steroidogenesis, and signaling. The latter is probably mediated by production of reactive oxygen species (ROS). Production of superoxide at complexes I and III of the electron transport chain is considered to be responsible for approximately 2% of mitochondrial oxygen consumption in healthy cells. As will be discussed later, production of ROS increases significantly during sepsis and may be responsible for mediating many of the pathological effects seen in this syndrome.

Mitochondrial ATP production is a highly sophisticated and regulated process (Fig. 1). It was first described as the chemiosmotic proposal (the coupling of biological electron transfer to ATP synthesis) by Peter Mitchell in the 1960s. Substrate is provided by oxidation of glucose (glycolysis), fats, and amino acids (notably alanine) from which acetyl co-enzyme A (acetyl CoA) is produced within the mitochondrion. This is incorporated within the tricarboxylic acid (Krebs') cycle, generating reducing equivalents in the form of NADH and $FADH_2$. These molecules provide electrons to complexes I and II, respectively, of the electron transport chain. Passage of electrons from NADH to complex I is considered the primary route. As electrons are passed down the chain to complexes III and IV, protons move across the inner mitochondrial membrane to generate a proton gradient that can drive ATP synthase to generate ATP from ADP. Complex IV (cytochrome oxidase) is the only point in the whole process where oxygen is consumed. For every glucose molecule metabolized, 2 molecules of ATP are generated during glycolysis, 2 in the Krebs' cycle, and approximately 25 in the electron transport chain.

Rich [7] assumed that if 90% of human power is provided by the protons transferred through ATP synthase, then the trans-membrane proton flux would have to represent roughly $3 \times 10^{21}$ protons per second and ATP would be reformed at a rate of around $9 \times 10^{20}$ molecules per second. This is equivalent to an ATP turnover rate of 65 kg per day, a figure that would rise considerably during periods of activity. He further calculated that to support an average adult oxygen consumption rate of 380 liters $O_2$ per day, $2 \times 10^{19}$ molecules of cytochrome oxidase are needed. The amount of inner mitochondrial membrane necessary to hold this amount of respiratory enzyme equates to a surface area of approximately 14,000 $M^2$.

## Mitochondria in Sepsis

Mitochondrial abnormalities – both biochemical and ultrastructural – have been recognized in *in vivo* and *in vitro* models of sepsis for more than 30 years. Of note, a systematic review of these models [8] showed variable findings in short-term models of varying severity lasting several hours, with increased, decreased, or unaltered mitochondrial function being reported. However, when the study duration exceeded 16 hours, dysfunction and/or injury were consistent features. Corresponding functional changes were noted that supported the concept of mitochondrial dysfunction. For example, Rosser et al. found that maximal oxygen consumption was markedly increased in a hepatocyte cell line exposed to endotoxin after six hours, but was significantly depressed by 24 hours [9]. In a patient study, Kreymann et al. noted that increasing sepsis severity was associated with progressive falls in oxygen consumption [10].

Human data are still relatively scanty. Initially, small case series reported decreases in ATP or decreased activity of various respiratory chain complexes [11–16]. A larger study published in 2002 consisted of a group of 28 patients in septic shock, and a control group of patients undergoing elective hip surgery [17]. A significant association was seen between sepsis severity and complex I inhibition in muscle biopsies taken within 24 hours of admission to intensive care. Interestingly, there was a clear delineation between subsequent survivors and non-survivors, with ATP levels being preserved in the former (compared to the orthopedic controls) and significantly reduced in the latter. This was found notwithstanding the lack of any clinical differentiation between the two septic groups at the time of biopsy. This human study prompted the development of a long-term (3-day) rat model of fecal peritonitis that remained adequately fluid resuscitated throughout to ensure an adequate circulating blood volume. This model mimics many of the physiological, biochemical, histological, and outcome characteristics of the human patient and enables comparison of muscle data with other 'vital', deeper organs, such as liver and kidney [18]. Mitochondrial results were comparable to the human muscle data in both liver and kidney with the more severely septic animals also demonstrating greater degrees of complex I inhibition and a fall in ATP levels. Importantly, recovery in mitochondrial function paralleled clinical and biochemical recovery. A crucial question that will be addressed later in this review is whether such mitochondrial recovery is fundamental to the restoration of organ function and, if so, how this could arise?

## Nitric Oxide: A Mechanism for Mitochondrial Inhibition

An important step in unraveling the mechanism of mitochondrial inhibition in sepsis arose from the discovery of nitric oxide (NO). This reactive species is produced in greater quantities in sepsis than in any other clinical condition and is largely responsible for the characteristic hypotension and vascular hyporeactivity (i. e., decreased responsiveness to vasoconstrictor catecholamines) of septic shock.

The subsequent recognition that NO and, more particularly, peroxynitrite (formed from the reaction between NO and superoxide), were potent inhibitors of the electron transport chain [19–21] suggested its likely relevance in sepsis. In both the septic patient and fecal peritonitis animal model studies described earlier [17,18], raised NO production (measured as tissue nitrite/nitrate) correlated with the degree of sepsis severity and complex I dysfunction. Glutathione, an endogenous mitochondrial antioxidant that protects complex I from nitrosative damage, was correspondingly reduced and the inability to reverse this inhibition with exogenous glutathione suggested nitration of the enzyme leading to a longer-lasting, if not irreversible, inhibition. In a macrophage cell line incubated with endotoxin [22], a progressive decrease in oxygen consumption and complex I inhibition was found. In conjunction with these findings, early nitrosylation was followed by a progressive increase in nitration which was accentuated in the presence of concurrent hypoxia. Similar findings have been reported in isolated rat aorta exposed to endotoxin and interferon (IFN)-γ where mild hypoxia significantly enhanced the damage induced by NO to the vessel [23].

If the above findings can be extrapolated to patients, coexisting tissue hypoxia (for example, due to delayed fluid resuscitation) would have a synergistic effect with systemic inflammation and would reduce the competition between NO and oxygen for the same binding site on cytochrome oxidase. Boulos et al. [24] incubated an endothelial cell line with plasma taken from septic patients and found a decrease in mitochondrial respiration and ATP levels compared to that seen following incubation with plasma from healthy controls. This depression could be reversed by inhibition of either NO synthase (NOS) or poly-ADP-ribose polymerase (PARP), a nuclear repair enzyme that depletes NAD stores yet also has anti-inflammatory actions. Excessive NO has also been implicated in the skeletal and cardiac muscle contractile failure seen in sepsis, for which a mitochondrial etiology has been suggested [25,26].

## Influence of Hormones on Mitochondrial Activity in Health and Sepsis

Numerous hormones impact on different aspects of mitochondrial function in health, for example, oxidative phosphorylation activity (insulin, thyroid, catecholamines), efficiency and uncoupling (thyroid, growth hormone, testosterone), free radical formation, and lipid peroxidation (insulin, dehydroepiandrosterone) and biogenesis (leptin).

During sepsis and other critical illness, there are well-recognized perturbations in endocrine, metabolic, and bioenergetic activity. For example, most patients develop the low T3 ('sick euthyroid') syndrome, the severity of which will distinguish eventual non-survivors from survivors, even on admission to intensive care [27]. As many of the actions of thyroid hormones on metabolism are mediated through their actions on mitochondrial activity, the low T3 syndrome in sepsis may also have direct implications on cellular respiration. Furthermore, thyroid status also has effects on NO production. In hypothyroidism, hypothalamic expression of NOS is significantly reduced [28], whereas liver and skeletal muscle mitochondrial NOS activities are significantly increased, correlating inversely with both serum T3 levels and oxygen uptake [29]. Adrenal insufficiency is also well recognized in sepsis, and corticosteroid replacement is now broadly applied to critically ill populations. However, while short-term dosing of corticosteroids increased rat skeletal muscle mitochondrial mass and respiratory complex activity [30], chronic administration had the opposite effect [31]. This may be pertinent in view of the critical illness myopathy that has been linked with steroid use. Yet another example of a hormonal perturbation in sepsis is that of leptin. Plasma leptin levels are increased in eventual survivors of sepsis [32]. As prolonged starvation is associated with marked decreases in leptin levels, fasted mice will show increased lethality to endotoxin which can be partly reversed by exogenous leptin administration [33]. We have reproduced this finding in a long-term mouse model and found an associated improvement in mitochondrial function (unpublished data).

## The Role of Mitochondria in Sepsis-induced Cell Death

Although most organs affected in sepsis demonstrate minimal, if any, evidence of cell death, a notable exception is the immune pathway. In post-mortem studies of patients dying from MOF, Hotchkiss et al. found evidence of increased apoptosis in spleen, lymphocytes, and gut epithelium [2]. In subsequent studies of isolated lymphocytes, they reported evidence of activation of mitochondrial cell death pathways [34]. Inhibition of caspase activation was related to improved outcomes in a mouse model of sepsis [35]. On the other hand, a number of investigations have shown that neutrophil apoptosis is profoundly depressed in sepsis [36] and burns [37]. Decreased activation of mitochondria-related death pathways was noted, with maintenance of mitochondrial transmembrane potential. Reasons for these contrasting responses in different immune cells need to be better understood, particularly in respect to potential application of therapies, e. g., caspase inhibitors that may affect both cell types. Increased lymphocyte apoptosis is associated with a shift in Th1:Th2 ratios and enhanced immunosuppression, whereas resolution of neutrophil (PMN)-mediated inflammation occurs through apoptosis.

Other specific cell types also show increased apoptosis. In one septic rat model [38], increased apoptosis was detected in neurons within the hippocampus, choroid plexus, and cerebellar Purkinje cells. Both mitochondrial Bax (a member of the pro-apoptotic Bcl-2 family) and cytochrome c were upregulated in the early stages of sepsis (6–12 hrs), but decreased later on (48–60 hrs). Increased neuronal and glial apoptosis was also found within the autonomic centers of the brain in post-mortem studies of patients dying of septic shock, and this was strongly associated with endothelial iNOS expression [39].

## Changes in Mitochondrial Phenotype

Other than direct inhibition of mitochondrial respiratory enzymes, recent data suggest that changes in phenotype during sepsis will also decrease the amount of mitochondrial protein expressed. In two related papers using a rat endotoxin model studied after 48 hours [40, 41], Callahan and Supinski described a down-regulation of genes encoding components of both the electron transport chain and glycolysis, with corresponding decreases in enzyme activities, mitochondrial oxygen consumption, and ATP formation. Calvano and colleagues [42] assessed changes in leukocyte gene expression patterns over a 24 hour period in volunteers given a single dose of endotoxin, thus allowing precise timing of the initiating inflammatory insult. Of 44,000 probe sets, the signal intensity of 5,093 probe sets (representing 3,714 unique genes) was significantly affected. A minority of probe sets was induced by 2 hours; over half showed reduced abundance at 2–9 hours but returned to baseline by 24 hours, while the remainder showed a delayed response, peaking at 4–9 hours but returning to baseline by 24 hours. Of note, these authors reported a suppression of ge nes involved in e ne rgy production (e. g., compone nts of mitochondrial respiratory chain complexes I, III, and V) with a concurrent down-regulation of genes encoding for both protein synthesis and protein degradation.

## Mitochondrial Recovery

In the afore-mentioned studies in septic shock patients [16] and in long-term rat fecal peritonitis [17], a decrease in complex I activity was noted, however complex IV activity showed a tendency to rise. This may be misleading, as rapid reversibility of competitive NO inhibition of this enzyme in the room air environment in which the *in vitro* assay was prepared and performed may belie any *in vivo* inhibition present in an environment where the oxygen tension is more than 20-fold lower. On the other hand, it may possibly represent a true result and be due to an increase in activity of the enzyme per unit mass due, for instance, to a conformational change. More likely, however, is the possibility that total enzyme protein has increased. Although other recent studies have reported a decrease in complex IV protein [43] and mitochondrial content [44], these were performed in severe, high mortality rodent models. On the other hand, Suliman et al. found that bacterial lipopolysaccharide (LPS, endotoxin) injected into rats produced early DNA damage followed by stimulation of new mitochondrial protein ('biogenesis') [45]. NO has been recently shown to be a crucial component in the production of new mitochondria [46, 47]. This is consistent with the finding of Elfering et al. [48] that nitration induced a greatly accelerated turnover in new mitochondrial protein. Thus, prolonged and excessive NO production may result in an initial inhibition of mitochondrial activity followed, if the organism survives, by a stimulation of recovery of function. This dual role is consistent with the notion we have proposed that MOF may actually represent a protective, adaptive response to a prolonged and severe inflammatory insult [49]. The acute phase of sepsis is marked by an abrupt rise in secretion of stress hormones with an associated increase in mito-chondrial and metabolic activity. The combination of severe inflammation, with excess ROS formation, and secondary changes in the endocrine profile and an alteration in phenotype, will then diminish energy production, metabolic rate, and normal cellular processes, leading to multiple organ dysfunction. However, reduced cellular metabolism could increase the chances of survival of cells, and thus organs, in the face of this overwhelming insult. This is analogous to hiberna-tion, estivation, and other environmental stressors. Levy and colleagues [50] have recently demonstrated biochemical, functional, and bioenergetic changes in septic hearts that reflect the hibernatory response to a cold environment.

## Mitochondrial Protection

If mitochondrial dysfunction and/or damage is central to the pathogenesis of MOF, strategies to protect the mitochondria may prevent the progression, or at least ameliorate, the development of organ failure.

An important advance in the clinical management of patients either with, or at high risk of developing sepsis, is the concept of intensive insulin therapy. The package of tight glycemic control (4.5–6.1 mmol/l) allied to additional insulin and glucose resulted in an impressive reduction in both mortality and morbidity [51]. A variety of putative mechanisms of action for the beneficial effects of intensive insulin therapy have been suggested. In an important follow-up paper examining liver and muscle biopsies taken soon after death [52], minimal cell death was seen in both intensive insulin therapy and conventionally-treated groups. However, inten-sive insulin therapy resulted in almost complete protection against the significant ultrastructural damage to liver mitochondria and the corresponding decrease in respiratory enzyme activity frequently seen in the control group. This suggests that better glycemic control, leading to reduced glycation of mitochondrial pro-tein, and/or additional insulin and glucose, enhancing glycolysis and having direct effects on mitochondrial function, represent potential protective mechanisms.

There are a number of other possible protective approaches to maintain mi-tochondrial function. As much of the injury to the organelle is considered to be mediated by reactive species, levels of intra-mitochondrial antioxidants, such as glutathione [53] or manganese superoxide dismutase [54], could be supplemented at an early stage. Melatonin is also an efficient scavenger of reactive oxygen and nitrogen species and will increase the mitochondrial glutathione pool. After sep-sis, administration of melatonin reduced expression and activity of the inducible isoform of NOS (iNOS) and improved mitochondrial function [55]. There may be a role for specific inhibitors of iNOS which have been shown to ameliorate cardiac depression and improve mitochondrial activity and structure in an endotoxic rat model [56].

Induction of heat shock protein (HSP) may also prove beneficial. A short period of hyperthermia 24 hours before a septic insult was protective for both heart [26] and liver [57] mitochondrial function. The precise mechanism(s) of action remains to be determined as the heat shock response offers broad cytoprotective properties with effects on apoptosis, NO production, and heme oxygenase induction. Among the various HSPs, HSP32 (heme oxygenase 1) has received considerable attention as its induction generates significant amounts of carbon monoxide and the potent antioxidant bilirubin which have been shown to have protective effects in a variety of shock models. Recently, hemin, a pharmacological inducer of heme oxygenase, was shown, in an endotoxic rat model, to increase tissue heme oxygenase levels, prevent alterations in mitochondrial function, and attenuate increases in plasma nitrite/nitrate levels and tissue markers of free radical generation [58].

PARP-1 is a DNA repair enzyme that is activated when nuclear damage occurs. It consumes NAD and may potentially deplete this vital electron carrier, and thus ATP production, within the mitochondria. PARP inhibitors were developed with the aim of preventing this energy depletion but, more recently, they have also been recognized to have potent anti-inflammatory properties. For example, in an oxidative stress model, PARP inhibition provided mitochondrial protection through inducing phosphorylation and activation of Akt [59]. In various septic models, PARP inhibition prevented mitochondrial dysfunction and improved outcomes [24,60].

In the situation of established sepsis, such protective strategies may prove less effective. Consideration should be given to approaches that provide substrate able to bypass the site of mitochondrial inhibition (e.g., succinate [61]) or stimulate recovery pathways such as accelerating mitochondrial biogenesis, e.g., through activation of the transcriptional coactivator, peroxisome proliferator-activated receptor gamma coactivator-1γ (PGC-1γ) [62]

## Conclusion

Prolonged sepsis will induce mitochondrial dysfunction and damage. As a consequence of decreased energy availability, metabolism must decrease or the cell will soon die. As cell death is not a major feature, it is thus feasible that the cells enter a hibernation-like state as a late protective response and this biochemical/physiological shutdown is manifest as multiple organ dysfunction/failure. Recovery would then be contingent upon restoration of mitochondrial function, either through repair of existing damaged mitochondria or production of new organelles. Excess production of NO and other reactive species appears likely to be the main 'culprit' of the initial injury and altered bioenergetics, yet, paradoxically, may provide the stimulus for eventual recovery of function. Therapeutic strategies could thus be geared towards mitochondrial protection or accelerating recovery.

# References

1. Martin GS, Mannino DM, Eaton S, Moss M (2003) The epidemiology of sepsis in the United States from 1979 through 2000. N Engl J Med 348:1546–1554
2. Hotchkiss RS, Swanson PE, Freeman BD, et al (1999) Apoptotic cell death in patients with sepsis, shock, and multiple organ dysfunction. Crit Care Med 27:1230–1251
3. Noble JS, MacKirdy FN, Donaldson SI, Howie JC (2001) Renal and respiratory failure in Scottish ICUs. Anaesthesia 56:124–129
4. VanderMeer TJ, Wang H, Fink MP (1995) Endotoxemia causes ileal mucosal acidosis in the absence of mucosal hypoxia in a normodynamic porcine model of septic shock. Crit Care Med 23:1217–1226
5. Rosser DM, Stidwill RP, Jacobson D, Singer M (1995) Oxygen tension in the bladder epithelium rises in both high and low cardiac output endotoxemic sepsis. J Appl Physiol 79: 1878–1882
6. Boekstegers P, Weidenhofer S, Pilz G, Werdan K (1991) Peripheral oxygen availability within skeletal muscle in sepsis and septic shock: comparison to limited infection and cardiogenic shock. Infection 19: 317–323
7. Rich P (2003) Chemiosmotic coupling: The cost of living. Nature 421:583
8. Singer M, Brealey D (1999) Mitochondrial dysfunction in sepsis. In: Brown GC, Nicholls DG, Cooper CE (eds) Mitochondria and Cell Death. Biochem Soc Symp No. 66. Portland Press, London, pp 149–166
9. Rosser DM, Manji M, Cooksley H, Bellingan G (1998) Endotoxin reduces maximal oxygen consumption in hepatocytes independent of any hypoxic insult. Intensive Care Med 24: 725–729
10. Kreymann G, Grosser S, Buggisch P, Gottschall C, Matthaei S, Greten H (1993) Oxygen consumption and resting metabolic rate in sepsis, sepsis syndrome, and septic shock. Crit Care Med 21:1012–1019
11. Bergstrom J, Bostrom H, Furst P, Hultman E, Vinnars E (1976) Preliminary studies of energy-rich phosphagens in muscle from severely ill patients. Crit Care Med 4:197–204
12. Poderoso JJ, Boveris A Jorge MA (1978) Function mitocondrial en el shock septico. Medicina 38:371–377
13. Liaw KY, Askanazi J, Michelson CB, Kantrowitz LR, Furst P, Kinney JM (1980) Effect of injury and sepsis on high-energy phosphates in muscle and red cells. J Trauma 20:755–759
14. Gasparetto A, Corbucci GG, Candiani A, Gohil K, Edwards RH (1983) Effect of tissue hypoxia and septic shock on human skeletal muscle mitochondria. Lancet ii:1486
15. Corbucci GG, Gasparetto A, Candiani A, et al (1985) Shock-induced damage to mitochondrial function and some cellular antioxidant mechanisms in humans. Circ Shock 15:15–26
16. Tresadern JC, Threlfall CJ, Wilford K, Irving MH (1988) Muscle adenosine 5'-triphosphate and creatine phosphate concentrations in relation to nutritional status and sepsis in man. Clin Sci 75:233–242
17. Brealey D, Brand M, Hargreaves I, et al (2002) Association between mitochondrial dysfunction and severity and outcome of septic shock. Lancet 360:219–223
18. Brealey D, Karyampudi S, Jacques TS, et al (2004) Mitochondrial dysfunction in a long-term rodent model of sepsis and organ failure. Am J Physiol Regul Integr Comp Physiol 286:R491–497
19. Heales SJ, Bolanos JP, Stewart VC, Brookes PS, Land JM, Clark JB (1999) Nitric oxide, mitochondria and neurological disease. Biochim Biophys Acta 1410:215–228
20. Beltran B, Mathur A, Duchen MR, Erusalimsky JD, Moncada S (2000) The effect of nitric oxide on cell respiration: A key to understanding its role in cell survival or death. Proc Natl Acad Sci USA 97:14602–14607
21. Borutaite V, Budriunaite A, Brown GC (2000) Reversal of nitric oxide-, peroxynitrite- and S-nitrosothiol-induced inhibition of mitochondrial respiration or complex I activity by light and thiols. Biochem Biophys Acta 1459:405–412

22. Frost MT, Wang Q, Moncada S, Singer M (2005) Hypoxia accelerates nitric oxide-dependent inhibition of mitochondrial complex I in activated macrophages. Am J Physiol Regul Integr Comp Physiol 288:R394–400
23. Borutaite V, Moncada S, Brown GC (2005) Nitric oxide from inducible nitric oxide synthase sensitizes the inflamed aorta to hypoxic damage via respiratory inhibition. Shock 23:319–323
24. Boulos M, Astiz ME, Barua RS, Osman M (2003) Impaired mitochondrial function induced by serum from septic shock patients is attenuated by inhibition of nitric oxide synthase and poly(ADP-ribose) synthase. Crit Care Med 31:353–358
25. Lanone S, Mebazaa A, Heymes C, et al (2000) Muscular contractile failure in septic patients: role of the inducible nitric oxide synthase pathway. Am J Respir Crit Care Med 162:2308–2315
26. Chen HW, Hsu C, Lu TS, Wang SJ, Yang RC (2003) Heat shock pretreatment prevents cardiac mitochondrial dysfunction during sepsis. Shock 20:274–279
27. Kaptein EM, Weiner JM, Robinson WJ, et al (1982) Relationship of altered thyroid hormone indices to survival in nonthyroidal illnesses. Clin Endocrinol 16:565–574
28. Ueta Y, Levy A, Chowdrey HS, Lightman SL (1995) Hypothalamic nitric oxide synthase gene expression is regulated by thyroid hormones. Endocrinology 136:4182–4187
29. Carreras MC, Peralta JG, Converso DP, et al (2001) Modulation of liver mitochondrial NOS is implicated in thyroid-dependent regulation of O2 uptake. Am J Physiol Heart Circ Physiol 281:H2282–2288
30. Weber K, Bruck P, Mikes Z, Kupper JH, Klingenspor M, Wiesner RJ (2002) Glucocorticoid hormone stimulate mitochondrial biogenesis specifically in skeletal muscle. Endocrinology 143:177–184
31. Mitsui T, Azuma H, Nagasawa M, et al (2002) Chronic corticosteroid administration causes mitochondrial dysfunction in skeletal muscle. J Neurol 249:1004–1009
32. Bornstein SR, Licinio J, Tauchnitz R, et al (1998) Plasma leptin levels are increased in survivors of acute sepsis: associated loss of diurnal rhythm, in cortisol and leptin secretion. J Clin Endocrinol Metab 83:280–283
33. Faggioni R, Moser A, Feingold KR, Grunfeld C (2000) Reduced leptin levels in starvation increase susceptibility to endotoxic shock. Am J Pathol 156:1781–1787
34. Hotchkiss RS, Osmon SB, Chang KC, Wagner TH, Coopersmith CM, Karl IE (2005) Accelerated lymphocyte death in sepsis occurs by both the death receptor and mitochondrial pathways. J Immunol 174:5110–5118
35. Hotchkiss RS, Chang KC, Swanson PE, et al (2000) Caspase inhibitors improve survival in sepsis: a critical role of the lymphocyte. Nat Immunol 1:496–501
36. Taneja R, Parodo J, Jia SH, Kapus A, Rotstein OD, Marshall JC (2004) Delayed neutrophil apoptosis in sepsis is associated with maintenance of mitochondrial transmembrane potential and reduced caspase-9 activity. Crit Care Med 32:1460–1469
37. Hu Z, Sayeed MM (2004) Suppression of mitochondria-dependent neutrophil apoptosis with thermal injury. Am J Physiol Cell Physiol 286: C170–178
38. Messaris E, Memos N, Chatzigianni E, et al (2004) Time-dependent mitochondrial-mediated programmed neuronal cell death prolongs survival in sepsis. Crit Care Med 32:1764–1770
39. Sharshar T, Gray F, Lorin de la Grandmaison G, et al (2003) Apoptosis of neurons in cardiovascular autonomic centres triggered by inducible nitric oxide synthase after death from septic shock. Lancet 362:1799–1805
40. Callahan LA, Supinski GS (2005) Downregulation of diaphragm electron transport chain and glycolytic enzyme gene expression in sepsis. J Appl Physiol 99:1120–1126
41. Callahan LA, Supinski GS (2005) Sepsis induces diaphragm electron transport chain dysfunction and protein depletion. Am J Respir Crit Care Med 172:861–868
42. Calvano SE, Xiao W, Richards DR, et al (2005) A network-based analysis of systemic inflammation in humans. Nature 437:1032–1037
43. Levy RJ, Vijayasarathy C, Raj NR, Avadhani NG, Deutschman CS (2004) Competitive and noncompetitive inhibition of myocardial cytochrome C oxidase in sepsis. Shock 21:110–114

44. Watts JA, Kline JA, Thornton LR, Grattan RM, Brar SS (2004) Metabolic dysfunction and depletion of mitochondria in hearts of septic rats. J Mol Cell Cardiol 36:141–150
45. Suliman HB, Welty-Wolf KE, Carraway M, Tatro L, Piantadosi CA (2004) Lipopolysaccharide induces oxidative cardiac mitochondrial damage and biogenesis. Cardiovasc Res 64:279–288
46. Nisoli E, Clementi E, Paolucci C, et al (2003) Mitochondrial biogenesis in mammals: the role of endogenous nitric oxide. Science 299:896–899
47. Nisoli E, Falcone S, Tonello C, et al (2004) Mitochondrial biogenesis by NO yields functionally active mitochondria in mammals. Proc Natl Acad Sci USA 101:16507–16512
48. Elfering SL, Haynes VL, Traaseth NJ, Ettl A, Giulivi C (2004) Aspects, mechanism, and biological relevance of mitochondrial protein nitration sustained by mitochondrial nitric oxide synthase. Am J Physiol Heart Circ Physiol 286:H22–29
49. Singer M, De Santis V, Vitale D, Jeffcoate W (2004) Multiorgan failure is an adaptive, endocrine-mediated, metabolic response to overwhelming systemic inflammation. Lancet 364:545–548
50. Levy RJ, Piel DA, Acton PD, et al (2005) Evidence of myocardial hibernation in the septic heart. Crit Care Med 33:2752–2756
51. van den Berghe G, Wouters P, Weekers F, et al (2001) Intensive insulin therapy in the critically ill patients. N Engl J Med 345:1359–1367
52. Vanhorebeek I, De Vos R, Mesotten D, Wouters PJ, De Wolf-Peeters C, Van den Berghe G (2005) Protection of hepatocyte mitochondrial ultrastructure and function by strict blood glucose control with insulin in critically ill patients. Lancet 365:53–59
53. Clementi E, Brown GC, Feelisch M, Moncada S (1998) Persistent inhibition of cell respiration by nitric oxide: crucial role of S-nitrosylation of mitochondrial complex I and protective action of glutathione. Proc Natl Acad Sci USA 95:7631–7636
54. Salvemini D, Riley DP, Cuzzocrea S (2002) SOD mimetics are coming of age. Nat Rev Drug Discov 1:367–374
55. Lopez LC, Escames G, Tapias V, Utrilla P, Leon J, Acuna-Castroviejo D (2006) Identification of an inducible nitric oxide synthase in diaphragm mitochondria from septic mice. Its relation with mitochondrial dysfunction and prevention by melatonin. Int J Biochem Cell Biol 38:267–278
56. Tatsumi T, Akashi K, Keira N, et al (2004) Cytokine-induced nitric oxide inhibits mitochondrial energy production and induces myocardial dysfunction in endotoxin-treated rat hearts. J Mol Cell Cardiol 37:775–784
57. Chen HW, Kuo HT, Lu TS, Wang SJ, Yang RC (2004) Cytochrome c oxidase as the target of the heat shock protective effect in septic liver. Int J Exp Pathol 85:249–256
58. Supinski GS, Callahan LA (2006) Hemin prevents cardiac and diaphragm mitochondrial dysfunction in sepsis. Free Radic Biol Med 40:127–137
59. Tapodi A, Debreceni B, Hanto K, et al (2005) Pivotal role of Akt activation in mitochondrial protection and cell survival by poly(ADP-ribose)polymerase-1 inhibition in oxidative stress. J Biol Chem 280:35767–35775
60. Szabo C, Zingarelli B, Salzman AL (1996) Role of poly-ADP ribosyltransferase activation in the vascular contractile and energetic failure elicited by exogenous and endogenous nitric oxide and peroxynitrite. Circ Res 78:1051–1063
61. Ferreira FL, Ladriere L, Vincent JL, Malaisse WJ (2000) Prolongation of survival time by infusion of succinic acid dimethyl ester in a caecal ligation and perforation model of sepsis. Horm Metab Res 32:335–336
62. Irrcher I, Adhihetty PJ, Sheehan T, Joseph AM, Hood DA (2003) PPARgamma coactivator-1alpha expression during thyroid hormone- and contractile activity-induced mitochondrial adaptations. Am J Physiol Cell Physiol 284:C1669–1677

# Metabolic Pathways

O. Rooyackers and J. Wernerman

## Introduction

With a better understanding of sepsis induced organ dysfunctions, metabolic oriented treatments as well as the metabolic effects of currently available treatments are coming into focus. Good examples of this are tight glucose control with feeding and insulin treatment, as well as intravenous glutamine supplementation [1, 2]. Understanding of metabolic pathways is therefore crucial in optimizing treatment in sepsis. In all phases of sepsis this is obvious – resuscitation, low flow phases as well as high flow phases, multiple organ failure (MOF), and during recovery. However, timing and relation to nutrition are important, and, therefore, insights into metabolic derangements in relation to nutrition may help to improve outcomes. Energy metabolism in sepsis is mainly characterized by an increase in insulin resistance. In addition, lipid oxidation is increased, and in protein metabolism it is the increase in net protein degradation that dominates. This overview will focus on protein metabolism, glutamine metabolism, glutathione metabolism, and finally mitochondrial metabolism.

## Protein Metabolism

In sepsis, a large proportion of the whole body energy expenditure is used on protein metabolism [3, 4]. This is particularly true in patients with MOF when several organ functions are more or less managed by external medical support, such as ventilators, dialysis machines and blood transfusions. Nevertheless, whole body expenditure is often elevated above the expected level of basal energy expenditure. Also, when techniques are used to estimate the whole body turnover of a labeled amino acid (usually leucine or phenylalanine) in order to estimate whole body protein turnover, values above what are found in healthy individuals are seen. In the basal state, humans are able to adapt to under-nutrition or starvation by decreasing energy expenditure, which mainly reflects a decrease in protein metabolism. This is, unfortunately, not an option for the septic patient. If the septic patient is undernourished, no such adaptation is seen. Therefore an under-nourished patient is rapidly energy depleted and the incidence and seriousness of complications that ensue are related to this energy deficit [5–7].

So far there is no direct evidence that failure of protein metabolism is related to such under-nutrition. It is more likely that prioritized protein synthesis is maintained at the expense of endogenous protein mainly in skeletal muscle, which continues as long as there are any endogenous reserves. On the other hand, there is some evidence that over-nutrition is harmful. Over-nutrition is a situation where calories are given in excess of the actual energy expenditure, and/or when large quantities of proteins or amino acids are administered. Employing enteral feeding usually eliminates the danger of over-feeding; however the concept of enteral feeding does not eliminate the risk of *under*-feeding. These aspects are related to the general success rate of enteral feeding, which is typically around 60% of the prescribed amount.

Protein depletion is a strong predictor of outcome in sepsis. Attenuation of ongoing protein depletion in septic states is, therefore, a cornerstone in treatment. In general terms, during sepsis this protein depletion is the result of increased protein synthesis in combination with an even greater increased protein degradation at the whole body level [8]. This is perhaps not the case during the initial low flow phase, a period not very well characterized in clinical studies. However, later on during the high flow phase and MOF this mechanism is definitely true. It is also well known that these changes in protein metabolism are not equally distributed between organs and tissues, and that in individual organs or tissues the *de novo* synthesis and degradation of individual proteins is altered in a non-uniform way [9]. The complexity of these changes has encouraged modern techniques to be used in this field. Genomics and proteomics provide information regarding genetic regulation of protein metabolism as well as the presence or absence of individual proteins. This information gives insight into how these processes are regulated at a tissue level as well as a cellular level. However, these measures should ideally be combined with quantification of the related metabolic pathways. Quantitative estimates are possible at the whole body level, at the tissue level and at the level of individual proteins.

It is generally recognized that liver protein synthesis is enhanced in septic patients. This enhancement is usually attributed to the so-called 'acute phase' reaction, involving proteins that appear in increased concentrations in the serum, which are synthesized in increased amounts, and which have functions in the acute inflammatory reaction. In contrast, the plasma concentration of albumin decreases. This decrease is, however, not a reflection of low albumin synthesis (Fig. 1). On the contrary, albumin synthesis is elevated and there are even indices that albumin synthesis is increased to a maximum in these situations [10,11]. The low plasma concentration of albumin is rather related to capillary leakage and to the degradation of albumin. The latter is a process not very well characterized and its assessment carries considerable methodological problems. In addition, increased protein synthesis rates are seen in circulating immune cells in septic patients (Fig. 1) [12, 13]. This is no surprise, as these cells are supposed to be activated, to produce export proteins and to undergo cell division.

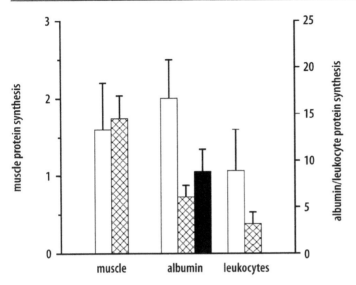

**Fig. 1.** Fractional synthesis rate (%/24 hours) in skeletal muscle proteins [16,51], albumin [11,52, 53], and proteins of circulating leukocytes [13,54] in sepsis (open bars), healthy controls (hatched bars), and during cholecystitis (filled bars). In muscle there is no change, while in albumin and leukocyte proteins a considerable increase is seen. For albumin the increase is much larger in sepsis than that seen in an acute inflammatory state such as cholecystitis. Values are given as means ± SD

Muscle tissue undergoes considerable wasting in septic patients. This is related to physical inactivity, but also to metabolism, which places muscle as a provider and net exporter of free amino acids. This is particularly true for alanine and glutamine, which will be elaborated on below. The amino acids are produced from a net degradation of muscle proteins. Muscle tissue decreases rapidly in the septic patient related to this export of amino acids, even in the fully fed state [14]. This is quite different from the situation in healthy individuals, who have a net uptake of amino acids in the fed state. In septic patients, protein synthesis is unaltered and degradation of muscle is increased [12,15–20]. The unaltered rate of muscle protein synthesis is a bit unexpected, as the protein synthesis rate in muscle decreases following elective surgery trauma [21]. However, it seems that with increasing size of trauma, protein synthesis in muscle moves from being decreased to being unaltered [22]. In septic patients, however, it remains unaltered (Fig. 1), and in some individuals it is actually markedly increased [23]. Protein degradation, on the other hand is generally increased. Due to methodological difficulties, quantification of this increase in degradation is still problematic, but qualitative assays clearly indicate that proteasome activity is increased, that the synthesis of proteasome subunits increased, and that the *de novo* synthesis and gene expression of ubiquitin is increased [15,17–20]. The few quantitative estimates on muscle protein degradation in septic patients further confirm this pattern [24]. Techniques used to investigate protein degradation quantitatively, involve the incorporation and/or balance of labeled amino acids across tissues. This opens the possibility of evaluating the natural course of seps is as well as the effects of treatments in the septic patient. The initial phase of sepsis may be studied in man by the use of an endotoxic challenge in healthy volunteers. During the initial 4 hours following endotoxemia, protein metabolism mainly displays a low flow phase with decreases rather than increases in muscle protein synthesis and protein degradation [25]. This is a pattern that does not correspond to what is seen later on during MOF.

## Glutamine Metabolism

Among the amino acids, glutamine has a special role. It is a non-essential amino acid, but there are indices that endogenous production is insufficient during critical illness and also that exogenous intravenous supplementation has beneficial effects on outcome. In general terms, glutamine has a central role in amino acid metabolism and in the interface between amino acids and carbohydrate metabolism. It is a main transporter of carbon skeletons as well as amino groups between skeletal muscle and the 'central' organs in the splanchnic area. The carbon skeleton of glutamine, $\alpha$-ketoglutarate, is also a constituent of Kreb's cycle and consequently is involved in energy production. In addition, glutamine is the precursor for nucleotide synthesis, and the availability of glutamine is crucial when cell division is prioritized. Cells that are rapidly dividing commonly utilize glutamine as an energy substrate, such as cells in the intestinal mucosa and immune cells. The slight disadvantage in terms of moles ATP per mole substrate in comparison with glucose is easily counterbalanced by the opportunity of having a substrate flow which can be turned easily into nucleotide synthesis when necessary. It is well documented that in various stressed states, cells are more likely to use glutamine as an energy substrate. In the basal state, endogenous glutamine production is 50–70 grams per 24 hours, mainly taking place in muscle tissue [26,27]. Glutamine is constantly exported from muscle and taken up in the splanchnic area, preferably as an energy substrate where the amino groups are transaminated to other amino acids or turned into urea in the liver. In sepsis, this turnover of glutamine is not changed [28–30]. However, it does not increase either, although the demand for glutamine may be elevated. This is the situation where availability of glutamine may be a limiting factor.

In the early phase of sepsis, as reproduced by an endotoxin challenge in healthy volunteers, glutamine plasma concentration decreases, free glutamine concentration in muscle decreases, and the export of glutamine from muscle increases [31]. Later on during MOF, the export of glutamine from muscle is relatively constant, while the concentrations of glutamine in plasma and in muscle tissue stay low [30,32]. The uptake of glutamine across the splanchnic area is related to plasma concentration. Plasma glutamine concentration on admission to the ICU is a prognostic factor [33]; a low value indicates a much worse prognosis. This factor is unrelated to the prognostic elements summarized in the APACHE II score. Intravenous glutamine supplementation can normalize plasma glutamine level in all patients [16]. An exogenous supply of amino acids does not increase the endogenous production of glutamine [29,34]. On the other hand, an exogenous supply of intravenous glutamine does not suppress *de novo* production but makes more glutamine available [28]. For muscle tissue, a short term exogenous glutamine supply does not restore the intracellular glutamine depletion and the efflux of glutamine from muscle is also unaltered [16,29,35]. Exogenous glutamine supplementation, therefore, does not *per se* save muscle protein, but makes more glutamine available for other organs. On a long term perspective, glutamine may also be beneficial in terms of saving muscle protein, but this remains to be demonstrated in septic patients. The clinical evidence for a beneficial effect of glutamine on mortality is so far limited to studies of intravenous supplementation of glutamine to patients with MOF [36,37]. The effects of enteral supplementation during earlier phases of sepsis are less well documented, but there are several reports of beneficial effects on morbidity [1]. There are also animal studies showing beneficial effects of glutamine supplementation during resuscitation [38]. Furthermore, the expression and production of heat shock proteins are enhanced in response to exogenous glutamine supplementation [38,39]. The clinical relevance of these findings is still not settled, however.

To evaluate the need for glutamine supplementation, as well as the optimal dose and the best route of administration, it is necessary to be able to measure endogenous glutamine production. This is best done as a measurement of the rate of appearance of glutamine. The conventional technique is to give a primed constant infusion of isotopically labeled glutamine and estimate the rate of appearance at steady state [27,34]. An alternative approach is to use the decay curve, which can also be obtained after a single injection of glutamine [26,29,40]. This latter approach avoids the problem related to the large distribution volume of glutamine, and also makes it possible to do estimates when a steady state is not possible. This technique has enabled us to estimate the rate of appearance of glutamine, and will also make it possible to evaluate glutamine supplementation by the entral route.

## Glutathione Metabolism

Glutathione is a tri-peptide (glutamyl–cysteinyl–glycine) that is synthesized in all cells. As a thiol it appears in a reduced and an oxidized form. The oxidized form is a dimer, with the residues are connected via sulfhydryl bonds. Glutathione has many functions, but the most important is attributed to its ability to remove reactive oxygen species (ROS) as an antioxidant. In this capacity, glutathione is quantitatively the most important antioxidant in man. In plasma, the glutathione concentration is very low, but intracellularly it appears in mmole concentrations in all tissues. The reduced form of glutathione is the dominant form representing > 80% of the glutathione in most tissues.

In sepsis, glutathione depletion is seen in erythrocytes as well as in muscle tissue (Fig. 2) [41–43]. In addition to a low concentration, the redox status of glutathione is altered into a more oxidized state. In erythrocytes, these changes are constant over time during MOF [42]. In acute sepsis, as represented by an endotoxin challenge to healthy volunteers, there is no immediate change in glutathione concentration or glutathione redox status in the erythrocytes. In muscle, glutathione is also left unaffected by an endotoxin challenge in the acute phase, but on admission to the ICU, septic patients show reduced glutathione concentrations and an altered redox status with a more oxidized state. The extent of this depletion is associated with short-term mortality [44]. Those surviving the acute phase of sepsis and developing MOF, show a gradual normalization of glutathione concentration in muscle over subsequent weeks (Fig. 2) [43]. The more oxidized state of glutathione, however, remains throughout the ICU stay. These are descriptive findings, which cannot be explained by a shortage of the constituent amino acids, in particular not by a shortage of cysteine [43, 45]. If anything, glutathione depletion is statistically correlated to simultaneous glutamate depletion. On the other hand, although glutamate concentrations are low, it is still quite abundant. Following elective surgery, a similar decrease in glutathione is seen on the first and third post-operative days [46]. This finding applies to the reduced form of glutathione only, with the redox status being unaffected. In addition, the decrease in glutathione concentration is statistically related to a decrease in free glutamate. Supplementation with intravenous glutamine counteracts the glutathione deple-

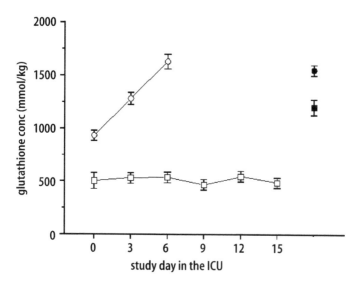

**Fig. 2.** Reduced glutathione concentrations in muscle (circles) [43] and in whole blood (squares) [42] over time in septic patients during their ICU stay (open symbols). Values are compared to those of controls (closed symbols). Initially, a decrease is seen in muscle as well as in erythrocytes. During the late course of sepsis a normalization is seen in muscle but not in erythrocytes. Values are given as means ± SD

tion to some degree following surgical trauma [47]. When patients with MOF in the ICU are given extra glutamine, the low glutathione concentration seen in muscle is not restored in response to this supplementation [16].

In addition to the obvious anti-oxidative effects of glutathione, a role in the overall regulation of protein metabolism has been suggested. In particular there is evidence from animal studies concerning the level of protein degradation [48]. However, the exact function of glutathione in this setting remains to be established.

## Mitochondrial Metabolism

Mitochondrial metabolism is mainly energy production, although active protein synthesis also occurs in the mitochondrion. The majority of proteins in the mitochondrion, however, are synthesized within the cellular cytoplasm encoded for by the cellular genome and not by mitochondrial DNA. These proteins are actively transported into the mitochondrion, and they are, for example, necessary for protein degradation in the mitochondrion. In sepsis, reduced mitochondrial function is described in the acute phase as well as during MOF [44, 49]. In the acute phase, it is potentially difficult to distinguish between a shortage of oxygen at the tissue level or at the mitochondrial level and functional impairment of the mitochondrion. In man, these pathways have been most extensively studied in skeletal muscle. In the acute phase, failure in energy production has been attributed to reduced function of complexes I and IV within the respiratory chain [44]. The reduced function is usually expressed as *in vitro* activity of complexes I and IV related to citrate synthase activity as an index of mitochondrial mass. If this functional depression is not reversed, energy collapse ensues and mortality is very high. Septic patients who develop MOF have reduced mitochondrial content in terms of a low citrate synthase activity related to DNA or protein content [49]. This decrease progresses with time [50]. In this situation, in the phase of MOF, the activity of the mitochondrial complexes I and IV as related to citrate synthase activity is not different from that in healthy controls. This is true for thigh muscle as well as for intercostal muscle. It can be hypothesized that this reduction in mitochondrial metabolism and the consequent decrease in energy-rich phosphates during MOF is related to muscle fatigue [49]. Hence, the underlying mechanism of reduced mitochondrial function in terms of energy production seems to be different in the acute phase of sepsis and in the later phase involving MOF.

## Conclusion

The understanding of sepsis-induced organ dysfunction has advanced considerably over the last few years. The interaction between signaling systems and metabolic pathways is a particularly 'hot' area of ongoing research. Energy production and the availability of substrates in the acute phase seem to have a crucial impact on the course of sepsis and on mortality and morbidity. Later on, during MOF, the same metabolic pathways determine outcome, but the mechanisms and clinical picture are different. Knowledge of these mechanisms is, therefore, necessary for optimal clinical practice.

## References

1. Novak F, Heyland DK, Avenell A, Drover JW, Su X (2002) Glutamine supplementation in serious illness: a systematic review of the evidence. Crit Care Med 30:2022–2029
2. Van den Berghe G, Wouters P, Weekers F, et al (2001) Intensive insulin therapy in the critically ill patients. N Engl J Med 345:1359–1367
3. Garlick PJ (1986) Protein synthesis and energy expenditure in relation to feeding. Int J Vitam Nutr Res 56:197–200
4. McClave SA, Snider HL (2001) Dissecting the energy needs of the body. Curr Opin Clin Nutr Metab Care 4:143–147
5. Dvir D, Cohen J, Singer P (2006) Computerized energy balance and complications in critically ill patients: An observational study. Clin Nutr 25:37–44
6. Reid CL, Campbell IT, Little RA (2004) Muscle wasting and energy balance in critical illness. Clin Nutr 23:273–280
7. Villet S, Chiolero RL, Bollmann MD, et al (2005) Negative impact of hypocaloric feeding and energy balance on clinical outcome in ICU patients. Clin Nutr 24:502–509
8. Arnold J, Campbell IT, Samuels TA, et al (1993) Increased whole body protein breakdown predominates over increased whole body protein synthesis in multiple organ failure. Clin Sci (Lond) 84:655–661
9. Garlick PJ, McNurlan MA (1998) Measurement of protein synthesis in human tissues by the flooding method. Curr Opin Clin Nutr Metab Care 1:455–460
10. Barle H, Januszkiewicz A, Hallstrom L, et al (2002) Albumin synthesis in humans increases immediately following the administration of endotoxin. Clin Sci (Lond) 103:525–531
11. Barle H, Gamrin L, Essen P, McNurlan MA, Garlick PJ, Wernerman J (2001) Growth hormone does not affect albumin synthesis in the critically ill. Intensive Care Med 27:836–843
12. Essen P, McNurlan MA, Gamrin L, et al (1998) Tissue protein synthesis rates in critically ill patients. Crit Care Med 26:92–100
13. Januszkiewicz J, Klaude M, Loré K, et al (2005) In vivo protein synthesis in immune cells of ICU patients. Clin Nutr 24:575 (abst)
14. Wernerman J, Vinnars E (1987) The effect of trauma and surgery on interorgan fluxes of amino acids in man. Clin Sci (Lond) 73:129–133
15. Klaude M, Hammarqvist F, Wemerman J (2005) An assay of microsomal membrane-associated proteasomes demonstrates increased proteolytic activity in skeletal muscle of intensive care unit patients. Clin Nutr 24:259–265
16. Tjader I, Rooyackers O, Forsberg AM, Vesali RF, Garlick PJ, Wernerman J (2004) Effects on skeletal muscle of intravenous glutamine supplementation to ICU patients. Intensive Care Med 30:266–275
17. Biolo G, Bosutti A, Iscra F, Toigo G, Gullo A, Guarnieri G (2000) Contribution of the ubiquitin-proteasome pathway to overall muscle proteolysis in hypercatabolic patients. Metabolism 49:689–691
18. Tiao G, Hobler S, Wang JJ, et al (1997) Sepsis is associated with increased mRNAs of the ubiquitin-proteasome proteolytic pathway in human skeletal muscle. J Clin Invest 99:163–168
19. Mansoor O, Beaufrere B, Boirie Y, et al (1996) Increased mRNA levels for components of the lysosomal, Ca2+-activated, and ATP-ubiquitin-dependent proteolytic pathways in skeletal muscle from head trauma patients. Proc Natl Acad Sci USA 93:2714–2718

20. Klaude M, Fredriksson K, Hammarqvist F, Ljungqvist O, Wernerman J, Rooyackers O (2005) Proteasome proteolytic activity increases in leg and intercostal muscle during critical illness. Clin Nutr 24:572 (abst)
21. Biolo G, Fleming RY, Maggi SP, Nguyen TT, Herndon DN, Wolfe RR (2002) Inverse regulation of protein turnover and amino acid transport in skeletal muscle of hypercatabolic patients. J Clin Endocrinol Metab 87:3378–3384
22. Tjader I, Essen P, Garlick PJ, McMnurlan MA, Rooyackers O, Wernerman J (2004) Impact of surgical trauma on human skeletal muscle protein synthesis. Clin Sci (Lond) 107:601–607
23. Tjader I, Rooyackers O, Klaude M, Nennesmo I, Wernerman J (2005) Reproducibility of skeletal muscle protein synthesis rate in intensive care patients. Clin Nutr 24:611 (abst)
24. Biolo G, Williams BD, Fleming RY, Wolfe RR (1999) Insulin action on muscle protein kinetics and amino acid transport during recovery after resistance exercise. Diabetes 48:949–957
25. Vesali RF, Klaude M, Rooyackers O, Wernerman J (2005) Muscle protein turnover in muscle following an endotoxin challenge to healthy volunteers. Clin Nutr 24:608–609
26. Rooyackers O, Prohn M, Van Riel N, Wernerman J (2005) Bolus injection on 13C-glutamine to study glutamine metabolism in humans. Clin Nutr 24:575–576
27. Van Acker BA, Hulsewe KW, Wagenmakers AJ, et al (1998) Absence of glutamine isotopic steady state: implications for the assessment of whole-body glutamine production rate. Clin Sci (Lond) 95:339–346
28. Jackson NC, Carroll PV, Russell-Jones DL, Sonksen PH, Treacher DF, Umpleby AM (2000) Effects of glutamine supplementation, GH, and IGF–I on glutamine metabolism in critically ill patients. Am J Physiol Endocrinol Metab 278:E226–233
29. Berg A, Gamrin L, Martling CR, Rooyackers O, Wernerman J (2004) Effect of glutamine supplementation on muscle glutamine release in ICU patients during continous renal replacement therapy (CRRT). Clin Nutr 23:845 (abst)
30. Vesali RF, Klaude M, Rooyackers OE, Tjader I, Barle H, Wernerman J (2002). Longitudinal pattern of glutamine/glutamate balance across the leg in long-stay intensive care unit patients. Clin Nutr 21:505–514
31. Vesali RF, Klaude M, Rooyackers O, Wernerman J (2005) Amino acid metabolism in leg muscle after an endotoxin injection in healthy volunteers. Am J Physiol Endocrinol Metab 288:E360–364
32. Gamrin L, Andersson K, Hultman E, Nilsson E, Essen P, Wernerman J (1997) Longitudinal changes of biochemical parameters in muscle during critical illness. Metabolism 46:756–762
33. Oudemans-van Straaten HM, Bosman RJ, Treskes M, van der Spoel HJ, Zandstra DF (2001) Plasma glutamine depletion and patient outcome in acute ICU admissions. Intensive Care Med 27:84–90
34. van Acker BA, Hulsewe KW, Wagenmakers AJ, Soeters PB, von Meyenfeldt MF (2000) Glutamine appearance rate in plasma is not increased after gastrointestinal surgery in humans. J Nutr 130:566–1571
35. Rooyackers O, Prohn M, Van Riel N, Wernerman J (2005) Effect of parenteral alanyl-glutamine on glutamine production rate. Intensive Care Med 31:S33 (abst)
36. Goeters C, Wenn A, Mertes N, et al (2002) Parenteral L-alanyl-L-glutamine improves 6-month outcome in critically ill patients. Crit Care Med 30:2032–2037
37. Griffiths RD, Jones C, Palmer TE (1997) Six-month outcome of critically ill patients given glutamine-supplemented parenteral nutrition. Nutrition 13:295–302
38. Wischmeyer PE (2002) Glutamine and heat shock protein expression. Nutrition 18:225–228
39. Ziegler TR, Ogden LG, Singleton KD, et al (2005) Parenteral glutamine increases serum heat shock protein 70 in critically ill patients. Intensive Care Med 31:1079–1086
40. Berg A, Rooyackers O, Norberg A, Wernerman J (2005) Elimination kinetics of L-alanyl-L-glutamine in ICU patients. Amino Acids 29:221–228
41. Hammarqvist F, Luo JL, Cotgreave IA, Andersson K, Wernerman J (1997) Skeletal muscle glutathione is depleted in critically ill patients. Crit Care Med 25:78–84

42. Flaring UB, Rooyackers OE, Hebert C, Bratel T, Hammarqvist F, Wernerman J (2005) Temporal changes in whole-blood and plasma glutathione in ICU patients with multiple organ failure. Intensive Care Med 31:1072–1078
43. Flaring UB, Rooyackers OE, Wernerman J, Hammarqvist F (2003) Temporal changes in muscle glutathione in ICU patients. Intensive Care Med 29:2193–2198
44. Brealey D, Brand M, Hargreaves I, et al (2002) Association between mitochondrial dysfunction and severity and outcome of septic shock. Lancet 360:219–223
45. Rutten EP, Engelen MP, Schols AM, Deutz NE (2005) Skeletal muscle glutamate metabolism in health and disease: state of the art. Curr Opin Clin Nutr Metab Care 8:41–51
46. Luo JL, Hammarqvist F, Andersson K, Wernerman J (1998) Surgical trauma decreases glutathione synthetic capacity in human skeletal muscle tissue. Am J Physiol 275:E359–365
47. Flaring UB, Rooyackers OE, Wernerman J, Hammarqvist F (2003) Glutamine attenuates post-traumatic glutathione depletion in human muscle. Clin Sci (Lond) 104:275–282
48. Tischler ME, Fagan JM (1982) Relationship of the reduction-oxidation state to protein degradation in skeletal and atrial muscle. Arch Biochem Biophys 217:191–201
49. Fredriksson K, Hammarqvist F, Ljungqvist O, Wernerman J, Rooyackers O (2005) Derangements in energy metabolism in leg and intercostal muscle of critically ill patients. Clin Nutr 24:612 (abst)
50. Radell P, Ahlbeck K, Rooyackers O, Fredriksson K, Eriksson L (2005) Repeated measurement of neuromuscular function in ICU patients during prolonged mechanical ventilation. Anesthesiology 103:A1124 (abst)
51. McNurlan MA, Essen P, Heys SD, Buchan V, Garlick PJ, Wernerman J (1991) Measurement of protein synthesis in human skeletal muscle: further investigation of the flooding technique. Clin Sci (Lond) 81:557–564 (abst)
52. Barle H, Nyberg B, Essen P, et al (1997) The synthesis rates of total liver protein and plasma albumin determined simultaneously in vivo in humans. Hepatology 25:154–158
53. Barle H, Nyberg B, Ramel S, et al (1999) Inhibition of liver protein synthesis during laparoscopic surgery. Am J Physiol 277:E591–596
54. Januszkiewicz A, Klaude M, Lore K, et al (2005) Determination of in vivo protein synthesis in human palatine tonsil. Clin Sci (Lond) 108:179–184

# Cell Death and Acute Lung Injury

T.R. Martin, N. Hagimoto, and G. Matute-Bello

## Introduction

Life and death are inextricably intertwined and homeostasis in adult organisms depends on death and renewal of tissues throughout the body. In normal cells, death occurs by two different processes, necrosis and apoptosis. Necrosis is an unregulated form of cell death that results in cell lysis and the escape of intracellular constituents into the surrounding environment. In contrast, apoptosis is a regulated form of cell death mediated by a series of cysteine proteases called 'caspases', that ultimately results in DNA cleavage [1]. Necrotic cell death is both inflammatory and toxic to surrounding cells, depending on what is released from the dying cells. In contrast, apoptosis is characterized by cellular involution and ingestion of the apoptotic cell by nearby leukocytes or other cells [2]. Apoptosis and necrosis overlap to some extent, as apoptotic cells can undergo secondary necrosis, so the dividing line is not always clear. Additional mechanisms of cell death have been described in neoplastic cells [3].

Cell death has important consequences in the lungs, particularly in the gas exchange parenchyma. The alveolar membrane is a simple structure, consisting at the minimum of a flattened Type I alveolar epithelial cell covering an intermediate layer of connective tissue matrix, which in turn overlies a flattened capillary endothelial cell. The alveolar membrane spreads approximately 95% of the right ventricular output over a very large surface, permitting rapid oxygen uptake and carbon dioxide elimination. Injury to endothelial or epithelial cells poses a major problem, as airspaces flood with plasma, inactivating surfactant and causing alveolar collapse. The consequent ventilation-perfusion ($V_A/Q$) imbalance causes life-threatening hypoxemia. The way in which cellular injuries lead to the death of the epithelium and endothelium is not well understood, but accumulating evidence suggests that apoptosis and necrosis are both important.

## Epithelial Function in the Lungs

Epithelial and endothelial function are critical for normal lung function. The pulmonary epithelium consists of the mucociliary epithelium in the nasopharynx and tracheobronchial tree, and the specialized alveolar epithelium, which is the largest surface area in the body that is in contact with the outside environment.

A great deal of progress has been made in clarifying the physiological role of alveolar epithelial cells in homeostasis [4]. The Type I alveolar epithelial barrier differs from the endothelial barrier, because it is nearly impermeable to water and its permeability is not regulated. By contrast, the capillary endothelium is more permeable, and endothelial cells undergo rapid and reversible changes in cell shape in response to thrombin and other pro-inflammatory stimuli, permitting plasma to move through intracellular gap junctions into the interstitium of the lungs. If interstitial pressures are moderate and the Type I alveolar epithelium is intact, the extracellular fluid is cleared via lymphatic channels along bronchovascular bundles to the hila of the lungs. Interstitial and lymphatic fluid accumulation can alter ventilation/perfusion relationships, with concomitant hypoxemia, but these changes are reversible if endothelial permeability reverses and the interstitial fluid is cleared from the lungs.

When fluid accumulates in the airspaces, as in hydrostatic pulmonary edema, alveolar water is absorbed across the Type I cell epithelium through specialized water channel proteins, named aquaporins, aquaporin V being the primary aquaporin in the alveolar epithelium [5]. Paracellular water transport also occurs, and helps to explain why aquaporin V knockout mice do not have a prominent lung phenotype [6]. Type I epithelial cell injury leads to the destruction of this tight epithelial boundary layer, and interstitial fluid floods into alveolar spaces at low interstitial pressures. Type II pneumocytes secrete surfactant, which stabilizes alveolar units at low lung volumes, and also contain specialized ion transport channels, which reabsorb sodium and chloride through catecholamine sensitive apical and basolateral transporters [7]. Separate protein transport systems also exist in the alveolar epithelium, but protein reabsorption is much slower than water and electrolyte reabsorption. Because the intact alveolar epithelium reabsorbs fluid more rapidly than protein, the protein concentration in intra-alveolar fluid rises with time, when alveolar fluid clearance is normal. Clinical studies in intubated patients with lung injury have shown that patients whose alveolar protein concentration rises over the first 6 hours after the onset of clinical acute lung injury (ALI) have a significantly better prognosis than patients whose protein concentration does not change, supporting the idea that intact alveolar epithelial function is a prognostic marker in patients with ALI [8,9].

## Alveolar Membrane Damage in Acute Lung Injury

Ultrastructural studies by Bachofen and Weibel showed that patients who died following ALI had evidence of epithelial and endothelial injury in the lungs, although the epithelial injury appeared to be more severe, with many areas of exposed alveolar basement membrane visible by electron microscopy [10]. Endothelial damage and areas of microvascular thrombosis also occur but are not as prominent [11]. Light microscopic studies of injured lungs commonly show fibrinous alveolar infiltrates, alveolar hemorrhage, and acute neutrophilic inflammation in the first

2–3 days after the onset of ALI. At later times, the pathology is characterized by mononuclear cell infiltrates, the proliferation of Type II pneumocytes, and intra-alveolar fibrosis.

Morphologic studies showing alveolar membrane damage are supported by functional studies showing that there is a major increase in alveolar protein concentration, with a loss of the normal sieving characteristics of the alveolar membrane, and an acute inflammatory profile in bronchoalveolar lavage (BAL) fluid [12]. The BAL protein and cell concentrations are elevated at the onset of acute respiratory distress syndrome (ARDS), remain elevated for at least three days, and then fall with time in patients who remain mechanically ventilated [13–15].

The cause of the alveolar membrane injury is not clear, but necrosis and apoptosis are both likely to be involved [16,17]. Necrosis can occur when alveolar epithelial cells are ruptured by shear and/or distending forces due to relative over ventilation of the injured lungs. When a standard tidal volume (e. g., 10 ml/kg) is introduced into injured lungs, which have heterogeneous areas of alveolar flooding and/or atelectasis, the open alveolar units receive much larger tidal volumes than anticipated, resulting in large local shear and distending forces [18–22]. These forces can rupture the alveolar walls; studies by Dreyfuss et al., showed ultrastructural evidence of alveolar epithelial rupture in an animal model of ventilator-induced lung injury (VILI) [23] (reviewed in [22]). The NIH ARDSnet trial of low tidal volume in ARDS is consistent with the interpretation that lower distending and shear forces reduce injury to the alveolar epithelium [24]. While this ARDSnet trial was a major advance, the mortality in the treatment group in this and a subsequent ARDSnet clinical trial ranged from 25-31%, providing clear evidence that new ideas and approaches are still needed to further reduce mortality [24,25].

## Apoptosis and Inflammation in ALI.

Evidence from BAL fluid studies of patients with ARDS shows that apoptotic pathways are activated in the lungs, suggesting that apoptosis is an important determinant of the fate of the epithelium, in addition to stress failure and necrosis [26]. Apoptosis in lung cells can be initiated by at least two different routes, receptor-mediated and mitochondrial pathways (Fig. 1) [reviewed in [27–29]]. A family of 'death' receptors can be triggered by protein ligands either on the surface of effector cells, or in the soluble phase of extracellular fluids [1,28]. Fas (CD95) is a membrane receptor protein that mediates apoptosis via activation of a series of intracellular cysteine proteases (caspases), resulting in the cleavage of nuclear DNA [1,30]. Ligation of membrane Fas activates the death pathway by clustering the intracellular tails of adjacent Fas molecules and recruiting molecules with the Fas-associated death domain (FADD). This growing complex recruits molecules of pro-caspase-8 from the cytoplasm, which dimerize and autoactivate to yield active caspase-8. Caspase-8 activates caspase-3, which in turn activates distal caspases-6 and -7, leading to DNA fragmentation. The caspases can be grouped into three

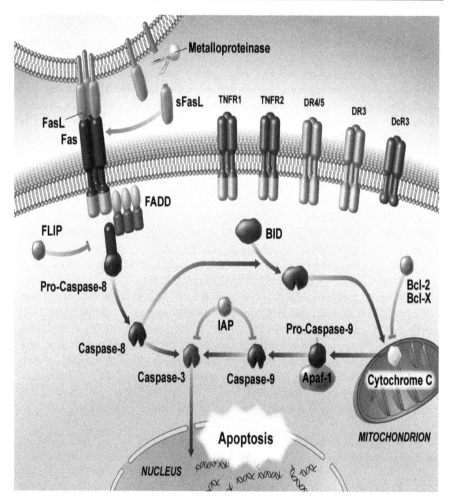

**Fig. 1.** Simplified view of receptors and pathways mediating cellular apoptosis. From [17] with permission

groups: the initiator caspases, which include caspases-8 and -9; the effector caspases, which include caspases-3, -6, and -7; and the inflammatory caspases. The inflammatory caspases, of which caspase-1 is the prototype, activate interleukin (IL)-1$\beta$ and IL-18. The caspase family of proteins was discovered as part of efforts to understand how IL-1$\beta$ was activated in inflammatory cells. The caspases are homologous to proteins in *Caenorhabditis elegans* that mediate cell death during development. Caspases exist as pro-forms in the cytoplasm, which prevents accidental activation. Once activated, caspases are regulated by specific inhibitor of apoptosis (IAP) proteins. The Bcl family members are mitochondrial membrane proteins that inhibit the mitochondrial apoptosis pathway [31]. The Fas-ligand (FasL) inhibitory proteins are proximal regulators of Fas activation [32].

FasL is a membrane protein on effector lymphocytes and other cells that accumulates in extracellular fluids when it is shed from cell membranes by activated metalloproteinases (soluble FasL, sFasL) [33, 34]. Monomeric sFasL is a relatively inefficient activator of membrane Fas, but multimeric forms of sFasL activate Fas and initiate intracellular signaling *in vitro* [35, 36]. Fine et al. reported that Fas is detectable on airway epithelial cells (Clara cells) and alveolar type II cells in rodents, and that activation of membrane Fas caused apoptosis of murine Type II cells *in vivo* [37, 38]. Other apoptosis pathways also exist, as Wang et al. have found that angiotensin peptides produced by fibroblasts from fibrotic human lungs (but not normal lungs) initiate apoptosis of alveolar epithelial cells via the angiotensin II receptor [39, 40]. Mice with deletion of angiotensin converting enzyme (ACE) develop less severe ALI in a sepsis model, whereas mice deficient in ACEII, which destroys ACEI, are relatively protected [41]. Mechanical stretch and major changes in oxygen concentration also induce apoptosis in lung epithelial cells and fibroblasts [42–46]. The effects of hyperoxia and hypoxia are mediated largely by the mitochondrial death pathway in epithelial and endothelial cells, with the release of mitochondrial cytochrome c and activation of caspase-9, which in turn activates the terminal caspases -3, -6, and -7 [45, 47–49]. Our own studies have indicated that sFasL is present in the BAL fluid of many patients with ARDS in a biologically active form which induces apoptosis of primary human lung epithelial cells *in vitro* (Fig. 2) [16]. Albertine, et al. confirmed and extended these findings by showing that sFasL is detectable in the pulmonary edema fluids of patients with ALI, and that membrane Fas appears to be upregulated on the alveolar epithelium of patients with ARDS who do not survive [50]. Soluble FasL also has been detected in the BAL fluid of patients with pulmonary fibrosis, as well as patients with chronic organizing pneumonia [51]. The intratracheal or endobronchial instillation of recombinant human sFasL causes lung injury and epithelial apoptosis in rabbits, and activation of membrane Fas in mouse lungs using a specific anti-Fas monoclonal antibody (JO-2) causes injury and epithelial apoptosis that is followed by fibrosis in the lungs [52–54].

We and others have found that activation of Fas pathways in the lungs is pro-inflammatory *in vivo*, consistent with experimental studies showing that Fas pathway intermediates like caspase-8 are linked to nuclear factor-kappa B (NF-κB) activation [55–57]. For example, instillation of human sFasL into rabbit lungs caused the production of IL-8 by alveolar macrophages [54], and activation of Fas in the lungs of mice caused histologic evidence of acute inflammation, with the production of macrophage inflammatory protein (MIP)-2 [53]. Park et al. showed that human monocyte-derived macrophages do not undergo apoptosis when stimulated with sFasL, even though they express the membrane Fas receptor. Instead, they become pro-inflammatory, releasing substantial quantities of IL-8 and tumor necrosis factor (TNF)-α [58] Normal alveolar macrophages have the

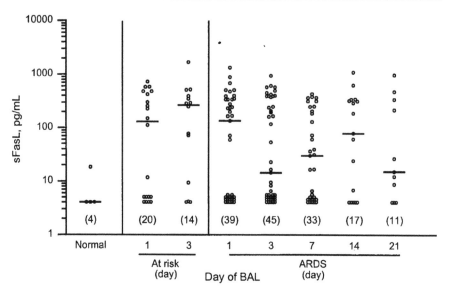

**Fig. 2.** Soluble Fas ligand (sFasL) in bronchoalveolar lavage (BAL) fluid from patients before and after the onset of lung injury, measured by ELISA. From [16] with permission

same characteristics, producing IL-8, a potent chemoattractant for neutrophils, when stimulated with sFasL *in vivo* [54].

## Experimental Links between Pro-Apoptotic Pathways and Fibrosis

Several different observations provide clues about the links between apoptosis, inflammation, and fibrosis. As cells become apoptotic, they become less adherent to the underlying matrix in the alveolar wall. Apoptotic Type I and Type II pneumocytes loosen, or 'fall away' (Greek, *apoptosis*), from the alveolar basement membrane, thereby exposing underlying matrix components in the alveolar wall. Because stimulation of Fas on monocyte/macrophages and human alveolar macrophages is pro-inflammatory, the accumulation of sFasL in the alveolar spaces is likely to create a pro-inflammatory phenotype in alveolar macrophages and newly recruited monocyte/macrophages in the airspaces [58]. The pro-inflammatory effects of Fas activation are evident in epithelial cells as well as alveolar macrophages, providing several different routes by which Fas activation can generate or amplify neutrophilic inflammation in the lungs [59]. Oxidants produced by activated polymorphonuclear cells (PMN) in the airspaces directly trigger mitochondrial death pathways, providing a means of amplifying apoptotic cell death at sites of inflammation [60,61]. Metalloproteinases and their natural inhibitors are known to accumulate in the BAL fluid of patients with ARDS [62–64], and activated alveolar macrophages release several different metalloproteinases which can degrade the basement membrane and interstitial components of the alveolar walls [65, 66]. The macrophage specific metalloproteinase, MMP-12, attacks elastin in alveolar walls [65]. Growth factors released by activated alveolar macrophages, such as transforming growth factor (TGF)-α and TGF-β, are also detectable in BAL fluid from ARDS patients [67]. These cytokines stimulate fibroblast proliferation and collagen production and have been linked with experimental lung injury [67–69].

Hagimoto et al. showed that repeatedly stimulating Fas by exposing mice to aerosols of the JO-2 mAb (which aggregates membrane Fas) every other day for 14 days resulted in increased lung hydroxyproline production and histological evidence of fibrosis [52]. Treatment of mice with intratracheal bleomycin causes Fas-dependent fibrosis, because fibrosis is markedly reduced in *lpr* mice, a naturally occurring strain in which membrane Fas is inactive [70]. The macrophage product, TGF-β enhances sFasL-dependent apoptosis of primary lung epithelial cells *in vitro* [71], and TGF-β is activated in bleomycin-induced fibrosis [72, 73].

Thus, accumulating evidence suggests that the Fas pathway triggers lung macrophage activation *in vitro* and *in vivo*, and that Fas activation in the lungs of mice causes delayed fibrosis. More information is needed about the specific mechanisms involved in this process so that specific steps in this pathway can be targeted in order to reduce or prevent some of the fibrotic consequences of ALI.

## Endothelial Cell Apoptosis

Endothelial cell death in the lungs also is likely to be important in the pathogenesis of ALI, but little specific information is available about endothelial cell apoptosis in the lungs. Endothelial apoptosis has a role in the systemic circulation and has been implicated in atherosclerosis and vascular remodeling, and it may also be important in sepsis (reviewed in [74, 75]). Like alveolar epithelial cells, apoptotic endothelial cells loosen from attachments in vessel walls, exposing the thrombogenic surface of underlying matrix. Because apoptotic endothelial cells lose intracellular adherens junctions, the apoptotic death of only a small number of endothelial cells could have a significant effect on microvascular permeability. Apoptotic endothelial cells become adhesive for platelets and leukocytes and promote coagulation, consistent with the microvascular thrombotic lesions seen in the lungs of patients dying following ALI [13, 76, 77]. As with lung epithelial cells and other types of cells, ligation of membrane death receptors on endothelial cells by TNF-α and related peptides kills endothelial cells *in vitro*. Although some endothelial cells are relatively resistant to Fas ligation *in vitro*, ligation of Fas *in vivo* using either an agonistic anti-Fas mAb, or aggregated sFasL, caused diffuse endothelial apoptosis in mice, and the lesions were preventable by an inhibitor of caspase-8, confirming that the Fas-dependent death pathway was involved [78]. Activation of Toll-like receptor 4 (TLR4) by bacterial lipopolysaccharide (LPS) and TLR2 by bacterial lipoproteins causes endothelial apoptosis *in vitro*, linking activation of innate immunity and endothelial cell death [79].

Endothelial cells are protected from apoptosis *in vitro* by growth and an-giogenic factors such as vascular endothelial growth factor (VEGF), fibroblast growth factor-2, hepatocyte growth factor, and others that activate the phospho-inositide 3-OH kinase (PI3-K)/AKT pathway, which leads to phosphorylation and inactivation of caspase-9 and other proapoptotic intermediates [75, 80]. Some types of endothelial cell have a constitutive anti-apoptotic pathway which pro-tects against LPS-induced apoptosis via activation of FLIP (FLICE-like inhibitory protein), which blocks NF-κB activation [81,82].

The role of endothelial cell apoptosis in sepsis is still being defined, because it has been difficult to detect apoptotic endothelial cells in vascular walls of patients dying with sepsis, or in mice following cecal ligation and puncture [83,84]. Apop-totic endothelial cells may be difficult to detect *in vivo* because they detach from vessel walls and are cleared in the circulation. Apoptosis of capillary endothelial cells in the lung was detectable but infrequent in mice with pseudomonas pneu-monia [85]. Treatment of septic animals with caspase inhibitors improves survival and reduces lung injury, but it is not clear whether this effect involves protection from endothelial apoptosis, or lymphocyte apoptosis, or both [86,87]. Overexpres-sion of the anti-apoptotic protein, Bcl-2, protects mice from death following cecal ligation and puncture, possibly by reducing endothelial cell apoptosis [88]. The importance of endothelial cell apoptosis in the pulmonary circulation in patients with ALI and in animal models of lung injury needs to be defined, and there is no information linking endothelial cell apoptosis with the delayed consequences of lung injury.

## Should Epithelial and Endothelial Apoptosis be Inhibited?

If apoptosis is part of normal tissue development and plays a role in repair and regeneration of injured tissues, then a major unanswered question is whether apoptotic pathways should be inhibited in ALI, and if so, for how long? The obser-vation that sFasL is present and biologically active in the lungs of patients at the onset of ALI suggests that sFasL has an important initial role in the injury [16]. Experimental evidence that Fas activation in the lungs is associated with delayed fibrosis, and that injury from agents such as bleomycin is associated with apoptosis and fibrosis suggests that inhibiting apoptosis pathways might limit fibrosis. How-ever, these findings are limited to very specific experimental models, and questions remain about the mechanistic importance of apoptosis in clinical settings that are significant risk factors for ALI, such as mechanical ventilation, bacterial pneumo-nias, sepsis, and trauma. Inhibition of apoptosis pathways improves survival in several different murine models of sepsis [86,87]. In the cecal ligation and punc-ture model, 'knock down' of either membrane Fas or caspase-8 using systemic administration of specific small interfering RNAs (siRNAs) *in vivo* improved sur-vival, but whether this strategy would modify the long term effects of lung injury in surviving animals is difficult to determine [89]. Rabbits treated with injurious mechanical ventilation developed lung injury and renal dysfunction associated with apoptosis of renal tubular epithelium, suggesting that blockade of apoptosis pathways might limit secondary renal injury in the setting of VILI [90]. In order to support the rationale for anti-apoptotic treatments in ALI, more information is needed about the relative contributions of apoptosis and necrosis to acute and delayed outcomes in different experimental models. While methods exist to measure apoptosis in tissues and individual cells *in vivo*, accurate methods to measure necrosis with the same level of detail are lacking. Because apoptosis is regulated, it makes sense to target key intermediates in apoptosis pathways, such as caspases. Studies of the effects of inhibiting apoptosis pathways *in vivo* must include measurement of organ-specific physiological endpoints and evidence of apoptosis in tissues, in order to prove that observed changes in outcome are actually linked to changes in apoptosis in tissue and to relevant physiological functions.

Although experimental evidence suggests that inhibition of apoptosis in some clinical settings might be beneficial, the possible adverse effects of inhibiting cell death also need to be considered. Apoptosis pathways in the lungs may be critical in the repair phase after ALI, as Fas pathways are likely to be involved in clearing proliferating Type II pneumocytes, as well as fibroblasts that accumulate during the repair phase [91,92]. Some evidence suggests that repair processes begin almost immediately after the onset of ALI, as the collagen precursor pro-collagen III is detectable in the lungs at the onset as well as during the course of ALI [93,94]. Early inhibition of these repair processes could have adverse consequences, which must be evaluated carefully when apoptosis is inhibited in animal models of lung injury.

## Conclusion

The concept that apoptosis pathways are involved in the onset and long-term consequences of lung injury is important, but significant questions remain. More information is needed about the factors that control the balance between tissue injury and tissue repair in the lungs. For example, we need to know more about what determines when the Fas pathway leads to tissue injury versus when Fas activation leads to the orderly removal of excess tissue at sites of tissue repair. Cell death pathways are complex and interlocking, and more information is needed about how different cellular activation pathways interact either to enhance or inhibit cell death in the lungs. Activation of innate immunity via TLR receptors modulates Fas pathway activity, and more information is needed about the mechanisms involved. At inflammatory sites, it seems likely that receptor-mediated death pathways and mitochondrial death pathways are activated almost simultaneously, and it is not clear whether strategies to inhibit one of the death pathways will be successful without simultaneously modulating all other death pathways. Importantly, it is not clear how long apoptosis pathways should be inhibited. Nevertheless, new ideas are needed to further reduce mortality in patients with ALI. Because apoptosis pathways are a tightly regulated mode of cell death, targeting specific control points in these pathways offers new opportunities to reduce the initial severity of ALI and improve long-term outcomes.

*Acknowledgement.* Supported in part by the Medical Research Service of the Department of Veterans Affairs, and by grants HL69852 and HL073996 from the National Institutes of Health.

# References

1.  Hengartner MO (2000) The biochemistry of apoptosis. Nature 407:770–776
2.  Henson PM, Bratton DL, Fadok VA (2001) Apoptotic cell removal. Curr Biol 11:R795–R805
3.  Okada H, Mak TW (2004) Pathways of apoptotic and non-apoptotic death in tumour cells. Nat Rev Cancer 4:592–603
4.  Matthay MA, Folkesson HG, Clerici C (2002) Lung epithelial fluid transport and the resolution of pulmonary edema. Physiol Rev 82:569–600
5.  Dobbs LG, Gonzalez R, Matthay MA, Carter EP, Allen L, Verkman AS (1998) Highly water-permeable type I alveolar epithelial cells confer high water permeability between the airspace and vasculature in rat lung. Proc Natl Acad Sci USA 95:2991–2996
6.  Ma T, Fukuda N, Song Y, Matthay MA, Verkman AS (2000) Lung fluid transport in aquaporin-5 knockout mice. J Clin Invest 105:93–100
7.  Matthay MA, Folkesson HG, Clerici C (2002) Lung epithelial fluid transport and the resolution of pulmonary edema. Physiol Rev 82:569–600
8.  Matthay MA, Wiener-Kronish JP (1990) Intact epithelial barrier function is critical for the resolution of alveolar edema in humans. Am Rev Respir Dis 142:1250–1257
9.  Ware LB, Matthay MA (2001) Alveolar fluid clearance is impaired in the majority of patients with acute lung injury and the acute respiratory distress syndrome. Am J Respir Crit Care Med 163:1376–1383
10. Bachofen A, Weibel ER (1982) Structural alterations of lung parenchyma in the adult respiratory distress syndrome. Clin Chest Med 3:35–56
11. Tomashefski JF Jr, Davies P, Boggis L, et.al (1983) The pulmonary vascular lesions of the adult respiratory distress syndrome. Am J Pathol 112:112–126
12. Holter JF, Weiland JE, Pacht ER, Gadek GE, Davis WB (1986) Protein permeability in the adult respiratory distress syndrome. Loss of size selectivity of the alveolar epithelium. J Clin Invest 78:1513–1522
13. Steinberg KP, Milberg JA, Martin TR, Maunder RJ, Cockrill BA, Hudson LD (1994) Evolution of bronchoalveolar cell populations in the adult respiratory distress syndrome. Am J Respir Crit Care Med 150:113–122
14. Goodman RB, Strieter RM, Steinberg KP, et al (1996) Inflammatory cytokines in patients with persistence of the acute respiratory distress syndrome. Am J Respir Crit Care Med 154:602–611
15. Park WY, Goodman RB, Steinberg KP, et al (2001) Cytokine balance in the lungs of patients with acute respiratory distress syndrome. Am J Respir Crit Care Med 164:1896–1903
16. Matute-BelloG, Liles WC, Steinberg KP, et al (1999) Soluble Fas-Ligand induces epithelial cell apoptosis in humans with acute lung injury (ARDS). J Immunol 163:2217–2225
17. Martin TR, Hagimoto N, Nakamura M, Matute-Bello G (2005) Apoptosis and epithelial injury in the lungs. Proc Am Thorac Soc 2:214–220
18. Dreyfuss D, Saumon G (1998) Ventilator-induced lung injury: lessons from experimental studies. Am J Respir Crit Care Med 157:294–323

19. Matthay MA, Bhattacharya S, Gaver D, et al (2002) Ventilator-induced lung injury: in vivo and in vitro mechanisms. Am J Physiol Lung Cell Mol Physiol 283:L678–L682

20. Plotz FB, Slutsky AS, van Vught AJ, Heijnen CJ (2004) Ventilator-induced lung injury and multiple system organ failure: a critical review of facts and hypotheses. Intensive Care Med 30:1865–1872

21. Vlahakis NE, Hubmayr RD (2003) Response of alveolar cells to mechanical stress. Curr Opin Crit Care 9:2–8

22. Vlahakis NE, Hubmayr RD (2005) Cellular stress failure in ventilator-injured lungs. Am J Respir Crit Care Med 171:1328–1342

23. Dreyfuss D, Soler P, Basset G, Saumon G (1988) High inflation pressure pulmonary edema. Respective effects of high airway pressure, high tidal volume, and positive end-expiratory pressure. Am Rev Respir Dis 137:1159–1164

24. The Acute Respiratory Distress Syndrome Network (2000) Ventilation with lower tidal volumes as compared with traditional tidal volumes for acute lung injury and the acute respiratory distress syndrome. N Engl J Med 342:1301–1308

25. Brower RG, Lanken PN, MacIntyre N, et al (2004) Higher versus lower positive end-expiratory pressures in patients with the acute respiratory distress syndrome. N Engl J Med 351:327–336

26. Matute-Bello G, Winn RK, Jonas M, Chi EY, Martin TR, Liles WC (1999) Activation of Fas (CD95) induces lung injury and apoptosis of type I and II pneumocytes in mice. Am J Respir Crit Care Med 159:A697 (abst)

27. Fine A, Janssen-Heininger Y, Soultanakis RP, Swisher SG, Uhal BD (2000) Apoptosis in lung pathophysiology. Am J Physiol Lung Cell Mol Physiol 279:L423–L427

28. Kuwano K, Hara N (2000) Signal transduction pathways of apoptosis and inflammation induced by the tumor necrosis factor receptor family. Am J Respir Cell Mol Biol 22:147–149

29. Rieux-Laucat F, Fischer A, Deist FL (2003) Cell-death signaling and human disease. Curr Opin Immunol 15:325–331

30. Riedl SJ, Shi Y (2004) Molecular mechanisms of caspase regulation during apoptosis. Nat Rev Mol Cell Biol 5:897–907

31. Cory S, Huang DC, Adams JM (2003) The Bcl-2 family: roles in cell survival and oncogenesis. Oncogene 22:8590–8607

32. Tschopp J, Irmler M, Thome M (1998) Inhibition of fas death signals by FLIPs. Curr Opin Immunol 10:552–558

33. Matsuno H, Yudoh K, Watanabe Y, Nakazawa F, Aono H, Kimura T (2001) Stromelysin-1 (MMP-3) in synovial fluid of patients with rheumatoid arthritis has potential to cleave membrane bound Fas ligand. J Rheumatol 28:22–28

34. Powell WC, Fingleton B, Wilson CL, Boothby M, Matrisian LM (1999) The metalloproteinase matrilysin proteolytically generates active soluble Fas ligand and potentiates epithelial cell apoptosis. Curr Biol 9:1441–1447

35. Schneider P, Holler N, Bodmer JL, et al (1998) Conversion of membrane-bound Fas (CD95) ligand to its soluble form is associated with downregulation of its proapoptotic activity and loss of liver toxicity. J Exp Med 187:1205–1213

36. Holler N, Tardivel A, Kovacsovics-Bankowski M, et al (2003) Two adjacent trimeric Fas ligands are required for Fas signaling and formation of a death-inducing signaling complex. Mol Cell Biol 23:1428–1440

37. Fine A, Anderson NL, Rothstein TL, Williams MC, Gochuico BR (1997) Fas expression in pulmonary alveolar type II cells. Am J Physiol Lung Cell Mol Physiol 273:L64–L71

38. Gochuico BR, Miranda KM, Hessel EM, et al (1998) Airway epithelial Fas ligand expression: potential role in modulating bronchial inflammation. Am J Physiol 274:L444–L449

39. Wang R, Zagariya A, Ang E, Ibarra-Sunga O, Uhal BD (1999) Fas-induced apoptosis of alveolar epithelial cells requires ANG II generation and receptor interaction. Am J Physiol 277:L1245–L1250

40. Wang R, Ramos C, Joshi I, et al (1999) Human lung myofibroblast-derived inducers of alveolar epithelial apoptosis identified as angiotensin peptides. Am J Physiol 277:L1158–L1164

41. Imai Y, Kuba K, Rao S, et al (2005) Angiotensin-converting enzyme 2 protects from severe acute lung failure. Nature 436:112–116
42. Chandel NS, Sznajder JI (2000) Stretching the lung and programmed cell death. Am J Physiol Lung Cell Mol Physiol 279:L1003–L1004
43. Edwards YS, Sutherland LM, Murray AW (2000) NO protects alveolar type II cells from stretch-induced apoptosis. A novel role for macrophages in the lung. Am J Physiol Lung Cell Mol Physiol 279:L1236–L1242
44. O'Reilly MA, Staversky RJ, Watkins RH, Maniscalco WM, Keng PC (2000) p53-independent induction of GADD45 and GADD153 in mouse lungs exposed to hyperoxia. Am J Physiol Lung Cell Mol Physiol 278:L552–L559
45. Budinger GR, Tso M, McClintock DS, Dean DA, Sznajder JI, Chandel NS (2002) Hyperoxia-induced apoptosis does not require mitochondrial reactive oxygen species and is regulated by Bcl-2 proteins. J Biol Chem 277:15654–15660
46. Wang X, Ryter SW, Dai C, et al (2003) Necrotic cell death in response to oxidant stress involves the activation of the apoptogenic caspase-8/bid pathway. J Biol Chem 278:29184–29191
47. McClintock DS, Santore MT, Lee VY, et al (2002) Bcl-2 family members and functional electron transport chain regulate oxygen deprivation-induced cell death. Mol Cell Biol 22:94–104
48. Santore MT, McClintock DS, Lee VY, Budinger GR, Chandel NS (2002) Anoxia-induced apoptosis occurs through a mitochondria-dependent pathway in lung epithelial cells. Am J Physiol Lung Cell Mol Physiol 282:L727–L734
49. Madesh M, Hawkins BJ, Milovanova T, et al (2005) Selective role for superoxide in InsP3 receptor-mediated mitochondrial dysfunction and endothelial apoptosis. J Cell Biol 170:1079–1090
50. Albertine KH, Soulier MF, Wang Z, et al (2002) Fas and fas ligand are up-regulated in pulmonary edema fluid and lung tissue of patients with acute lung injury and the acute respiratory distress syndrome. Am J Pathol 161:1783–1796
51. Kuwano K, Kawasaki M, Maeyama T, et al (2000) Soluble form of fas and fas ligand in BAL fluid from patients with pulmonary fibrosis and bronchiolitis obliterans organizing pneumonia. Chest 118:451–458
52. Hagimoto N, Kuwano K, Miyazaki H, et al (1997) Induction of apoptosis and pulmonary fibrosis in mice in response to ligation of Fas antigen. Am J Respir Cell Mol Biol 17:272–278
53. Matute-Bello G, Winn RK, Jonas M, Chi EY, Martin TR, Liles WC (2001) Fas (CD95) induces alveolar epithelial cell apoptosis in vivo: implications for acute pulmonary inflammation. Am J Pathol 158:153–161
54. Matute-Bello G, Liles WC, Frevert CW, et al (2001) Recombinant human Fas ligand induces alveolar epithelial cell apoptosis and lung injury in rabbits. Am J Physiol Lung Cell Mol Physiol 281:L328–L335
55. Chaudhary PM, Eby MT, Jasmin A, Kumar A, Liu L, Hood L (2000) Activation of the NF-kappaB pathway by caspase 8 and its homologs. Oncogene 19:4451–4460
56. Kreuz S, Siegmund D, Rumpf JJ, et al (2004) NFkappaB activation by Fas is mediated through FADD, caspase-8, and RIP and is inhibited by FLIP. J Cell Biol 166:369–380
57. Imamura R, Konaka K, Matsumoto N, et al (2004) Fas ligand induces cell-autonomous NF-kappaB activation and interleukin-8 production by a mechanism distinct from that of tumor necrosis factor-alpha. J Biol Chem 279:46415–46423
58. Park DR, Thomsen AR, Frevert CW, et al (2003) Fas (CD95) induces pro-inflammatory cytokine responses by human monocytes and monocyte-derived macrophages. J Immunol 170:6209–6216
59. Matute-Bello G, Lee JS, Liles WC, et al (2005) Fas-mediated acute lung injury requires Fas expression on nonmyeloid cells of the lung. J Immunol 175:4069–4075
60. Yin L, Stearns R, Gonzalez-Flecha B (2005) Lysosomal and mitochondrial pathways in H2O2-induced apoptosis of alveolar type II cells. J Cell Biochem 94:433–445

61. Ruchko M, Gorodnya O, LeDoux SP, Alexeyev MF, Al-Mehdi AB, Gillespie MN (2005) Mitochondrial DNA damage triggers mitochondrial dysfunction and apoptosis in oxidant-challenged lung endothelial cells. Am J Physiol Lung Cell Mol Physiol 288:L530–L535

62. Ricou B, Nicod L, Lacraz S, Welgus HG, Suter PM, Dayer JM (1996) Matrix metalloproteinases and TIMP in acute respiratory distress syndrome. Am J Respir Crit Care Med 154:346–352

63. Torii K, Iida K, Miyazaki Y, et al (1997) Higher concentrations of matrix metalloproteinases in bronchoalveolar lavage fluid of patients with adult respiratory distress syndrome. Am J Respir Crit Care Med 155:43–46

64. Lanchou J, Corbel M, Tanguy M, et al (2003) Imbalance between matrix metalloproteinases (MMP-9 and MMP-2) and tissue inhibitors of metalloproteinases (TIMP-1 and TIMP-2) in acute respiratory distress syndrome patients. Crit Care Med 31:536–542

65. Belaaouaj A, Shipley JM, Kobayashi DK, et al (1995) Human macrophage metalloelastase. Genomic organization, chromosomal location, gene linkage, and tissue-specific expression. J Biol Chem 270:14568–14575

66. Parks WC, Wilson CL, Lopez-Boado YS (2004) Matrix metalloproteinases as modulators of inflammation and innate immunity. Nat Rev Immunol 4:617–629

67. Madtes DK, Klima LD, Rubenfeld G, et al (1998) Elevated transforming growth factor-a levels in bronchoalveolar lavage fluid in patients with acute respiratory distress syndrome. Am J Respir Crit Care Med 158:424–430

68. Pittet JF, Griffiths MJ, Geiser T, et al (2001) TGF-beta is a critical mediator of acute lung injury. J Clin Invest 107:1537–1544

69. Fahy RJ, Lichtenberger F, McKeegan CB, Nuovo GJ, Marsh CB, Wewers MD (2003) The acute respiratory distress syndrome: a role for transforming growth factor-beta 1. Am J Respir Cell Mol Biol 28:499–503

70. Kuwano K, Hagimoto N, Kawasaki M, et al (1999) Essential roles of the Fas-Fas ligand pathway in the development of pulmonary fibrosis. J Clin Invest 104:13–19

71. Hagimoto N, Kuwano K, Inoshima I, et al (2002) TGF-beta 1 as an enhancer of Fas-mediated apoptosis of lung epithelial cells. J Immunol 168:6470–6478

72. Hagimoto N, Kuwano K, Nomoto Y, Kunitake R, Hara N (1997) Apoptosis and expression of Fas/Fas ligand mRNA in bleomycin-induced pulmonary fibrosis in mice. Am J Respir Cell Mol Biol 16:91–101

73. Kaminski N, Allard JD, Pittet JF, et al (2000) Global analysis of gene expression in pulmonary fibrosis reveals distinct programs regulating lung inflammation and fibrosis. Proc Natl Acad Sci USA 97:1778–1783

74. Mallat Z, Tedgui A (2000) Apoptosis in the vasculature: mechanisms and functional importance. Br J Pharmacol 130:947–962

75. Winn RK, Harlan JM (2005) The role of endothelial cell apoptosis in inflammatory and immune diseases. J Thromb Haemost 3:1815–1824

76. Bombeli T, Karsan A, Tait JF, Harlan JM (1997) Apoptotic vascular endothelial cells become procoagulant. Blood 89:2429–2442

77. Bombeli T, Schwartz BR, Harlan JM (1999) Endothelial cells undergoing apoptosis become proadhesive for nonactivated platelets. Blood 93:3831–3838

78. Janin A, Deschaumes C, Daneshpouy M, et al (2002) CD95 engagement induces disseminated endothelial cell apoptosis in vivo: immunopathologic implications. Blood 99:2940–2947

79. Bannerman DD, Goldblum SE (2003) Mechanisms of bacterial lipopolysaccharide-induced endothelial apoptosis. Am J Physiol Lung Cell Mol Physiol 284:L899–L914

80. Downward J (2004) PI 3-kinase, Akt and cell survival. Semin Cell Dev Biol 15:177–182

81. Bannerman DD, Tupper JC, Ricketts WA, Bennett CF, Winn RK, Harlan JM (2001) A constitutive cytoprotective pathway protects endothelial cells from lipopolysaccharide-induced apoptosis. J Biol Chem 276:14924–14932

82. Bannerman DD, Eiting KT, Winn RK, Harlan JM (2004) FLICE-like inhibitory protein (FLIP) protects against apoptosis and suppresses NF-kappaB activation induced by bacterial lipopolysaccharide. Am J Pathol 165:1423–1431

83. Hotchkiss RS, Swanson PE, Freeman BD, et al (1999) Apoptotic cell death in patients with sepsis, shock, and multiple organ dysfunction. Crit Care Med 27:1230–1251
84. Hotchkiss RS, Tinsley KW, Swanson PE, Karl IE (2002) Endothelial cell apoptosis in sepsis. Crit Care Med 30:S225–S228
85. Hotchkiss RS, Dunne WM, Swanson PE, et al (2001) Role of apoptosis in Pseudomonas aeruginosa pneumonia. Science 294:1783
86. Kawasaki M, Kuwano K, Hagimoto N, et al (2000) Protection from lethal apoptosis in lipopolysaccharide-induced acute lung injury in mice by a caspase inhibitor. Am J Pathol 157:597–603
87. Hotchkiss RS, Chang KC, Swanson PE, et al (2000) Caspase inhibitors improve survival in sepsis: a critical role of the lymphocyte. Nat Immunol 1:496–501
88. Iwata A, Stevenson VM, Minard A, et al (2003) Over-expression of Bcl-2 provides protection in septic mice by a trans effect. J Immunol 171:3136–3141
89. Wesche-Soldato DE, Chung CS, Lomas-Neira J, Doughty LA, Gregory SH, Ayala A (2005) In vivo delivery of caspase-8 or Fas siRNA improves the survival of septic mice. Blood 106:2295–2301
90. Imai Y, Parodo J, Kajikawa O, et al (2003) Injurious mechanical ventilation and end-organ epithelial cell apoptosis and organ dysfunction in an experimental model of acute respiratory distress syndrome. JAMA 289:2104–2112
91. Bardales RH, Xie SS, Schaefer RF, Hsu SM (1996) Apoptosis is a major pathway responsible for the resolution of Type II pneumocytes in acute lung injury. Am J Pathol 149:845–852
92. Polunovsky VA, Chen B, Henke C, et al (1993) Role of mesenchymal cell death in lung remodeling after injury. J Clin Invest 92:388–397
93. Clark JG, Milberg JA, Steinberg KP, Hudson LD (1995) Type III procollagen peptide in the adult respiratory distress syndrome: association of increased peptide levels in bronchoalveolar lavage fluid with increased risk for death. Ann Intern Med 122:17–23
94. Chesnutt AN, Matthay MA, Tibayan FA, Clark JG (1997) Early detection of type III procollagen peptide in acute lung injury: pathogenetic and prognostic significance. Am J Respir Crit Care Med 156:840–845

# Mechanisms of Immunodepression after Central Nervous System Injury

C. Meisel and H.-D. Volk

## Introduction

Infections are a leading cause of death in patients suffering from acute central nervous system (CNS) injury, such as stroke, traumatic brain injury, or spinal cord injury. Infections not only increase morbidity and mortality after CNS trauma but also worsen the neurological recovery of affected patients. Several risk factors have been attributed to the increased susceptibility to infections after CNS injury, including the exposure of patients to invasive medical procedures and hospitalization, and the loss of protective reflexes leading to bladder dysfunction, dysphagia, and aspiration. However, experimental and clinical studies have also demonstrated profound suppression of immune responsiveness after brain injury. It has become evident that CNS injury induces a disturbance of the normally well balanced interplay between the CNS and the immune system. As a result, CNS injury leads to secondary immunodeficiency (CNS injury-induced immunodepression, CIDS) and infection.

The CNS senses inflammation in the body through the autonomic nervous system, and mounts a strong counterregulatory response in case of infection and severe injury. This acute response is anti-inflammatory in nature, and can be considered adaptive, as it helps contain infection and injury-induced inflammation when they occur in the periphery. Brain or spinal cord injury can lead to the production of inflammatory mediators within the CNS, or disruption of signaling within the control circuitry of neural-immune interactions, both of which may also lead to systemic downregulation of innate and adaptive immunity. In the absence of immune stimulation by peripheral inflammation, however, this leads to profound deficiencies of the body's defense systems, leaving the host vulnerable to invading microorganisms.

## Infections after CNS Injury

Infection is a frequent medical complication in patients suffering from stroke, traumatic brain or spinal cord injuries. The most common infectious complications after CNS injury are pneumonia and urinary tract infections [1–4]. Between 10 and 60% of patients with injuries of the CNS develop nosocomial infections, with a particularly high prevalence in patients requiring mechanical ventilation after neurotrauma [2–7]. The incidence of infections in patients with CNS injury is thus significantly higher than the general prevalence of hospital acquired infections (4% to 9% of all hospitalized patients) and that reported among surgical patients (3%) [8]. Infectious complications frequently occur within the first days after CNS injury [1,3,6,7]. However, the increased risk of infections persists beyond the acute phase and infections are common complications also during the rehabilitation phase [4,5].

Infections are a major determinant of outcome after CNS injury. Although early mortality in brain injured patients is due to direct complications of CNS and other organ system dysfunction, infections are the leading cause of death in the post-acute phase of CNS injury. In stroke patients, the 30-day mortality in patients who developed pneumonia was increased up to three fold compared to patients not suffering from pneumonia [9]. Reines and Harris [10] reported an attributable mortality rate of 11% for patients with spinal cord injury due to pulmonary complications, and pneumonia was the leading cause of death over a period of 12 years after injury [11]. In addition, pneumonia is associated with fever, hypoxemia, arterial hypotension, and intracranial hypertension, which are known to worsen the neurological outcome of patients with brain injury [6]. In summary, there is ample evidence that CNS injury is associated with a high risk of infections that, in turn, have profound consequences for patient outcome.

Why are patients with CNS injury at such a high risk of infection? They often have complicating peripheral injury (polytrauma), undergo invasive medical treatment (surgery, catheterization, mechanical ventilation), may be immobilized and exposed to various multiple drug resistant bacteria, and may have CNS lesions that specifically impair their ability to swallow, leading to aspiration. These factors, alone or in combination, seem sufficient to explain a high incidence of infections. In particular, aspiration is the commonly cited explanation for pneumonia in patients with CNS injury. However, aspiration alone is not sufficient to induce pneumonia; approximately half of all healthy adults aspirate during sleep without developing pneumonia [12].

## Impaired Cell-mediated Immune Responses after CNS Injury

A host of studies have demonstrated immune dysfunction after CNS injury [13–16]. While the initial local response to brain damage is pro-inflammatory and accompanied by a systemic response comprising features of the systemic inflammatory response syndrome (SIRS), patients with CNS injury concurrently show signs of systemic immunodepression. Commonly reported defects in immune functions in patients after stroke, traumatic brain injury, or spinal cord injury, include reduced peripheral blood lymphocyte counts and impaired T- and natural killer (NK) cell activity. It has been demonstrated that peripheral blood T-lymphocytes obtained from patients with CNS injury show reduced mitogen-induced cytokine production and proliferation in vitro [13,14,17,18]. The rate of anergic delayed-type hypersensitivity (DTH) skin test responses to recall antigens in brain trauma patients was found to correlate with trauma severity [18, 19]. Moreover, decreased NK cell counts and cytotoxic activity was observed in these patients [13, 20]. In contrast to impaired T and NK cell functions, humoral immune responses seem less affected after CNS injury [17, 20]. Trauma-induced immunodepression is also reflected by impaired phagocytotic activity of granulocytes and by monocyte deactivation [16, 21, 22]. Circulating monocytes from patients with acute brain injury have decreased major histocompatibility complex (MHC) class II expression and a profoundly reduced capacity to produce pro-inflammatory cytokines after *ex vivo* stimulation with endotoxin [16, 22]. Impaired monocyte functions result in insufficient antigen-presentation and decreased expression of secreted or membrane-bound co-stimulatory molecules and, therefore, may contribute to reduced lymphocyte responses [23]. In general, changes in cellular immune responses correlate with severity of brain injury. They occur rapidly within hours after the injurious insult and can last for up to several weeks [13, 14, 17]. In addition, the extent and duration of impaired cell-mediated immune responses in CNS injured patients correlated to an increased risk of infections and poor outcome [16, 24].

In summary, substantial clinical evidence points towards a major role of impaired cell-mediated immune responses in the high incidence of infectious complications after CNS injury. To understand how and why CNS injury induces immunodepression, we have to explore the mechanisms by which the immune system and the CNS interact.

## Communication Between the CNS and Immune System

The nervous and immune systems are engaged in intense bidirectional communication to response to environmental challenges. The basis for this interaction is provided by the rich innervation of lymphoid tissues and visceral organs by the autonomous nervous system as well as by the expression of receptors for neurotransmitters, endocrine hormones, and cytokines on both CNS and immune cells. Sensors within the peripheral and central autonomic nervous systems relay information on the status of the immune system in response to environmental stressors. This input is processed by the CNS and results in homeostatic signals via three major thoroughfares of neuroimmunomodulation: the hypothalamo-pituitary adrenal (HPA) axis, the sympathetic and the parasympathetic nervous systems [25–27].

### Sensing of Inflammation by the CNS

There are at least two major afferent pathways by which the brain senses inflammation: a neural (mainly by the vagus nerve) and a humoral pathway [28, 29]. Activation of innate immune cells in response to invading pathogens or tissue trauma leads to the release of cytokines (e.g., interleukin [IL]-1β, tumor necrosis factor [TNF]-α), which activate afferent sensory fibers of the vagus nerve located in the vicinity [30]. Afferent vagal fibers predominantly terminate in the nucleus tractus solitarius (NTS), from which signals are relayed through neural projections to other brain sites, including the paraventricular nucleus (PVN) of the hypothalamus, the rostral ventrolateral medulla (RVM), and the locus coeruleus, that modulate the activity of the HPA axis and the sympathetic nervous system.

The second, humoral pathway of immune-to-brain communication, which may be primarily operational during systemic inflammatory responses, involves the transportation of cytokines via the circulation into the brain. Cytokines in the blood stream may bind to receptors on brain endothelial cells, where they induce the abluminal release of diffusible mediators, such as nitric oxide (NO) and prostaglandin $E_2$ ($PGE_2$). $PGE_2$ has bee nsuggested to act as a central mediator of fever and HPA axis activation. Alternatively, cytokines may enter the brain either actively through carrier mediated mechanisms [31], or passively through the capillary endothelium of circumventricular organs which lack blood-brain barrier properties [32]. The circumventricular organs include the pineal gland, the subfornical organ, the median eminence, the neural lobe of the pituitary, the subcommissural organ, the area postrema, and the organum vasculosum of the lamina terminalis (OLVT) [33]. The circumventricular organs, in particular the area postrema and OLVT have been suggested as central relays of cytokine-to-brain signaling, through which information is fed into hypothalamic, sympathetic, and parasympathetic processing.

Cytokines arising from injury-induced inflammation within the CNS may access control centers of neural-immune interaction via diffusion in the extracellular space and cerebrospinal fluid (CSF), or indirectly via the bloodstream. In general, cytokine receptors relevant for CNS-immune communication in the brain are preferentially located in the circumventricular organs and the medial preoptic area, from which the signal is relayed to the paraventricular nucleus of the hypothalamus through neural projections [34]. In addition to signals through neural connections, hypothalamic neurons can directly respond to cytokines. Through the release of corticotropin releasing factor (CRF) from specialized neurons in the PVN, the hypothalamus modulates the HPA axis and the sympathetic nervous system. In addition, descending projections from the PVN to brain stem centers (e.g., NTS) also affect vagal output.

## Modulation of Immune Responses by the CNS

Immune responses are modulated by the CNS through at least three major efferent pathways: the HPA axis, the sympathetic nervous system, and the cholinergic anti-inflammatory pathway. High circulating levels of glucocorticoids and catecholamines, the end products of the HPA axis and the sympathetic nervous system, respectively, mobilize leukocytes from the marginal pool within the vasculature, thereby rapidly increasing the number of available immune cells to enter infected tissues and potentially reducing the migration of these cells into uninflamed tissue. Glucocorticoids and catecholamines downregulate inflammatory responses by suppressing the production of many pro-inflammatory mediators including cytokines (IL-1$\beta$, TNF-$\alpha$), and by enhancing the release of anti-inflammatory mediators such as IL-10 [16,35–37].

Glucocorticoids also enhance the resolution of inflammation by stimulating the production of acute phase reactants and by promoting antigen uptake by phagocytes [38–40]. On the other hand, glucocorticoids and catecholamines can decrease the capacity of antigen-presenting cells to induce antigen-specific T cell responses by downregulating the expression of MHC class II and co-stimulatory molecules (e.g., CD86) [41,42]. Moreover, they can alter the balance of type 1/type 2 T helper (Th) cell responses. Glucocorticoids and catecholamines suppress the production of IL-12 and enhance the release of IL-10 from monocyte/macrophages and dendritic cells, thereby preferentially inhibiting the induction of Th1 responses [43,44]. In addition, catecholamines can directly inhibit cytokine production by Th1 cells by binding to the $\beta$2-adrenoreceptor which is expressed on Th1, but not Th2 cells [45]. Glucocorticoids and catecholamines can also induce apoptosis in lymphocytes [46].

The cholinergic anti-inflammatory pathway is a recently described neural-based circuit that can rapidly downregulate the activation of resident macrophages [28,47]. Increased activity of efferent vagus nerve fibers leads to a local release of acetylcholine, the principal neurotransmitter of the parasympathetic nervous system that binds to specific nicotinic receptors on macrophages and inhibits the release of pro-inflammatory cytokines, such as TNF-$\alpha$. While these observations indicate that the mediators of the HPA axis, sympathetic and parasympathetic nervous systems have predominantly anti-inflammatory effects, substantial experimental evidence suggests that the actions of these mediators can be sometimes pro-inflammatory depending on the context, the site of release, and their concentration. It should also be mentioned that various other neurotransmitters and neuroendocrine mediators, including the sensory neuropeptides, calcitonin gene-related peptide (CGRP), substance P, neuropeptide Y (NPY), vasoactive peptide (VIP), CRF, and $\alpha$-melanocyte-stimulating hormone ($\alpha$-MSH) have been found to modulate immune responses by binding to specific receptors expressed on immune cells.

## Immunodepression as a Result of CNS Injury

The release of pro-inflammatory cytokines in response to endogenous or exogenous stressors plays a central role in bacterial defense and tissue regeneration. However, excessive production of pro-inflammatory cytokines can lead to an overwhelming systemic inflammatory response which may result in shock and multiple organ failure (MOF). As mentioned above, in addition to autoregulatory mechanisms of immune cells, the CNS mounts a counterregulatory anti-inflammatory response to control inflammation (compensatory anti-inflammatory response syndrome, CARS). Ideally, inflammatory and anti-inflammatory responses to stress are balanced to allow containment of pathogens and wound healing, while preventing hyperinflammation. A well balanced anti-inflammatory action of the nervous system therefore appears to be beneficial to overcome the injurious insult and to restore homeostasis. An excessive neuroendocrine response particularly when triggered in the absence of systemic inflammation, may be detrimental, shutting down defense mechanisms and rendering the organism susceptible to infection. As described earlier, patients with acute CNS injury often demonstrate profound suppression of cell-mediated immune responses associated with an increased risk of infectious complications.

Clinical and experimental studies have provided evidence for the involvement of neuroendocrine pathways in the immunodepressive alterations after CNS injury. High plasma levels of adrenocorticotropic hormone (ACTH) and cortisol have been found in patients with traumatic brain injury, cerebral ischemic stroke, spinal cord injury, and neurosurgical patients [13,48–50]. Activation of the HPA axis was associated with decreased lymphocyte functions, monocyte deactivation (downregulation of monocytic human leukocyte antigen [HLA]-DR and secretion capacity of pro-inflammatory cytokines), and increased susceptibility to infections [13,50]. In a rat model of acute brain injury, Woiciechowsky et al. [16] demonstrated that sympathetic activation after brain injury triggers the rapid systemic release of IL-10, a cytokine with potent immunosuppressive activities. In the same study, brain injured patients showed strong signs of sympathetic activation associated with increased IL-10 plasma levels and strongly reduced monocytic HLA-DR expression. In accordance with marked signs of immunodepression, the majority of these patients developed severe infections [16]. Direct evidence for a causative link between a CNS injury-induced suppression of cell-mediated responses and the development of bacterial infections was recently provided in a mouse model of focal cerebral ischemia [51]. All mice spontaneously developed pneumonia and bacteremia about 3 days after cerebral ischemia. Infections were preceded by signs of profound inhibition of cell-mediated immunity which were observed as early as 12 hours after ischemia. Stroke induced a rapid and extensive apoptotic loss of lymphocytes in lymphoid organs and peripheral blood. Suppression of cellular immune functions was evident by decreased lymphocytic interferon-γ (IFNγ) and monocyte/macrophage TNF-α production. Adoptive transfer of IFNγ-producing lymphocytes (i.e., T and NK, but not B cells) from healthy littermates or treatment with recombinant IFNγ greatly diminished bacterial burden. Importantly, the defective IFNγ response and the occurrence of bacterial infections were prevented by blocking the sympathetic nervous system, but not the HPA axis, suggesting that a catecholamine-mediated lymphocyte dysfunction plays a major role in the impaired antibacterial defense after CNS injury. In summary, substantial clinical and experimental data support the notion that CNS injury-induced immunodepression is caused by an excessive neuroendocrine stress response, and that this is the major mechanism by which CNS injury results in infection (Fig. 1).

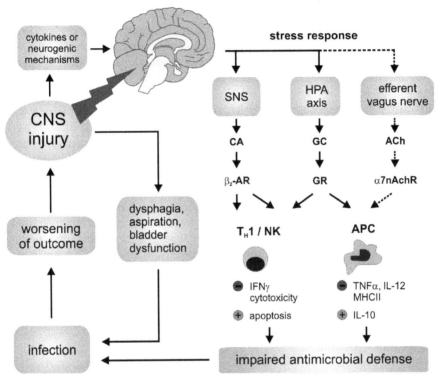

**Fig. 1.** Mechanisms of CNS injury-induced immunodepression and increased risk of infection after CNS injury. CNS injury induces a disturbance of the normally well balanced interplay between the immune system and the CNS. CNS injury leads to the release of inflammatory cytokines (e.g., interleukin [IL]-1β) in the damaged tissue, or the activation of 'neurogenic' mechanisms, resulting in the activation of the hypothalamo-pituitary-adrenal (HPA) axis and the sympathetic nervous system (SNS). Through the release of glucocorticoids and catecholamines, a systemic anti-inflammatory response is mounted that severely impairs antimicrobial defenses and results in increased risk of infections. Additional factors including the loss of protective reflexes leading to dysphagia, aspiration, and bladder dysfunction, and invasive medical procedures (e.g., catheters, mechanical ventilation) increase the risk of infection further. Systemic infection increases morbidity and mortality in patients with CNS injury, and leads to worsening of outcome. Although not yet proven by experimental evidence, it is proposed that the parasympathetic nervous system may be an important contributor to CNS injury-induced immunodepression. CNS injury may also result in enhanced activation of efferent vagus nerve fibers, leading to the release of acetylcholine and inhibition of macrophage function through binding to specific nicotinic acetylcholine receptors. CA: catecholamines; GC: glucocorticoids; Ach: acetylcholine; GR: glucocorticoid receptor; β2-AR: beta-2 adrenoreceptor; α7nAChR: alpha-7 subunit-containing nicotinic acetylcholine receptors; $T_H1$: type 1 T helper cell; NK: natural killer cell; APC: antigen-presenting cell; TNF-α: tumor necrosis factor-α; IFNγ: interferon-γ; MHCII: major histocompatibility class II molecules

A disturbance of the normally well balanced interplay between the CNS and the immune system may also contribute to the pathophysiology of other medical conditions, including severe sepsis and major surgery. Impaired CNS-mediated anti-inflammatory mechanisms would favor excessive production of pro-inflammatory mediators, resulting in shock, MOF, and death. In line with this, disruption of the HPA axis by hypophysectomy, or ablation of the cholinergic anti-inflammatory pathway by vagotomy, significantly increases the sensitivity of animals to the lethal effects of endotoxin due to enhanced production of pro-inflammatory cytokines [52]. On the other hand, an excessive stimulation of counterregulatory efferent CNS pathways in response to overwhelming systemic inflammation may result in severe immunodepression, rendering the host unable to mount an efficient antibacterial defense. Patients after major surgery or persistent sepsis, in which neuroendocrine activation is common, frequently show signs of temporary immunodepression including monocyte deactivation, lymphopenia, and impaired antigen-specific T cell responses [23, 53–55]. In its severest form, this immunodepression has been described as 'immunoparalysis', which is associated with an unfavorable outcome [56].

## Induction of CNS Injury-induced Immunodepression by Humoral Signaling?

The mechanisms by which CNS injury triggers SIRS remain to be elucidated. Several lines of clinical and experimental evidence indicate that pro-inflammatory cytokines produced within the damaged brain tissue can directly induce HPA axis and sympathetic nervous system activation. Increased levels of cytokines like IL-1$\beta$, TNF-$\alpha$, and IL-6 in brain parenchyma and CSF have been found in various brain disorders including trauma, subarachnoid hemorrhage, and ischemia [57]. In patients with brain injury or stroke, elevated levels of IL-6 released into the CSF and plasma have been shown to correlate with increased plasma ACTH and cortisol concentrations [48, 58, 59]. Intracerebroventricular administration of IL-1$\beta$ results in rapid increases in plasma ACTH, glucocorticoid, and catecholamine levels in rats and primates [60, 61]. Furthermore, various cellular immune responses including NK cell activity, mitogen-induced T-cell proliferation and cytokine production, as well as monocyte/macrophage functions, were found to be suppressed after administration of IL-1$\beta$ into the brain [60–63]. The partial or total prevention of IL-1$\beta$ induced changes by adrenalectomy, hypophysectomy, or $\beta_2$-adrenoceptor antagonists demonstrates the involvement of HPA axis and sympathetic nervous system activation in brain IL-1$\beta$-induced systemic immunosuppressive effects [60, 62, 63]. While these findings confirm the ability of raised intracerebral pro-inflammatory cytokine levels to activate the sympathetic nervous system and HPA axis, formal proof that pro-inflammatory cytokines are the primary trigger of immunodepression after CNS injury is lacking so far.

## Induction of CNS Injury-induced Immunodepression by 'Neurogenic' Mechanisms?

As outlined above, the release of pro-inflammatory cytokines within the CNS in the course of injury may result in CNS injury-induced immunodepression. Thus, the mechanisms for triggering CNS injury-induced immunodepression considered so far are very similar to those responsible for triggering anti-inflammatory responses when injury or infection occurs outside the CNS (CARS). In contrast to CARS, however, there may be additional, alternative pathways by which anti-inflammatory response and immunodepression are induced after CNS injury, pathways which do not rely on cytokine signaling. Damage to sites within the nervous system controlling neural-immune interactions (e.g., the hypothalamus) may lead to 'neurogenic' anti-inflammatory signals, without initial involvement of immune mechanisms.

As the autonomous system of the CNS is 'hard wired' with secondary lymphoid organs, it comes without surprise that interruption of these circuitries can result in immune dysfunction. Most types of CNS injury can lead to direct damage of sympathetic CNS structures involved in neuroimmunomodulation. These are located in the brain (frontal pre-motor cortex, thalamus, hypothalamus, formatio reticularis, hippocampus, cerebellum and brain stem) and spinal cord (columna lateralis and nucleus intermediolateralis). Sympathetic neurons in the spinal cord innervate the adrenal medulla, thymus, spleen and lymph-nodes [64]. Damage of sympathetic control centers in the spinal cord may directly affect immunity: After spinal cord injury the peripheral vegetative nervous system may escape supraspinal control and display segmental sympathetic autonomy. This results in a 'sympathetic reflex-like condition', which, for example, may give rise to hypertensive episodes, headache, or even cardiac arrest [65]. These symptoms of autonomic dysfunction result from stimulation of the sympathetic nervous system below the level of injury and are a consequence of pre-ganglionic injury, resulting in deafferentation of the CNS from the peripheral vegetative nervous system [65]. As sympathetic mediators can downregulate innate and adaptive immune responses, autonomic dysfunction may be accompanied by immunodepression. Thus, disruption of pre-ganglionic sympathetic pathways may cause 'reflex-like' sympathetic outflow to the lymphatic organs, resulting in immunodepression. This may not only apply to spinal cord injury, as autonomic dysfunction also occurs by similar mechanisms following stroke or transient ischemic attacks when brainstem or midbrain structures of sympathetic control are affected [66,67]. For example, because the direct neural connection from the medial preoptic area to the paraventricular nucleus is inhibitory [68], a lesion of the preoptic area or its fibers is predicted to trigger the release of CRF from the PVN, with resultant HPA and sympathetic nervous system activation and reduction in cellular immunity.

Further support for the concept of the neurogenic nature of CNS injury-induced immunodepression comes from studies on the lateralization of the autonomic nervous system within the brain. Lateralization of the structures of the vegetative nervous system [69,70] might serve to explain some localization dependent effects of neural-immune interactions subsequent to a brain lesion [71,72]. Furthermore, lateralization is also reflected in vegetative dysfunction following stroke [73,74]. Interestingly, post-injury activation of the sympathetic nervous system was most pronounced when the insular cortex of the right-hemisphere was affected [67].

The insular cortex receives projections from the NTS of the dorsal vagal complex in the medulla oblongata and sends fibers to the amygdala and lateral hypothalamus. The insular cortex thereby plays an important role in the higher control of the autonomic nervous system [75]. Thus, localization (e.g., insular infarction) and, to a lesser extent, size of infarction may differentially affect the degree and type of autonomic dysfunction in stroke patients [76]. Similarly, following spinal cord injury, the extent of vegetative dysfunction and corresponding immunodeficiency, which depends on lesion level, is correlated with the extent of sympathetic outflow deafferentation [65,77]. Spinal cord injury above thoracic level 6 results in marked reduction of intact sympathetic fibe is and supraspinal control of the spleen, as well as the vasculature of the lower extremity [65]. With regards to the immune system, complete tetraplegics, who are injured above the level of sympathetic outflow tracts, show a pronounced reduction in lymphocyte proliferation, responsiveness, and NK cell function. Moreover, the degree of immune dysfunction in spinal cord injury patients correlated well with the extent of deafferentation of the sympathetic outflow, with higher injuries inducing more severe immune dysfunction [21].

Only a few studies have directly addressed the issue of neurogenic mechanisms by which CNS lesions affect immune function. However, the existing evidence suggests that damage to vegetative control structures in the CNS may play an important role in the induction of CNS injury-induced immunodepression.

## How to Measure Immunodepression?

Because temporary immunodepression by itself does not present with clinical symptoms, paraclinical parameters are required for its early diagnosis. Several markers, including soluble plasma mediators (e.g., the ratio between pro- and anti-inflammatory cytokines), functional tests (e.g., endotoxin-induced cytokine production in whole blood, mitogen-induced T cell cytokine production and proliferation), and cell surface markers (e.g., HLA-DR expression on monocytes), have been evaluated for monitoring temporary immunodepression in critically ill patients. In particular, monocytic HLA-DR expression has been found to be a promising diagnostic tool for assessing the magnitude and persistence of immunodepression [54–56,78].

HLA-DR belongs to the family of MHC II molecules constitutively expressed on antigen presenting cells, including monocytes. The level of HLA-DR expression on monocytes is influenced by immuno-stimulatory and -inhibitory mediators. For example, it is increased by the immunostimulatory cytokine IFNγ and downregulated by anti-inflammatory mediators, such as IL-10, and the stress hormones glucocorticoids and catecholamines. Diminished monocytic HLA-DR expression has been shown to correlate with impaired cellular functions (particularly pro-inflammatory cytokine secretion capacity and induction of antigen-specific Th cell responses), indicating that monocytic HLA-DR expression may serve as a global marker for immunodepression/immunoparalysis [23]. Diminished monocytic HLA-DR expression was found to correlate with an increased risk of infections, for example, in patients with severe burns [78], following cardiopulmonary bypass (CBP) surgery [55], and in neurosurgical patients [50]. Ongoing studies in patients with cerebral ischemia from our laboratory also indicate that low monocytic HLA-DR early after stroke (i.e., already on day 1 after ischemia) can predict the development of infectious complications (unpublished results, C. Meisel, 2006). However, other studies have failed to demonstrate a prognostic value for HLA-DR in predicting secondary infections [79]. Similarly, many sepsis patients show severely reduced monocytic HLA-DR expression as a sign of immunoparalysis, but this only predicts poor outcome if persistent for more than 3 days [56].

Several reasons may explain the conflicting results regarding the predictive value of monocytic HLA-DR in critically ill patients. First, the consequences of immunodepression for clinical outcome of these patients appear to depend on the magnitude of immunodepression, its time course, and the underlying trigger. For example, at early time points following CPB surgery, all patients presented with low monocytic HLA-DR expression indicating severe immunodepression [55]. Whereas most patients recovered within 2 to 3 days after surgery without infectious complications, some patients showed persistent signs of severe immunodepression, leading to the development of infection. Secondly, all above mentioned studies were single center studies. In fact, no multicenter trials have been performed so far to ascertain the diagnostic value of monocytic HLA-DR expression, because of the lack of a standardized flow-cytometric assay. Differences in the pre-analytical handling of samples, the use of different HLA-DR antibodies, different flow cytometer and instrument settings, and different quantification strategies (HLA-DR levels expressed as either percentage of positive monocytes or mean fluorescence intensity) have made it difficult to compare the results of the various studies.

In collaboration with Becton Dickinson (Franklin Lakes, NJ, USA), our laboratory has recently developed a standardized assay for the quantification of monocytic HLA-DR expression, independent of the flow cytometer and instrument settings [80]. A multicenter comparison demonstrated excellent interassay and interlaboratory coefficients of variance of less than 10 and 25%, respectively [80]. The availability of a standardized assay for HLA-DR quantification will permit multicenter trials to further evaluate the diagnostic value of monocytic HLA-DR to predict infectious complications and outcome in critically ill patients.

## Conclusion

CNS injury is associated with an increased risk of infectious complications, which are important contributors to outcome in patients suffering from CNS injury. Clinical and experimental studies over recent years have provided substantial evidence that CNS injury downregulates the immune system through neural and neuroendocrine mechanisms, a mechanism which at least in part underlies the increased susceptibility to infections. Although the concept that brain-immune interactions after CNS injury have serious clinical implications is supported by increasingly more substantive data, many questions remain unanswered. For example, what are the mediators, receptors, anatomical structures, and pathways by which the CNS senses that it is injured? Does the parasympathetic nervous system contribute to CNS injury-induced immunodepression? Does CNS injury-induced immunodepression protect the CNS against autoaggressive immune responses by invading immune cells? Which parameters are useful in monitoring immunodepression and in predicting infectious complications in patients with CNS injury? How can we prevent or treat CNS injury-induced immunodepression without doing harm? CNS injury-induced immunodepression is a prototypical example for pathological brain-immune interactions. CNS injury-induced immunodepression after experimental stroke, traumatic brain injury, or spinal cord injury may also serve as a model to study the mechanisms and mediators by which the brain controls immunity during other pathophysiological conditions. A better understanding of CNS injury-induced immunodepression may eventually result in effective strategies that can improve outcome after CNS damage.

## References

1. Davenport RJ, Dennis MS, Wellwood I, Warlow CP (1996) Complications after acute stroke. Stroke 27:415–420
2. Johnston KC, Li JY, Lyden PD, et al (1998) Medical and neurological complications of ischemic stroke: experience from the RANTTAS trial. RANTTAS Investigators. Stroke 29:447–453
3. Fabregas N, Torres A (2002) Pulmonary infection in the brain injured patient. Minerva Anestesiol 68:285–290
4. Waites KB, Canupp KC, Chen Y, DeVivo MJ, Moser SA (2001) Bacteremia after spinal cord injury in initial versus subsequent hospitalizations. J Spinal Cord Med 24:96–100
5. Kalra L, Yu G, Wilson K, Roots P (1995) Medical complications during stroke rehabilitation. Stroke 26:990–994
6. Bronchard R, Albaladejo P, Brezac G, et al (2004) Early onset pneumonia: risk factors and consequences in head trauma patients. Anesthesiology 100:234–239
7. Woratyla SP, Morgan AS, Mackay L, Bernstein B, Barba C (1995) Factors associated with early onset pneumonia in the severely brain-injured patient. Conn Med 59:643–647
8. Prass K, Meisel C, Wolf T, Volk HD, Dirnagl U, Meisel A (2003) Striking the immune system – Stroke-induced immune depression. In: Krieglstein T (ed) Pharmacology of Cerebral Ischemia. Medpharm, Stuttgart, pp 217–221

9. Katzan IL, Cebul RD, Husak SH, Dawson NV, Baker DW (2003) The effect of pneumonia on mortality among patients hospitalized for acute stroke. Neurology 60:620–625
10. Reines HD, Harris RC (1987) Pulmonary complications of acute spinal cord injuries. Neurosurgery 21:193–196
11. DeVivo MJ, Black KJ, Stover SL (1993) Causes of death during the first 12 years after spinal cord injury. Arch Phys Med Rehabil 74:248–254
12. Marik PE (2001) Aspiration pneumonitis and aspiration pneumonia. N Engl J Med 344:665–671
13. Cruse JM, Lewis RE, Bishop GR, Kliesch WF, Gaitan E (1992) Neuroendocrine-immune interactions associated with loss and restoration of immune system function in spinal cord injury and stroke patients. Immunol Res 11:104–116
14. Czlonkowska A, Cyrta B, Korlak J (1979) Immunological observations on patients with acute cerebral vascular disease. J Neurol Sci 43:455–464
15. Quattrocchi KB, Frank EH, Miller CH, Amin A, Issel BW, Wagner FC, Jr. (1991) Impairment of helper T-cell function and lymphokine-activated killer cytotoxicity following severe head injury. J Neurosurg 75:766–773
16. Woiciechowsky C, Asadullah K, Nestler D, et al (1998) Sympathetic activation triggers systemic interleukin-10 release in immunodepression induced by brain injury. Nat Med 4:808–813
17. Meert KL, Long M, Kaplan J, Sarnaik AP (1995) Alterations in immune function following head injury in children. Crit Care Med 23:822–828
18. Quattrocchi KB, Frank EH, Miller CH, Dull ST, Howard RR, Wagner FC Jr (1991) Severe head injury: effect upon cellular immune function. Neurol Res 13:13–20
19. Imhoff M, Gahr RH, Hoffmann P (1990) Delayed cutaneous hypersensitivity after multiple injury and severe burn. Ann Ital Chir 61:525–528
20. Miller CH, Quattrocchi KB, Frank EH, Issel BW, Wagner FC Jr (1991) Humoral and cellular immunity following severe head injury: review and current investigations. Neurol Res 13:117–124
21. Campagnolo DI, Bartlett JA, Keller SE, Sanchez W, Oza R (1997) Impaired phagocytosis of Staphylococcus aureus in complete tetraplegics. Am J Phys Med Rehabil 76:276–280
22. Huschak G, Zur NK, Stuttmann R, Riemann D (2003) Changes in monocytic expression of aminopeptidase N/CD13 after major trauma. Clin Exp Immunol 134:491–496
23. Wolk K, Docke WD, von Baehr V, Volk HD, Sabat R (2000) Impaired antigen presentation by human monocytes during endotoxin tolerance. Blood 96:218–223
24. Asadullah K, Woiciechowsky C, Docke WD, et al (1995) Immunodepression following neurosurgical procedures. Crit Care Med 23:1976–1983
25. Elenkov IJ, Wilder RL, Chrousos GP, Vizi ES (2000) The sympathetic nerve – an integrative interface between two supersystems: the brain and the immune system. Pharmacol Rev 52:595–638
26. Pavlov VA, Tracey KJ (2004) Neural regulators of innate immune responses and inflammation. Cell Mol Life Sci 61:2322–2331
27. Steinman L (2004) Elaborate interactions between the immune and nervous systems. Nature Immunology 5:575–581
28. Pavlov VA, Wang H, Czura CJ, Friedman SG, Tracey KJ (2003) The cholinergic anti-inflammatory pathway: a missing link in neuroimmunomodulation. Mol Med 9:125–134
29. Mulla A, Buckingham JC (1999) Regulation of the hypothalamo-pituitary-adrenal axis by cytokines. Baillieres Best Pract Res Clin Endocrinol Metab 13:503–521
30. Goehler LE, Gaykema RP, Hansen MK, Anderson K, Maier SF, Watkins LR (2000) Vagal immune-to-brain communication: a visceral chemosensory pathway. Auton Neurosci 85:49–59
31. Banks WA, Kastin AJ, Broadwell RD (1995) Passage of cytokines across the blood-brain barrier. Neuroimmunomodulation 2:241–248

32. Buller KM (2001) Role of circumventricular organs in pro-inflammatory cytokine-induced activation of the hypothalamic-pituitary-adrenal axis. Clin Exp Pharmacol Physiol 28:581–589
33. Weindl A (1973) Neuroendocrine aspects of circumventricular organs. In: Ganong WF, Martini L (eds) Frontiers in Neuroendocrinology. Oxford University Press, New York, pp 3–32
34. Haddad JJ, Saade NE, Safieh-Garabedian B (2002) Cytokines and neuro-immune-endocrine interactions: a role for the hypothalamic-pituitary-adrenal revolving axis. J Neuroimmunol 133:1–19
35. Elenkov IJ, Papanicolaou DA, Wilder RL, Chrousos GP (1996) Modulatory effects of glucocorticoids and catecholamines on human interleukin-12 and interleukin-10 production: clinical implications. Proc Assoc Am Physicians 108:374–381
36. Van der PT, Coyle SM, Barbosa K, Braxton CC, Lowry SF (1996) Epinephrine inhibits tumor necrosis factor-alpha and potentiates interleukin 10 production during human endotoxemia. J Clin Invest 97:713–719
37. Hodge S, Hodge G, Flower R, Han P (1999) Methyl-prednisolone up-regulates monocyte interleukin-10 production in stimulated whole blood. Scand J Immunol 49:548–553
38. Cowan HB, Vick S, Conary JT, Shepherd VL (1992) Dexamethasone up-regulates mannose receptor activity by increasing mRNA levels. Arch Biochem Biophys 296:314–320
39. Liu Y, Cousin JM, Hughes J et al. (1999) Glucocorticoids promote nonphlogistic phagocytosis of apoptotic leukocytes. J Immunol 162:3639–3646
40. Wilckens T, De Rijk R (1997) Glucocorticoids and immune function: unknown dimensions and new frontiers. Immunol Today 18:418–424
41. Pan J, Ju D, Wang Q et al. (2001) Dexamethasone inhibits the antigen presentation of dendritic cells in MHC class II pathway. Immunol Lett 76:153–161
42. Schwiebert LM, Schleimer RP, Radka SF, Ono SJ (1995) Modulation of MHC class II expression in human cells by dexamethasone. Cell Immunol 165:12–19
43. Panina-Bordignon P, Mazzeo D, Lucia PD, et al (1997) Beta2-agonists prevent Th1 development by selective inhibition of interleukin 12. J Clin Invest 100:1513–1519
44. Blotta MH, DeKruyff RH, Umetsu DT (1997) Corticosteroids inhibit IL-12 production in human monocytes and enhance their capacity to induce IL-4 synthesis in CD4+ lymphocytes. J Immunol 158:5589–5595
45. Sanders VM, Baker RA, Ramer-Quinn DS, Kasprowicz DJ, Fuchs BA, Street NE (1997) Differential expression of the beta2-adrenergic receptor by Th1 and Th2 clones: implications for cytokine production and B cell help. J Immunol 158:4200–4210
46. Tuosto L, Cundari E, Montani MS, Piccolella E (1994) Analysis of susceptibility of mature human T lymphocytes to dexamethasone-induced apoptosis. Eur J Immunol 24:1061–1065
47. Tracey KJ (2002) The inflammatory reflex. Nature 420:853–859
48. Woiciechowsky C, Schoning B, Cobanov J, Lanksch WR, Volk HD, Docke WD (2002) Early IL-6 plasma concentrations correlate with severity of brain injury and pneumonia in brain-injured patients. J Trauma 52:339–345
49. Fassbender K, Schmidt R, Mossner R, Daffertshofer M, Hennerici M (1994) Pattern of activation of the hypothalamic-pituitary-adrenal axis in acute stroke. Relation to acute confusional state, extent of brain damage, and clinical outcome. Stroke 25:1105–1108
50. Asadullah K, Woiciechowsky C, Docke WD et al. (1995) Very low monocytic HLA-DR expression indicates high risk of infection–immunomonitoring for patients after neurosurgery and patients during high dose steroid therapy. Eur J Emerg Med 2:184–190
51. Prass K, Meisel C, Hoflich C, et al (2003) Stroke-induced immunodeficiency promotes spontaneous bacterial infections and is mediated by sympathetic activation reversal by poststroke T helper cell type 1-like immunostimulation. J Exp Med 198:725–736
52. Borovikova LV, Ivanova S, Zhang M, et al (2000) Vagus nerve stimulation attenuates the systemic inflammatory response to endotoxin. Nature 405:458–462

53. Hotchkiss RS, Karl IE (2003) The pathophysiology and treatment of sepsis. N Engl J Med 348:138–150
54. Monneret G, Finck ME, Venet F, et al (2004) The anti-inflammatory response dominates after septic shock: association of low monocyte HLA-DR expression and high interleukin-10 concentration. Immunol Lett 95:193–198
55. Strohmeyer JC, Blume C, Meisel C, et al (2003) Standardized immune monitoring for the prediction of infections after cardiopulmonary bypass surgery in risk patients. Cytometry B Clin Cytom 53:54–62
56. Volk HD, Reinke P, Docke WD (2000) Clinical aspects: from systemic inflammation to 'immunoparalysis'. Chem Immunol 74:162–77
57. Feuerstein GZ, Liu T, Barone FC (1994) Cytokines, inflammation, and brain injury: role of tumor necrosis factor-alpha. Cerebrovasc Brain Metab Rev 6:341–360
58. Johansson A, Olsson T, Carlberg B, Karlsson K, Fagerlund M (1997) Hypercortisolism after stroke–partly cytokine-mediated? J Neurol Sci 147:43–47
59. Szczudlik A, Dziedzic T, Bartus S, Slowik A, Kieltyka A (2004) Serum interleukin-6 predicts cortisol release in acute stroke patients. J Endocrinol Invest 27:37–41
60. Brown R, Li Z, Vriend CY, et al (1991) Suppression of splenic macrophage interleukin-1 secretion following intracerebroventricular injection of interleukin-1 beta: evidence for pituitary-adrenal and sympathetic control. Cell Immunol 132:84–93
61. Sullivan GM, Canfield SM, Lederman S, Xiao E, Ferin M, Wardlaw SL (1997) Intracerebroventricular injection of interleukin-1 suppresses peripheral lymphocyte function in the primate. Neuroimmunomodulation 4:12–18
62. Sundar SK, Becker KJ, Cierpial MA, et al (1989) Intracerebroventricular infusion of interleukin 1 rapidly decreases peripheral cellular immune responses. Proc Natl Acad Sci USA 86:6398–6402
63. Woiciechowsky C, Schoning B, Daberkow N, et al (1999) Brain-IL-1beta induces local inflammation but systemic anti-inflammatory response through stimulation of both hypothalamic-pituitary-adrenal axis and sympathetic nervous system. Brain Res 816:563–571
64. Stevens-Felten SY, Bellinger DL (1997) Noradrenergic and peptidergic innervation of lymphoid organs. Chem Immunol 69:99–131
65. Teasell RW, Arnold JM, Krassioukov A, Delaney GA (2000) Cardiovascular consequences of loss of supraspinal control of the sympathetic nervous system after spinal cord injury. Arch Phys Med Rehabil 81:506–516
66. Chesnut RM, Gautille T, Blunt BA, Klauber MR, Marshall LF (1998) Neurogenic hypotension in patients with severe head injuries. J Trauma 44:958–963
67. Meyer S, Strittmatter M, Fischer C, Georg T, Schmitz B (2004) Lateralization in autonomic dysfunction in ischemic stroke involving the insular cortex. Neuroreport 15:357–361
68. Saphier D, Feldman S (1986) Effects of stimulation of the preoptic area on hypothalamic paraventricular nucleus unit activity and corticosterone secretion in freely moving rats. Neuroendocrinology 42:167–173
69. Harper RM, Bandler R, Spriggs D, Alger JR (2000) Lateralized and widespread brain activation during transient blood pressure elevation revealed by magnetic resonance imaging. J Comp Neurol 417:195–204
70. Kalogeras KT, Nieman LK, Friedman TC, et al (1996) Inferior petrosal sinus sampling in healthy subjects reveals a unilateral corticotropin-releasing hormone-induced arginine vasopressin release associated with ipsilateral adrenocorticotropin secretion. J Clin Invest 97:2045–2050
71. Meador KJ, Loring DW, Ray PG, Helman SW, Vazquez BR, Neveu PJ (2004) Role of cerebral lateralization in control of immune processes in humans. Ann Neurol 55:840–844
72. Tarkowski E, Jensen C, Ekholm S, Ekelund P, Blomstrand C, Tarkowski A (1998) Localization of the brain lesion affects the lateralization of T-lymphocyte dependent cutaneous inflammation. Evidence for an immunoregulatory role of the right frontal cortex-putamen region. Scand J Immunol 47:30–36

73. Robinson RG (1979) Differential behavioral and biochemical effects of right and left hemispheric cerebral infarction in the rat. Science 205:707–710
74. Tarkowski E, Naver H, Wallin BG, Blomstrand C, Tarkowski A (1995) Lateralization of T-lymphocyte responses in patients with stroke. Effect of sympathetic dysfunction? Stroke 26:57–62
75. Cechetto DF, Chen SJ (1990) Subcortical sites mediating sympathetic responses from insular cortex in rats. Am J Physiol 258:R245-R255
76. Sander D, Klingelhofer J (1995) Changes of circadian blood pressure patterns and cardiovascular parameters indicate lateralization of sympathetic activation following hemispheric brain infarction. J Neurol 242:313–318
77. Popovich PG (2000) Immunological regulation of neuronal degeneration and regeneration in the injured spinal cord. Prog Brain Res 128:43–58
78. Sachse C, Prigge M, Cramer G, Pallua N, Henkel E (1999) Association between reduced human leukocyte antigen (HLA)-DR expression on blood monocytes and increased plasma level of interleukin-10 in patients with severe burns. Clin Chem Lab Med 37:193–198
79. Oczenski W, Krenn H, Jilch R, et al (2003) HLA-DR as a marker for increased risk for systemic inflammation and septic complications after cardiac surgery. Intensive Care Med 29:1253–1257
80. Docke WD, Hoflich C, Davis KA, et al (2005) Monitoring temporary immunodepression by flow cytometric measurement of monocytic HLA-DR expression: a multicenter standardized study. Clin Chem 51:2341–2347

# Organ-specific Mechanisms of Dysfunction

# Pulmonary Dysfunction

N.S. MacCallum, G.J. Quinlan, and T.W. Evans

## Introduction

### Definitions

The host response to infection and other forms of tissue injury has been termed the systemic inflammatory response syndrome (SIRS). Although controversy exists concerning the optimal defining criteria for SIRS, traditionally these have reflected changes in thermoregulation (body temperature > 38 °C or < 36 °C), cardiovascular (heart rate > 90 beats/min) and respiratory (tachypnea > 20 breaths/min) stability, and alterations in white blood cell count (> 12,000 cells/mm$^3$, < 4,000 cells/mm$^3$ or the presence of > 10% immature forms) [2]. When SIRS is attributable to an identifiable infectious process, it is termed sepsis. Sepsis complicated by predefined organ system dysfunction, through tissue or systemic hypotension, is regarded as severe [1]. Together, SIRS, sepsis, and septic shock have been termed the 'sepsis syndromes'.

### SIRS, Sepsis, and Severe Sepsis: Precipitating Factors

SIRS is seen in association with a wide variety of non-infectious insults, including major trauma and surgery [3]. The incidence of SIRS is high, and may affect up to 33% of all patients requiring hospital admission. It is also insult-dependent, and is particularly common following surgery. There is a progression between the different stages of the sepsis syndromes. Thus, the prevalence of infection and bacteremia increase with the number of SIRS criteria fulfilled, and some 30% and 25% of cases eventually evolve to meet the defining criteria for sepsis and severe sepsis, respectively [4].

## Incidence, Morbidity, and Mortality of Sepsis

### Incidence and Characteristics of Sepsis

In the USA, the national estimate of the incidence of severe sepsis was recently estimated to be 300 per 100,000 population per year, with a projected annual increase of 1.5% per annum [5]. In a parallel retrospective study, an annualized increase in incidence from 82.7 to 240.4 cases per 100,000 population was identified over a 22 year period. Although in-hospital mortality fell during the accounting period (from 27.8% to 17.9%), the total number of deaths rose [6]. Published statistics for the United Kingdom (UK), albeit for patients with severe sepsis cared for within intensive care units (ICUs), reveal a similar pattern. Thus, 27.1% of adult ICU admissions met the defining criteria for severe sepsis in the first 24 hours, producing an overall incidence of 51 cases per 100,000 population per year [7].

## Organ Failure in Sepsis

Patients with sepsis syndromes are characterized clinically by reduced systemic vascular resistance that is refractory to pressor agents, and display diminished cardiac compliance. Tissue hypoperfusion ensues, with cellular hypoxia and metabolic dysfunction. Consequently, the majority of patients with SIRS and its sequelae who fail to survive succumb to multiple organ dysfunctions. Indeed, multiple organ dysfunction contributes cumulatively to mortality in patients with sepsis in that some 15% of patients without organ failure die compared to 70% of those with 3 or more failing organs. The proportion of patients with organ failure complicating sepsis increased from 19.1–30.2% over the preceding 22 years from 1979–2000 [6].

## Lung Failure in Sepsis

The increased metabolic rate associated with sepsis necessitates a high minute volume requirement. The compliance of the respiratory system is diminished. Airway resistance is increased and muscle efficiency impaired [8]. Consequently, approximately 85% of patients with severe sepsis and septic shock require mechanical ventilatory support, typically for 7 to 14 days [9]. Such pulmonary dysfunction can be 'primary', resulting from, for example, a respiratory tract infection; or 'secondary' following some distant, non pulmonary infective insult and is classified by severity as acute lung injury (ALI) or its more extreme manifestation the acute respiratory distress syndrome (ARDS) (Table 1). ALI is characterized by increased pulmonary capillary permeability, and is defined clinically by arterial hypoxemia refractory to oxygen therapy alone ($PaO_2/FiO_2$ ratio $\leq 300$ mmHg) and on chest radiography by diffuse bilateral chest abnormalities indicative of alveolar edema. Patients with ARDS have more severe hypoxemia ($PaO_2/FiO_2 \leq 200$ mmHg) [1]. The lung is the most frequently failing organ in sepsis [10,11]; some 50% of patients suffering from sepsis complicated by respiratory failure meet the defining criteria for ARDS [12, 13]. Although functional impairment can take months to resolve and sub-clinical spirometric changes are sometimes permanent, unremitting lung failure is uncommon [14].

Table 1. Definitions of acute lung injury (ALI) and the acute respiratory distress syndrome (ARDS) [2]

| Timing | • acute onset |
|---|---|
| Oxygenation | • **ALI: PaO$_2$/FiO$_2$ ≤ 300 mmHg   (40 kPa)**<br>• **ARDS: PaO$_2$/FiO$_2$ ≤ 200 mmHg   (26.7 kPa)** |
| Chest radiograph | • **bilateral infiltrates seen on frontal chest radiograph,**<br>**(consistent with pulmonary edema)** |
| Pulmonary artery occlusion pressure | • **≤ 18 mmHg when measured or no clinical evidence**<br>**of left atrial hypertension** |

ALI is defined as a syndrome of inflammation and increased permeability associated with clinical, physiological and radiological abnormalities that cannot be explained, but may coexist with, left atrial or pulmonary capillary hypertension. ALI is acute in onset and persistent, characterized by refractory hypoxemia resistant to oxygen therapy alone and associated with diffuse radiological infiltrates.

## Pathophysiology of Sepsis

### The Dysfunctional Inflammatory Response

The precise pathophysiology of the sepsis syndromes remains unclear. However, evidence from a large number of sources and using a variety of experimental systems, indicates that both physical and infective insults lead initially to leukocyte recruitment to inflammatory foci. Leukocyte recruitment is mediated via the concerted action of adhesion molecules and chemo-attractants, termed chemokines, which provide a directional cue. How this host response is controlled once activated is less clear. Thus, individual cells possess the unique and altruistic ability to initiate self-destruction if their continued presence proves detrimental to the organism as a whole. Evidence suggests that this highly conserved process of self-initiated death, or apoptosis, is delayed in neutrophils taken from patients with sepsis [15, 16]. Thus, in patients undergoing rapid post-mortem examination following death attributable to the septic syndromes these processes are demonstrable in lung and other tissues [17], although the results are inconsistent. The relative contribution of apoptotic cell loss to pulmonary and other organ dysfunction is not known. Indeed, apoptosis may even be protective, by removing the potential of injured cells to necrose and further propagate the inflammatory response. Thus, an excessive and prolonged inflammatory host response is thought to lead to the vascular and cellular dysfunction and tissue hypoxia that characterizes the sepsis syndromes.

## Reactive Oxygen Species and the Inflammatory Response

The term reactive oxygen species (ROS) defines oxygen free radicals and related oxidizing/reducing oxygen intermediates. The production of such species in biological systems, whilst known to be essential for aerobic life, can lead to deleterious consequences when they are inadequately controlled. Indeed, the manifestation and accumulation of oxidative damage to biological molecules attributable to ROS has been shown in association with numerous inflammatory disease states [18]. Such findings have led to the hypothesis that excessive production of ROS, at levels that overwhelm endogenous (antioxidant) protective substances and stratagems, plays a causative role in the onset and progression of a range of conditions. Specifically, clear associations have been identified between a range of markers of oxidative stress and morbidity and mortality amongst the critically ill. More recently, these hypotheses have evolved beyond the concept that ROS are responsible for direct, oxidant-mediated cytotoxicity alone (reviewed in [19,20]). Rather, it is now recognized that the production of ROS at subtoxic levels signals a variety of changes in cell function. This so-called 'redox signaling' function of ROS has been linked to the regulation of the inflammatory response, with significant implications for both the development and resolution of inflammation (Fig. 1).

## Role of ROS, Cytotoxicity, Iron, and Cell Signaling in the Pathophysiology of the Sepsis Syndromes and Lung Failure

For some years, it has been known that free iron can catalyze the formation of ROS, but it has also recently been shown to play a crucial role in modulating cell-signaling, either directly or via a modulating effect on redox regulation. Indeed, oxidant/anti-oxidant imbalance, redox signaling, and iron-mediated catalytic reactions are now implicated in the inflammatory processes that characterize the sepsis syndromes. Thus, plasma concentrations of thiobarbituric acid reactant substances (TBARS), an index of oxidative stress, have been shown to correlate positively with rising severity of illness scores (e. g., Sequential Organ Failure Assessment [SOFA]) in the critically ill. TBARS were significantly higher in those with organ system failure. Moreover, the duration of SIRS was significantly associated with the percentage increase in plasma TBARS concentration [21]. Second, neutrophil accumulation in patients with SIRS and ALI complicating surgery involving cardiopulmonary bypass (CPB) is associated with elevated indices of neutrophil-derived pro-oxidant activity [22]. Third, dynamic changes in the regulation of iron metabolism significantly influence morbidity and mortality in patients with sepsis, SIRS, and ALI/ARDS and are associated with oxidative damage to proteins and lipids (reviewed in [23]), and changes to redox-regulated cell signaling moieties. Fourth, the role of oxidative stress in the pathogenesis of ALI/ARDS attributable to a wide variety of infective and non-infective insults now seems established. Thus, oxidative damage to plasma proteins and lipids is detectable, and a mortality predictor, in patients with established ARDS [24–27]. Deficiencies in anti-oxidant

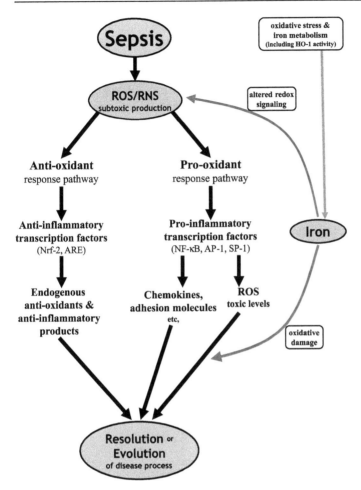

**Fig. 1.** The role of reactive oxygen (ROS) and nitrogen (RNS) species in the inflammatory response. ROS/RNS initiate pro and anti-oxidant responses, the equilibrium of which determines redox balance, which in turn affects the outcome of the disease process. Nrf-2: NF-E2-related factor 2; ARE: anti-oxidant response elements; NF-κB: nuclear factor kappa B; AP-1: activator protein 1; SP-1: stimulating transcription factor 1

protection against the catalytic effects of iron in these patients have been demonstrated [28]. Fifth, plasma iron mobilization is significantly associated with the development of ALI in patients with SIRS following CPB surgery [29]. Such patients had low molecular mass redox active iron detectable in plasma as a result of the surgical procedure [30]. Significant associations between iron levels and the specific marker of lipid oxidation 4-hydroxy-2-nonenal have also been shown in these patients [31], a result strongly indicative of pronounced iron-catalyzed oxidative stress. Indeed, low molecular mass iron is measurable in plasma from patients with sepsis and ARDS [32]. Sixth, markers of hydroxyl-radical mediated oxidative damage (peroxynitrite and hypochlorous acid) were detectable in bronchoalveo-lar lavage (BAL) fluid from patients with ARDS [33,34]. Moreover, aberrant iron chemistry and significantly increased levels of non-heme iron was demonstrated in BAL from those who failed to survive [35].

Indeed, iron mobilization before and during critical illness appears to form a key part of the susceptibility to, and pathogenesis and clinical manifestations of, the sepsis syndromes. Why such pronounced alterations in body iron mobilization and chemistry occur during the onset of acute inflammatory episodes is unclear, but may represent a defensive need to limit microbial invasion and virulence; iron being an absolute requirement for bacterial growth. The anti-microbial properties of blood and other tissues cannot be maintained unless there are exceptionally low levels of iron available. An atypical availability of iron is responsible for fatal septicemia, due to inundation of the phagocytic system by rapidly multiplying organisms when iron is freely available [36,37].

Results obtained from observational studies in patients with the sepsis syndromes 'at risk' of, and with established ALI/ARDS, indicate that the formation of ROS occurs in these populations at levels that overwhelm endogenous antioxidant defenses. They also suggest that iron mobilization before and during critical illness contributes to these processes and forms a key part of the susceptibility to, and pathogenesis and clinical manifestations of, the sepsis syndromes (Fig. 2).

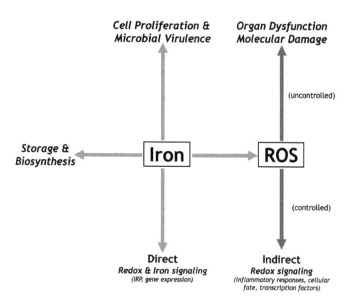

Fig. 2. Key biologic roles of iron. Iron can signal directly via iron regulatory protein (IRP) activity, be stored and used for biosynthesis, or effect cell proliferation and act as a microbial virulence factor. Iron can also act indirectly via redox signaling potentially causing organ dysfunction and damage, but in controlled signaling events it may have beneficial effects. ROS: reactive oxygen species

## Trials of Anti Oxidants in Patients with ALI/ARDS

In promising early studies, n-acetylcysteine (NAC) improved static lung compliance, pulmonary vascular resistance, and chest X-ray scores as well as reducing the number of days that patients suffered from a low $PaO_2/FiO_2$ ratio [38]. Patients with mild to moderate lung injury showed similar improvements [39], although no difference was found in mortality, length of ventilatory support, or improvement in oxygenation in those with established ARDS [40–43]. A large phase III trial of procysteine was stopped early due to concern over mortality in the treatment arm of the study. Currently, there is little evidence that intravenous NAC or procysteine are of benefit to patients with ARDS. This lack of a survival advantage may reflect naivety in terms of the nature and dose of the interventions employed, and concerning their ability to modify both the cytotoxic consequences of pro-oxidant stress, and the influence of redox imbalance on cell signaling processes.

## Direct and Indirect Iron-Regulated Cell Signaling Mechanisms: Role of Iron Regulatory Proteins and Hemoxygenases

### Direct Mechanisms

Recently, interest in the role of ROS and reactive nitrogen species (RNS) at subtoxic levels and their subsequent involvement in redox signaling has increased substantially. Indeed, the expression of numerous substances implicated in the inflammatory response, including apoptosis, may be regulated by such mechanisms (reviewed in [44, 45]. Low molecular mass iron is a key signaling determinant for the activity of the iron regulatory proteins (IRP-1,2) that control the expression of synthesis proteins containing iron-responsive elements, and in particular transferrin receptors and ferritin, both of which are intimately involved in cellular iron uptake and storage.

Associations between iron-signaling and the onset and progression of critical illness are emerging. Specifically, there may be circumstances in which the heme oxygenases (HO)-1 and -2, known enzymatic sources of low molecular mass iron, initiate regulatory responses in the IRPs via an iron-signaling mechanism. Catabolism of heme by the HOs produces iron, carbon monoxide and bilirubin. To date, little research effort has centered on investigating the role of iron produced by HOs in directing functional changes in cell signaling moieties. Constitutive enzymatic activity and iron-production by HO-2 may be significant in this regard, but the upregulation of (inducible) HO-1, which is now known to occur in critical illness, is likely the primary mediator in this process (Fig. 3).

HO-1 induced by oxidative stress as part of the inflammatory response is usually considered to be cytoprotective [46], but can produce lung injury in animal models relevant to critical illness by mechanisms related to the formation of low molecular mass redox active iron [47]. HO-1 is upregulated in rats subjected to

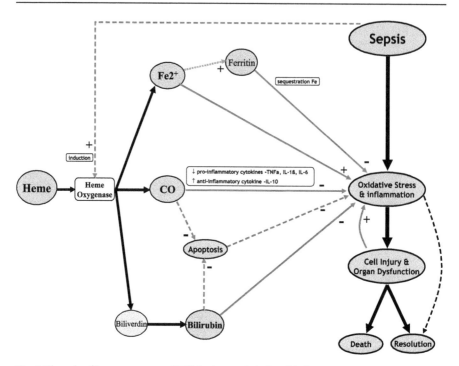

**Fig. 3.** The role of heme oxygenase (HO) in the sepsis induced inflammatory process. HO generates bilverdin, carbon monoxide (CO) and ferrous iron (Fe2$^{+}$) in equimolar amounts from the oxidation of heme. Positive and negative signs denote stimulation and inhibition of processes. CO downregulates pro-inflammatory cytokines, tumor necrosis factor (TNF)-$\alpha$, interleukin (IL)-1$\beta$, IL-6, and upregulates anti-inflammatory cytokine, IL-10. Fe2$^{+}$ induces the synthesis of ferritin, which it in turn sequesters, representing a possible anti-inflammatory role for ferritin

iron overload, and more rapidly in lung than in other organs [48]. Further, organ-specific regulation of ferritin and transferrin receptor synthesis occurs in response to challenge with lipopolysaccharide (LPS). In this rodent model, HO inhibition or iron chelation had pronounced effects on steady state IRP activity. In terms of enzymatic activity, the iron-mediated pro oxidant affects of HO outweighed its anti-oxidant effects.

Upregulation of such cellular iron accumulation mechanisms could have pro-oxidant implications specific to the lung which is exposed to the external environment of microbes and toxins, with a mandatory requirement for anti-oxidant and anti-microbial defenses. In this context, elevated HO-1 protein has been demonstrated in lung tissue and plasma of patients with ARDS compared with controls. Moreover, a significant association between iron mobilization and HO-1 levels, and HO-1 and ferritin or soluble transferrin receptors can be demonstrated in BAL fluid from patients with established ARDS [49] (Fig. 4).

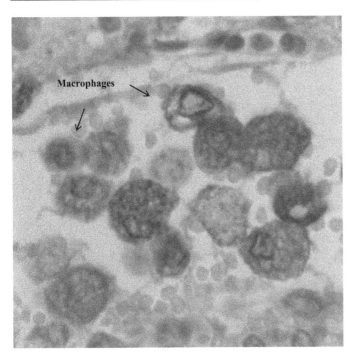

**Fig. 4.** Intense heme oxygenase HO-1 staining in macrophages from a patient with acute respiratory distress syndrome (ARDS) (40x magnification). (Reproduced courtesy of Dr. R.L. Upton [78])

## Iron-regulated Cell Signaling Moieties

Some such signaling responses are mediated via the effects of iron on redox-sensitive signaling processes [23, 50]. Indeed, the activity of several transcription factors can be regulated by iron of various forms under particular circumstances and in specific cell types. For instance, the activity of nuclear factor-kappa B (NF-κB) [51–53], activator protein (AP)-1 and specificity protein (SP)-1 [54, 55] can be influenced either through increasing the supply of iron or restricting the use of chelators. Iron availability also regulates activity of the nuclear transcription factor, hypoxia inducible factor (HIF). The hypoxia response pathway senses levels of ambient oxygen and responds to low oxygen tensions by upregulating the transcription of numerous genes including vascular endothelial growth factor (VEGF), erythropoietin and HO-1. HIF activation is now recognized to direct these transcriptional events leading to the expression of a variety of bio-active substances and the regulation of functional aspects including apoptosis. HIF is itself regulated by the hydroxylation of key prolyl residues which, when hydroxylated, inhibit transcription activity and lead to proteasomal destruction. This regulatory action is an enzyme-driven process catalyzed by key prolyl hydroxylases with an absolute requirement for 2-oxoglutarate and ferrous iron [56]. HIF is often described as an oxygen sensing transcription factor, but could equally be regarded as an iron sensing moiety.

HIF is likely to be key in regulating the cellular response to inflammation in critical illness, given that a redistribution of microcirculatory perfusion and tissue hypoxia characterize the sepsis syndromes [57]. Second, cyclical stretch in endothelial and epithelial cells, as occurs in the pulmonary circulation during mechanical ventilation, is now known to influence HIF activity [58]. Iron availability may also impact on the anti-oxidant response pathway, as it is also regulated by ROS/RNS (see Fig. 1).

### Substrate Availability and Cell Signaling Processes

Evidence suggests that a number of cellular iron-signaling processes implicated in the inflammatory response are regulated by the HOs. Substrate availability for these enzymes is likely to be of key importance in determining the nature of the response. Exposure of isolated healthy human neutrophils to hemin or oxyhemoglobin, over a biologically relevant dose range for 24 hours, results in significantly decreased levels of apoptosis [59]. Results obtained are comparable to those achieved using granulocyte macrophage stimulating factor (GM-CSF). Further, neutrophil persistence is associated with increased expression of (inducible) HO-1, a known anti-apoptotic factor [60].

A diverse array of heme containing substances are potential substrates for the HOs. Extracellular sources include hemoglobin, myoglobin, myeloperoxidase, and free heme, and intracellular sources include cytochrome c, catalase, and an array of other heme containing proteins. The conditions and clinical scenarios under which substrates are presented for heme catabolism are equally diverse, but all represent a significant risk for the onset and progression of ALI.

Such data have profound implications for the sepsis syndromes and their sequelae, in that neutrophil longevity has been linked with the development of SIRS and sepsis, and has adverse prognostic significance in patients with ARDS [61]. These experimental and clinical data suggest an important relationship between HO-1 induction, and iron availability and regulation in the lungs of patients with the sepsis syndromes complicated by ARDS. The ability of HO-1 and HO-2 to produce ROS and oxidative damage via iron catalysis clearly demonstrates the potential for this enzymatic pathway to influence redox signaling processes via an indirect iron-signaling mechanism. Moreover, the ability of HOs to regulate the IRP network strongly suggests that this pathway also has the ability to signal regulatory change directly via iron.

## Endothelial and Epithelial Dysfunction

### Loss of Barrier Function

The consequence of the pathophysiological mechanisms outlined above is increased permeability of the alveolar-capillary membrane, which is composed of the microvascular endothelium and the alveolar epithelium. The epithelium, which serves as a barrier to the systemic circulation and regulates both formation and removal of fluid in the lung, is less permeable than the endothelium. It is composed of type I flat cells and type II cuboidal cells, constituting 90% and 10% of the alveolar surface area, respectively. Type II cells, which are easily injured in comparison to the more resistant type I cells, are responsible for surfactant production, ion transport, proliferation, and differentiation into type I cells. Damage and repair of the alveolar epithelium is important in both the development of and recovery from lung injury [62–64]. Indeed, the degree of alveolar injury is a key predictor of outcome [65, 66]. Loss of epithelial integrity and injury to type II cells disrupts normal epithelial fluid transport, impairing removal of edema fluid from the alveolar space contributing to alveolar flooding. Additionally, injury to type II cells reduces production and turnover of surfactant [67, 68]. Disorganized and insufficient epithelial repair leads to fibrosis in cases where epithelial injury is severe.

Endothelial injury results in increased vascular permeability, resulting in the influx of protein rich edema fluid into alveolar airspaces and interstitium during the acute phase of ALI [69]. Initially this is balanced by an increase in alveolar fluid clearance, potentially allowing recovery from the initial precipitant of lung injury. Patients with higher alveolar fluid clearance in ALI have improved survival [70,71]. However, loss of this steady state leads to formation of pulmonary edema, which can be compounded by elevated pulmonary vascular volume and pressure. There is a current NHLBI trial investigating whether lowering lung vascular pressures in patients with ALI/ARDS improves outcome by reducing extravasated protein-rich edema fluid.

## Loss of Pulmonary Vascular Control

Patients with ARDS demonstrate refractory hypoxemia. Under physiological circumstances, the distribution of pulmonary blood flow is regulated by a local action of alveolar oxygen tension on pre-capillary pulmonary vessels. Thus, the reflex of hypoxic pulmonary vasoconstriction ensures that blood flow is diverted away from areas of damaged lung, thereby preserving the matching of ventilation (V) and perfusion (Q). However, patients with ARDS demonstrate diminished hypoxic pulmonary vasoconstriction leading to adverse changes in V/Q matching, which accounts in substantial degree for the refractory hypoxemia which characterizes the clinical syndrome [72]. This is thought due at least in part to an imbalance in the release of endothelially-derived vasodilator (e. g., NO) and vasoconstrictor (e. g., endothelins) substances [73]. It is possible that changes in redox balance also modulate hypoxic pulmonary vasoconstriction.

## Repair and Fibrosis

The reparative or fibroproliferative phase of ARDS is characterized by histological evidence of fibrosis with acute and chronic inflammatory cellular infiltration
and partial resolution of pulmonary edema. Newly formed blood vessels, mesenchymal cells, and their products fill the alveolar spaces. There is accumulation
of collagen and fibronectin in the lung. Transforming growth factor-$\beta$ (TGF-$\beta$)
is capable of enhancing mesenchymal cell proliferation and extracellular matrix
formation. Three isoforms have been identified in humans, of which TGF-$\beta$1 is
most associated with the development of pulmonary fibrosis. Functionally active
TGF-$\beta$1 has been documented within the first 24 hours of diagnosis of ARDS [74].
Macrophages are also able to release a variety of cytokines capable of regulating the
fibrotic process. Macrophage-produced platelet derived growth factor (PDGF) is
a potent mitogen and chemoattractant of fibroblasts and smooth muscle cells, and
is capable of stimulating collagen synthesis. Insulin like growth factor-1 (IGF-1)
increases fibroblast proliferation. Tumor necrosis factor (TNF)-$\alpha$ is responsible for
the production of IGF-1 and TGF-$\beta$ [75,76]. There is also collagen deposition early
in the evolution of lung injury. BAL fluid from patients with ARDS contains elevated levels of type I pro-collagen coupled with a decrease in markers of collagen
degradation, favoring net type I collagen deposition [77]. Fibrosis and elevated
levels of pro-collagen III peptide are associated with an increased mortality.

## Conclusion

Sepsis is increasing in incidence and is commonly complicated by organ failure, of which the lung is the most common. Pronounced changes in cellular iron
regulation occur in such patients, leading to dysregulation of the inflammatory
response through the regulation of pro-oxidant potential and apoptotic function.
The availability of heme substrate determines the nature of a range of responses
to pro-inflammatory stimuli, especially in endothelial cells and neutrophils. HO-1
expression accompanies these changes and early indications suggest that fluxes in
cellular iron levels direct the responses. Clinically relevant mechanical and biological stimuli result in similar pro-inflammatory responses in alveolar epithelial
(like) cells, suggesting that a common signaling pathway directs iron-mediated
responses. Finally, damage to alveolar epithelial cell and the microvascular endothelium leads to changes in pulmonary structure and function that characterize
ALI/ARDS.

## References

1. Levy MM, Fink MP, Marshall JC, et al (2003) 2001 SCCM/ESICM/ACCP/ATS/SIS International
   Sepsis Definitions Conference. Crit Care Med 31:1250–1256

2. Bernard GR, Artigas A, Brigham KL, et al (1994) Report of the American-European Consensus conference on acute respiratory distress syndrome: definitions, mechanisms, relevant outcomes, and clinical trial coordination. Consensus Committee. J Crit Care 9:72–81
3. Brun-Buisson C (2000) The epidemiology of the systemic inflammatory response. Intensive Care Med 26 (Suppl 1):S64–74
4. Rangel-Frausto MS, Pittet D, Costigan M, Hwang T, Davis CS, Wenzel RP (1995) The natural history of the systemic inflammatory response syndrome (SIRS). A prospective study. JAMA 273:117–123
5. Angus DC, Linde-Zwirble WT, Lidicker J, Clermont G, Carcillo J, Pinsky MR (2001) Epidemiology of severe sepsis in the United States: analysis of incidence, outcome, and associated costs of care. Crit Care Med 29:1303–1310
6. Martin GS, Mannino DM, Eaton S, Moss M (2003) The epidemiology of sepsis in the United States from 1979 through 2000. N Engl J Med 348:1546–1554
7. Padkin A, Goldfrad C, Brady AR, Young D, Black N, Rowan K (2003) Epidemiology of severe sepsis occurring in the first 24 hrs in intensive care units in England, Wales, and Northern Ireland. Crit Care Med 31:2332–2338
8. Field S, Kelly SM, Macklem PT (1982) The oxygen cost of breathing in patients with cardiorespiratory disease. Am Rev Respir Dis 126:9–13
9. Wheeler AP, Bernard GR (1999) Treating patients with severe sepsis. N Engl J Med 340:207–214
10. Finfer S, Bellomo R, Lipman J, French C, Dobb G, Myburgh J (2004) Adult-population incidence of severe sepsis in Australian and New Zealand intensive care units. Intensive Care Med 30:589–596
11. Brun-Buisson C, Meshaka P, Pinton P, Vallet B (2004) EPISEPSIS: a reappraisal of the epidemiology and outcome of severe sepsis in French intensive care units. Intensive Care Med 30:580–588
12. Bernard GR, Wheeler AP, Russell JA, et al (1997) The effects of ibuprofen on the physiology and survival of patients with sepsis. The Ibuprofen in Sepsis Study Group. N Engl J Med 336:912–918
13. Wheeler AP, Christma B, Swindell B, et al (1998) Lung dysfunction in sepsis: impact of ibuprofen. Am J Respir Crit Care Med 157 (Suppl):A115 (abst)
14. Suntharalingam G, Regan K, Keogh BF, Morgan CJ, Evans TW (2001) Influence of direct and indirect etiology on acute outcome and 6-month functional recovery in acute respiratory distress syndrome. Crit Care Med 29:562–566
15. Mahidhara R, Billiar TR (2000) Apoptosis in sepsis. Crit Care Med 28 (Suppl4):N105–113
16. Oberholzer C, Oberholzer A, Clare-Salzler M, Moldawer LL (2001) Apoptosis in sepsis: a new target for therapeutic exploration. Faseb J 15:879–892
17. Hotchkiss RS, Swanson PE, Freeman BD, et al (1999) Apoptotic cell death in patients with sepsis, shock, and multiple organ dysfunction. Crit Care Med 27:1230–1251
18. Gutteridge JM (1993) Free radicals in disease processes: a compilation of cause and consequence. Free Radic Res Commun 19:141–158
19. Forman HJ, Fukuto JM, Torres M (2004) Redox signaling: thiol chemistry defines which reactive oxygen and nitrogen species can act as second messengers. Am J Physiol Cell Physiol 287:C246–256
20. Haddad JJ (2003) Science review: redox and oxygen-sensitive transcription factors in the regulation of oxidant-mediated lung injury: role for hypoxia-inducible factor-1alpha. Crit Care 7:47–54
21. Motoyama T, Okamoto K, Kukita I, Hamaguchi M, Kinoshita Y, Ogawa H (2003) Possible role of increased oxidant stress in multiple organ failure after systemic inflammatory response syndrome. Crit Care Med 31:1048–1052
22. Sinclair DG, Haslam PL, Quinlan GJ, Pepper JR, Evans TW (1995) The effect of cardiopulmonary bypass on intestinal and pulmonary endothelial permeability. Chest 108:718–724

23. Quinlan GJ, Chen Y, Evans TW, Gutteridge JM (2001) Iron signalling regulated directly and through oxygen: implications for sepsis and the acute respiratory distress syndrome. Clin Sci (Lond) 100:169–182

24. Quinlan GJ, Evans TW, Gutteridge JM (1994) Linoleic acid and protein thiol changes suggestive of oxidative damage in the plasma of patients with adult respiratory distress syndrome. Free Radic Res 20:299–306

25. Quinlan GJ, Evans TW, Gutteridge JM (1994) Oxidative damage to plasma proteins in adult respiratory distress syndrome. Free Radic Res 20:289–298

26. Quinlan GJ, Evans TW, Gutteridge JM (1994) 4-hydroxy-2-nonenal levels increase in the plasma of patients with adult respiratory distress syndrome as linoleic acid appears to fall. Free Radic Res 21:95–106

27. Quinlan GJ, Lamb NJ, Evans TW, Gutteridge JM (1996) Plasma fatty acid changes and increased lipid peroxidation in patients with adult respiratory distress syndrome. Crit Care Med 24:241–246

28. Gutteridge JM, Quinlan GJ, Mumby S, Heath A, Evans TW (1994) Primary plasma antioxidants in adult respiratory distress syndrome patients: changes in iron-oxidizing, iron-binding, and free radical-scavenging proteins. J Lab Clin Med 124:263–273

29. Messent M, Sinclair DG, Quinlan GJ, Mumby SE, Gutteridge JM, Evans TW (1997) Pulmonary vascular permeability after cardiopulmonary bypass and its relationship to oxidative stress. Crit Care Med 25:425–429

30. Pepper JR, Mumby S, Gutteridge JM (1994) Transient iron-overload with bleomycin-detectable iron present during cardiopulmonary bypass surgery. Free Radic Res 21:53–58

31. Quinlan GJ, Mumby S, Pepper J, Gutteridge JM (1994) Plasma 4-hydroxy-2-nonenal levels during cardiopulmonary bypass, and their relationship to the iron-loading of transferrin. Biochem Mol Biol Int 34:1277–1282

32. Gutteridge JM, Quinlan GJ, Evans TW (1994) Transient iron overload with bleomycin detectable iron in the plasma of patients with adult respiratory distress syndrome. Thorax 49:707–710

33. Lamb NJ, Quinlan GJ, Westerman ST, Gutteridge JM, Evans TW (1999) Nitration of proteins in bronchoalveolar lavage fluid from patients with acute respiratory distress syndrome receiving inhaled nitric oxide. Am J Respir Crit Care Med 160:1031–1034

34. Lamb NJ, Gutteridge JM, Baker C, Evans TW, Quinlan GJ (1999) Oxidative damage to proteins of bronchoalveolar lavage fluid in patients with acute respiratory distress syndrome: evidence for neutrophil-mediated hydroxylation, nitration, and chlorination. Crit Care Med 27:1738–1744

35. Gutteridge JM, Mumby S, Quinlan GJ, Chung KF, Evans TW (1996) Pro-oxidant iron is present in human pulmonary epithelial lining fluid: implications for oxidative stress in the lung. Biochem Biophys Res Commun 220:1024–1027

36. Bullen JJ, Ward CG, Rogers HJ (1991) The critical role of iron in some clinical infections. Eur J Clin Microbiol Infect Dis 10:613–617

37. Patruta SI, Horl WH (1999) Iron and infection. Kidney Int Suppl 69:S125–130

38. Bernard GR (1991) N-acetylcysteine in experimental and clinical acute lung injury. Am J Med 91:54S–59S

39. Ortolani O, Conti A, De Gaudio AR, Masoni M, Novelli G (2000) Protective effects of N-acetylcysteine and rutin on the lipid peroxidation of the lung epithelium during the adult respiratory distress syndrome. Shock 13:14–18

40. Suter PM, Domenighetti G, Schaller MD, Laverriere MC, Ritz R, Perret C (1994) N-acetylcysteine enhances recovery from acute lung injury in man. A randomized, double-blind, placebo-controlled clinical study. Chest 105:190–194

41. Jepsen S, Herlevsen P, Knudsen P, Bud MI, Klausen NO (1992) Antioxidant treatment with N-acetylcysteine during adult respiratory distress syndrome: a prospective, randomized, placebo-controlled study. Crit Care Med 20:918–923

42. Domenighetti G, Suter PM, Schaller MD, Ritz R, Perret C (1997) Treatment with N-acetylcysteine during acute respiratory distress syndrome: a randomized, double-blind, placebo-controlled clinical study. J Crit Care 12:177–182

43. Bernard GR, Wheeler AP, Arons MM, et al (1997) A trial of antioxidants N-acetylcysteine and procysteine in ARDS. The Antioxidant in ARDS Study Group. Chest 112:164–172

44. Kamata H, Hirata H (1999) Redox regulation of cellular signalling. Cell Signal 11:1–14

45. Mates JM, Sanchez-Jimenez FM (2000) Role of reactive oxygen species in apoptosis: implications for cancer therapy. Int J Biochem Cell Biol 32:157–170

46. Jin Y, Choi AM (2005) Cytoprotection of heme oxygenase-1/carbon monoxide in lung injury. Proc Am Thorac Soc 2:232–235

47. Dennery PA, Visner G, Weng YH, et al (2003) Resistance to hyperoxia with heme oxygenase-1 disruption: role of iron. Free Radic Biol Med 34:124–133

48. Anning PB, Chen Y, Lamb NJ, et al (1999) Iron overload upregulates haem oxygenase 1 in the lung more rapidly than in other tissues. FEBS Lett 447:111–114

49. Mumby S, Upton RL, Chen Y, et al (2004) Lung heme oxygenase-1 is elevated in acute respiratory distress syndrome. Crit Care Med 32:1130–1135

50. Kotamraju S, Kalivendi SV, Konorev E, Chitambar CR, Joseph J, Kalyanaraman B (2004) Oxidant-induced iron signaling in Doxorubicin-mediated apoptosis. Methods Enzymol 378:362–382

51. Lin M, Rippe RA, Niemela O, Brittenham G, Tsukamoto H (1997) Role of iron in NF-kappa B activation and cytokine gene expression by rat hepatic macrophages. Am J Physiol 272:G1355–1364

52. Jeong HJ, Chung HS, Lee BR, et al (2003) Expression of proinflammatory cytokines via HIF-1alpha and NF-kappaB activation on desferrioxamine-stimulated HMC-1 cells. Biochem Biophys Res Commun 306:805–811

53. Xiong S, She H, Takeuchi H, et al (2003) Signaling role of intracellular iron in NF-kappaB activation. J Biol Chem 278:17646–17654

54. Kramer-Stickland K, Edmonds A, Bair WB, 3rd, Bowden GT (1999) Inhibitory effects of deferoxamine on UVB-induced AP-1 transactivation. Carcinogenesis 20:2137–2142

55. Tsuji Y, Torti SV, Torti FM (1998) Activation of the ferritin H enhancer, FER-1, by the cooperative action of members of the AP1 and Sp1 transcription factor families. J Biol Chem 273:2984–2992

56. Hewitson KS, McNeill LA, Elkins JM, Schofield CJ (2003) The role of iron and 2-oxoglutarate oxygenases in signalling. Biochem Soc Trans 31:510–515

57. Sair M, Etherington PJ, Peter Winlove C, Evans TW (2001) Tissue oxygenation and perfusion in patients with systemic sepsis. Crit Care Med 29:1343–1349

58. Mumby SP, Griffiths L, Callister MJD, et al (2004) Cyclical stretch of A549 cells increases HIF-1 DNA binding activity. Am J Respir Crit Care Med 169:A737 (abst)

59. Melley DD, deSouza PM, Quinlan GJ, Evans TW (2004) Hemoglobin delays apoptosis in isolated human neutrophils. Am J Respir Crit Care Med 169 (Suppl 7):A65 (abst)

60. Melley DD, Bettinson HV, Quinlan GJ, Evans TW (2004) Hemin and hemoglobin induce the enzyme heme oxygenase 1 in isolated human neutrophils. Am J Respir Crit Care Med 167 (Suppl 7):A415 (abst)

61. Aggarwal A, Baker CS, Evans TW, Haslam PL (2000) G-CSF and IL-8 but not GM-CSF correlate with severity of pulmonary neutrophilia in acute respiratory distress syndrome. Eur Respir J 15:895–901

62. Pittet JF, Mackersie RC, Martin TR, Matthay MA (1997) Biological markers of acute lung injury: prognostic and pathogenetic significance. Am J Respir Crit Care Med 155:1187–1205

63. Wiener-Kronish JP, Albertine KH, Matthay MA (1991) Differential responses of the endothelial and epithelial barriers of the lung in sheep to Escherichia coli endotoxin. J Clin Invest 88:864–875

64. Martin TR, Hagimoto N, Nakamura M, Matute-Bello G (2005) Apoptosis and epithelial injury in the lungs. Proc Am Thorac Soc 2:214–220

65. Matthay MA, Wiener-Kronish JP (1990) Intact epithelial barrier function is critical for the resolution of alveolar edema in humans. Am Rev Respir Dis 142:1250–1257
66. Ware LB, Matthay MA (1999) Maximal alveolar epithelial fluid clearance in clinical acute lung injury: an excellent predictor of survival and duration of mechanical ventilation. Am J Respir Crit Care Med 159 (Suppl):A694 (abst)
67. Gregory TJ, Longmore WJ, Moxley MA, et al (1991) Surfactant chemical composition and biophysical activity in acute respiratory distress syndrome. J Clin Invest 88:1976–1981
68. Greene KE, Wright JR, Steinberg KP, et al (1999) Serial changes in surfactant-associated proteins in lung and serum before and after onset of ARDS. Am J Respir Crit Care Med 160:1843–1850
69. Pugin J, Verghese G, Widmer MC, Matthay MA (1999) The alveolar space is the site of intense inflammatory and profibrotic reactions in the early phase of acute respiratory distress syndrome. Crit Care Med 27:304–312
70. Ware LB, Matthay MA (2001) Alveolar fluid clearance is impaired in the majority of patients with acute lung injury and the acute respiratory distress syndrome. Am J Respir Crit Care Med 163:1376–1383
71. Saldias FJ, Comellas A, Ridge KM, Lecuona E, Sznajder JI (1999) Isoproterenol improves ability of lung to clear edema in rats exposed to hyperoxia. J Appl Physiol 87:30–35
72. Dantzker DR, Brook CJ, Dehart P, Lynch JP, Weg JG (1979) Ventilation-perfusion distributions in the adult respiratory distress syndrome. Am Rev Respir Dis 120:1039–1052
73. Curzen NP, Griffiths MJ, Evans TW (1994) Role of the endothelium in modulating the vascular response to sepsis. Clin Sci (Lond) 86:359–374
74. Fahy RJ, Lichtenberger F, McKeegan CB, Nuovo GJ, Marsh CB, Wewers MD (2003) The acute respiratory distress syndrome: a role for transforming growth factor-beta 1. Am J Respir Cell Mol Biol 28:499–503
75. Krein PM, Winston BW (2002) Roles for insulin-like growth factor I and transforming growth factor-beta in fibrotic lung disease. Chest 122 (Suppl 6):289S–293S
76. Shimabukuro DW, Sawa T, Gropper MA (2003) Injury and repair in lung and airways. Crit Care Med 31 (Suppl 8):S524–531
77. Armstrong L, Thickett DR, Mansell JP, et al (1999) Changes in collagen turnover in early acute respiratory distress syndrome. Am J Respir Crit Care Med 160:1910–1915
78. Upton RL (2004) Inducible Haem Oxygenase as a Key Mediator of Iron-Signalling Processes: Implications for Critical Illness. Imperial College, University of London, London

# The Gut

M.P. Fink

## Introduction

The gut probably participates in the pathogenesis of the multiple organ dysfunction syndrome (MODS) in many different ways. In order to keep this chapter focused and concise, the author will focus on three potential mechanisms: 1) alterations in intestinal epithelial permeability, leading to the systemic absorption of pro-inflammatory mediators or toxins derived from luminal microbes; 2) release into the lymphatic drainage from the gut of toxic materials; 3) release from enterocytes of pro-inflammatory cytokines, especially high mobility group box 1 (HMGB1).

## Intestinal Epithelial Permeability is Increased in Critically Ill Patients

Alterations in the barrier function of the intestinal epithelium could permit the leakage of bacteria or microbial products, such as lipopolysaccharide (LPS) or exotoxin A (ETA), from the lumen of the gut into the systemic compartment, leading to the initiation or amplification of a deleterious inflammatory response and/or direct toxic effects on distant tissues. The notion that this process actually occurs in patients with MODS is supported by results from a number of clinical studies, which have documented increases in intestinal epithelial permeability in a variety of acute conditions that are associated with systemic inflammation [1–7]. Moreover, in several recent studies, increased intestinal permeability in critically ill patients has been shown to be associated with an increased risk of complications, MODS, or even mortality [3,4,7–9].

The strong association between increased gut mucosal permeability and MODS and mortality in critical illness suggests the existence of a causal linkage: i. e., the gut is the 'motor' that drives development of MODS [10]. There is, however, another, equally plausible, possibility. According to this second notion, altered gut mucosal permeability during critical illness is just one aspect of a more generalized phenomenon that affects epithelial barrier function in a variety of organs, including the lungs, liver, and kidneys [11]. This more global view suggests the pathophysiological mechanisms that are responsible for the derangements in gut barrier function also pertain to epithelia in other organs. Moreover, this view suggests that many of the clinical features of MODS, such as alveolar flooding in the lung, cholestatic jaundice, and azotemia, can be explained – at least in part –

by a single unifying cellular mechanism: impaired expression and/or targeting of some or all of the proteins that form the tight junctions (see below) between adjacent epithelial cells.

## Alterations in Intestinal Epithelial Permeability

The normal functioning of the lungs, liver, kidneys, and intestine, among other organs, depends on the establishment and maintenance of compositionally distinct compartments that are lined by sheets of epithelial cells. An essential element in this process is the formation of tight junctions between adjacent cells making up the epithelial sheet. The tight junction serves as a fence that differentiates the cytosolic membrane into apical and basolateral domains. This fence function preserves cellular polarity and, in combination with transcellular vectorial transport processes, generates distinct internal environments in the opposing compartments that are formed by the epithelial sheet. In addition, the tight junction acts as a regulated semi-permeable barrier that limits the passive diffusion of solutes across the paracellular pathway between adjacent cells. Thus, the barrier function of the tight junction is necessary to prevent dissipation of the concentration gradients that exist between the two compartments defined by the epithelium. In some organs, notably the gut and the lung, this barrier function is also important to prevent systemic contamination by microbes and toxins that are present in the external environment [12].

## Multiple Proteins are Necessary for the Assembly and Function of Tight Junctions

The formation of tight junction involves the assembly of at least nine different peripheral membrane proteins and at least three different integral membrane proteins [13]. Among the peripheral membrane proteins associated with tight junctions are the membrane-associated guanylate kinase-like (MAGUK) proteins, ZO-1, ZO-2, and ZO-3. The integral membrane proteins involved in tight junction formation include, but are not limited to, occludin, and members of a large class of proteins called claudins. Both occludin and the claudins contain four transmembrane domains and are thought to be the actual points of cell-cell contact within the tight junction [14]. ZO-1 has been shown to interact with the cytoplasmic tails of occludin and the claudins [15]. In addition, ZO-1 interacts with ZO-2 and ZO-3, which then interact with various actin-binding proteins, such as pp120$^{CAS}$ [16, 17], thereby linking the tight junction with the cytoskeleton. Studies of mouse embryos indicate that ZO-1 localizes in plasma membrane plaques well before occludin is incorporated [18, 19], suggesting that ZO-1 probably plays a central role in the assembly of mature tight junctions.

## Nitric Oxide (NO) and/or Peroxynitrite (ONOO⁻) Are Involved in the Regulation of Tight Junction Protein Expression and Function

We [20–22] and others [23–25] have shown that the permeability of cultured epithelial monolayers increases when the cells are incubated with various pro-inflammatory cytokines. The mechanisms responsible for cytokine-induced epithelial hyperpermeability are incompletely understood. It is known, however, that compounds that spontaneously release NO increase the permeability of cultured intestinal epithelial cell monolayers [26,27]. This observation is pertinent, since incubating Caco-2 human enterocyte-like cells with the pro-inflammatory cytokine, interferon (IFN)-γ, or a mixture of the pro-inflammatory cytokines, IFNγ + tumor necrosis factor (TNF) and interleukin (IL)-1β, leads to increased expression of inducible NO synthase (iNOS) and increased production of NO [21, 28, 29]. Moreover, compounds that inhibit iNOS have been shown to ameliorate the development of hyperpermeability induced by exposing Caco-2 cells to IFNγ [21] or 'cytomix' (IFN-γ + TNF + (IL)-1β) [29]. Similarly, L-N(6)-(1-iminoethyl)lysine (L-NIL), an isoform-selective iNOS inhibitor, blocks the development of hyperpermeability when Calu-3 (human alveolar epithelial) monolayers are incubated with cytomix [30]. Thus, IFN-γ or cytomix appear to increase intestinal epithelial permeability, at least in part, by increasing the production of NO by enterocytes.

NO reacts rapidly with superoxide ($O_2^-$) to form the potent oxidizing and nitrating species, ONOO⁻ [31, 32]. Several lines of evidence support the view that ONOO⁻ (or some related species) rather than NO *per se* is responsible for the deleterious effects of NO on intestinal epithelial barrier function. Thus, when Caco-2 monolayers are incubated with the NO donor, SNAP, permeability is significantly increased, but the magnitude of the effect is small [27]. Furthermore, the permeability of Caco-2 monolayers is not affected when the cells are incubated with pyrogallol, a compound that spontaneously generates $O_2^-$ in aqueous solutions [27]. However, if Caco-2 cells are co-incubated with both SNAP and pyrogallol, then epithelial permeability is dramatically increased [27]. SNAP-induced hyperpermeability is also markedly enhanced by co-incubating the cells with diethyldithiocarbamate, a compound that is known to inactivate Cu-Zn superoxide dismutase and would thereby be expected to increase the concentration of endogenously generated $O_2^-$ [27]. Taken together, these findings support the view that NO-induced hyperpermeability is enhanced by the simultaneous availability of $O_2^-$; i.e., conditions favoring the formation of ONOO⁻. Since ONOOH is a weak acid (pKa~6.8) and many of the effects of ONOO⁻ are thought to be mediated by an unstable form of the protonated species, studies from our group showing that NO-induced hyperpermeability is enhanced under mildly acidic conditions further support the notion that ONOO⁻/ONOOH is the responsible moiety [20,33].

The mechanism(s) responsible for NO- or ONOO⁻-mediated intestinal epithelial hyperpermeability remain to be elucidated. However, our laboratory reported that NO generated endogenously as the result of iNOS expression induced by incubating Caco-2 cells with cytomix, or exogenously from the NO donor DETA-NONOate [(Z)-1-[2(2-aminoethyl)-N-(2-ammonioethyl) amino]diazen-1-

ium-1,2-diolate] decreased the expression and impaired proper localization of the tight junction proteins, ZO-1, ZO-3, and occludin [22]. We also showed that incubating Caco-2 cells with either DETA-NONOate or cytomix increases the expression of another key tight junction protein, claudin-1, and promotes the accumulation of this protein in what appear to be vesicles within the cells. These findings support the view that NO (or a related reactive species) increases epithelial permeability by causing derangements in the expression and/or localization of several key tight junction proteins.

## NO-dependent Changes in $Na^+,K^+$-ATPase Activity can Affect Tight Junction Assembly and Function

Sugi et al. proposed that one way that NO might alter the expression or localization of various tight junction proteins is by modulating the activity of the membrane pump, $Na^+,K^+$-ATPase [34]. In a series of studies using monolayers of T84 enterocyte-like cells, these investigators reported that intracellular sodium concentration and cell volume increase following exposure to the pro-inflammatory cytokine, IFNγ. Additionally, Sugi et al. showed that incubating T84 cells with either NO or IFNγ decreases the expression and activity of $Na^+,K^+$-ATPase. Remarkably, growing the monolayers in medium with low sodium concentration inhibits the development of hyperpermeability following exposure to IFNγ and also prevents IFNγ-induced alterations in occludin expression. These findings suggest a pathway that involves the following steps: IFNγ (and/or other pro-inflammatory cytokines) → iNOS induction → NO production → inhibition of $Na^+,K^+$-ATPase expression and function → cell swelling → altered expression and/or targeting of tight junction proteins (e. g., occludin) → hyperpermeability.

Qayyum et al. reported that treatment of rat brain membranes with $ONOO^-$ *in vitro* decreases the activity of the $Na^+,K^+$-ATPase, and hypothesized that this effect may be caused by nitration of the $Na^+,K^+$-ATPase [35]. However, these authors did not demonstrate that $ONOO^-$ actually modifies the $Na^+,K^+$-ATPase. In an earlier report, the same authors also implicated lipid peroxidation in the inactivation of the $Na^+, K^+$-ATPase [36], but only showed an association between lipid peroxidation and altered $Na^+,K^+$-ATPase activity in their studies. However, these authors convincingly showed that ROS decrease the affinity of the $Na^+,K^+$-ATPase for $Na^+$ and $K^+$, inhibiting transport of these ions [35,36]. Taken together, these results support the notion that oxidative or nitrosative post-translational modifications of $Na^+,K^+$-ATPase can lead to decreased epithelial barrier function.

## Functional iNOS Expression is Essential for LPS-induced Alterations in Intestinal Permeability in Mice

Several years ago, our laboratory showed that gut mucosal permeability to a fluorescent macromolecule, fluorescein isothiocyanate-labeled dextran (molecular mass, 4 kDa; FD4), was increased 24 hours after injecting rats with a low dose of

LPS [37]. However, when rats were treated with either of two chemically dissimilar isoform-selective iNOS inhibitors, aminoguanidine or S-methylisothiourea, the injection of LPS failed to increase gut mucosal permeability.

In a more recent study, the biochemical basis for the increase in gut mucosal permeability was investigated by our laboratory. Specifically, C57Bl/6J mice were injected with a sublethal (2 mg/kg) dose of E. coli LPS, and ileal mucosal permeability to FD4 was assessed 18 hours later [38]. Although mucosal permeability increased significantly when mice were injected with LPS, treatment with L-NIL, an isoform-selective iNOS inhibitor [39], reversed this effect. Basal ileal mucosal permeability in control (PBS-treated) iNOS knockout (iNOS$^{-/-}$) mice on a C57Bl/6J background was greater than that measured in control (wild-type) iNOS$^{+/+}$ mice, a finding that is consistent with reports that basal levels of NO are required for normal gut homeostasis [40, 41]. Despite a basal defect in intestinal barrier function in iNOS$^{-/-}$ mice, permeability to FD4 failed to increase further when these mice were challenged with LPS.

In these studies [38], we used a portion of ileal tissue to prepare total and NP-40 (detergent)-insoluble protein extracts, the latter being enriched for tight junction-associated and other cytoskeletal proteins [42]. Total protein extracts were subjected to immunoblotting. NP-40 insoluble proteins were first solubilized with detergent-containing buffer and concentrated by immunoprecipitation prior to immunoblotting. The expression of occludin in NP-40 insoluble extracts was decreased in samples obtained 6 hours after injecting mice with LPS [38]. Occludin expression in NP-40 insoluble extracts decreased still further at 12 hours, but was starting to return toward normal 18 hours after LPS challenge. In total protein extracts, changes in occludin levels were less dramatic, and the maximal decrease was observed at 12 hours. ZO-1 expression decreased slightly in total protein extracts from ileal mucosa of mice exposed to LPS. However, there was a large decrease in ZO-1 levels in the NP-40 insoluble fraction. This finding suggests that the ZO-1 that is present in the cells of endotoxemic animals is unable to assemble into tight junctions. Consistent with our observations obtained using the Caco-2 system [22], claudin-1 expression increased in total protein extracts prepared from ileal mucosa. Immunoblotting total protein extracts for actin revealed equivalent loading of the samples in these gels. As expected, iNOS protein expression increased in total protein extracts from ileal mucosa of LPS-treated mice.

## Endotoxemia is Associated with Derangements in Ileal Mucosal Tight Junction Protein Localization

Immunohistochemical studies of ileal tissue from endotoxemic mice were performed using samples harvested 12 hours after injection of LPS. ZO-1 formed a continuous staining pattern around the enterocyte layer near the apical region of the lateral membrane of crypt and villous cells of the epithelium and the endothelium of the lamina propria from normal mice. Following injection of mice with LPS, ZO-1 staining was maintained in the crypts, but staining progressively decreased over the tips of the villi. In sections from endotoxemic mice, the staining patterns for ZO-1 were disrupted only in focal regions of the ileum; approximately 60% of the villi in a given section stained normally. If the endotoxemic mice were treated with L-NIL to pharmacologically block iNOS-dependent NO production, then the correct targeting of ZO-1 in the ileal mucosa was preserved. Similar findings were obtained when staining was carried out for occludin instead of ZO-1.

Parallel experiments were performed using iNOS$^{-/-}$ mice. The levels of occludin and ZO-1 in ileal mucosa from control iNOS$^{-/-}$ mice (i. e., those not challenged with LPS) were reproducibly lower than the levels of these proteins in control iNOS$^{+/+}$ mice. To some extent, these basal differences in occludin and ZO-1 expression confounded interpretation of the results obtained in LPS-challenged animals. Nevertheless, it was apparent that injecting iNOS$^{-/-}$ mice with LPS failed to cause a further decrease in the expression of ZO-1 or occludin in ileal mucosa. The localization of ZO-1 and occludin was preserved in ileal sections prepared from LPS-treated iNOS$^{-/-}$ mice, being essentially unchanged from what was observed in sections from iNOS$^{-/-}$ animals injected with vehicle.

## Surgical Stress Leads to Systemic Absorption of Gut-derived Toxins

Dating back to the era of Jacob Fine [43, 44], investigators have recognized that the gut represents a huge reservoir of bacteria-derived products, especially LPS, and that derangements in gut barrier function might lead to systemic absorption of these agents. Although Moore et al. were unable to detect LPS in the portal venous or peripheral venous blood samples obtained from critically ill trauma victims [45], other clinical and laboratory findings provide strong support for the notion that LPS can be systemically absorbed in patients or animals with acute conditions, such as hemorrhagic shock [46], necrotizing pancreatitis [5–7], or cardiopulmonary bypass [47, 48], that are associated with derangements in gut mucosal permeability.

Despite its other name, endotoxin, LPS is not really a toxin in the true sense of the word. Rather LPS is toxic because it is capable of activating intracellular signaling pathways in a variety of cell types, leading to the production of a variety of potentially cytotoxic mediators, including ROS and cytokines, such as TNF. However, in addition to releasing LPS and other pro-inflammatory molecules, many bacteria also produce extremely potent true toxins. For example, *Pseudomonas aeruginosa* are known to secrete at least 19 different soluble exoproteins, including several exotoxins (A, S, U and Y), elastase, staphylolytic protease, lipase, and phospholipase C. ETA is distantly related to diphtheria toxin produced by *Corynebacterium diphtheriae* [49]. Both ETA and diphtheria toxin kill the eukaryotic cells of the host by promoting mono-ADP-ribosylation and, thereby, inactivation of a key protein, translation elongation factor 2 (eEF2), which is essential for protein synthesis [49]. ETA is an extremely potent toxin, possessing a LD50 (dose that kills 50% of treated animals) of 0.2 g/kg following intraperitoneal injection into mice [49].

Based on a remarkable series of publications from Alverdy and colleagues at the University of Chicago as well as other investigators, data have accumulated to support the hypothesis that surgical stress (or presumably other forms of critical illness) lead to two synergistic gut-related consequences that promote development of distant organ dysfunction and even mortality. First, *P. aeruginosa* within the gut lumen respond to signals from the host, such as the cytokine, IFNγ [50], other factors released by hypoxic enterocytes [51], or norepinephrine [52]. In response to these signals, the bacteria increase their expression of virulence proteins, such as the PA-I lectin, a protein that is capable of causing derangements in gut epithelial permeability. Second, when *P. aeruginosa* are incubated under hypoxic conditions, secretion of ETA increases substantially [53]. It is likely that IFNγ also increases ETA secretion by *P. aeruginosa,* although this hypothesis remains to be tested. Thus, through a variety of mechanisms, critical illness can both increase elaboration within the gut lumen of a very potent toxin (ETA) and increase the permeability of the intestinal epithelium, permitting systemic absorption of this protein. The validity of this concept has been directly verified in a series of elegant *in vivo* studies using mice [52].

## Release of Toxic Materials into the Lymphatic Drainage from the Gut

Although many lines of investigation suggested that the gut might be the "motor of multiple organ system failure" [10], the failure in some key clinical studies to observe clear evidence of LPS in portal venous blood [45] or bacteria in mesenteric lymph nodes [54] in trauma victims led to skepticism about this concept. Nevertheless, two research groups, one directed by Deitch in Newark and another directed by Moore in Denver, formulated a novel hypothesis to explain the data: rather than the portal venous system, the draining mesenteric lymphatics might be the source of key gut-derived factors that promote distant organ dysfunction in critical illness [55,56]. Over the past few years, an impressive body of evidence, obtained mostly by studying rat models of hemorrhagic shock or burn injury, has accumulated in support of this concept. Briefly, it has been shown that post-shock (but not control) mesenteric lymph primes or activates neutrophils *in vitro* [56,57], and is toxic to various cell types in culture [57]. Furthermore, ligation of the main draining mesenteric lymphatic in rats ameliorates hemorrhagic shock- or burn-induced distant organ injury [55,56,58]. Finally, administration of post-shock (but not control) mesenteric lymph is capable of inducing distant organ dysfunction in rodents [55].

The precise nature of the factor (or factors) in post-shock lymph that is responsible for its deleterious actions remains elusive. Both lipophilic [59–61] and hydrophilic [61,62] factors have been implicated. One of the factors may be a peptide, derived from the action of serine proteases on albumin [61,63].

## Release from Enterocytes of Pro-inflammatory Cytokines

The gastrointestinal tract is the largest immune organ in the body. Numerous specialized lymphocytes, intraepithelial lymphocytes (IELs), reside between adjacent enterocytes within the epithelium. Plasma cells, lymphocytes, macrophages, mast cells, and neutrophils are present within the lamina propria even under basal conditions, and, following the induction of a local or systemic inflammatory response, many more immune cells migrate into this layer of the bowel wall as well as into the muscularis propria. These immune cells are capable of producing a wide array of cytokines and other mediators, such as platelet activating factor (PAF) and histamine.

Although they are not 'professional' immune cells, enterocytes making up the epithelial layer of the gut are capable of secreting chemokines [64, 65], cytokines [66, 67] and other pro-inflammatory mediators [68]. Recent data from our laboratory suggest that HMGB1, a recently discovered cytokine-like protein, is among the pro-inflammatory substances that are released by immunostimulated enterocytes.

High-mobility group proteins are small DNA-binding proteins that serve an important role in transcriptional regulation [69]. One of these proteins, HMGB1, has been identified as a late-acting mediator of LPS- [70] or sepsis-induced [71] lethality in mice. HMGB1 also has been implicated as a mediator LPS- [72] or hemorrhagic shock-induced acute lung injury (ALI) in mice [73]. Additionally, our laboratory showed that adding recombinant HMGB1 to the culture medium for Caco-2 human enterocyte-like monolayers increases the permeability of the epithelial barrier to a fluorescent macromolecule, fluorescein isothiocyanate-labeled dextran with an average molecular mass of 4,000 Da (FD4) [74]. Moreover, we showed that injecting mice with HMGB1 induces gut mucosal hyperpermeability to FD4 and promotes bacterial translocation to mesenteric lymph nodes [74]. Additional studies have documented that HMGB1 is a cytokine-like molecule that can promote TNF release from mononuclear cells [75].

HMGB1 also has been implicated in the pathogenesis of human disease. In the original report describing HMGB1 as a mediator of LPS-induced lethality, Abraham et al. reported that circulating levels of this protein are increased in patients with severe sepsis [72]. Shortly thereafter, Ombrellino and co-workers described a patient with high circulating levels of HMGB1 following an episode of hemorrhagic shock [76]. More recently, increased levels of HMGB1 mRNA have been detected in whole blood samples from patients with septic shock, particularly among non-survivors [77]. Similarly, persistently high serum levels of HMGB1 protein have been detected in patients with septic shock [78]

HMGB1 is actively secreted by immunostimulated macrophages [70, 79–81], natural killer cells [82], and pituicytes [83]. This protein is also released by necrotic, but not apoptotic, cells [84]. Because HMGB1 has been shown to modulate intestinal epithelial barrier function [74], we hypothesized that active secretion by enterocytes might be yet another source for this cytokine-like protein. Recently, we reported that stimulating either Caco-2 cells or primary cultures of murine enterocytes with cytomix induced secretion of HMGB1 [85]. Additionally, we showed that addition of a neutralizing polyclonal anti-HMGB1 antibody partially blocked the increase in permeability caused by incubating Caco-2 monolayers with cytomix [85]. The data also indicate that HMGB1 is secreted in soluble form as well as a particulate form that is sequestered within exosomes. These data support the view that enterocyte-derived HMGB1 may be an autocrine amplifier of derangements in epithelial barrier function initiated by other pro-inflammatory stimuli.

## References

1. Langkamp-Henken B, Donovan TB, Pate LM, Maull CD, Kudsk KA (1995) Increased intestinal permeability following blunt and penetrating trauma. Crit Care Med 23:660–664
2. Pape H-C, Dwenger A, Regel G, et al (1994) Increased gut permeability after multiple trauma. Br J Surg 81:850–852
3. Kompan L, Kremzar B, Gadzijev E, Prosek M (1999) Effects of early enteral nutrition on intestinal permeability and the development of multiple organ failure after multiple injury. Intensive Care Med 25:157–161
4. Faries PL, Simon RJ, Martella AT, Lee MJ, Machiedo GW (1998) Intestinal permeability correlates with severity of injury in trauma patients. J Trauma 44:1031–1036
5. Penalva JC, Martinez J, Laveda R, et al (2004) A study of intestinal permeability in relation to the inflammatory response and plasma endocab IgM levels in patients with acute pancreatitis. J Clin Gastroenterol 38:512–517
6. Ammori BJ, Fitzgerald P, Hawkey P, McMahon MJ (2003) The early increase in intestinal permeability and systemic endotoxin exposure in patients with severe acute pancreatitis is not associated with systemic bacterial translocation: molecular investigation of microbial DNA in the blood. Pancreas 26:18–22
7. Ammori BJ, Leeder PC, King RFGJ, et al (1999) Early increase in intestinal permeability in patients with severe acute pancreatitis: correlation with endotoxemia, organ failure, and mortality. J Gastrointest Surg 3:252–262
8. Doig CJ, Sutherland LR, Sandham JD, Fick GH, Verhoef M, Meddings JB (1998) Increased intestinal permeability is associated with the development of multiple organ dysfunction syndrome in critically ill ICU patients. Am J Respir Crit Care Med 158:444–451
9. Oudemans-van Straaten HM, Jansen PG, Hoek FJ, et al (1996) Intestinal permeability, circulating endotoxin, and postoperative systemic responses in cardiac surgery patients. J Cardiothorac Vasc Anesth 10:187–194
10. Carrico CJ, Meakins JL, Marshall JC, Fry D, Maier RV (1985) Multiple-organ-failure syndrome. Arch Surg 121:196–208
11. Fink MP, Delude RL (2005) Epithelial barrier dysfunction: a unifying theme to explain the pathogenesis of multiple organ dysfunction at the cellular level. Crit Care Clin 21:177–196
12. Stevenson BR (1999) Understanding tight junction clinical physiology at the molecular level. J Clin Invest 104:3–4
13. Tsukita S, Furuse M, Itoh M (2001) Multifunctional strands in tight junctions. Nat Rev Mol Cell Biol 2:285–293
14. Tsukita S, Furuse M (2000) The structure and function of claudins, cell adhesion molecules at tight junctions. Ann NY Acad Sci 915:129–135
15. Furuse M, Itoh M, Hirase T, Nagafuchi A, Yonemura S, Tsukita S (1994) Direct association of occludin with ZO-1 and its possible involvement in the localization of occludin in tight junctions. J Cell Biol 127:1617–1626

16. Fanning AS, Jameson BJ, Jesaitis LA, Anderson JM (1998) The tight junction protein ZO-1 establishes a link between the transmembrane protein occludin and the actin cytoskeleton. J Biol Chem 273:29745–29753
17. Itoh M, Nagafuchi A, Moroi S, Tsukita S (1997) Involvement of ZO-1 in cadherin-based cell adhesion through its direct binding to alpha catenin and actin filaments. J Cell Biol 138:181–192
18. Sheth B, Fesenko I, Collins JE, et al (1997) Tight junction assembly during mouse blastocyst formation is regulated by late expression of ZO-1 alpha+ isoform. Development 124:2027–2937
19. Sheth B, Moran B, Anderson JM, Fleming TP (2000) Post-translational control of occludin membrane assembly in mouse trophectoderm: a mechanism to regulate timing of tight junction biogenesis and blastocyst formation. Development 127:831–840
20. Unno N, Hodin RA, Fink MP (1999) Acidic conditions exacerbate interferon-gamma-induced intestinal epithelial hyperpermeability: role of peroxynitrous acid. Crit Care Med 27:1429–1436
21. Unno N, Menconi MJ, Smith M, Fink MP (1995) Nitric oxide mediates interferon-gamma-induced hyperpermeability in cultured human intestinal epithelial monolayers. Crit Care Med 23:1170–1176
22. Han X, Fink MP, Delude RL (2003) Proinflammatory cytokines cause NO·-dependent and independent changes in expression and localization of tight junction proteins in intestinal epithelial cells. Shock 19:229–237
23. Adams RB, Planchon SM, Roche JK (1993) IFN-γ modulation of epithelial barrier function: time course, reversibility, and site of cytokine binding. J Immunol 150:2356–2363
24. Planchon SM, Martins CAP, Guerrant RL, Roche JK (1994) Regulation of intestinal epithelial barrier function by TGF-b1. Evidence for its role in abrogating the effects of T cell cytokine. J Immunol 153:5730–5739
25. Madara JL, Stafford J (1989) Interferon-γ directly affects barrier function of cultured intestinal epithelial monolayers. J Clin Invest 83:724–727
26. Salzman AL, Menconi MJ, Unno N, et al (1995) Nitric oxide dilates tight junctions and depletes ATP in cultured Caco-2BBe intestinal epithelial monolayers. Am J Physiol 268:G361–G373
27. Menconi MJ, Unno N, Smith M, Aguirre DE, Fink MP (1998) The effect of nitric oxide donors on the permeability of cultured intestinal epithelial monolayers: role of superoxide, hydroxyl radical, and peroxynitrite. Biochem Biophys Acta 1425:189–203
28. Chavez A, Morin MJ, Unno N, Fink MP, Hodin RA (1999) Acquired interferon-γ responsiveness during Caco-2 cell differentiation: effects on iNOS gene expression. Gut 44:659–665
29. Chavez A, Menconi MJ, Hodin RA, Fink MP (1999) Cytokine-induced epithelial hyperpermeability: role of nitric oxide. Crit Care Med 27:2246–2251
30. Han X, Fink MP, Uchiyama T, Delude RL (2004) Increased iNOS activity is essential for the development of pulmonary epithelial tight junction dysfunction in endotoxemic mice. Am J Physiol Lung Cell Mol Physiol 286:L259–L267
31. Wink DA, Mitchell JB (1998) Chemical biology of nitric oxide: insights into regulatory, cytotoxic, and cytoprotective mechanisms of nitric oxide. Free Radical Biol Med 25:434–456
32. Pryor WA, Squadrito GL (1995) The chemistry of peroxynitrite: a product from the reaction of nitric oxide with superoxide. Am J Physiol 268:L699–L722
33. Unno N, Menconi MJ, Smith M, Aguirre DG, Fink MP (1997) Hyperpermeability of intestinal epithelial monolayers is induced by NO: effect of low extracellular pH. Am J Physiol 272:G923–G934
34. Sugi K, Musch MW, Field M, Chang EB (2001) Inhibition of Na$^+$,K$^+$-ATPase by interferon gamma down-regulates intestinal epithelial transport and barrier function. Gastroenterology 120:1393–1403

35. Qayyum I, Zubrow AB, Ashraf QM, Kubin J, Delivoria-Papadopoulos M, Mishra OP (2001) Nitration as a mechanism of Na+, K+-ATPase modification during hypoxia in the cerebral cortex of the guinea pig fetus. Neurochem Res 26:1163–1169

36. Mishra OP, Delivoria-Papadopoulos M, Cahillane G, Wagerle LC (1989) Lipid peroxidation as the mechanism of modification of the affinity of the Na+, K+-ATPase active sites for ATP, K+, Na+, and strophanthidin in vitro. Neurochem Res 14:845–851

37. Unno N, Wang H, Menconi MJ, et al (1997) Inhibition of inducible nitric oxide synthase ameliorates lipopolysaccharide-induced gut mucosal barrier dysfunction in rats. Gastroenterology 113:1246–1257

38. Han X, Fink MP, Yang R, Delude RL (2004) Increased iNOS activity is essential for intestinal epithelial tight junction dysfunction in endotoxemic mice. Shock 21:261–270

39. Moore WM, Webber RK, Jerome GM, Tjong FS, Misko TP, Currie MG (1994) L-N6-(1-iminoethyl)lysine: A selective inhibitor of inducible nitric oxide synthase. J Med Chem 37:3886–3888

40. Kubes P (1993) Ischemia-reperfusion in the feline small intestine: a role for nitric oxide. Am J Physiol 264:G143–G149

41. Kubes P (1992) Nitric oxide modulates epithelial permeability in the feline small intestine. Am J Physiol 262:G1138–G1142

42. Sakakibara A, Furuse M, Saitou M, Ando-Akatsuka Y, Tsukita S (1997) Possible involvement of phosphorylation of occludin in tight junction formation. J Cell Biol 137:1393–1401

43. Ravin HA, Rowley D, Jenkins C, Fine J (1960) On the absorption of bacterial endotoxin from the gastro-intestinal tract of the normal and shocked animal. J Exp Med 112:783–792

44. Fine J, Frank ED, Rutenberg SH, Schweinburg FB (1959) The bacterial factor in traumatic shock. N Engl J Med 260:214–216

45. Moore FA, Moore EE, Poggetti R, et al (1991) Gut bacterial translocation via the portal vein: a clinical perspective with major torso trauma. J Trauma 31:629–638

46. Luyer MD, Buurman WA, Hadfoune M, et al (2004) Pretreatment with high-fat enteral nutrition reduces endotoxin and tumor necrosis factor-alpha and preserves gut barrier function early after hemorrhagic shock. Shock 21:65–71

47. Wan S, LeClerc JL, Huynh CH, et al (1999) Does steroid pretreatment increase endotoxin release during clinical cardiopulmonary bypass? J Thorac Cardiovasc Surg 117:1004–1008

48. Martinez-Pellus AE, Merino P, Bru M, et al (1993) Can selective digestive decontamination avoid the endotoxemia and cytokine activation promoted by cardiopulmonary bypass. Crit Care Med 21:1684–1691

49. Yates SP, Jorgensen R, Andersen GR, Merrill AR (2006) Stealth and mimicry by deadly bacterial toxins. Trends Biochem Sci 31:123–133

50. Wu L, Estrada O, Zaborina O, et al (2005) Recognition of host immune activation by *Pseudomonas aeruginosa*. Science 309:774–747

51. Kohler JE, Zaborina O, Wu L, et al (2005) Components of intestinal epithelial hypoxia activate the virulence circuitry of Pseudomonas. Am J Physiol Gastrointest Liver Physiol 288:G1084–G1054

52. Alverdy J, Holbrook C, Rocha F, et al (2000) Gut-derived sepsis occurs when the right pathogen with the right virulence genes meets the right host: evidence for In vivo virulence expression in pseudomonas aeruginosa. Ann Surg 232:480–489

53. Gaines JM, Carty NL, Colmer-Hamood JA, Hamood AN (2005) Effect of static growth and different levels of environmental oxygen on toxA and ptxR expression in the Pseudomonas aeruginosa strain PAO1. Microbiology 151:2263–2275

54. Peitzman AB, Udekwu AO, Ochoa J, Smith S (1991) Bacterial translocation in trauma patients. J Trauma 31:1083–1087

55. Magnotti LJ, Upperman JS, Xu D-Z, Lu Q, Deitch EA (1998) Gut-derived mesenteric lymph but not portal blood increases endothelial cell permeability and promotes lung injury after hemorrhagic shock. Ann Surg 228:518–527

56. Zallen G, Moore EE, Johnson JL, Tamura DY, Ciesla DJ, Silliman CC (2006) Posthemorrhagic shock mesenteric lymph primes circulating neutrophils and provokes lung injury. J Surg Res 83:83–88
57. Upperman JS, Deitch EA, Guo W, Lu Q, Xu D (1998) Post-hemorrhagic shock mesenteric lymph is cytotoxic to endothelial cells and activates neutrophils. Shock 10:407–414
58. Magnotti LJ, Xu DZ, Lu Q, Deitch EA (1999) Gut-derived mesenteric lymph: a link between burn and lung injury. Arch Surg 134:1333–1340
59. Gonzalez RJ, Moore EE, Ciesla DJ, Meng X, Biffl WL, Silliman CC (2001) Post-hemorrhagic shock mesenteric lymph lipids prime neutrophils for enhanced cytotoxicity via phospholipase A2. Shock 16:218–222
60. Gonzalez RJ, Moore EE, Ciesla DJ, Biffl WL, Offner PJ, Silliman CC (2001) Phospholipase A(2)–derived neutral lipids from posthemorrhagic shock mesenteric lymph prime the neutrophil oxidative burst. Surgery 130:198–203
61. Kaiser VL, Sifri ZC, Dikdan GS, et al (2005) Trauma-hemorrhagic shock mesenteric lymph from rat contains a modified form of albumin that is implicated in endothelial cell toxicity. Shock 23:417–425
62. Dayal SD, Hauser CJ, Feketeova E, et al (2002) Shock mesenteric lymph-induced rat polymorphonuclear neutrophil activation and endothelial cell injury is mediated by aqueous factors. J Trauma 52:1048–1055
63. Deitch EA, Shi HP, Lu Q, Feketeova E, Xu DZ (2003) Serine proteases are involved in the pathogenesis of trauma-hemorrhagic shock-induced gut and lung injury. Shock 19:452–456
64. Eckmann L, Jung HC, Schurer-Maly C, Panja A, Morzycka-Wroblewska E, Kagnoff MF (1993) Differential cytokine expression by human intestinal epithelial cell lines. Gastroenterology 105:1689–1697.
65. Kim JM, Kim JS, Jun HC, Oh YK, Song IS, Kim CY (2002) Differential expression and polarized secretion of CXC and CC chemokines by human intestinal epithelial cancer cell lines in response to Clostridium difficile toxin A. Microbiol Immunol 46:333–342
66. Taylor CT, Fueki N, Agah A, Hershberg RM, Colgan SP (1999) Critical role of cAMP response element binding protein expression in hypoxia-elicited induction of epithelial tumor necrosis factor-alpha. J Biol Chem 274:19447–19454
67. Jung HC, Eckmann L, Yang SK, et al (1995) A distinct array of proinflammatory cytokines is expressed in human colon epithelial cells in response to bacterial invasion. J Clin Invest 95:55–65
68. Eckmann L, Stenson WF, Savidge TC, et al (1997) Role of intestinal epithelial cells in the host secretory response to infection by invasive bacteria. Bacterial entry induces epithelial prostaglandin H synthase-2 expression and prostaglandin E2 and F2 production. J Clin Invest 100:296–309
69. Bustin M, Lehn DA, Landsman D (1990) Structural features of the HMG chromosomal proteins and their genes. Biochim Biophys Acta 1049:231–243
70. Wang H, Bloom O, Zhang M, et al (1999) HMG-1 as a late mediator of endotoxin lethality in mice. Science 285:248–251
71. Yang H, Ochani M, Li J, et al (2004) Reversing established sepsis with antagonists of endogenous HMGB1. Proc Natl Acad Sci USA 101:296–301
72. Abraham E, Arcaroli J, Carmody A, Wang H, Tracey KJ (2000) HMG-1 as a mediator of acute lung inflammation. J Immunol 165:2950–2954
73. Kim JY, Park JS, Strassheim D, et al (2005) HMGB1 contributes to the development of acute lung injury after hemorrhage. Am J Physiol Lung Cell Mol Physiol 288:L958–L965
74. Sappington PL, Yang R, Yang H, Tracey KJ, Delude RL, Fink MP (2002) HMGB1 B box increases the permeability of Caco-2 enterocytic monolayers and impairs intestinal barrier function in mice. Gastroenterology 123:790–802
75. Andersson U, Wang H, Palmblad K, et al (2001) High mobility group 1 protein (HMG-1) stimulates proinflammatory cytokine synthesis in human monocytes. J Exp Med 192:565–570

76. Ombrellino M, Wang H, Ajemian MS, et al (1999) Increased serum concentrations of high-mobility-group protein 1 in haemorrhagic shock. Lancet 354:1446–1447
77. Pachot A, Monneret G, Voirin N, et al (2005) Longitudinal study of cytokine and immune transcription factor mRNA expression in septic shock. Clin Immunol 114:61–69
78. Sunden-Cullberg J, Norrby-Teglund A, Rouhianen A, et al (2005) Persistent elevation of high mobility group box-1 protein (HMGB1) in patients with severe sepsis and septic shock. Crit Care Med 33:564–573
79. Rendon-Mitchell B, Ochani M, Li J, et al (2003) IFN-gamma induces high mobility group box 1 protein release partly through a TNF-dependent mechanism. J Immunol 170:3890–3897
80. Gardella S, Andrei C, Ferrera D, et al (2002) The nuclear protein HMGB1 is secreted by monocytes via a non-classical, vesicle-mediated secretory pathway. EMBO Rep 3:995–1001
81. Bonaldi T, Talamo F, Scaffidi P, et al (2003) Monocytic cells hyperacetylate chromatin protein HMGB1 to redirect it towards secretion. EMBO J 22:5551–5560
82. Semino C, Angelini G, Poggi A, Rubartelli A (2005) NK/iDC interaction results in IL-18 secretion by DCs at the synaptic cleft followed by NK cell activation and release of the DC maturation factor HMGB1. Blood 106:609–616
83. Wang H, Vishnubhakat JM, Bloom O, et al (2002) Proinflammatory cytokines (tumor necrosis factor and interleukin 1) stimulate release of high mobility group protein-1 by pituicytes. Surgery 126:389–392
84. Scaffidi P, Misteli T, Bianchi ME (2002) Release of chromatin protein HMGB1 by necrotic cells triggers inflammation. Nature 418:191–195
85. Liu S, Stolz DB, Sappington PL, et al (2006) HMGB1 is secreted by immunostimulated enterocytes and contributes to cytomix-induced hyperpermeability of Caco-2 monolayers. Am J Physiol Cell Physiol 290:C990–999

# Endogenous Danger Signals in Liver Injury: Role of High Mobility Group Box Protein-1

A. Tsung, G. Jeyabalan, and T.R. Billiar

## Introduction

The liver is a central regulator of the systemic immune response following acute traumatic or surgical insult. It is the primary site for clearance of bacterial endotoxin and is also subject to injury and dysfunction during sepsis or following local insults such as warm ischemia/reperfusion. Recent advances in the study of mechanisms for the activation of the innate immune system have pointed to the Toll-like receptors (TLRs) as a common pathway for immune recognition of microbial invasion and tissue injury. By recognizing either microbial products or endogenous molecules, the TLR system is capable of alerting the host of danger by activating the innate immune system. Initially, this is manifested by the production of inflammatory mediators and the rapid uptake of invading microbes and their products. When excessive, this inflammatory response can contribute to organ damage and dysfunction. In this chapter, we will discuss the role of endogenous danger signals, specifically high mobility group box ptotein-1 (HMGB1), as a signaling molecule that activates inflammatory pathways in a TLR-dependent manner in response to liver injury.

## Endogenous Proteins and Toll-like Receptors

Innate immunity typically refers to the initial pro-inflammatory response that occurs in response to an invading microorganism. This response serves as the front-line defense mechanism against infection. Tissue injury activates many of the same inflammatory pathways. This observation, among others, led to the hypothesis proposed by Polly Matzinger [1, 2] that the immune system is designed to recognize any substance that is potentially dangerous to the host. In this scenario, both pathogens and tissue damage represent a threat that leads to disruption of homeostasis. Recent observations show that both microbial products (pathogen-associated molecular patterns [PAMPs]) or endogenous molecules (damage-associated molecular patterns [DAMPs]) can be recognized through the TLRs, a family of receptors crucial to the innate immune system [3–8].

To date, 13 TLRs have been described in mice, and 10 in humans [9]. TLRs are a family of proteins which are mammalian homologs to the *Drosophila* Toll, a protein that functions in development and immunity [10]. The cytoplasmic portion of

TLRs is similar to that of the interleukin (IL)-1 receptor (IL-1R) family and is called the Toll/IL-1 receptor (TIR) domain. Unlike the IL-1 receptor extracellular portion that consists of an immunoglobulin-like domain, the TLR have leucine-rich repeats in their extracellular portion [11]. The TLR have many structural similarities both extracellularly and intracellularly, but they differ from each other in ligand specificities, expression patterns, and with some variability in the signaling pathways they activate [12].

Perhaps more than any of the other TLR family members, TLR4 sits at the interface of microbial and sterile inflammation. It is required for signal initiation for both bacterial endotoxin and many DAMPs. Whereas the role of TLR4 in the recognition of lipopolysaccharide (LPS) is well established [10], only recently has it become apparent that TLR4 also participates in the recognition of DAMPs. *In vivo* evidence for TLR4-mediated danger signaling comes from studies of acute tissue injury in hemorrhagic shock [13] as well as cardiac [14], renal [14, 15], and hepatic [7, 16] ischemia/reperfusion models. In each case, TLR4-mutant animals exhibited reduced injury or inflammation compared to wild-type controls. We [7] and others [16] recently reported that liver damage following warm ischemia/reperfusion was markedly decreased in TLR4-mutant animals. Furthermore, HMGB1, a nuclear protein released after necrotic cell death, has been identified as one of the mediators of this TLR4-dependent activation of the innate immune responses.

Danger signals or DAMPs can be classified as normal cell constituents released by damage or dying cells or components of the extracellular matrix, released by the action of proteases at the site of tissue damage. These molecules are recognized by antigen-presenting cells which can become activated and initiate primary immune responses. Endogenous danger signals can be divided into those that serve as primary initiators of the immune response and those that act as feedback signals. Furthermore, some of these signals can function both as initiators and as positive-feedback mediators.

Much of the work on activation of the immune system by endogenous molecules has been with immune cells, specifically dendritic cells. The activation of TLRs on dendritic cells by danger signals may be partly responsible for the induction of cytokine and chemokine production as well as the maturation of this cell population. Substances released by necrotic, but not apoptotic, cell death appear to be primarily responsible for interacting with resting dendritic cells in various tissues [17–19]. Dendritic cells initiate adoptive immune responses through antigen presentation in the setting of co-stimulation. Whereas DAMPs can activate dendritic cells for antigen presentation, a process important to adoptive microbial defenses, antigen presentation does not appear to be part of the typical tissue injury response. Instead the lack of antigen may lead to a state of immune depression. In a variety of cell systems, TLR4-dependent signaling has been observed following exposure to heat shock proteins (HSPs) [8], fibrinogen [5], hyaluronic acid [3], heparin sulfate [4], and HMGB1 [6, 7]. Concerns over the possible contribution of contaminating LPS linger [20], but the data for the LPS-independent activation of TLR4-signaling by these proteins are becoming more convincing. HSPs are one of the most extensively studied endogenous danger signals and can serve as both constitutive and inducible danger signals. Various forms of constitutively active or stress-induced HSPs are released from different cellular compartments during necrotic cell death and activate resting dendritic cells via different receptors, including the TLR family [8]. As mentioned before, certain cellular adhesion molecules on dendritic cells can become activated when bound to the degradation products of their normal ligands. An example is the extracellular matrix glycosaminoglycan, hyaluronan, which is seen in the course of both normal matrix turnover of lung epithelium and in acute lung injury (ALI). Pro-inflammatory cytokine production and immune cell activation can occur through interaction of hyaluronan and its degradation products with TLRs as part of the innate immune response [21].

## High Mobility Group Box Protein-1:
## Mediator of Inflammation in Liver Ischemia/Reperfusion

HMGB1 is a fascinating protein with multiple functions. Evolutionarily ancient, HMGB1 predates speciation and is highly conserved across species [22]. It was initially identified in 1973, and the early studies focused on its role as a DNA-binding, nuclear protein that co-purified with chromosomal DNA since HMGB1 is loosely bound to chromatin (unlike the more tightly bound histones) [23, 24]. HMGB1 is present in almost all eukaryotic cells, functions to stabilize nucleosomes, and acts as a transcription factor that regulates the expression of several genes [25, 26]. During the course of experiments to identify late-acting mediators of endotoxemia and sepsis, HMGB1 was discovered to be secreted by activated macrophages [27]. HMGB1 release occurred significantly later than macrophage secretion of the classical early pro-inflammatory mediators, TNF and IL-1 [28]. In an endotoxemia model in mice, serum HMGB1 levels begin to increase 12-18 hours after the peak of TNF, which occurs at 2 hours, and of IL-1 (4–6 hours) [29]. Neutralizing HMGB1 markedly improved survival in these septic mice. HMGB1 is also readily released from necrotic or damaged cells and serves as a signal for inflammation [30, 31]. Thus, HMGB1, in addition to its nuclear role, is a critical mediator of the response to infection, injury, and inflammation.

Whereas HMGB1 is a late mediator of systemic inflammation in sepsis, recent studies from our laboratory demonstrate that HMGB1 also acts as an endogenous danger signal, serving as a key link between the initial damage to cells and the activation of inflammatory signaling. This role of HMGB1 as an early mediator of inflammation is in clear contrast to sepsis where the action of HMGB1 is delayed. We utilized a model of warm, partial hepatic ischemia/reperfusion in mice previously characterized in our laboratory to study the role of HMGB1 in the setting of acute, local organ damage [32]. Ischemia/reperfusion is a pathophysiologic process whereby hypoxic organ damage is accentuated following return of blood flow and oxygen delivery. Transient episodes of hepatic ischemia are encountered during solid organ transplantation, trauma, hypovolemic shock, and elective liver resection, when inflow occlusion or total vascular exclusion is used to minimize blood loss. In our model, hepatic ischemia is initiated with the occlusion of only the left hepatic artery and left branches of the portal vein, preserving flow though the right side and avoiding intestinal venous congestion. We have found that marked hepatic injury to the ischemic lobes becomes apparent at 3–6 h of reperfusion following 45–60 min of ischemia [32].

The pathophysiology of liver ischemia/reperfusion injury includes both direct cellular damage as the result of the ischemic insult as well as delayed dysfunction and damage resulting from activation of inflammatory pathways [33,34]. Although the distal cascade of inflammatory responses resulting in organ damage after ischemia/reperfusion injury has been studied extensively, the extent to which the initial cellular injury contributes to activation of the inflammatory response and leads to further tissue damage is poorly understood. We hypothesized that the key link between the initial damage to cells and the activation of inflammatory signaling involves release of HMGB1 from ischemic cells. This was based on initial observations that following 60 minutes of hepatic ischemia, HMGB1 protein expression was upregulated as early as 1 hour after reperfusion and then increased in a time-dependent manner up to 24 hours. Previous studies have shown that HMGB1 localizes predominantly in the nucleus of macrophages [31]. Thus, to determine the cellular localization of HMGB1 in the liver, we performed immunofluorescence staining in normal livers and in livers undergoing ischemia and reperfusion. As expected, expression of HMGB1 was noted predominantly in the nucleus of hepatocytes in normal livers. However, after ischemia and reperfusion, HMGB1 expression was found to be enhanced in the nucleus as well as the cytoplasm of hepatocytes. Similar findings of HMGB1 being upregulated by stress was also seen *in vitro*. Since hypoxia is believed to be the initiating event in the ischemia/reperfusion insult, we assessed the expression of HMGB1 in cultured hepatocytes exposed to hypoxia. Primary hepatocytes exposed to normoxia (21% oxygen) have a basal level of HMGB1 expression which did not change significantly up to 24 hours of incubation. However, exposure of the hepatocytes to hypoxia (1% oxygen) resulted in a time-dependent increase in cellular HMGB1 expression as well as increased HMGB1 release into the media. The findings that HMGB1 is rapidly upregulated in hepatocytes in hepatic ischemia/reperfusion and in hepatocytes made ischemic *in vitro*, suggested that stressed or damaged hepatocytes in hepatic ischemia/reperfusion provide the danger signal to the neighboring immune cells in the liver. Further support for the role of HMGB1 in the inflammation and injury seen after hepatic ischemia/reperfusion included studies demonstrating that inhibition of HMGB1 activity with neutralizing antibody significantly decreased liver damage after ischemia/reperfusion while administration of recombinant HMGB1 worsened ischemia/reperfusion injury.

To investigate the mechanism by which local injury is sensed by the liver, TLR4- and CD14-deficient mouse strains were subjected to ischemia/reperfusion. The CD14 knockout-($CD14^{-/-}$) mouse strain did not exhibit a reduction in ischemia/reperfusion-induced damage compared to wild-type controls. The results using the CD14$^{-/-}$ mice were of particular importance because they argued against a role for intestinal derived LPS in the early ischemia/reperfusion-induced inflammation. In contrast to the results obtained with CD14$^{-/-}$ mice, TLR4-mutant (C3H/HeJ) or deficient (TLR4$^{-/-}$) mice exhibited a dramatic reduction in ischemia/reperfusion-induced damage and cytokine production. These results were similar to those reported by Zhai et al. who also showed that TLR4, but not TLR2, was required for hepatic ischemia/reperfusion injury [16].

We hypothesized that if TLR4 was involved in the recognition of HMGB1 and that the HMGB1 neutralizing antibody functioned by preventing TLR4-mediated HMGB1 signaling, then the antibody should provide no further protection in the TLR4-mutant mice; this indeed was the case. Although the ischemia/reperfusion-induced damage in TLR4-mutant mice was only 40% of wild-type mice, anti-HMGB1 treatment afforded no additional protection in the TLR4-mutant mice while reducing damage in the wild-type mice to a level similar to that seen in the mutant animals. Further proof that HMGB1 is recognized via a TLR4-dependent mechanism came from an experiment showing that exogenous recombinant HMGB1 worsened the ischemia/reperfusion-induced damage only in wild-type and not in TLR4-mutant mice. Taken together, these results demonstrate that HMGB1 is an early mediator of injury and inflammation in liver ischemia/reperfusion and implicates TLR4 as one of the receptors involved in the process.

## Sensing the Danger in the Liver

As previously described, TLR4 appears to respond to both bacterial endotoxin and multiple other endogenous ligands, including hyaluronic acid [3], heparin sulphate [4], fibrinogen [5], HMGB1 [6,7], and HSPs [8]. In addition, both inflammation and injury responses in warm hepatic ischemia/reperfusion are partially TLR4 dependent [7,16]. The liver is well equipped to respond to these potential endogenous ligands. The liver consists of parenchymal cells (hepatocytes) and non-parenchymal cells, including Kupffer cells, sinusoidal endothelial cells, stellate cells, and hepatic dendritic cells. TLR4 is present on both hepatocytes and non-parenchymal cells and both cell populations possess intact TLR4 signaling pathways [35,36]. Our above studies [7] suggested a central role for HMGB1 in the TLR4 dependent component associated with hepatocyte damage and the resultant enhanced inflammation associated with hepatic ischemia/reperfusion injury. Our working hypothesis was that endogenous danger signals such as HMGB1 are released from stressed and injured hepatocytes, and in the context of ischemia and reperfusion, these molecules activate phagocytic cells via TLR4 for inflammatory mediator production. Thus, the next question we sought to answer was which cell type in the liver expressing TLR4 was required for ischemia/reperfusion-induced injury.

To elucidate the cell type mediating the TLR4-dependent inflammatory response after hepatic ischemia/reperfusion, we needed to be able to differentiate between the responses of hepatocytes and non-parenchymal cells in the intact liver. To do this, we turned to a chimeric mouse model in which recipient mice receive lethal irradiation to eradicate bone marrow cells, followed by bone marrow transplantation [37]. This procedure allowed for the reconstitution of the bone marrow with syngeneic bone marrow from mice with mutations in specific components of the TLR4 response system. After 8–10 weeks, the immune cells within the liver were replaced with the cells expressing the new bone marrow's phenotype, while the long-lived parenchymal cells retained the host's phenotype. Our experiments required two test groups and two control groups. Control groups included wild-type (WT:WT, host:bone marrow) and TLR4-mutant (Mutant:Mutant) strains. In these studies, the host mouse received bone marrow identical to the host to control for the experimental manipulation. Test groups included wild-type mice receiving TLR4-mutant bone marrow (WT:Mutant) and TLR4-mutant mice receiving wild-type bone marrow (Mutant:WT).

After confirming that the administration of bone marrow resulted in a conversion of the non-parencyhmal cells to the donor phenotype in our chimeric mice, we subjected these animals to our model of partial hepatic warm ischemia/reperfusion. In agreement with previous studies, WT:WT mice exhibited significant hepatocellular damage after ischemia/reperfusion where as Mutant:Mutant mice were protected from injury [37]. Interestingly, Mutant:WT mice exhibited similar damage to the wild-type control group and WT:Mutant mice were protected from ischemia/reperfusion injury. Thus, functional TLR4 on non-parenchymal cells, regardless of hepatocyte phenotype, was required for inflammation and organ damage after ischemia/reperfusion.

To further characterize the non-parenchymal cell type responsible for TLR4-mediated injury, we performed phagocytic depletion studies. Gadolinium chloride (GdCl$_3$) pretreatment is toxic to phagocytic cells in the liver, thereby eradicating Kupffer cells and dendritic cells [38]. To determine if these cells accounted for the TLR4-dependent responses in hepatic ischemia/reperfusion, wild type and TLR4-deficient mice were treated with GdCl$_3$ prior to hepatic ischemia/reperfusion. GdCl$_3$ markedly reduced ischemia/reperfusion-induced damage in wild-type mice but afforded no further protection in the TLR4-mutant mice. Taken together, our results indicated that TLR4 signaling in non-parenchymal cells, most likely Kupffer and dendritic cells, is required for the ischemia/reperfusion-induced injury and inflammation.

## Conclusion

The liver is a complex organ with an extraordinary spectrum of functions. Although the TLR system equips the liver to sense and clear bacteria, this system also participates in the inflammatory response to local liver injury through the recognition

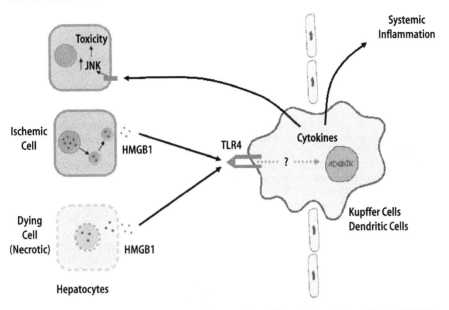

**Fig. 1.** Model for Toll-like receptor 4 (TLR4) activation in liver ischemia/reperfusion. HMGB1: high mobility group box protein 1

of endogenous danger molecules such as HMGB1. Figure 1 outlines our current view of the role of the HMGB1-TLR4 pathway in the hepatic ischemia/reperfusion response. Ischemic stress leads to passive HMGB1 release from injured cells or to active secretion. Both are likely to occur but the specific pathways leading to HMGB1 release remain unknown. HMGB1 is then recognized by TLR4 through a CD14-independent mechanism by Kupffer cells and dendritic cells. Park et al. have recently reported that HMGB1 directly interacts with TLR4 and TLR2 [39]. Since TLR2 knockout mice show no reduction in injury or inflammation, the key interaction in liver ischemia/reperfusion is through TLR4. The recognition of HMGB1 by TLR4 leads to production of pro-inflammatory mediators in the context of ischemia/reperfusion and these mediators lead to activation of toxic signaling pathways in stressed hepatocytes. Many steps in these series of events remain to be defined. In addition, several simultaneous signaling events clearly take place and may serve as the key co-signaling events that amplify or even permit HMGB1 recognition. This paradigm suggests that HMGB1 and TLR4 are potential targets for therapeutic intervention in both acute liver injury and ischemia/reperfusion insults.

# References

1. Gallucci S, Matzinger P (2001) Danger signals: SOS to the immune system. Curr Opin Immunol 13:114–119
2. Matzinger P (2002) The danger model: a renewed sense of self. Science 296:301–305
3. Termeer C, Benedix F, Sleeman J, et al (2002) Oligosaccharides of Hyaluronan activate dendritic cells via toll-like receptor 4. J Exp Med 195:99–111
4. Johnson GB, Brunn GJ, Kodaira Y, Platt JL (2002) Receptor-mediated monitoring of tissue well-being via detection of soluble heparan sulfate by Toll-like receptor 4. J Immunol 168:5233–5239
5. Smiley ST, King JA, Hancock WW (2001) Fibrinogen stimulates macrophage chemokine secretion through toll-like receptor 4. J Immunol 167:2887–2894
6. Park JS, Svetkauskaite D, He Q, et al (2004) Involvement of toll-like receptors 2 and 4 in cellular activation by high mobility group box 1 protein. J Biol Chem 279:7370–7377
7. Tsung A, Sahai R, Tanaka H, et al (2005) The nuclear factor HMGB1 mediates hepatic injury after murine liver ischemia-reperfusion. J Exp Med 201:1135–1143
8. Vabulas RM, Ahmad-Nejad P, Ghose S, Kirschning CJ, Issels RD, Wagner H (2002) HSP70 as endogenous stimulus of the Toll/interleukin-1 receptor signal pathway. J Biol Chem 277:15107–15112
9. Palsson-McDermott EM, O'Neill LA (2004) Signal transduction by the lipopolysaccharide receptor, Toll-like receptor-4. Immunology 113:153–162
10. Poltorak A, He X, Smirnova I, et al (1998) Defective LPS signaling in C3H/HeJ and C57BL/10ScCr mice: mutations in Tlr4 gene. Science 282:2085–8
11. Akira S, Takeda K (2004) Toll-like receptor signalling. Nat Rev Immunol 4:499–511
12. Medzhitov R, Janeway CA (2002) Decoding the patterns of self and nonself by the innate immune system. Science 296:298–300
13. Barsness KA, Arcaroli J, Harken AH, et al (2004) Hemorrhage-induced acute lung injury is TLR-4 dependent. Am J Physiol Regul Integr Comp Physiol 287:R592–R599
14. Oyama J, Blais C Jr, Liu X, et al (2004) Reduced myocardial ischemia-reperfusion injury in toll-like receptor 4-deficient mice. Circulation 109:784–789
15. Wolfs TG, Buurman WA, van Schadewijk A, et al (2002) In vivo expression of Toll-like receptor 2 and 4 by renal epithelial cells: IFN-gamma and TNF-alpha mediated up-regulation during inflammation. J Immunol 168:1286–1293
16. Zhai Y, Shen XD, O'Connell R, et al (2004) Cutting edge: TLR4 activation mediates liver ischemia/reperfusion inflammatory response via IFN regulatory factor 3-dependent MyD88-independent pathway. J Immunol 173:7115–7119
17. Basu S, Binder RJ, Suto R, Anderson KM, Srivastava PK (2000) Necrotic but not apoptotic cell death releases heat shock proteins, which deliver a partial maturation signal to dendritic cells and activate the NF-kappa B pathway. Int Immunol 12:1539–1546
18. Gallucii S, Lolkema M, Matzinger P (1999) Natural adjuvants: endogenous activators of dendritic cells. Nat Med 5:1249–1255
19. Sauter B, Albert ML, Francisco L, Larsson M, Somersan S, Bhardwaj N (2000) Consequences of cell death: exposure to necrotic tumor cells, but not primary tissue cells or apoptotic cells, induces the maturation of immunostimulatory dendritic cells. J Exp Med 191:423–434
20. Tsan MF, Gao B (2004) Endogenous ligands of Toll-like receptors. J Leukoc Biol 76:514–519
21. Jiang D, Liang J, Fan J, et al (2005) Regulation of lung injury and repair by Toll-like receptors and hyaluronan. Nat Med 11:1173–1179
22. Yotov WV, St-Arnaud R (1992) Nucleotide sequence of a mouse cDNA encoding the nonhistone chromosomal high mobility group protein-1 (HMG1). Nucleic Acids Res 20:3516
23. Bustin M, Hopkins RB, Isenberg I (1978) Immunological relatedness of high mobility group chromosomal proteins from calf thymus. J Biol Chem 253:1694–1699
24. Javaherian K, Liu JF, Wang JC (1978) Nonhistone proteins HMG1 and HMG2 change the DNA helical structure. Science 199:1345–1346

25. Park JS, Arcaroli J, Yum HK, et al (2003) Activation of gene expression in human neutrophils by high mobility group box 1 protein. Am J Physiol Cell Physiol 284:870–879
26. West KL, Castellini MA, Duncan MK, Bustin M (2004) Chromosomal proteins HMGN3a and HMGN3b regulate the expession of glycine transporter 1. Mol Cell Biol 24:3747–3756
27. Wang H, Bloom O, Zhang M, et al (1999) HMG-1 as a late mediator of endotoxin lethality in mice. Science 285:248–251
28. Andersson U, Wang H, Palmblad K, et al (2000) High mobility group 1 protein (HMG-1) stimulates proinflammatory cytokine synthesis in human monocytes. J Exp Med 192:565–570
29. Yang H, Ochani M, Li J, et al (2004) Reversing established sepsis with antagonists of endogenous high-mobility group box 1. Proc Natl Acad Sci USA 101:296–301
30. Degryse B, Bonaldi T, Scaffidi P, et al (2001) The high mobility group (HMG) boxes of the nuclear protein HMG1 induce chemotaxis and cytoskeleton reorganization in rat smooth muscle cells. J Cell Biol 152:1197–1206
31. Scaffidi P, Misteli T, Bianchi ME (2002) Release of chromatin protein HMGB1 by necrotic cells triggers inflammation. Nature 418:191–195
32. Lee VG, Johnson ML, Baust J, Laubach VE, Watkins SC, Billiar TR (2001) The roles of iNOS in liver ischemia-reperfusion injury. Shock 16:355–360
33. Fondevila C, Busuttil RW, Kupiec-Weglinski JW (2003) Hepatic ischemia/reperfusion injury—a fresh look. Exp Mol Pathol 74:86–93
34. Selzner N, Rudiger H, Graf R, Clavien PA (2003) Protective strategies against ischemic injury of the liver. Gastroenterology 125:917–36
35. Liu S, Gallo DJ, Green AM, et al (2002) Role of toll-like receptors in changes in gene expression and NF-kappa B activation in mouse hepatocytes stimulated with lipopolysaccharide. Infect Immun 70:3433–3442
36. Su GL, Klein RD, Aminlari A, et al (2000) Kupffer cell activation by lipolysaccharide in rats: role for lipopolysaccharide binding protein and toll-like receptor 4. Hepatology 31:932–936
37. Tsung A, Hoffman RA, Izuishi K, et al (2005) Hepatic ischemia/reperfusion injury invovles functional TLR4 signaling in nonparenchymal cells. J Immunol 175:7661–7668
38. Jaeschke H, Farhood A (1991) Neutrophil and Kupffer cell-induced oxidant stress and ischemia-reperfusion injury in rat liver. Am J Physiol 260:G355–G362
39. Park JS, Gamboni-Robertson F, He Q, et al (2005) High mobility group box 1 protein (HMGB1) interacts with multiple Toll like receptors. Am J Physiol Cell Physiol 290:C917–924

# Sepsis-induced Acute Renal Failure and Recovery

M. Raghavan, R. Venkataraman, and J.A. Kellum

## Introduction

Acute renal failure remains a common syndrome in the setting of critical illness, and is associated with a high risk of death. Approximately 1–25% of patients in the intensive care unit (ICU) develop acute renal failure depending on the criteria used to define its presence [1]. Severe sepsis plays a major factor in the development of acute renal failure in the ICU. The mortality from sepsis-induced acute renal failure remains high despite our increasing ability to support vital organs. Unfortunately our understanding of the pathogenesis of sepsis-induced renal dysfunction is quite limited. It is, therefore, very important for critical care physicians to have an appreciation of what is known and not known about this condition in order to implement rational therapies.

## Epidemiology of Sepsis-induced Acute Renal Failure in the ICU

Sepsis and severe sepsis are currently the major contributing factors in the evolution of acute renal failure in ICU patients and account for nearly 50% of acute renal failure observed in the ICU [2]. Acute renal failure occurs in approximately 19% of patients with moderate sepsis, 23% with severe sepsis, and 51% with septic shock when blood cultures are positive [3]. Despite considerable improvements in medical treatment of various critical illnesses over the last three decades, the therapy of acute renal failure is rather disappointing and mortality rates due to acute renal failure exceed 60% in many published series [2]. It remains unclear, however, whether acute renal failure plays a significant role in the subsequent development of multiple organ failure (MOF) through its effects on metabolic homeostasis, or if acute renal failure is merely a manifestation of MOF. Patients who develop acute renal failure in the setting of sepsis are more likely to die than dialysis-dependent patients with sepsis admitted to the ICU [4]. This suggests that new onset acute renal failure during critical illness by itself has an 'attributable' mortality, and that the poor outcome associated with the development of new onset renal dysfunction is independent of the poor outcome associated with sepsis syndrome [5].

# Pathophysiology of Sepsis-induced Acute Renal failure: 'Time for a Paradigm Shift'

In the past, acute renal failure during critical illness was essentially considered a 'hemodynamic disease' caused by renal ischemia, a view largely influenced by findings in animal models, at least some of which had questionable relevance to the clinical state. Indeed, most models inducing so-called acute tubular necrosis (ATN) are based on ischemia/reperfusion (e. g., renal artery clamping). Such models produce very different physiology compared to the high cardiac output, low systemic vascular resistance state typically seen during human sepsis. Recent research however, underscores the importance of other mechanisms of renal injury such as acute renal tubular cell apoptosis [6,7], renal tubular epithelial barrier dysfunction [8], and endothelial dysfunction [9] in the pathogenesis of sepsis-induced acute renal failure. These concepts fit well with the typical paucity of histologic findings seen in ATN and with growing evidence of varying mechanisms of organ injury during sepsis and inflammation in general [8, 10]. Thus, the pathophysiologic mechanisms whereby sepsis-induced acute renal failure occur can be divided into four broad areas: 1. renal perfusion; 2. inflammation; 3. cellular mechanisms; and 4. coagulation.

## Renal Perfusion

The concept of renal hypoperfusion as the primary cause of acute renal failure is so thoroughly engrained in the literature of critical care and nephrology as to elevate to the status of dogma. Even the terms that we use, (e. g. acute tubular necrosis) suggest an ischemic etiology. For many years, empiric treatment of renal hypoperfusion with dopamine, a renal vasodilator, was seen as standard care not only for patients with acute renal failure but even for patients thought to be at high risk of acute renal failure. This practice has largely ceased after evidence accrued that dopamine is not helpful [11, 12] but other vasodilators (e. g., fenoldopam) are still being investigated. Furthermore, many clinicians shun agents such as norepinephrine over concerns that renal vasoconstriction will result in further deterioration in renal function. In this context, it is perhaps important to recall that blood flow to the kidneys is normally many times greater than metabolic need. This is because total or 'global' renal blood flow is in the service of glomerular filtration rather than oxygen delivery.

### Global Renal Blood Flow

Traditionally, the observation of an association between acute renal failure and 'low flow' states, such as cardiogenic, hemorrhagic, or even septic shock, led to the belief that renal ischemia plays a key role in the evolution of acute renal failure. This construct implies that restoration and maintenance of adequate renal blood flow should therefore be the primary target for renal protection in the critically ill. Several experimental studies of sepsis-induced acute renal failure have shown that global renal blood flow declines after induction of sepsis or endotoxemia [3,13,14]. Current evidence, however, suggests that most of sepsis-induced acute renal failure arises not due to renal hypoperfusion but indeed in the setting of adequate, or even increased renal perfusion [15]. Therefore, while renal hypoperfusion might be important in 'low flow' shock states, it is unlikely to play a key role in the development of acute renal failure during hyperdynamic states such as sepsis. The observation of acute renal failure in hyperdynamic models of septic shock suggests that renal blood flow-independent mechanisms of renal injury must exist and may be more important in the pathogenesis of sepsis-induced acute renal failure.

## Intrarenal Hemodynamics

It is possible that even though there is preserved or increased global renal blood flow during sepsis, regional redistribution of blood flow favoring the cortex, so-called 'cortico-medullary redistribution', may occur [16]. However recent studies by Di Giantomasso and colleagues found that both cortical and medullary blood flows remain unchanged in sheep with hyperdynamic septic shock, conditions closely resembling those of clinical sepsis [17]. Interestingly, the administration of norepinephrine resulted in a significant increase in flow to both regions. These observations challenge the view that the medulla is ischemic during hyperdynamic sepsis but simultaneously highlight that hemodynamic factors are indeed at work, and can be modified by interventions that affect systemic blood pressure and cardiac output. Furthermore, although cortico-medullary redistribution could be an important mechanism of renal injury in certain settings, it is likely to represent only one of the potential mechanisms responsible for loss of renal function. Although these studies do not completely discount the possible role of regional hypoperfusion (particularly in the microcirculation) in the pathophysiology of sepsis-induced acute renal failure, they do suggest that other factors, such as mediators of cellular injury, rather than lack of blood flow, may be closer to center stage in this unfolding drama [6].

## Inflammation

Since neither global renal hemodynamic changes nor intrarenal hemodynamic changes have been consistently shown to be predominant contributors to sepsis-induced acute renal failure, there must, therefore, be other mechanisms at work during the evolution of sepsis-induced acute renal failure that are not hemodynamic in nature. Sepsis is characterized by the release of a vast array of inflammatory cytokines, arachidonate metabolites, vasoactive substances, thrombogenic agents, and other biologically active mediators. A large body of experimental data suggests that these various mediators, along with neuroendocrine mechanisms, might be involved in the pathogenesis of organ dysfunction in sepsis [10].

## Cytokines

Cellular and humoral factors are integral to organ dysfunction in sepsis syndrome, with the kidney being especially vulnerable to cytokine-mediated injury. The mesangial cells are capable of expressing multiple pro-inflammatory cytokines and chemokines, such as interleukin (IL)-1, IL-6, tumor necrosis factor (TNF), and platelet activating factor (PAF) (Fig. 1). Tubular cells are also capable of releasing pro-inflammatory cytokines after stimulation by lipopolysaccharide (LPS) [18]. Studies of isolated kidneys perfused *ex vivo* with LPS do not demonstrate a decrease in glomerular filtration rate (GFR) despite increased mRNA expression for pro-inflammatory cytokines. However, *in vivo* experiments involving LPS stimulation demonstrate the expected renal dysfunction, suggesting that the acute renal failure in this setting involves host factors outside the renal parenchyma [19,20].

Major mediators of cytokine-induced renal injury include TNF and IL-1, both of which promote further cytokine release, induce vasoconstriction, neutrophil aggregation, production of reactive oxygen species (ROS), and induction of tissue factor and promotion of thrombosis [21]. TNF is produced and circulated systemically, whereas IL-1 is expressed in the glomerular endothelial cells early in animal models of sepsis. In the kidney, endotoxin also stimulates release of TNF from glomerular mesangial cells [22]. When infused into animal models, TNF and IL-1 result in renal damage and decreased renal blood flow and GFR [23]. Messmer et al. [24] have shown that TNF and LPS elicit apoptotic cell death of cultured bovine glomerular endothelial cells, which is time and concentration dependent. The effect of these compounds was characterized by an increase in proapoptotic proteins and a decrease in antiapoptotic proteins such as Bcl-xL. Furthermore, these pleiotropic cytokines are capable of inducing mesangial and endothelial production of PAF, endothelin, adenosine, nitric oxide (NO), and prostaglandin E2.

More recently, the direct toxic role of TNF to the kidney has been become evident. Knotek et al. [25] using soluble TNF receptor 55 (TNFsRp55)-based neutralization of TNF, achieved protection against LPS-induced renal failure in wild-type mice. With pretreatment using TNFsRp55, GFR decreased by only 30%, compared with a 75% decrease without TNF neutralization, suggesting that TNF plays an important role in sepsis-induced acute renal failure. Furthermore, van Lanschot et al. [26] infused TNF in sublethal doses in dogs. TNF induced an increase in water and sodium excretion, an effect that could be prevented by prior cyclooxygenase inhibition, suggesting that vasodilatory prostaglandins mediated some of the renal response to sublethal TNF in this model. Cunningham and colleagues [27] used *Escherichia coli* LPS as an intraperitoneal injection to establish a mice model of sepsis, and showed that LPS-induced acute renal failure can be attributed to TNF acting directly on its receptor, TNF Receptor-1 (TNFR1), in the kidney. Mice deficient in TNF receptor were resistant to LPS-induced renal failure, had less tubular

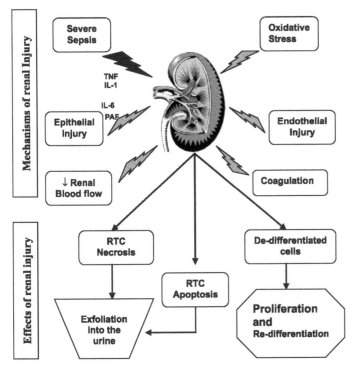

**Fig. 1.** Pathophysiology of acute renal failure and recovery during sepsis. Sepsis induces renal injury by a variety of mechanisms. Injured cells may recover promptly or undergo apoptosis or, rarely, necrosis. They may undergo de-differentiation and proliferation to replace lost cells. Control over these processes is complex and involves numerous factors. RTC: renal tubular cells; TNF: tumor necrosis factor; IL: interleukin; PAF: platelet activating factor; RBF: renal blood flow

apoptosis, and had fewer infiltrating neutrophils. Although TNF receptor-negative mice implanted with TNF receptor-positive kidneys developed LPS-induced renal failure, TNF-positive mice implanted with TNF receptor-negative kidneys did not. TNF thus seems to be an important direct mediator of endotoxin's effects during sepsis-induced acute renal failure. However, despite all the above findings, TNF blockade with monoclonal antibodies fails to protect animal or kidney during endotoxemia [28]. These observations suggest that toxic/immunologic mechanisms are important in mediating renal injury during sepsis.

### Nitric Oxide

During hyperdynamic septic shock renal blood flow is preserved, with apparent redistribution of flow from cortex to medulla, maintaining oxygen delivery to the most vulnerable portions of the renal parenchyma, while also decreasing the work of the tubules. This redistribution of blood flow coincides with an increase in NO in the medulla [29]. Inducible NO synthase (iNOS) can be expressed locally, in glomerular mesangial cells and endothelial cells, after stimulation with pro-inflammatory cytokines, including TNF and IL-1, and endotoxin [30]. Nonselective or selective blockade of iNOS decreases renal blood flow while increasing mean arterial pressure (MAP). This suggests that iNOS plays a role in maintaining renal blood flow in the setting of shock through its vasodilatory effects at the afferent arteriole. The mechanism of vasodilation by NO is dependent on the synthesis of cyclic guanosine monophosphate (cGMP) by soluble guanylate cyclase. Studies of LPS stimulation in mice leading to shock and acute renal failure have demonstrated a decrease in cGMP to basal levels at 24 hours, despite an early rise in and sustained iNOS levels, suggesting that desensitization of soluble guanylate cyclase results in loss of regulatory vasodilation in the kidney [31]. NOS inhibition in animal models of endotoxemia results in glomerular thrombosis and decline in creatinine clearance. The glomerular thrombosis in the setting of NOS inhibition seems related to the antithrombotic qualities of NOS, by inhibiting leukocyte interactions with endothelial cells and inhibiting platelet aggregation [32].

## Endothelins

The production of endothelins, which are potent vasoconstrictors, by endothelial, mesangial, and tubular cells is stimulated by pro-inflammatory cytokines, including TNF. The vasoconstrictors, vasopressin and angiotensin II, also stimulate endothelin release. Endothelins cause vigorous constriction of the afferent and efferent arterioles, and mesangial cell contraction. The effects of endothelin may be secondary to its induction of PAF synthesis in the mesangium or thromboxane A2 by the endothelium. PAF is a vasoconstrictor that additionally is chemotactic for activated inflammatory cells, including neutrophils. Increases in PAF lead to a reduction in GFR. Blockade of PAF receptors lessens the deterioration of renal function in animal models of endotoxemia [33].

Additionally, endothelin also induces some vasodilators, counteracting its vasoconstricting effect, including prostacyclin, NO, and prostaglandin E2. Two endothelin receptors are active in the renal parenchyma: the endothelin-A receptor is found mainly in the vascular compartment, and the endothelin-B receptor is found mainly in the tubular compartment. In an animal model of glycerol-mediated toxic renal injury, selective antagonism of the endothelin-A receptor lessened the reduction in GFR [34]. Preliminary evidence suggested that the endothelin-B receptor is integral to clearing endothelin-1, and probably plays a beneficial role in ischemia. Studies of selective endothelin-A receptor blockade and nonselective endothelin receptor blockade (both endothelin-A receptor and endothelin-B receptor) demonstrated improved outcomes only for the selective blockade in a chronic ischemia animal model, further supporting the beneficial effects of intact endothelin-B receptor function [35].

## Oxidative Stress

Endotoxemia is known to be associated with the generation of reactive oxygen radicals and thus may contribute to oxidative renal injury [3, 36, 37]. Endogenous scavengers of ROS have been shown to attenuate renal tubular injury during endotoxemia. During endotoxemia, levels of endogenous scavengers of ROS such as extracellular superoxide dismutase, which is found predominantly in blood vessels and the kidney, have been noted to be decreased [36]. In a murine model of septic shock and acute renal failure, administration of a superoxide dismutase mimetic that had properties of oxygen-radical scavengers decreased deaths in the animals [36]. Oxygen radicals also scavenge NO to produce peroxynitrite, an injurious ROS. This excess burden of protein oxidation is significantly greater in patients with acute renal failure as compared with critically ill patients with preserved renal function. The levels of protein oxidation are improved by dialysis, but only transiently, and oxidized proteins continue to accumulate during the intradialytic period [37]. The oxidative burden in patients who have acute renal failure in the setting of critical illness may be a target for potential therapies to decrease the excess mortality in these patients.

## Cellular Mechanisms

### Epithelial Dysfunction

The clinical syndrome of acute renal failure in the setting of sepsis manifests itself by a decreasing urine output and rising serum creatinine. It is highly improbable that loss of cell mass *per se* (eithe r by necrosis or apoptosis) accounts for the development of renal dysfunction. Since the histopathology of acute renal failure in humans is remarkably bland, the final step in the development of acute renal failure is probably the widespread dysfunction of renal tubular epithelial cells as a result of the deleterious effects of a poorly controlled sepsis-induced inflammatory response [8]. An important step in this process is the dysfunction of specialized structures in tubular epithelial cells namely the tight junctions [38]. During the evolution of sepsis-induced acute renal failure, dysfunction of tight junctions leads to backleakage of tubular fluid across the epithelium [8, 39]. Loss of cell adhesion to the tubular basement membrane and subsequent shedding into the lumen results in denuded cells appearing in the urine as tubular epithelial cell casts. Such casts may cause micro-obstruction to urine flow. The damaged tubular basement membrane may fill with cast material, cellular debris, and Tamm-Horsfall protein. Sublethal injury results in loss of the brush border, which is the site of much energy consuming metabolic activity. All of the above mechanisms collectively induce renal dysfunction in the absence of overt histological features of renal tubular cell loss.

### The Endothelium

Endothelial activation induced by circulating cytokines and activated complement is likely a key instigator in the evolution of sepsis-induced acute renal failure.

The changes induced in endothelial function by this stimulation enhance the inflammatory process by increasing the production of inflammatory mediators. Endothelial activation is an early host response to circulating pathogens, and likely is triggered by activated and adherent neutrophils and their degradation products. The dysfunctional endothelium is more severely damaged and results in the leaky capillaries associated with sepsis. The process by which endothelium evolves from activated and physiologic to damaged and dysfunctional is relatively unknown and represents a key area for research and a potential target for therapy.

## Apoptosis

Cells can die by one of two pathways: necrosis or apoptosis. Apoptosis is an energy-requiring form of cell death that is mediated by a genetically determined biochemical pathway and is characterized morphologically by cell shrinkage, plasma membrane blebbing, chromatin condensation, and nuclear fragmentation [6,7,40]. Necrosis, however, results from severe ATP depletion and leads to uncoordinated and rapid collapse of cellular homeostasis. Because apoptosis does not result in the release of intracellular material into the extracellular space, it does not result in an inflammatory response [7]. Apoptotic cells are present in tissue sections for a very short period of time ($1\pm3$ hours) before being phagocytosed and destroyed. By contrast, it may take days for histologic evidence of cell necrosis to resolve. Therefore, counting the number of apoptotic and necrotic cells in tissue sections is likely to substantially underestimate the contribution of apoptosis to cell death [7]. Current evidence suggest that human renal tubular cells die by apoptosis as well as necrosis in patients with acute renal failure [41]. Apoptosis is more commonly seen in distal tubular cells, both in animals and in allografts of patients with biopsy-confirmed ATN [42]. It is not yet possible, however, to quantify the relative contributions made by necrosis and apoptosis during acute renal failure *in vivo*.

Schumer et al. [43] have demonstrated that after a very brief period of ischemia (5 minutes), apoptotic bodies could be found 24 hours and 48 hours after reperfusion, and without any evidence of necrosis. After more prolonged periods of ischemia, areas of necrosis became evident, but substantial numbers of apoptotic bodies were still seen after 24 to 48 hours of reperfusion. Until recently the mode of cell necrosis following ischemia was thought to be entirely related to the severity of ATP depletion [40]. Dagher and colleagues [44] however, have shown that ischemia causes depletion of ATP as well as guanine triphosphate (GTP) in cultured renal tubular cells and in the ischemic kidney *in vivo*. Using selective depletion techniques of either ATP or GTP these authors showed that isolated ATP depletion induces necrosis and GTP depletion induces apoptosis. Although GTP supplementation has been shown to reduce apoptosis and ameliorate ischemic renal dysfunction, the mechanisms responsible for the differences in the mode of cell death induced by ATP and GTP depletion remains to be elucidated [45]. The evidence of whether apoptosis plays an important role in tubular injury *in vivo* remains controversial. Particularly controversial is whether renal cell apoptosis occurs in any large measure during sepsis.

'Death Receptors'

The most extensively characterized 'death receptors' belong to the TNF receptor family and include CD95 (Fas) and TNFR-1 [46]. The intracellular domains of these receptors contain 'death domains'. The binding of Fas ligand (FasL) and TNF to their respective receptors, Fas and TNFR-1, leads to oligomerization of the receptors and subsequent activation of caspase 8. While renal tubular cells constitutively express Fas and TNFR-1 [47, 48], they are normally relatively resistant to FasL- and TNF-induced apoptosis. However, during sepsis and endotoxemia renal tubular cells are exposed to inflammatory cytokines or to ATP depletion (which induces cytokine release from these cells) [49], the expression of Fas/FasL and TNF-α/TNFR-1 is upregulated, and the cells become sensitized to Fas and TNF mediated apoptosis [48]. Jo et al. [50] have recently shown that apoptosis of tubular cells by inflammatory cytokines and LPS is a possible mechanism of renal dysfunction in endotoxemia. They found that if high-dose TNF was added to cultured kidney proximal tubular cells, there was increased expression of Fas mRNA, the Fas associated death domain protein, as well as increased DNA fragmentation.

These findings suggest that constitutively expressed death receptors, FasL and TNFR-1, are provided with their appropriate ligand during acute renal injury, and therefore may contribute to apoptosis of renal tubular cells in acute renal failure. Interestingly, increased production of TNF by renal tubular cells during ischemia appears to be mediated by activation of p38, a member of the mitogen-activated protein kinase (MAPK) family of kinases [48]. Almost all current evidence to support a role for Fas and TNF in acute renal failure is derived from studies *in vitro* in cultured renal tubular cells. More studies using experimental models of acute renal failure are needed to firmly establish the importance of FasL and TNFR-1 in acute renal failure *in vivo* during sepsis.

## Coagulation

The activation of coagulation and deposition of fibrin in the tissues is a well-defined component of sepsis-related MOF. Increased expression of tissue factor in response to LPS and TNF stimulation of inflammatory and endothelial cells may contribute to organ injury in sepsis, including renal injury. Tissue factor binds activated factor VII. This complex activates factor X, which cleaves prothrombin to thrombin, which in turn cleaves fibrinogen to fibrin. The activation of the coagulation cascade increases the tissue inflammatory response. Fibrin is often deposited in the intravascular space in animal models of sepsis, including the glomerular capillaries. For these reasons, anticoagulant therapies, or therapies that interfere with initiation of coagulation, are of potential interest in ameliorating organ dysfunction, including renal failure. In a primate model of sepsis, animals were treated with site-inactivated factor VIIa, which serves as a competitive inhibitor of tissue factor, to block the initiation of the coagulation cascade. The treated animals showed preserved renal function at 48 hours, less metabolic acidosis, and better urine output. Histologic examination of the kidneys demonstrated less tubular injury and inflammatory cell infiltration, and fewer fibrin clots than in untreated animals [51]. Activated protein C improves outcomes in sepsis, and it is currently unclear whether it also attenuates sepsis-associated acute renal failure [52].

## Renal Recovery following Acute Renal Failure

Following sub-lethal cell injury, renal tubular cells undergo repair, regeneration, and proliferation (Fig. 1). The first phase of this regeneration process consists of the death and exfoliation of irreversibly injured cells and is characterized by stress response gene expression and infiltration by mononuclear cells [53]. Subsequently many quiescent renal tubular cells enter the cell cycle and undergo either repair or death. This decision point is carefully regulated and cyclin-dependent kinase inhibitors, especially p21, play an important role [54]. Growth factors may play a role in determining the fate of the epithelial cells and may contribute to the generation of signals that result in neutrophil and monocyte infiltration. In the second phase, poorly differentiated epithelial cells appear, which are believed to represent a population of stem cells residing in the kidney [55]. This stage is a dedifferentiation stage. In the third phase, a marked increase in proliferation of the surviving proximal tubule cells is evident and here growth factors may play an important role in this response [56]. In this last phase, the regenerative tubular cells regain their differentiated character and produce a normal proximal tubule epithelium.

A number of growth factors that have anti-apoptotic as well as pro-proliferation effects have been evaluated in acute renal failure. Unfortunately, early clinical trials have not yielded consistent results. However, two agents, bone morphogenic protein-7 (BMP-7) and erythropoietin, have promising, albeit largely hypothetical, effects on renal tubular cells [57]. Recent stem cell research shows that hematopoietic stem cells and other tissue specific stem cells are capable of crossing tissue and even germ-line barriers and can give rise to a remarkable range of cell types [58]. This plasticity of stem cells is thought to be useful in therapeutic strategies designed to enhance tissue regeneration after severe organ injury. Traditionally, stem cells were believed to be organ specific. However, experiments with whole-bone marrow transplantation de monstrated that bone marrow-derived ste mcells could populate the renal tubular epithelium [59]. More recently, injection of mesenchymal stem cells of bone marrow origin has been shown to protect from severe tubular injury and subsequent renal failure in animal models of acute renal failure [60].

## Conclusion

Development of acute renal failure during sepsis syndrome is common and portends a poor outcome. The interplay between systemic host responses, local insults in the kidney, vascular bed, and immune system, all play a role in the development of sepsis-induced acute renal failure. Despite advances in critical care, mortality rates have remained high for sepsis-associated acute renal failure. This may be, in part, a function of our poor understanding of the mechanisms of sepsis-induced acute renal failure, leading to misguided management strategies for acute renal failure. Improved understanding of various emerging mechanisms of sepsis-induced acute renal failure such as epithelial barrier dysfunction, apoptosis, and cytokine-mediated injury, should open newer avenues of therapeutic targets in this field. As has often been the case in the study of sepsis, simple universal mechanisms such as tissue perfusion, have failed to explain the diverse and complex clinical response, and therapeutic strategies aimed at single mechanisms have not been successful. The pathophysiologic mechanisms now understood to be operative in sepsis-induced acute renal failure overlap and interact at many levels. Therefore, therapeutic strategies to prevent acute renal failure or to facilitate recovery will likely need to be multifaceted.

## References

1. de Mendonca A, Vincent JL, Suter PM, et al (2000) Acute renal failure in the ICU: risk factors and outcome evaluated by the SOFA score. Intensive Care Med 26:915–921
2. Uchino S, Kellum JA, Bellomo R, et al (2005) Acute renal failure in critically ill patients: a multinational, multicenter study. JAMA 294:813–818
3. Schrier RW, Wang W (2004) Acute renal failure and sepsis. N Engl J Med 351:159–169
4. Clermont G, Acker CG, Angus DC, Sirio CA, Pinsky MR, Johnson JP (2002) Renal failure in the ICU: comparison of the impact of acute renal failure and end-stage renal disease on ICU outcomes. Kidney Int 62:986–996
5. Kellum JA, Angus DC (2002) Patients are dying of acute renal failure. Crit Care Med 30:2156–2157
6. Wan L, Bellomo R, Di Giantomasso D, Ronco C (2003) The pathogenesis of septic acute renal failure. Curr Opin Crit Care 9:496–502
7. Bonegio R, Lieberthal W (2002) Role of apoptosis in the pathogenesis of acute renal failure. Curr Opin Nephrol Hypertens 11:301–308
8. Fink MP, Delude RL (2005) Epithelial barrier dysfunction: a unifying theme to explain the pathogenesis of multiple organ dysfunction at the cellular level. Crit Care Clin 21:177–196
9. Messmer UK, Briner VA, Pfeilschifter J (2000) Basic fibroblast growth factor selectively enhances TNF-alpha-induced apoptotic cell death in glomerular endothelial cells: effects on apoptotic signaling pathways. J Am Soc Nephrol 11:2199–2211
10. Marshall JC, Vincent JL, Fink MP, et al (2003) Measures, markers, and mediators: toward a staging system for clinical sepsis. A report of the Fifth Toronto Sepsis Roundtable, Toronto, Ontario, Canada, October 25-26, 2000. Crit Care Med 31:1560–1567
11. Kellum JA, Decker M (2001) Use of dopamine in acute renal failure: a meta-analysis. Crit Care Med 29:1526–1531
12. Bellomo R, Chapman M, Finfer S, Hickling K, Myburgh J (2000) Low-dose dopamine in patients with early renal dysfunction: a placebo-controlled randomised trial. Australian and New Zealand Intensive Care Society (ANZICS) Clinical Trials Group. Lancet 356:2139–2143
13. Kikeri D, Pennell JP, Hwang KH, Jacob AI, Richman AV, Bourgoignie JJ (1986) Endotoxemic acute renal failure in awake rats. Am J Physiol 250:F1098–F1106

14. Badr KF (1992) Sepsis-associated renal vasoconstriction: potential targets for future therapy. Am J Kidney Dis 20:207–213
15. Langenberg C, Bellomo R, May C, Wan L, Egi M, Morgera S (2005) Renal blood flow in sepsis. Crit Care 9:R363–R374
16. Brezis M, Rosen S (1995) Hypoxia of the renal medulla–its implications for disease. N Engl J Med 332:647–655
17. Di Giantomasso D, Morimatsu H, May CN, Bellomo R (2003) Intrarenal blood flow distribution in hyperdynamic septic shock: Effect of norepinephrine. Crit Care Med 31:2509–2513
18. Camussi G, Ronco C, Montrucchio G, Piccoli G (1998) Role of soluble mediators in sepsis and renal failure. Kidney Int Suppl 66:S38–S42
19. Linas SL, Whittenburg D, Repine JE (1991) Role of neutrophil derived oxidants and elastase in lipopolysaccharide-mediated renal injury. Kidney Int 39:618–623
20. Xia Y, Feng L, Yoshimura T, Wilson CB (1993) LPS-induced MCP-1, IL-1 beta, and TNF-alpha mRNA expression in isolated erythrocyte-perfused rat kidney. Am J Physiol 264:F774–F780
21. Thijs A, Thijs LG (1998) Pathogenesis of renal failure in sepsis. Kidney Int Suppl 66:S34–S37
22. Baud L, Oudinet JP, Bens M, et al (1989) Production of tumor necrosis factor by rat mesangial cells in response to bacterial lipopolysaccharide. Kidney Int 35:1111–1118
23. Kohan DE (1994) Role of endothelin and tumour necrosis factor in the renal response to sepsis. Nephrol Dial Transplant 9 Suppl 4:73–77
24. Messmer UK, Briner VA, Pfeilschifter J (1999) Tumor necrosis factor-alpha and lipopolysaccharide induce apoptotic cell death in bovine glomerular endothelial cells. Kidney Int 55:2322–2337
25. Knotek M, Rogachev B, Wang W, et al (2001) Endotoxemic renal failure in mice: Role of tumor necrosis factor independent of inducible nitric oxide synthase. Kidney Int 59:2243–2249
26. van Lanschot JJ, Mealy K, Jacobs DO, Evans DA, Wilmore DW (1991) Splenectomy attenuates the inappropriate diuresis associated with tumor necrosis factor administration. Surg Gynecol Obstet 172:293–297
27. Cunningham PN, Dyanov HM, Park P, Wang J, Newell KA, Quigg RJ (2002) Acute renal failure in endotoxemia is caused by TNF acting directly on TNF receptor-1 in kidney. J Immunol 168:5817–5823
28. Rodriguez-Wilhelmi P, Montes R, Matsukawa A, et al (2003) Tumor necrosis factor-alpha inhibition reduces CXCL-8 levels but fails to prevent fibrin generation and does not improve outcome in a rabbit model of endotoxic shock. J Lab Clin Med 141:257–264
29. Cohen RI, Hassell AM, Marzouk K, Marini C, Liu SF, Scharf SM (2001) Renal effects of nitric oxide in endotoxemia. Am J Respir Crit Care Med 164:1890–1895
30. Spain DA, Wilson MA, Garrison RN (1994) Nitric oxide synthase inhibition exacerbates sepsis-induced renal hypoperfusion. Surgery 116:322–330
31. Knotek M, Esson M, Gengaro P, Edelstein CL, Schrier RW (2000) Desensitization of soluble guanylate cyclase in renal cortex during endotoxemia in mice. J Am Soc Nephrol 11:2133–2137
32. Zimmerman GA, Prescott SM, McIntyre TM (1992) Endothelial cell interactions with granulocytes: tethering and signaling molecules. Immunol Today 13:93–100
33. Wang J, Dunn MJ (1987) Platelet-activating factor mediates endotoxin-induced acute renal insufficiency in rats. Am J Physiol 253:F1283–F1289
34. Shimizu T, Kuroda T, Ikeda M, Hata S, Fujimoto M (1998) Potential contribution of endothelin to renal abnormalities in glycerol-induced acute renal failure in rats. J Pharmacol Exp Ther 286:977–983
35. Forbes JM, Hewitson TD, Becker GJ, Jones CL (2001) Simultaneous blockade of endothelin A and B receptors in ischemic acute renal failure is detrimental to long-term kidney function. Kidney Int 59:1333–1341
36. Wang W, Jittikanont S, Falk SA, et al (2003) Interaction among nitric oxide, reactive oxygen species, and antioxidants during endotoxemia-related acute renal failure. Am J Physiol Renal Physiol 284:F532–F537

37. Himmelfarb J, McMonagle E, Freedman S, et al (2004) Oxidative stress is increased in critically ill patients with acute renal failure. J Am Soc Nephrol 15:2449–2456
38. Stevenson BR (1999) Understanding tight junction clinical physiology at the molecular level. J Clin Invest 104:3–4
39. Lechner J, Pfaller W (2001) Interferon alpha2b increases paracellular permeability of renal proximal tubular LLC-PK1 cells via a mitogen activated protein kinase signaling pathway. Ren Fail 23:573–588
40. Lieberthal W, Menza SA, Levine JS (1998) Graded ATP depletion can cause necrosis or apoptosis of cultured mouse proximal tubular cells. Am J Physiol 274:F315–F327
41. Kaushal GP, Basnakian AG, Shah SV (2004) Apoptotic pathways in ischemic acute renal failure. Kidney Int 66:500–506
42. Oberbauer R, Rohrmoser M, Regele H, Muhlbacher F, Mayer G (1999) Apoptosis of tubular epithelial cells in donor kidney biopsies predicts early renal allograft function. J Am Soc Nephrol 10:2006–2013
43. Schumer M, Colombel MC, Sawczuk IS, et al (1992) Morphologic, biochemical, and molecular evidence of apoptosis during the reperfusion phase after brief periods of renal ischemia. Am J Pathol 140:831–838
44. Dagher PC (2000) Modeling ischemia in vitro: selective depletion of adenine and guanine nucleotide pools. Am J Physiol Cell Physiol 279:C1270–C1277
45. Kelly KJ, Plotkin Z, Dagher PC (2001) Guanosine supplementation reduces apoptosis and protects renal function in the setting of ischemic injury. J Clin Invest 108:1291–1298
46. Leist M, Jaattela M (2001) Four deaths and a funeral: from caspases to alternative mechanisms. Nat Rev Mol Cell Biol 2:589–598
47. Lorz C, Ortiz A, Justo P, et al (2000) Proapoptotic Fas ligand is expressed by normal kidney tubular epithelium and injured glomeruli. J Am Soc Nephrol 11:1266–1277
48. Meldrum KK, Meldrum DR, Hile KL, et al (2001) p38 MAPK mediates renal tubular cell TNF-alpha production and TNF-alpha-dependent apoptosis during simulated ischemia. Am J Physiol Cell Physiol 281:C563–C570
49. Feldenberg LR, Thevananther S, del Rio M, de Leon M, Devarajan P (1999) Partial ATP depletion induces Fas- and caspase-mediated apoptosis in MDCK cells. Am J Physiol 276:F837–F846
50. Jo SK, Cha DR, Cho WY, et al (2002) Inflammatory cytokines and lipopolysaccharide induce Fas-mediated apoptosis in renal tubular cells. Nephron 91:406–415
51. Carraway MS, Welty-Wolf KE, Miller DL, et al (2003) Blockade of tissue factor: treatment for organ injury in established sepsis. Am J Respir Crit Care Med 167:1200–1209
52. Bernard GR, Vincent JL, Laterre PF, et al (2001) Efficacy and safety of recombinant human activated protein C for severe sepsis. N Engl J Med 344:699–709
53. Lameire N (2005) The pathophysiology of acute renal failure. Crit Care Clin 21:197–210
54. Price PM, Megyesi J, Saf Irstein RL (2004) Cell cycle regulation: repair and regeneration in acute renal failure. Kidney Int 66:509–514
55. Al Awqati Q, Oliver JA (2002) Stem cells in the kidney. Kidney Int 61:387–395
56. Hammerman MR, Miller SB (1994) Therapeutic use of growth factors in renal failure. J Am Soc Nephrol 5:1–11
57. Kellum JA (2004) What can be done about acute renal failure? Minerva Anestesiol 70:181–188
58. Rookmaaker MB, Verhaar MC, van Zonneveld AJ, Rabelink TJ (2004) Progenitor cells in the kidney: biology and therapeutic perspectives. Kidney Int 66:518–522
59. Poulsom R, Forbes SJ, Hodivala-Dilke K, et al (2001) Bone marrow contributes to renal parenchymal turnover and regeneration. J Pathol 195:229–235
60. Lange C, Togel F, Ittrich H, et al (2005) Administered mesenchymal stem cells enhance recovery from ischemia/reperfusion-induced acute renal failure in rats. Kidney Int 68:1613–1617

# Sepsis-Induced Brain Dysfunction

C. Guidoux, T. Sharshar, and D. Annane

## Introduction

The central nervous system (CNS) controls a wide range of physiological functions [1, 2] that are crucial to maintain homeostasis and to orchestrate the host response to stress at behavioral, neuroendocrine, and autonomic levels [2]. Interactions between the immune system and the CNS are considered to play a major role in the host response in septic shock. It is well established that brain centers involved in neuroendocrine [3] and autonomic control, wakefulness, awareness, and behavior are signaled during sepsis. This signaling, which involves various inflammatory mediators and neurotransmitters, can foster an adaptive response, optimizing the host response to stress, but also a maladaptive one, through inappropriate activity or damage to these centers. It has been shown that encephalopathy, and neuroendocrine or autonomic dysfunction, occur frequently during septic shock and may contribute to organ dysfunction and death.

## Definition

Sepsis is defined as infection with systemic inflammation, consisting of two or more of the following: increased or decreased temperature, increased or decreased leukocyte count, tachycardia, and rapid breathing [4]. Septic shock is sepsis with hypotension that persists after resuscitation with intravenous fluid. Normally, the immune and neuroendocrine systems control the local inflammatory process to eradicate pathogens. When this local control mechanism fails, systemic inflammation occurs, allowing the progression from infection to sepsis, severe sepsis, and septic shock.

## Cerebral Mechanisms Involved During Sepsis

### Brain Structures

Multiple brain structures orchestrate the responses to a stressful challenge (Fig. 1). The systemic response to infection depends on a complex, organized, and coherent interaction between immune, autonomic, neuroendocrine, and behavioral systems [3, 5, 6]. The main brain structures involved in this response are, briefly:

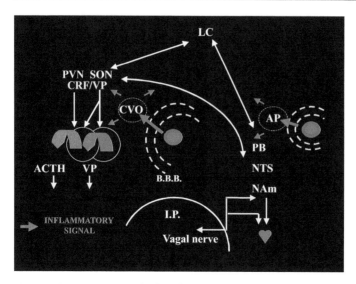

**Fig. 1.** Brain structures involved in the response to inflammation. PVN: parvocellular nucleus; SON: supraoptic nucleus; CRF: corticotropin releasing factor; VP: vasopressin; ACTH: adrenocorticotropin hormone; CVO: circum ventricular ovale; BBB: blood-brain barrier; AP: area postrema; PB: parabrachial nucleus; NTS: nucleus tractus solitarius; Nam: nucleus ambiguus

1. The medullary autonomic nuclei (i. e., solitary tract nuclei, the dorsal motor nucleus of the vagus, and the nucleus ambiguus), which control parasympathetic output directly and sympathetic activity indirectly, through the intermedio-lateral cell column in the thoracic spinal cord. These nuclei are controlled by the parabrachial nuclei, A5 cell group, and the area postrema, which are located in the brainstem and control the medullary autonomic nuclei.

2. The reticular formation which contains various nuclei that are the core of the specific neurotransmitter network involved in the control of sleep and arousal. Thus, midbrain raphe nuclei, the basal Meynert nuclei, and the locus coeruleus are the core of the serotonergic, cholinergic, and noradrenergic networks. The locus coeruleus is connected to the hypothalamus and to the medullar autonomic nuclei.

3. The hypothalamus and pituitary gland. The hypothalamic paraventricular and supraoptic nuclei play an important role in the stress response as they synthesize and release corticotrophin-releasing factor (CRF) and vasopressin. These hypothalamic nuclei are linked directly or indirectly to the brainstem nuclei, locus coeruleus, and the amygdala, which is located in the hippocampus and connected to the limbic system [3].

## Neuroendocrine Mechanisms

The stress response includes, among others, activation of the renin–angiotensin system and activation of the hypothalamic–pituitary–adrenocortical axis. A typical neuroendocrine response is characterized by [3]:

- within seconds, an increase in the secretion of catecholamines (epinephrine and norepinephrine) from the sympathetic nervous system and adrenal medulla, the release of CRF and vasopressin from parvicellular neurons into the portal circulation, and the secretion of oxytocin from the neural lobe of the pituitary
- 5–10 seconds later, the secretion of pituitary ACTH
- a few seconds later, decreased secretion of pituitary gonadotropins and increased secretion of prolactin and growth hormone (in primates) from the anterior pituitary, as well as increased secretion of renin and glucagon from the kidneys and pancreas, respectively.
- a few minutes later, an increase in the plasma levels of glucocorticoids and inhibition of the secretion of gonadal steroids.

Various neuropeptides and neurotransmitters regulate the stress response in a coordinated way, each following a particular time course and being specific for a given stressor. These neuropeptides comprise in the main vasopressin, serotonin, norepinephrine, vasoactive intestinal polypeptide, neuropeptide Y, substance P, and estrogen.

## The Immune System

The immune system can be considered as a diffuse sensory system, which informs the brain of the presence of microorganism constituents or inflammation through three main pathways: [2–7]:

1. cerebral structures which are deprived of the blood-brain barrier so that microorganisms and inflammatory components can easily diffuse into the brain. These structures are the circumventricular organs, which include, at the level of the fourth ventricle, the area postrema, and at the level of the third ventricle, the median eminence, neurohypophysis, pineal gland, subfornical organ, and lamina terminalis. These structures are strategically located as they are very close to the autonomic or neuroendocrine centers.
2. the vagus nerve, which acts as a reflex loop as it senses peripheral inflammation (presumably through cytokine receptors on the nerve surface), conveys immune-related information to the medulla, and then suppresses the inflammatory response at the site of infection (through nicotinic acetylcholine receptors on the monocyte surface).
3. endothelial activation and leakage, which enables release or passive diffusion of mediators.

The brain is, therefore, physiologically signaled during sepsis because it is reached by constituents of microorganisms and inflammatory mediators and because it is able to detect these molecules through specific receptors. Physiologically, there is in fact a sort of inflammatory signal (so-called migratory pattern of brain activation) that is characterized by expression of mediators and their receptors, and that originates from vagus nerve nuclei, from the blood-brain barrier-deprived structures, or from activated endothelial cells, and spreads to deeper brain areas controlling neuroendocrine and autonomic functions, involving both glial cells and neurons. Alteration of the blood-brain barrier, which may occur during sepsis, favors brain edema and inflammation.

## Blood-brain Barrier

The blood-brain barrier is a diffusion barrier [8], controlling entry of plasma substances. It is composed of endothelial cells, astrocyte end-feet, and pericytes. The tight junctions between the cerebral endothelial cells form a diffusion barrier, which selectively excludes most blood-borne substances from entering the brain.

Diffuse endothelial activation or 'panendothelitis' is a hallmark of septic shock. Lipopolysaccharide (LPS) and pro-inflammatory cytokines induce expression of CD40 [9], and of adhesion molecules by endothelial cells from human brain. They also cause transcriptional activation of the cyclooxygenase 2 gene and stimulation of the I$\kappa$B-$\alpha$/nuclear factor-$\kappa$B (NF-$\kappa$B) pathway. Although brain endothelial cells do not express surface CD14, LPS triggers the mitogen-activated protein kinase (MAPK) cascade through soluble CD14. LPS-activated brain endothelial cells exhibit interleukin (IL)-1 and tumor necrosis factor (TNF)-$\alpha$ receptors; produce IL-1$\beta$, TNF-$\alpha$, and IL-6; and exhibit endothelial and inducible nitric oxide synthase (NOS). These mediators are able to interact with surrounding brain cells, relaying the inflammatory response into the brain. Septic shock-induced endothelial activation may result in alteration in the blood-brain barrier and cerebrovascular dysfunction, an effect which is attenuated by glial cells, dexamethasone, or NOS inhibition. Nevertheless, contradictory results have been obtained in animal and human studies that have assessed cerebral blood flow, endothelial reactivity, and oxygen consumption during sepsis.

## Apoptosis

Inflammatory signals may result in neuronal and glial apoptosis [10]. Indeed, TNF-$\alpha$ and NO, which are expressed in the brain during sepsis, are pro-apoptotic factors. Apoptotic neurons and microglial cells have been found in neuroendocrine and autonomic nuclei of patients who have died from septic shock. The intensity of apoptosis is correlated with iNOS expression in endothelial cells. This result suggests that sepsis-induced activation of astro- and microglia in the brain and subsequent production of NO initiates apoptosis and necrosis of neurons and glial cells. However, it cannot be inferred that apoptosis is detrimental, even if it has been reported that it correlates with antemortem duration of hypotension in humans. For example, neuronal cytochrome C, which is a pro-apoptotic factor, might favor survival of rats with sepsis. Further studies are needed to assess the mechanisms and consequences of apoptosis and the pathogenic role of NO and other inflammatory mediators in sepsis-related encephalopathy, neuroendocrine and autonomic dysfunction. It remains speculative to claim that strategies based on NO inhibition or apoptosis prevention will be neuroprotective.

## Neuropathology

In a prospective autopsy study of 23 patients who had died from septic shock [11], various lesions were found, including ischemia (in all cases), hemorrhage (in 26% of cases), micro-thrombi (in 9%), micro-abscesses (in 9%) and multifocal necrotizing leukoencephalopathy (in 9%), which were associated with both local expression and high circulating levels of pro-inflammatory cytokines. The latter finding demonstrates that the brain can be damaged through pure inflammatory processes during septic shock and not only through ischemia or coagulation disturbances. However, the incidence and features of brain lesions in the ante-mortem period and in patients surviving septic shock remain to be explored.

## Clinical Features: Sepsis-associated Encephalopathy

## Introduction

Sepsis and its complications are the leading causes of mortality accounting for 10 to 50% of intensive care unit (ICU) deaths [12]. The characterization of inflammatory cascades leading to multiple organ failure (MOF) and ultimately death has attracted much interest. Studies have mostly focused on peripheral organs such as the lung, liver, gut, and kidney, and much less on the brain whose role in the pathophysiological mechanisms of shock is far from fully understood.

Septic encephalopathy is the clinical manifestation of sepsis- or SIRS (systemic inflammatory response syndrome)-related brain dysfunction [13]. It is the most common cause of encephalopathy in the critically ill. The severity of encephalopathy correlates with the severity of illness, as assessed by the Acute Physiology and Chronic Health Evaluation (APACHE) II score or organ failure scores and mortality. Septic encephalopathy is an independent predictor of death.

The most immediate complication of septic encephalopathy is impaired consciousness, and the patient may require ventilation. The etiology of septic encephalopathy involves disruption of the blood-brain barrier as a result of the interaction of inflammatory mediators with the cerebrovascular endothelium, abnormal neurotransmitter composition of the reticular activating system, impaired astrocyte function and neuronal degeneration, reduced cerebral blood flow and oxygen extraction, and cerebral edema.

## Definition

Septic patients often develop encephalopathy, defined as a deterioration in mental status or level of consciousness. This encephalopathy may occur without evidence of bacterial blood stream invasion. Wilson and Young [14] prefer the term "sepsis-associated encephalopathy" rather than "septic encephalopathy", as it suggests a diffuse cerebral dysfunction induced by the systemic response to infection without clinical or laboratory evidence of direct infection of the CNS, whereas the latter signifies a cerebral infection.

## Clinical Features

Sepsis associated encephalopathy can be classified as 'early' or 'late' [1], depending on whether it occurs before or after development of MOF. Hepatic and renal failure may obviously exacerbate the brain dysfunction in advanced sepsis.

Neurological symptoms range, according to severity, from fluctuating confusion, inattention and inappropriate behavior, to delirium and then deterioration in conscious level or coma. Motor signs such as asterixis, myoclonus, or tremor, are rarely observed and more frequent in metabolic – than in septic-encephalopathy. More common is 'paratonic rigidity', which is a velocity dependent resistance to passive movements and requires moving the limbs rapidly in order to demonstrate it.

Seizures are uncommon in sepsis-associated encephalopathy and the cranial nerves are usually spared [14]. Neuroimaging is mandatory if focal neurological signs are present as they are exceptional in septic encephalopathy and suggest a cerebral lesion.

## Evaluation

Different scores can be used to assess the severity of encephalopathy induced by sepsis. The Glasgow Coma Scale (GCS) is certainly the most used [15] and is useful as it clearly correlates with mortality [16]. As the GCS score drops from 15 to below 8, the mortality rate increases from 16% to 63%. However, we believe that the Confusion Assessment Method for Intensive Care Unit (CAM-ICU) is more sensitive than the GCS to detect brain dysfunction, especially in mechanically ventilated patients.

## Investigations
### Electroencephalogram and Somatosensory Evoked Potentials

Electroencephalogram (EEG) is better than GCS for detecting sepsis-associated encephalopathy [17], as it may reveal mild diffuse reversible slowing in patients with normal neurological examination. Five classes of progressively worsening

EEG pattern have been identified: 1 = normal EEG; 2 = excessive theta; 3 = predominant delta; 4 = triphasic waves; 5 = suppression or burst suppression. The mortality rate is proportional to the severity of the EEG abnormality, ranging from 0 to 67% as EEG abnormalities progress from class 1 to 5. The bispectral index (BIS) of the EEG (a statistically derived variable that allows an easier interpretation of the EEG) might be useful for assessment of neurological status in non-sedated critically ill patients [18]. The main limitation of the EEG is that it cannot detect brain dysfunction in sedated patients.

In contrast, somatosensory evoked potentials (SEPs) are not affected by sedative drugs [19]. An increase in subcortical and cortical peak latencies of SEPs has been reported in patients with SIRS related or not to sepsis. The impairment of subcortical and cortical pathways was correlated with severity of illness, but did not differ between patients with severe sepsis and those with septic shock. In a pig model of pancreatitis-related SIRS [20], SEP amplitude attenuation preceded hemodynamic SIRS criteria by at least four hours.

## Magnetic Resonance Imaging (MRI)

No study has determined whether septic encephalopathy is associated with actual radiographic lesions. Computed tomography (CT) scan is limited for this purpose, with magnetic resonance imaging (MRI) being a better tool for screening early abnormalities. Indeed, the new sequences, such as diffusion-weight and apparent diffusion coefficients, are highly sensitive. The main limitation is that unstable and mechanically ventilated patients need to be transported to the MRI room.

## Biological Investigations

Cerebrospinal fluid (CSF) analysis is generally normal, except for an inconstant elevation in protein concentration. Neurone-specific enolase, a marker of brain injury, may be of some prognostic value in septic shock [21].

## Conclusion

Sepsis is often associated with CNS dysfunction that is frequently unrecognized. This dysfunction is not due to direct infection of the CNS, so is better termed 'sepsis-associated encephalopathy'. An altered mental status may be present in the early stage of sepsis, even preceding common clinical signs of sepsis. EEG and other neurophysiologic techniques may help to detect sub-clinical alterations and to establish clinical outcome. The pathophysiological mechanism of sepsis-associated encephalopathy is not perfectly understood and is very likely multifactorial, involving direct toxicity of microorganisms or byproducts, and the effects of inflammatory mediators, metabolic alterations, and impaired cerebral circulation. There are no specific or symptomatic treatments for sepsis-associated encephalopathy.

# References

1. Papadopoulos MC, Davies DC, Moss RF, Tighe D, Bennett ED (2000) Pathophysiology of septic encephalopathy: a review. Crit Care Med 28:3019–3024
2. Sharshar T, Hopkinson NS, Orlikowski O, Annane D (2005) Science review: The brain in sepsis – culprit and victim. Crit Care 9:37–44
3. Carrasco GA, Van de Kar LD (2003) Neuroendocrine pharmacology of stress. Eur J Phamarcol 463:235–272
4. Annane D, Bellissant E, Cavaillon JM (2005) Septic shock. Lancet 365:63–78
5. Spyer KM (1989) Neural mechanisms involved in cardiovascular control during affective behaviour. Trends Neurosci 12:506–513.
6. Chrousos GP (1995) The hypothalamic-pituitary-adrenal-axis and immune-mediated inflammation. N Engl J Med 332:1351–1362
7. Goehler LE, Gaykema RP, Hansen MK, Anderson K, Maier SF, Watkins LR (2000) Vagal immune-to-brain communication: a visceral chemosensory pathway. Auton Neurosci 85:49–59
8. Ballabh P, Braun A, Nedergaard M (2004) The blood–brain barrier: an overview: Structure, regulation, and clinical implications. Neurobiol Dis 16:1–13
9. Omari KM, Dorovini-Zis K (2003) CD40 expressed by human brain endothelial cells regulate CD4+ T cell adhesion to endothelium. J Neuroimmunol 134:166–178
10. Yuan J, Yankner BA (2000) Apoptosis in the nervous system. Nature 407:802–809
11. Sharshar T, Annane D, de la Grandmaison G, Brouland JP, Hopkinson NS, Gray F (2004) The neuropathology of septic shock. Brain Pathol 14:21–33
12. Barlas I, Oropello JM, Benjamin E (2001) Neurologic complications in intensive care Current Opinion in Critical Care 7:68–73
13. G. Consales, A.R. De Gaudio (2005) Sepsis associated encephalopathy. Minerva Anestesiol 71:39–52
14. Wilson JX, Young GB (2002) Sepsis-associated encephalopathy: evolving concepts. Can J Neurol Sci 30: 98–105
15. Cook R, Cook D, Tilley J, Lee K, Marshall J (2001) Multiple organ dysfunction: baseline and serial component scores. Crit Care Med 29:2046–2050
16. Russell JA, Singer J, Bernard GR, et al (2000) Changing pattern of organ dysfunction in early human sepsis is related to mortality. Crit Care Med 28:3405–3411
17. Young GB, Bolton CF, Archibald YM, Austn TW, Wells GA (1992) The electroencephalogram in sepsis-associated encephalopathy. J Clin Neurophysiol 9:145–152
18. Gilbert TT, Wagner MR, Halukurike V, Paz HL, Garland A (2001) Use of bispectral electroencephalogram monitoring to assess neurologic status in unsedated, critically ill patients. Crit Care Med 29:1996–2000
19. Zauner C, Gendo A, Kramer L, et al (2002) Impaired subcortical and cortical sensory evoked potential pathways in septic patients. Crit Care Med 30:1136–1139
20. Ohnesorge H, Bishoff P, Scholz J, Yekebas E, Schulte AM, Esch J (2003) Somatosensory evoked potentials as predictor of systemic response syndrome in pigs? Intensive Care Med 29:801–807
21. Weigand MA, Volkmann M, Scmidt H, Martin E, Bohrer H, Bardenheuer HU (2000) Neuron specific enolase as a marker of fatal outcome in patients with severe sepsis or septic shock. Anesthesiology 92:905–907

# Myocardial Depression in Sepsis and Septic Shock

A. Kumar and J.E. Parrillo

## Introduction

Sepsis and septic shock represent a major cause of mortality and morbidity in the developed world. The most widely accepted estimate of incidence of severe sepsis in the United States suggests 750,000 cases per year, with 215,000 annual deaths [1]. Over the past 40 years, the incidence of sepsis has increased at approximately 8.7% per year [2]. During the same time period, total mortality has increased, even though the overall mortality rate has fallen from 27.8% to 17.9% [2]. Age adjusted mortality has increased from 0.5–7 per 100,000 episodes of sepsis and septic shock. Much of that mortality occurs in the as many as 60% of severely septic patients who develop circulatory shock with organ failure and hypotension refractory to fluid resuscitation. In these patients, mortality may exceed 60%. Despite major advances in our understanding of the pathophysiology of septic shock, the associated mortality of septic shock appears not to have changed substantially over the past 40 years.

Sepsis has been defined as the systemic inflammatory response to infection [3]. The inciting focus of sepsis, via either exotoxins or a structural microbial component (endotoxin, teichoic acid, peptidoglycans, bacterial nucleic acids) causes local and systemic release of a wide variety of endogenous inflammatory mediators like tumor necrosis factor-$\alpha$ (TNF-$\alpha$), interleukin-1$\alpha$ (IL-1$\alpha$), platelet activating factor (PAF), oxygen free radicals, interferon gamma (IFN-$\gamma$) and arachidonic acid metabolites from monocytes/macrophages and other cells. In order to maintain homeostasis (and likely as part of a feedback mechanism), several anti-inflammatory mediators are also released, including IL-10, transforming growth factor-$\beta$ (TGF$\beta$) and IL-1 receptor antagonist (IL-1ra). If homeostasis cannot be maintained, there can be progressive and sequential dysfunction of various organ systems, termed the multiple organ dysfunction syndrome (MODS). If the inflammatory stimulus is particularly intense or if there is limited cardiovascular reserve, effects on the cardiovascular system as manifested by septic shock may dominate the clinical presentation. Sepsis-associated myocardial depression occurs as one manifestation of cardiovascular dysfunction in septic shock.

This chapter reviews the following aspects of septic myocardial dysfunction – right and left ventricular failure, systolic and diastolic dysfunction and cardiovascular prognosticating factors. Potential pathophysiologic mechanisms of myocardial depression from organ to molecular/cellular level are also examined.

# Clinical Manifestations of Cardiovascular Dysfunction

## Historical Perspectives

The last 30 years have yielded substantial information about the underlying abnormalities in septic shock, but many unanswered questions remain. Prior to the introduction of the balloon-tipped pulmonary artery catheter (PAC) to assess cardiovascular performance, much of our understanding of septic hemodynamics was based on clinical findings. There were two distinct clinical presentations of septic shock: warm shock characterized by high cardiac output, warm dry skin, and bounding pulses; and cold shock characterized by low cardiac output, cold clammy skin and diminished pulses [4]. Clowes et al. [5] described the relationship between warm and cold shock as a continuum in which either recovery or progression to death occurred. Other clinical studies also supported a correlation between survival and a high cardiac index (CI). The concept was further reinforced by experimental animal studies that demonstrated low CI in endotoxic shock. However, all the clinical studies used central venous pressure (CVP) as a reflection of left ventricular (LV) end-diastolic volume (LVEDV) and adequacy of resuscitation. Based on evidence collected over the past four decades, we now know that CVP is a poor measure of preload in critically ill patients, particularly septic patients [6]. With respect to the animal studies, endotoxic shock was found to be a poor model of the cardiovascular response to clinical infection with live organisms in a defined focus of infection. Prior to the widespread adoption of the PAC, the direct linkage between adequacy of intravascular volume and CI and their relationship to survival was suggested in only a handful of studies.

In addition to allowing the routine measurement of cardiac output, the introduction of the PAC enabled the routine measurement of preload as pulmonary artery occlusion pressure (PAOP). Human studies performed since the introduction of the PAC have consistently demonstrated that adequately volume resuscitated septic shock patients consistently manifest a hyperdynamic circulatory state with high cardiac output and reduced systemic vascular resistance (SVR), with this hyperdynamic profile usually persisting until death in non-survivors (Fig. 1) [7,8]. These findings have now been confirmed in several live infection animal models of sepsis.

In the years following the introduction of the PAC, radionuclide cineangiography (RNCA) and its application to critically ill patients have offered insight into the relative contribution of decreased contractility and compliance in myocardial depression. More recently, bedside transthoracic and transesophageal echocardiographic techniques have further expanded our understanding of cardiac dysfunction during sepsis and septic shock.

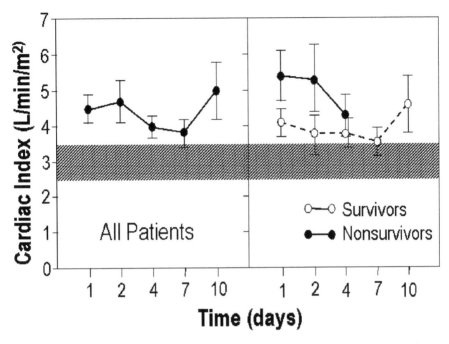

**Fig. 1.** The mean (SEM) cardiac index plotted against time for all patients, survivors, and non-survivors. The hatched areas show the normal range. All groups maintained an elevated cardiac index throughout the study period. The difference between the survivors and non-survivors was not statistically significant. Open circles, survivors; closed circles, non-survivors. From [11] with permission

## Ventricular Function

After the typical high cardiac output, low SVR pattern of septic shock was demonstrated, MacLean and colleagues [4] were among the first to argue that heart failure remained an issue during septic shock because metabolic demand exceeds myocardial performance. The concept of septic myocardial depression despite a hyperdynamic circulatory state was reinforced by both Weisel et al. [9] and Rackow et al. [10]. These groups examined responses to fluid resuscitation in septic shock patients using PACs. Each demonstrated similar evidence of myocardial depression in septic shock patients, showing decreased stroke work response to fluid resuscitation.

The two studies were hampered by inherent limitations in standard PAC-derived data. Changes in myocardial contractility or compliance can identically produce the depression of the Frank-Starling curve derived from PAC-derived filling pressures. This problem was solved by the application of RNCA to critically ill patients [11, 12].

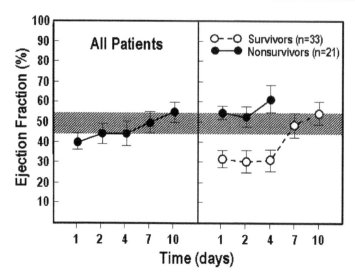

Fig. 2. The mean (*i* SEM) left ventricular ejection fraction (LVEF) plotted versus time for all patients, survivors, and non-survivors. Overall, septic shock patients showed a decreased LVEF at the time of initial assessment. This effect was due to marked early depression of LVEF among survivors that persisted for up to 4 days and returned to normal within 7 to 10 days. Non-survivors maintained LVEF in the normal range. The hatched area represents the normal range. Open circles, survivors; closed circles, nonsurvivors. From [11] with permission

## Left Ventricular Function

Systolic dysfunction has been shown to be impaired in septic patients in a number of studies. Parker et al. [11] demonstrated that septic shock survivors had decreased LV ejection fraction (LVEF) and acute LV dilatation evidenced by increased LVEDV index (LVEDVI) (Fig. 2) using RNCA. These changes in survivors corrected to baseline in 7–10 days. Non-survivors sustained normal LVEF and LVEDVI until death. Despite systolic dysfunction, septic shock patients maintained a high cardiac output and low SVR as shown by the PAC. In a late r study, Ognibene et al. compared LV performance curves (plotting LVSWI vs. LVEDVI) of septic and non-septic critically ill patients (Fig. 3). They showed a flattening of the curve in septic shock patients, with significantly smaller LVSWI increments in response to similar LVEDVI increments when compared to non-septic critically ill controls [13]. In the years since these observations, other studies have confirmed the presence of significant LV systolic dysfunction in septic patients using both RNCA and echocardiographic techniques [12,14,15]. Raper and colleagues in particular have confirmed myocardial depression in septic patients without shock [16].

LV diastolic dysfunction in septic patients is less clearly defined. The acute LV dilatation shown by Parker et al. [11] and a concordant relation between PAOP and LVEDV do not support the presence of significant diastolic dysfunction. However, Ellrodt and colleagues [12] suggested the possibility of significant variations of

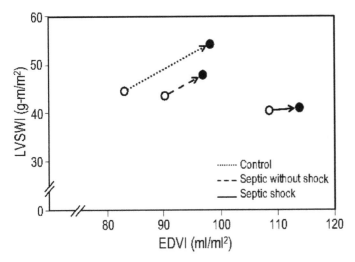

**Fig. 3.** Frank-Starling ventricular performance relationships for each of the 3 patient groups. Data points plotted represent the mean prevolume and postvolume infusion values of end-diastolic volume index (EDVI) and left ventricular stroke work index (LVSWI) for each patient group. Control patients showed a normal increase of EDVI and LVSWI in response to volume infusion. The absolute increases of EDVI and LVSWI in patients with sepsis without shock were less than those of control subjects, but the slope of the curve is similar to control patients. Patients with septic shock had a greatly diminished response and showed a marked rightward and downward shift of the Frank-Starling relationship. From [13] with permission

diastolic compliance in septic patients, based on a lack of correlation between measured PAOP and any parameter of LV performance or volume. Jafri et al. [17], using doppler echocardiographic techniques, demonstrated reduced rapidity of ventricular filling and greater reliance on atrial contributions to LVEDV in patients with either normotensive sepsis or septic shock, when compared with controls. Recently, using transesophageal echocardiography (TEE) of vasopressor-dependent septic shock, Poelaert and colleagues [18] demonstrated a continuum of LV pathophysiology ranging from isolated diastolic dysfunction to combined systolic and diastolic abnormalities. This was subsequently confirmed by Munt and colleagues who demonstrated aberrant LV relaxation by Doppler echocardiography in a group of patients with severe sepsis [19]. These investigators have further documented a more severe defect in non-survivors than in survivors of severe sepsis.

The concept of preload adaptation by acute LV dilatation in septic shock has been questioned by Jardin and colleagues in recent years [20]. TEE was performed in patients with septic shock following fluid and pressor resuscitation. LVEDV appeared to remain in normal range and low LVEF correlated with stroke index independently of LVEDV. A subsequent longitudinal echocardiographic study found significantly smaller LVEDV in non-survivors than in survivors [15]. Unfortunately, the authors did not utilize PAC monitoring as a measure of fluid loading so direct comparison with the series of studies by Parker and colleagues is difficult [11, 13]. However, differences in the two groups' observations may potentially be explained by more modest fluid loading in these recent echocardiographic studies [15, 20].

## Right Ventricular Function

Although the output of the ventricles cannot differ in the absence of anatomic cardiopulmonary shunts, the right ventricle may be subject to substantially different influences than the left ventricle particularly in pathophysiologic conditions such as shock. For that reason, right ventricular (RV) function in sepsis and septic shock cannot be assumed to closely parallel LV function. In the systemic circulation, septic shock is associated with a decreased vascular resistance and blood pressure, almost always resulting in decreased LV afterload which in turn tends to maintain or elevate cardiac output despite the presence of depressed LV contractility. In contrast, RV afterload is often elevated in sepsis and septic shock due to increases in pulmonary vascular resistance (PVR) associated with acute lung injury (ALI) and acute respiratory distress syndrome (ARDS), tending to decrease RV output. Further, it has also been suggested that differentially reduced RV perfusion and contractility could potentially result from a decrease in the RV perfusion gradient during septic shock associated with pulmonary hypertension.

Systolic RV dysfunction has been shown by decreased RVEF and RV dilatation in volume resuscitated patients. Kimchi et al. [21] and Parker et al. [22] showed that RV dysfunction can occur even in the absence of increased pulmonary artery pressures and PVR suggesting that increased RV afterload may not be the sole explanation for RV dysfunction in septic shock. Parker et al. [22] also showed that RV and LV function paralleled each other in dysfunction and recovery (Fig. 4). In this study, survivors showed RV dilatation and decreased RVEF and RVSWI which normalized in 7–14 days. As with the left ventricle, the right ventricle was only moderately dilated and RVEF marginally decreased; both persisted through their course of sepsis.

Since RV dysfunction occurred independently of changes in PVR and pulmonary artery pressures, increased RV afterload could not be the dominant cause of RV depression in human septic shock. Another hypothesis suggested that sepsis-associated RV dilation caused septal displacement (due to pericardial constraint) thereby decreasing LV compliance, preload, and performance. The study by Parker et al. [22] also argued against this proposal since biventricular dilation makes that possibility highly unlikely. Newer technologies, using newly developed PACs equipped with fast response thermistors coupled to computerized analytic equipment, have generated confirmatory data regarding RV dysfunction in sepsis.

Available evidence suggests that despite the differences between the ventricles in structure and function, RV dysfunction in septic shock closely parallels LV dysfunction. RV function in both sepsis and septic shock is characterized by ventricular dilation and decreased RVEF, changes that resolve over 7–14 days in septic

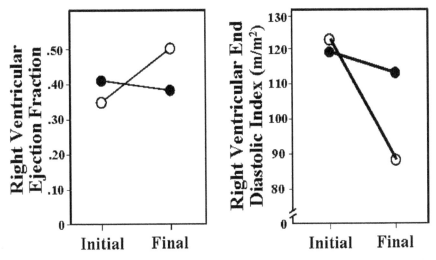

**Fig. 4.** Serial changes in right ventricular ejection fraction and end-diastolic volume index during septic shock in humans. (A) Mean initial and final right ventricular ejection fractions for survivors (closed circles, p<0.001) and non-survivors (open circles, p<0.001). (B) Mean initial and final right ventricular end-diastolic volume index for survivors (closed circles, p<0.05) and nonsurvivors (open circles, p = not significant). The right ventricle, similar to the left, undergoes dilation with a drop in ejection fraction with the acute onset of septic shock. In 7 to 10 days, right ventricular dilation and decreased ejection fraction revert to normal in survivors. From [87] with permission, data from [22]

shock survivors. The cardiovascular profiles of non-survivors are characterized by persistence of RV dysfunction.

Diastolic (compliance) dysfunction of the right ventricle has also been demonstrated in a number of studies. Kimchi et al. [21] noticed a lack of correlation between right atrial pressure and RVEDV, suggesting altered RV compliance. In another study, a subgroup of patients who were volume loaded demonstrated increase in CVP but not in RVEDVI [23]. As in the left ventricle, the relative contribution of systolic and diastolic dysfunction in the right ventricle is unknown.

## Cardiovascular Prognostic Factors in Septic Shock

CI appears not to be a reliable predictor of mortality in septic shock. Despite early evidence suggesting low CI as a poor prognostic factor [5], introduction of the PAC has shown that septic shock patients, both survivors and non-survivors, when adequately fluid-resuscitated have a high CI and low SVR. Armed with the PAC, other hemodynamic parameters were investigated as prognostic indicators.

Baumgartner et al. [24] recognized that patients with extremely high CI ($> 7.0 \, l/min/m^2$) and accordingly low SVR had poor outcomes. Groeneveld et al. also found that non-survivors had lower SVR than survivors after matching other characteristics, concluding that there may be a link between outcome in septic shock and the degree of peripheral vasodilation [25].

Parker et al. [7] reviewed hemodynamic data from septic shock patients on presentation and at 24 hours to identify prognostic value. On presentation, only heart rate < 106 beats/min suggested a favorable outcome. At 24 hours, heart rate< 95 beats/min, SVRI> 1,529 dynes/sec/cm$^5$/m$^2$, a decrease in heart rate> 18 beats/min and a decrease in CI > 0.5 l/min/m$^2$ all predicted survival. In a subsequent study [8], the same authors confirmed previous findings of decreased LVEF and increased LVEDVI in survivors of septic shock but not in non-survivors, a finding that has been confirmed by other groups [14, 15]. Although myocardial depression has been historically linked to increased mortality, these data may imply that depression, at least as manifested by decreased ejection fraction with ventricular dilatation, may actually represent an adaptive response to stress rather than a maladaptive manifestation of injury.

From the studies of Parker and Parillo [7, 8], it is apparent that, despite not developing significant LV dilatation overall, non-survivors can be divided into two patterns: those with progressively declining LVEDVI and CI, and those with incremental increases in LVEDVI while maintaining CI. Based on this, Parker et al. described different hemodynamic collapse profiles leading to death in septic shock [7, 8]. First, some patients die from refractory hypotension secondary to distributive shock with preserved or elevated CI. The other pattern consists of a cardiogenic form of septic shock with decreased CI and a mixture of cardiogenic and distributive shock patterns. The explanation of the two patterns came from a study by Parker et al. [8]. It appears that patients who cannot dilate their left ventricle (decreasing CI and LVEDVI) die from a cardiogenic form of septic shock. The other fatal pattern consists of those patients who can dilate their left ventricle and preserve CI (increase LVEDVI while maintaining CI) but eventually die of distributive shock

The prognostic value of RV hemodynamic parameters has been debated. A number of studies have shown that RV dilatation and decreased RVEF, if persistent, is associated with poor prognosis [22, 26]. However, Vincent et al. [26] suggested that high initial RVEF portends a good prognosis. On the other hand, Parker et al. [22] found that survivors had a lower RVEF. The answer to this question requires additional investigation.

The other prognostic parameter is response of hemodynamic parameters to dynamic challenges, namely dobutamine. Non-survivors of septic shock have a blunted response to dobutamine [27, 28], whereas survivors demonstrated increased SVI (stroke work index), increase mixed venous oxygen saturation (SvO$_2$), ventricular dilatation and a decrease in diastolic blood pressure after a dobutamine challenge. The above response to dobutamine predicts survival in patients with septic shock.

# Etiology of Myocardial Depression in Sepsis and Septic Shock

Two major theories regarding the nature of septic myocardial depression in humans and animals have existed in the past. The first theory, which held dominance for decades, suggested that sepsis was associated with globally decreased myocardial perfusion resulting in ischemic injury to the septic heart. This position was supported over the years by animal models of endotoxic shock (mostly canine) which had demonstrated evidence of global myocardial hypoperfusion [29]. However, it gradually became apparent that endotoxic shock was not the most appropriate model through which to study septic myocardial dysfunction. With this realization, the second major theory regarding the nature of myocardial depression in septic shock, that a circulating depressant substance was responsible, emerged [30]. The origins of this theory can be traced to Wiggers' classic 1947 report proposing the presence of a myocardial depressant factor in experimental hemorrhagic shock [31].

## Organ Level

### Myocardial Hypoperfusion

The potential of myocardial hypoperfusion leading to myocardial depression via global ischemia has been largely dismissed by a number of clinical studies. Cunnion et al. [32] placed thermodilution catheters into the coronary sinus of septic shock patients and measured serial coronary flow and metabolism (Fig. 5). Normal or elevated coronary flow was present in septic patients in comparison to normal controls with comparable heart rates. In addition, septic shock patient's hearts exhibited an absence of net lactate production. Dhainaut et al. [33] confirmed these findings while employing similar methods. In addition to human studies, myocardial high energy phosphates and oxygen utilization were preserved in a canine model of septic shock [34]. Other studies employing different models and methodologies have demonstrated similar results.

Despite these data, there is evidence for myocardial cell injury evidenced by increased troponin I levels in septic shock. Some initially took this to indicate evidence of myocardial hypoperfusion. A study by ver Elst et al. [35] examined levels of troponin I and T in patients with septic shock. A correlation between LV dysfunction and troponin I positivity (78% vs. 9% in troponin I negative patients $p<0.001$) existed. They also found that older patients with underlying cardiovascular disease more often had both troponin positivity and LV dysfunction. Similarly Mehta et al. [36] demonstrated that serum cardiac troponin I is elevated in 43% of patients with septic shock (without creatine kinase isoenzyme MB [CK-MB] elevation or ischemic electrocardiographic [EKG] changes). Serum cardiac troponin I correlated with LV dysfunction and was an independent predictor of need for inotropic/vasopressor support, adverse outcome and mortality in septic shock patients. Although troponin is used as a marker of myocardial injury particularly

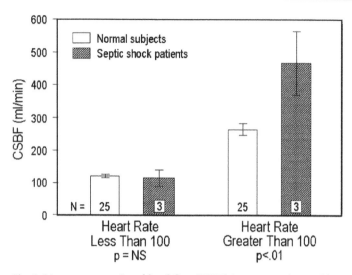

**Fig. 5.** Mean coronary sinus blood flow (CSBF) in seven patients with septic shock compared with normal subjects. Flow measurements were stratified into heart rates above and below 100 beats/min. Coronary blood flow in septic shock patients equaled (heart rate < 100/min) or exceeded (heart rate>100/min) coronary blood flow in control patients. From [32] with permission

in the context of myocardial ischemia, elevation of this marker does not specifically suggest myocardial hypoperfusion in other contexts. Increased troponin can occur as a consequence of myocardial injury from a variety of potential sources. Further, whether the clinically unapparent myocardial cell injury that is the source of elevated troponin contributes to or is a consequence of septic shock is yet to be determined.

In summary, myocardial perfusion and myocardial energetics studies argue against global myocardial ischemia and hypoperfusion despite that fact that myocardial troponins are clearly elevated in septic shock.

Myocardial Depressant Substances

The presence of a "myocardial depressant factor" as originally postulated by Wiggers [31] in 1947 in the context of hemorrhagic shock was supported by Brand and Lefer [37] in 1966. This work prompted extensive further research into septic myocardial depressant substances [37–44].

A number of exogenous and endogenous substances have been implicated as potential causes of septic myocardial depression. Among the exogenous substances, endotoxin stands out. Studies have associated endotoxemia with a lower mean LVEF, lower SVR, as well as increased mortality, and infusion of intravenous endotoxin in human volunteers has been shown to mimic the hemodynamic effects of spontaneous human sepsis [45,46]. Available data clearly support a central role for endotoxin in the pathogenesis of Gram-negative sepsis and septic shock.

There is much less compelling evidence for the role of endotoxin as a direct mediator of cardiovascular dysfunction in sepsis and septic shock. *In vitro* application of endotoxin, by itself, at high doses does not directly damage or otherwise adversely affect myocardial tissues, despite the fact that nanogram quantities of endotoxin have been shown to cause endotoxic shock in rats, guinea pigs and rabbits with *ex vivo* depression of contraction of isolated ventricular myocytes from these animals [47]. Of note, 1 ug/ml endotoxin does not directly depress cardiac myocyte contractility *in vitro* while far lower concentrations (0.1 ng/ml), when co-incubated with phorbol 12-myristate 13-acetate (PMA)-activated macrophages, result in a cellular culture supernatant that contains marked depressant activity [48].

The significant hemodynamic depressant effects of endotoxin when infused *in vivo* into animals but the lack of such effects on cardiovascular tissue exposed to endotoxin directly *in vitro* makes it clear that endogenously produced factors must mediate *in vivo* responses to endotoxin. A number of endogenous substances have been suggested as potential causes of septic myocardial depression. These have included estrogenic compounds, histamine, eicosanoids/prostaglandins and most recently, leukocyte lysozyme. However, a number of these apparent novel substances could never be effectively isolated [37–44, 49–51] (for review [52]) (Table 1).

In one of the seminal studies in the field, Parrillo et al. in 1985 [53] showed a link between myocyte depression and septic serum from a patient with sepsis associated myocardial depression. The serum from patients demonstrated concentration-dependent depression of *in vitro* myocyte contractility (Fig. 6). Parrillo et al. were also able to correlate a temporal and qualitative relationship between *in vivo* myocardial depression (decreased LVEF) and *in vitro* cardiac myocyte depression induced by serum from corresponding patients. In another study [54], investigators noted that higher levels of myocardial depressant activity correlated with higher peak serum lactate, increased ventricular filling pressures, increased LVEDVI, and mortality when compared with patients with lower or absent activity levels. Early filtration studies [54] found that the substance was water soluble, heat labile and greater than 10 kDa consistent with a protein or polypeptide including cytokines such as TNF-α and IL-1β.

TNF-α likely has a role as a myocardial depressant substance for a number of reasons. TNF-α shares the same biochemical profile as myocardial depressant substances [53]. Clinically, TNF-α is associated with fever, increased lactic acid, disseminated intravascular coagulation (DIC), ALI, and death. The hemodynamic (and metabolic) effects of TNF-α administered to animals and human are similar to septic shock with hypotension, increased cardiac output and low SVR. Experimentally, animal and human myocardial tissue exposed to increasing concentrations of TNF-α demonstrate a concentration dependent depression of contractility [39]. Kumar et al. [55] have shown that removal of TNF-α from the serum of patients with septic shock decreased the septic serum-induced myocardial depression. In addition, Vincent et al. [56] in a pilot study showed improved LVSWI with admin-

Table 1. Myocardial depressant substances in endotoxic and septic shock: Physical and biochemical characterization

| STUDY AUTHORS | SUBJECT MODEL | ASSAY | CONTROL | IN VIVO CORRELATION | ISOLATION |
|---|---|---|---|---|---|
| Wangensteen et al. [49] | canine | endotoxin bolus | cat papillary muscle | none | none | MW 800–1,000 Da peptide |
| Lovett et al. [41] | human | mixed septic and hemorragic shock | cat papillary muscle | serum from perioperative patients | none | MW 800–1,000 Da peptide |
| McConn et al. [50] | human | spontaneous sepsis | in vivo canine cardiac performance during coronary perfusion with septic plasma | yes, but nonseptic plasma caused depression | no formal comparison | multiple fractions MW < 1,000 Da MW 1,000–10,000 Da |
| Carli et al. [51] Benassayag et al. [42] | human | spontaneous septic shock | rat cardiomyocytes | serum from healthy donors | none | MW < 1,000 Da heat stable, lipid soluble estrogenic compound |
| Gomez et al. [43] Jha et al. [44] Gu et al. [39] Mink et al. [38] | canine | live E. Coli infusion | canine right ventricular trabeculae | plasma from nonendotoxic hypotensive dogs | change in in-vivo pressure volume curve correlated with in-vitro trabecular depression | MW 10,000–30,000 d heat labile, acetone insoluble proteinase senstive probable protein inconsistent with TNF alone identified as leukocyte lysozyme partially NO-dependent |
| Pathan et al. [60] Pathan et al. [61] | human | spontaneous meningococcal septic shock | rat cardiomyocytes | serum from healthy controls no critically ill controls | degree of myocyte depresion correlates with severity of illness score and pressor requirement | heat stable (57 °C), proteinaceious MW 10–25,000 d eliminated by immunoabsorption of IL-6; cGMP-independent |
| Parrillo et al. [53] Reilly et al. [54] Kumar et al. [55] Kumar et al. [74] | human | spontaneous mixed etiology septic shock | rat cardiomyocytes | serum from multiple controls including critically ill non-septic patients | degree of myocyte depression correlated to LVEF | min 2 fractions MW 500–5,000 Da MW > 10,000 Da heat labile (100 °C), ethylacetate insoluble; probable protein; activity eliminated by immunoabsorption of TNF and IL-1 NO-dependent |

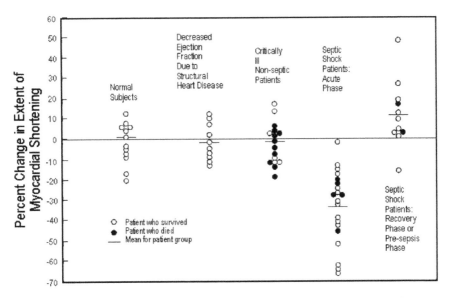

**Fig. 6.** The effect of serum from septic shock patients and control groups on the extent of myocardial cell shortening of spontaneously beating rat heart cells *in vitro*. Septic shock patients during the acute phase demonstrated a statistically significant lower extent of shortening (p<0.001) compared with any other group. Open circles, survivors; closed circles, non-survivors; horizontal line, mean for each group. From [53] with permission

istration of anti-TNF-α monoclonal antibody even though there was no survival benefit.

IL-1β produces similar hemodynamic responses to TNF-α. IL-1β levels are also elevated in sepsis and septic shock [57]. *In vitro* and *ex vivo* myocardial contractility is depressed when cardiac tissue is exposed to IL-1β [58]. Removal of IL-1β via immunoabsorption from septic human serum attenuates the depression of cardiac myocytes [55]. However, the effects of IL-1β antagonists on cardiac function and survival are unimpressive even though metabolic derangements are attenuated by IL-1β antagonists.

It is likely that cytokines such as TNF-α and IL-1, rather than working in isolation synergize to exert their depressant effects. In isolation, TNF-α and IL-1β require very high concentrations to induce *in vitro* rat myocyte depression [55]. However, when combined, they act synergistically and require concentrations 50–100 times lower than those required individually [55,59]. These concentrations are within the range of those found in septic shock patients.

Parallel to the earlier work of Parrillo and colleagues [53], Pathan and colleagues have confirmed the presence of a circulatory myocardial depressant substance in the blood of children with meningococcal septic shock [60]. Pathan and colleagues have strongly implicated circulating IL-6 as an important myocardial depressant substance in human meningococcal septic shock [60,61]. These investigators have demonstrated that meningococcal sepsis is associated with induction of IL-6 expression in blood mononuclear cells. In addition, they have shown that the level of serum IL-6 corresponds with the severity of illness (Pediatric Risk of Mortality [PRISM] score) and magnitude of pressor requirement in such patients. Degree of septic cardiac dysfunction (e.g., via echocardiography or radionuclide ventriculography) was not directly assessed in this study. Further, this group have recently shown that IL-6 depresses contractility of myocardial tissue *in vitro* and that neutralization of IL-6 in serum from patients with meningococcal septic shock neutralizes this effect [61]. In contrast to the work suggesting that synergistic activity of TNF-α and IL-1β drives septic myocardial depression, these findings implicating IL-6 may arise from the fact that meningococcal septic shock may be more physiologically analogous to endotoxic shock than the clinically and microbiologically mixed forms of septic shock assessed by Kumar et al. [55]

Evidence for other potential myocardial depressant substances continues to be developed. Recently, Mink et al. have implicated lysozyme c (consistent with that found in leukocytes in the spleen or other organs) as a potential myocardial depressant substance [38]. In a canine model of *E. coli* sepsis, lysozyme c caused myocardial depression and attenuated the response to beta-agonists [38]. The potential mechanism proposed was lysozyme binding or hydrolyzing the membrane glycoprotein of cardiac myocytes, thereby affecting signal transduction (linking physiologic excitation with physiologic contraction). The levels of lysozyme c were found to be elevated in the heart and spleen, but not in lymphocytes when compared to preseptic levels [38]. Mink et al. went on to show that pretreatment with an inhibitor of lysozyme (N,N′,N″-triacetylglucosamine) prevented myocardial depression in canine sepsis [62]. However, the effect of this lysozyme inhibitor was only seen in pretreatment and early treatment groups (1.5 hours after onset of septic shock) and not in late treatment groups (greater than 3.5 hours). The relevance of this work is limited by the fact that it has only been isolated to date in experimental endotoxin-equivalent canine models. Isolation of this substance during human septic shock will be required to ensure clinical relevance.

An important microbial factor that has recently been shown to potentially exert hemodynamic and myocardial depressant activity in sepsis and septic shock is bacterial nucleic acid. Several investigators have demonstrated that unique aspects of bacterial nucleic acid structure may allow bacterial DNA to generate a shock state similar to that produced by endotoxin [63]. Extending these observations, we have recently demonstrated depression of rat myocyte contraction with bacterial DNA and RNA [64]. This effect was more marked when DNA and RNA came from pathogenic strains of *S. aureus* and *E. coli*. These effects were not seen when the rat myocyte was pretreated with DNase and RNase. Again, the direct relevance to septic shock will not be defined until measurements of bacterial nucleic acid in the circulation can be made and, if present, the effect of elimination of these antigens assessed.

Other factors may also play a role in septic myocardial depression. Natriuretic peptides have emerged as valuable marker substances to detect LV dysfunction in heart failure of different origins including critical illness. Both brain natriuretic peptide (BNP) and atrial natriuretic peptide (ANP) have been found to be significantly elevated in patients with septic shock in comparison with controls [65]. Others have made similar observations for BNP in patients with severe sepsis or septic shock who have echocardiographic evidence of systolic myocardial dysfunction [66]. High plasma BNP levels appear to be associated with poor outcome of sepsis. Available evidence suggests that NT-proBNP (the N-terminal prohormone of BNP) could be an even more sensitive indicator of sepsis-induced ventricular dilatation [67]. Whether natriuretic peptides may have any kind of direct role in sepsis-induced myocardial dysfunction is entirely unknown.

## Cellular Level

The sequence of mechanisms leading from a circulating myocardial depressant substance to cellular dysfunction remains unclear. There are several potential mechanisms that may play a role at the cellular level. Overproduction of nitric oxide (NO) and derangements of calcium physiology in the myocardial cell are two non-exclusive potential cellular mechanisms.

*In vitro*, myocyte depression in response to inflammatory cytokines can be divided into early and late phases. Early depression of cardiac myocyte depression occurs within minutes of exposure to either TNF-$\alpha$, IL-1$\beta$, TNF-$\alpha$ and IL-1$\beta$ given together, or septic serum [55,68]. TNF-$\alpha$ also has the ability to cause rapid myocardial depression in dogs [69]. Besides the early effects, TNF-$\alpha$, IL-1$\beta$ and supernatants of activated macrophages also have a later, prolonged effect on *in vitro* myocardial tissue [58,70,71]. This late phase establishes within hours and lasts for days. This suggests the possibility of a different mechanism from early myocardial depression.

Production of NO may be a potential explanation for both early and late myocardial depression. NO is produced from conversion of L-arginine to L-citrulline by NO synthase (NOS). NOS has two forms: one is constitutive (cNOS) and the other is inducible (iNOS). NO produced by cNOS appears to have a regulatory role in cardiac contractility. However, when cardiac myocytes are exposed to supraphysiologic levels of NO or NO donors (nitroprusside and SIN-1) there is a reduction in myocardial contractility [72]. Paulus et al. [73] infused nitroprusside into coronary arteries which decreased intraventricular pressures and improved diastolic function.

Current evidence suggests that early myocyte dysfunction may occur through generation of NO and resultant cGMP via cNOS activation in cardiac myocytes and adjacent endothelium [59,68,74]. We have further demonstrated that the early phase may also involve an NO-independent defect of $\beta$-adrenoreceptor signal transduction [52,74–76]. Late myocardial depression appears to be secondary to induction of iNOS [58,68]. In addition, the generation of peroxynitrite via interaction of the free radical NO group and oxygen may also play a role in more prolonged effects [77]. Kinugawa et al. have shown that IL-6 can cause both early and late NO-mediated myocardial depression in an avian myocardial cell model via sequential activation of cNOS followed by induction of iNOS [78,79], a finding that could explain recent human data implicating IL-6 in meningococcal septic myocardial dysfunction [60,61]. These data suggest a role for sequential production of NO from cNOS and iNOS in the pathogenesis of myocardial depression from cytokines.

Although NO may be central, the biochemical mechanisms underlying septic myocardial depression are clearly complex with redundant, branching pathways. Some of these pathways may represent intermediate steps to NO generation. Others may be able to mediate myocardial depression entirely independently of NO. For example, the neutral sphingomyelinase pathway involving the sequential generation of ceramide and sphingosine in adult feline cardiac myocytes has been implicated in early TNF-α-induced cardiac myocyte depression [80]. Guinea pig cardiac myocyte depression by TNF-α appears to involve similar mechanisms although a role for NO in IL-6-mediated depression of contractility of avian and guinea pig cardiac myocytes has also been proposed [78,81]. In a study using human adult atrial tissue exposed to TNF-α, sphingosine and NO pathways were simultaneously implicated suggesting a mechanistic link [59]. Other data suggest that PAF, a phospholipid with marked activity in the cardiovascular system, may play an intermediate role between the depressant activity of TNF-α and NO [82]. Leukocyte lysozyme has also demonstrated some evidence of NO-dependent responses [38,62]. Cyclooxygenase products, leukotrienes, protein kinase C, altered energy metabolism, and impairment of sarcoplasmic reticulum function may also play a role in septic myocardial depression. Although human data have been contradictory, there is emerging evidence to suggest that a variety of transcription factors, adhesion molecules, and apoptotic mechanisms may also be involved in septic myocardial dysfunction. Marked increases in myocardial apoptosis, often in association with contractile dysfunction, have been documented in a variety of experimental endotoxic shock models. Neviere et al., utilizing an endotoxic shock model, observed an approximate 3-fold increase in rat myocyte apoptosis and activation of caspases 3, 8 and 9 [83]. Caspase inhibitors when administered 2 h after endotoxin challenge, improved endotoxin-induced myocardial dysfunction, reduced caspase activation and reduced myocyte apoptosis [84]. Stimulation of cardiac myocytes with pro-inflammatory cytokines (such as those produced in septic or endotoxic shock) results in myocyte apoptosis [85]. We have recently demonstrated that human septic serum with marked myocardial depressant activity activates the transcription factors signal transducers and activators of transcription 1 (STAT1), interferon regulatory factor-1 (IRF1) and nuclear factor-kappa B (NF-κB) in human fetal myocytes [86]. Both reporter and electrophoretic mobility shift assays demonstrated a substantial increase in activation of transcription factors STAT1, IRF1 and NF-κB in response to incubation with human septic serum. Further, addition of human septic serum to human fetal myocytes induced apoptosis in the myocytes.

Although overt increased apoptosis in the human heart has not been noted in spontaneous disease or in live infection models of sepsis and septic shock, pre-apoptotic signaling may occur in many cells of dysfunctional organs affected by sepsis including the heart. In this view of the pathophysiology of sepsis, widespread pre-apoptotic signaling leads to cellular dysfunction that can lead to organ failure including myocardial depression during septic shock and sepsis-associated multiple organ dysfunction.

## Conclusion

Myocardial dysfunction is an important component in the hemodynamic collapse induced by sepsis and septic shock. A series of inflammatory cascades triggered by the inciting infection generate circulatory myocardial depressant substances, including TNF-α, IL-1β, PAF and lysozyme. Current evidence suggests that septic myocardial depression in humans is characterized by reversible biventricular dilatation, decreased systolic contractile function, and decreased response to both fluid resuscitation and catecholamine stimulation, all in the presence of an overall hyperdynamic circulation. This phenomenon is linked to the presence of a circulating myocardial depressant substance or substances which probably represents low concentrations of pro-inflammatory cytokines including TNF-α, IL-1β and perhaps IL-6 acting in synergy. These effects are mediated through mechanisms that include but are not limited to NO and cGMP generation. The mechanism through which NO depresses cardiac contractility is largely unknown. Recent data suggest that pre-apoptotic signaling involving transcription factors STAT1, IRF1 and NF-κB leading to apoptotic pathways may play a role in septic myocardial depression related to inflammatory cytokines circulating during septic shock. Links between this response and NO generation are postulated but have not been fully delineated.

## References

1. Angus DC, Linde-Zwirble WT, Lidicker J, et al (2001) Epidemiology of severe sepsis in the United States: analysis of incidence, outcome, and associated costs of care. Crit Care Med 29:1303–1310
2. Martin GS, Mannino DM, Eaton S, Moss M (2003) The epidemiology of sepsis in the United States from 1979 through 2000. N Engl J Med 348:1546–1554
3. Bone RC, Balk R, Cerra FB, et al (1992) ACCP/SCCM Consensus Conference: Definitions for sepsis and organ failure and guidelines for use of innovative therapies in sepsis. Chest 101:1644–1655
4. MacLean LD, Mulligan WG, McLean APH, Duff JH (1967) Patterns of septic shock in man: A detailed study of 56 patients. Ann Surg 166:543–562
5. Clowes GHA, Vucinic M, Weidner MG (1966) Circulatory and metabolic alterations associated with survival or death in peritonitis. Ann Surg 163:866–844
6. Packman MI, Rackow EC (1983) Optimum left heart filling pressure during fluid resuscitation of patients with hypovolemic and septic shock. Crit Care Med 11:165–169
7. Parker MM, Shelhamer JH, Natanson C, et al (1987) Serial cardiovascular variables in survivors and nonsurvivors of human septic shock: Heart rate as an early predictor of prognosis. Crit Care Med 15:923–929

8. Parker MM, Suffredini AF, Natanson C, et al (1989) Responses of left ventricular function in survivors and non-survivors of septic shock. J Crit Care 4:19–25
9. Weisul RD, Vito L, Dennis RC, et al (1977) Myocardial depression during sepsis. Am J Surg 133:512–521
10. Rackow EC, Kaufman BS, Falk JL, et al (1987) Hemodynamic response to fluid repletion in patients with septic shock: evidence for early depression of cardiac performance. Circ Shock 22:11–22
11. Parker MM, Shelhamer JH, Bacharach SL, et al (1984) Profound but reversible myocardial depression in patients with septic shock. Ann Intern Med 100:483–490
12. Ellrodt AG, Riedinger MS, Kimchi A, et al (1985) Left ventricular performance in septic shock: Reversible segmental and global abnormalities. Am Heart J 110:402–409
13. Ognibene FP, Parker MM, Natanson C, et al (1988) Depressed left ventricular performance. Response to volume infusion in patients with sepsis and septic shock. Chest 93:903–910
14. Vieillard BA, Schmitt JM, Beauchet A, et al (2001) Early preload adaptation in septic shock? A transesophageal echocardiographic study. Anesthesiology 94:400–406
15. Jardin F, Fourme T, Page B, et al (1999) Persistent preload defect in severe sepsis despite fluid loading: A longitudinal echocardiographic study in patients with septic shock. Chest 116:1354–1359
16. Raper RF, Sibbald WJ, Driedger AA, Gerow K (1989) Relative myocardial depression in normotensive sepsis. J Crit Care 4:9–18
17. Jafri SM, Lavine S, Field BE, et al (1991) Left ventricular diastolic function in sepsis. Crit Care Med 18:709–714
18. Poelaert J, Declerck C, Vogelaers D, et al (1997) Left ventricular systolic and diastolic function in septic shock. Intensive Care Med 23:553–560
19. Munt B, Jue J, Gin K, et al (1998) Diastolic filling in human severe sepsis: An echocardiographic study. Crit Care Med 26:1829–1833
20. Jardin F, Valtier B, Beauchet A, et al (1994) Invasive monitoring combined with two-dimensional echocardiographic study in septic shock. Intensive Care Med 20:550–554
21. Kimchi A, Ellrodt GA, Berman DS, et al (1984) Right ventricular performance in septic shock: a combined radionuclide and hemodynamic study. J Am Coll Cardiol 4:945–951
22. Parker MM, McCarthy KE, Ognibene FP, Parrillo JE (1990) Right ventricular dysfunction and dilatation, similar to left ventricular changes, characterize the cardiac depression of septic shock in humans. Chest 97:126–131
23. Schneider AJ, Teule GJJ, Groeneveld ABJ, et al (1988) Biventricular performance during volume loading in patients with early septic shock, with emphasis on the right ventricle: a combined hemodynamic and radionuclide study. Am Heart J 116:103–112
24. Baumgartner J, Vaney C, Perret C (1984) An extreme form of hyperdynamic syndrome in septic shock. Intensive Care Med 10:245–249
25. Groeneveld ABJ, Nauta JJ, Thijs L (1988) Peripheral vascular resistance in septic shock: its relation to outcome. Intensive Care Med 14:141–147
26. Vincent JL, Reuse C, Frank N, et al (1989) Right ventricular dysfunction in septic shock: assessment by measurements of right ventricular ejection fraction using the thermodilution technique. Acta Anaesthesiol Scand 33:34–38
27. Rhodes A, Lamb FJ, Malagon R, et al (1999) A prospective study of the use of a dobutamine stress test to identify outcome in patients with sepsis, severe sepsis or septic shock. Crit Care Med 27:2361–2366
28. Kumar A, Schupp E, Bunnell E, et al (1994) The cardiovascular response to dobutamine in septic shock. Clin Invest Med 17: B18 (abst)
29. Hinshaw LB, Archer LT, Spitzer JJ, et al (1974) Effects of coronary hypotension and endotoxin on myocardial performance. Am J Physiol 227:1051–1057
30. Lefer AM, Martin J (1970) Origin of myocardial depressant factor in shock. Am J Physiol 218:1423–1427

31. Wiggers CJ (1947) Myocardial depression in shock. A survey of cardiodynamic studies. Am Heart J 33:633–650
32. Cunnion RE, Schaer GL, Parker MM, et al (1986) The coronary circulation in human septic shock. Circulation 73:637–644
33. Dhainaut JF, Huyghebaert MF, Monsallier JF, et al (1987) Coronary hemodynamics and myocardial metabolism of lactate, free fatty acids, glucose, and ketones in patients with septic shock. Circulation 75:533–541
34. Solomon MA, Correa R, Alexander HR, et al (1994) Myocardial energy metabolism and morphology in a canine model of sepsis. Am J Physiol 266:H757–H768
35. ver Elst KM, Spapen HD, Nguyen DN, et al (2000) Cardiac troponins I and T are biological markers of left ventricular dysfunction in septic shock. Clin Chem 46:650–657
36. Mehta NJ, Khan IA, Gupta V, et al (2004) Cardiac troponin I predicts myocardial dysfunction and adverse outcome in septic shock. Int J Cardiol 95:13-7
37. Lefer AM (1979) Mechanisms of cardiodepression in endotoxin shock. Circ Shock (suppl) 1:1–8
38. Mink SN, Jacobs H, Bose D, et al (2003) Lysozyme: a mediator of myocardial depression and adrenergic dysfunction in septic shock in dogs. J Mol Cell Cardiol 35:265–275
39. Gu M, Bose R, Bose D, et al (1998) Tumor necrosis factor-a but not septic plasma depresses cardiac myofilament contraction. Can J Anaesth 45:352–359
40. Maksad KA, Chung-Ja C, Clowes GHA, et al (1979) Myocardial depression in septic shock: physiologic and metabolic effects of a plasma factor on an isolated heart. Circ Shock 1:35–42
41. Lovett WL, Wangensteen SL, Glenn TM, Lefer AM (1971) Presence of a myocardial depressant factor in patients with circulatory shock. Surgery 70:223–231
42. Benassayag C, Christeff MC, Auclair MC, et al (1984) Early released lipid-soluble cardiodepressant factor and elevated oestrogenic substances in human septic shock. Eur J Clin Invest 14:288–294
43. Gomez A, Wang R, Unruh H, et al (1990) Hemofiltration reverses left ventricular dysfunction during sepsis in dogs. Anesthesiology 73:671–685
44. Jha P, Jacobs H, Bose D, et al (1993) Effects of E. coli sepsis and myocardial depressant factor on interval-force relations in dog ventricle. Am J Physiol 264:H1402–H1410
45. Suffredini AF, Fromm RE, Parker MM, et al (1989) The cardiovascular response of normal humans to the administration of endotoxin. N Engl J Med 321:280–287
46. Danner RL, Elin RJ, Hosseini JM, et al (1991) Endotoxemia in human septic shock. Chest 99:169–175
47. Parker JL, Adams HR (1981) Contractile dysfunction of atrial myocardium from endotoxin-shocked pigs. Am J Physiol 240:H954–H962
48. Kumar A, Kosuri R, Ginsburg B, et al (1994) Myocardial cell contractility is depressed by supernatants of endotoxin stimulated THP-1 cells. Crit Care Med 22:A118 (abst)
49. Wangensteen SL, Geissenger WT, Lovett WL, et al (1971) Relationship between splanchnic blood flow and a myocardial depressant factor in endotoxin shock. Surgery 69:410–418
50. McConn R, Greineder JK, Wasserman F, Clowes GHA (1979) Is there a humoral factor that depresses ventricular function in sepsis? Circ Shock 1:9–22
51. Carli A, Auclair MC, Vernimmen C, Jourdon P (1979) Reversal by calcium of rat heart cell dysfunction induced by human sera in septic shock. Circ Shock 6:147–157
52. Kumar A, Krieger A, Symeoneides S, et al (2001) Myocardial dysfunction in septic shock, Part II: Role of cytokines and nitric oxide. J Cardiovasc Thorac Anesth 15:485–511
53. Parrillo JE, Burch C, Shelhamer JH, et al (1985) A circulating myocardial depressant substance in humans with septic shock. Septic shock patients with a reduced ejection fraction have a circulating factor that depresses in vitro myocardial cell performance. J Clin Invest 76:1539–1553
54. Reilly JM, Cunnion RE, Burch-Whitman C, et al (1989) A circulating myocardial depressant substance is associated with cardiac dysfunction and peripheral hypoperfusion (lactic acidemia) in patients with septic shock. Chest 95:1072–1080

55. Kumar A, Thota V, Dee L, et al (1996) Tumor necrosis factor-alpha and interleukin-1 beta are responsible for depression of in vitro myocardial cell contractility induced by serum from humans with septic shock. J Exp Med 183:949–958
56. Vincent JL, Bakker J, Marecaux G, et al (1992) Administration of anti-TNF antibody improves left ventricular function in septic shock patients: Results of a pilot study. Chest 101:810–815
57. Hesse DG, Tracey KJ, Fong Y, et al (1988) Cytokine appearance in human endotoxemia and primate bacteremia. Surg Gynecol Obstet 166:147–153
58. Hosenpud JD, Campbell SM, Mendelson DJ (1989) Interleukin-1-induced myocardial depression in an isolated beating heart preparation. J Heart Transplant 8:460–464
59. Cain BS, Meldrum DR, Dinarello CA, et al (1999) Tumor necrosis factor – a and interleukin-1b synergistically depress human myocardial function. Crit Care Med 27:1309–1318
60. Pathan N, Sandiford C, Harding SE, Levin M (2002) Characterization of a myocardial depressant factor in meningococcal septicemia. Crit Care Med 30:2191–2198
61. Pathan N, Hemingway CA, Alizadeh AA, et al (2004) Role of interleukin 6 in myocardial dysfunction of meningococcal septic shock. Lancet 363:203–209
62. Mink SN, Jacobs H, Duke K, et al (2004) N,N′,N″-triacetylglucosamine, an inhibitor of lysozyme, prevents myocardial depression in Escherichia coli sepsis in dogs. Crit Care Med 32:184–93
63. Sparwasser T, Miethke T, Lipford G, et al (1997) Bacterial DNA causes septic shock. Nature 386:336–337
64. Paladugu B, Kumar A, Parrillo JE, et al (2004) Bacterial DNA and RNA induce rat cardiac myocyte contraction depression in-vitro. Shock 21:364–369
65. Witthaut R, Busch C, Fraunberger P, et al (2003) Plasma atrial natriuretic peptide and brain natriuretic peptide are increased in septic shock: impact of interleukin-6 and sepsis-associated left ventricular dysfunction. Intensive Care Med 39:1696–1702
66. Charpentier J, Luyt CE, Fulla Y, et al (2004) Brain natriuretic peptide: A marker of myocardial dysfunction and prognosis during severe sepsis. Crit Care Med 32:660–665
67. Chua G, Kang-Hoe L (2004) Marked elevations in N-terminal brain natriuretic peptide: a marker of myocardial dysfunction and prognosis during severe sepsis. Crit Care 8:R248–R250
68. Finkel MS, Oddis CV, Jacobs TD, et al (1992) Negative inotropic effects of cytokines on the heart mediated by nitric oxide. Science 257:387–389
69. Eichenholz PW, Eichacker PQ, Hoffman WD, et al (1992) Tumor necrosis factor challenges in canines: Patterns of cardiovascular dysfunction. Am J Physiol 263:H668–H675
70. Gulick T, Chung MK, Pieper SJ, et al (1989) Interleukin-1 and tumor necrosis factor inhibit cardiac myocyte adrenergic responsiveness. Proc Natl Acad Sci USA 86:6753–6757
71. Walley KR, Hebert PC, Wakai Y, et al (1994) Decrease in left ventricular contractility after tumor necrosis factor-a infusion in dogs. J Appl Physiol 76:1060–1067
72. Brady AJ, Poole-Wilson PA, Harding SE, Warren JB (1992) Nitric oxide production within cardiac myocytes reduces their contractility in endotoxemia. Am J Physiol 263:H1963–H1966
73. Paulus WJ, Vantrimpont PJ, Shah AM (1994) Acute effects of nitric oxide on left ventricular relaxation and diastolic distensability in humans. Assessment by bicoronary sodium nitroprusside infusion. Circulation 89:2070–2078
74. Kumar A, Brar R, Wang P, et al (1999) The role of nitric oxide and cyclic GMP in human septic serum-induced depression of cardiac myocyte contractility. Am J Physiol 276:R265–R276
75. Anel R, Paladugu B, Makkena R, et al (1999) TNFa induces a proximal defect of b-adrenoreceptor signal transduction in cardiac myocytes. Crit Care Med 27:A95 (abst)
76. Kumar A, Brar R, Sun E, Olson J, Parrillo JE (1996) Tumor necrosis factor (TNF) impairs isoproterenol-stimulated cardiac myocyte contractility and cyclic AMP producton via a nitric oxide-independent mechanism. Crit Care Med 24:A95 (abst)
77. Szabo C (1996) The pathophysiological role of peroxynitrite in shock, inflammation, and ischemia-reperfusion injury. Shock 6:79–88

78. Kinugawa K, Takahashi T, Kohmoto O, et al (1994) Nitric oxide-mediated effects of interleukin-6 on [Ca2+]i and cell contraction in cultured chick ventricular myocytes. Circ Res 75:285–295
79. Kinugawa KI, Kohmoto O, Yao A, et al (1997) Cardiac inducible nitric oxide synthase negatively modulates myocardial function in cultured rat myocytes. Am J Physiol. 272:H35–H47
80. Oral H, Dorn GW, Mann DL (1997) Sphingosine mediates the immediate negative inotropic effects of tumor necrosis factor-a in the adult mammalian cardiac myocyte. J Biol Chem 272:4836–4841
81. Sugishita K, Kinugawa K, Shimizu T, et al (1999) Cellular basis for the acute inhibitory effects of IL-6 and TNF – a on excitation-contraction coupling. J Mol Cell Cardiol 31:1457–1467
82. Alloatti G, Penna C, De Martino A, et al (1999) Role of nitric oxide and platelet-activating factor in cardiac alterations induced by tumor necrosis factor-alpha in the guinea-pig papillary muscle. Cardiovasc Res 41:611–619
83. Neviere R, Fauvel H, Chopin C, et al (2001) Caspase inhibition prevents cardiac dysfunction and heart apoptosis in a rat model of sepsis. Am J Respir Crit Care Med 163:218–225
84. Fauvel H, Marchetti P, Chopin C, et al (2001) Differential effects of caspase inhibitors on endotoxin-induced myocardial dysfunction and heart apoptosis. Am J Physiol Heart Circ Physiol 280:H1608–H1614
85. Krown KA, Page MT, Nguyen C, et al (1996) Tumor necrosis factor alpha-induced apoptosis in cardiac myocytes. Involvement of the sphingolipid signaling cascade in cardiac cell death. J Clin Invest 98:2854–2865
86. Kumar A, Kumar A, Michael P, et al (2005) Human serum from patients with septic shock activates transcription factors STAT1, IRF1 and NFkB and induces apoptosis in human cardiac myocytes. J Biol Chem 280:42619–42626
87. Parrillo JE, Parker MM, Natanson C, et al (1990) Septic shock in humans: Advances in the understanding of pathogenesis, cardiovascular dysfunction, and therapy. Ann Intern Med 113:227–242

# Skeletal Muscle

R.D. Griffiths, T. Bongers, and A. McArdle

## Introduction

Muscle weakness and muscle wasting are common and debilitating phenomena in intensive care and seen most profoundly in multiple organ failure (MOF) following severe sepsis and severe burn injuries. Intensive care clinicians recognize that muscle weakness contributes to prolonged mechanical ventilation, a prolonged ICU and hospital stay, and adds considerably to the cost of caring for these patients [1]. This dysfunction goes beyond fatigue and weakness of the muscle, and also includes changes in muscle metabolism, muscle as a nutrient store, and in the inflammatory state of the whole body. The last 25 years has brought a greater appreciation of the mechanisms, structural and metabolic characteristics, the consequences, and possible avenues for therapy of muscle dysfunction as a component of MOF.

## Contractile Dysfunction

Muscle contraction (force generation) is the final step in a complex chain of command that runs from the higher centers of the central nervous system (CNS) via the spinal cord and peripheral nerves to the muscle. From here an action potential must be generated, calcium released, and cross bridge cycling activated, resulting in muscle force generation via actin and myosin interactions. Loss of strength observed clinically can arise secondary to an interruption at any point in this chain, such as a loss of contractile proteins, reduced membrane excitability, or disturbance in neural signaling. Clinically, it is important not to consider dysfunction of muscle force generation separately from the existing activity level and the energy supply side since the endurance capacity of muscle with repetitive activity is thought to be determined by, at least in part, the number of mitochondria per unit mass of muscle [2]. A trained muscle may contain five times more mitochondria than a healthy sedentary subject and a low mitochondrial content is associated with lower ATP content, increased glycogen breakdown, and lactate production with limitations in performance.

The difficulty in understanding muscle dysfunction in the ICU is the contribution of disuse-mediated muscle loss to the overall muscle wasting and breakdown.

Inactivity is an abnormal, even 'diseased', state of muscle in man, with normal activity acting as a potent stimulus for metabolism and protein synthesis. The human genome developed over 10,000 years ago when it was associated with a cycle of hunting and rest, feasting and famine, such that muscle was structured as a cyclical organ, highly plastic to synthesis and degradation, storage and utilization. These changes can be very rapid with a 50% decline in peripheral insulin-stimulated glucose utilization after as little as 72 hrs of bed rest [3]. After 20 days of bed rest, maximal muscle blood flow is reduced [4]. Skeletal muscle shows an adaptive reductive remodeling with continued decreased usage (bed rest, spaceflight or old age) [5]. This is associated with a shift in myosin isoforms from slow (fibers that have more oxidative metabolism with more mitochondria) to faster isoforms (fibers that are more glycolytic with fewer mitochondria). This may also result in a shift in fuel metabolism away from lipids and towards glucose. Metabolically, this impacts on fuel utilization and is manifested in marked changes in hepatic metabolism with an increase in gluconeogenisis. Such an adaptive process produces a muscle capable of high-intensity, short duration activity at the expense of endurance, making the tissue easily fatigable. How much of this change is substrate or hormonal driven is unclear but the impairment in peripheral (skeletal muscle) insulin-mediated glucose uptake has become a significant target for management with insulin as shown in the 'Leuven study' [6]. During catabolic stress, the gluconeogenic potential (and hyperglycemia) arises from increased amino acids released by proteolysis but not efficiently reutilized [7]. In skeletal muscle, increased lactate production occurs through exaggerated glycolysis with septic stimulation of $Na^+$, $K^+$ ATPase activity [8]. Triglyceride accumulation is seen in muscle of ICU patients [9, 10]. The precise mechanisms for the fat accumulation, its lack of utilization, and insulin resistance remain unclear but may involve dysregulation of malonyl CoA and inhibition of carnitine palmitoyl transferase-1 preventing long chain fatty acids from entering mitochondria [11].

## Impairment of Muscle Metabolism in Sepsis

The debate of whether there is a primary defect in the microcirculation [12], with shunting [13] compromising oxygen energy substrate delivery, or a cellular mitochondrial dysfunction limiting utilization in muscle during sepsis, either as a result of toxic damage [14] (endotoxin mediated [15] or adaptive [16]), is probably best settled by accepting that both occur. Which of these occurs first and to what extent each contributes to the septic cascade is the challenging question. Skeletal muscle has a highly variable blood flow depending on the contractile state. The regulation and distribution of blood flow is disturbed in sepsis, affecting microcirculatory flow. Phase-modulated near-infrared spectroscopy (NIRS) in septic patients showed that while blood volume was increased, the oxygen content remained unchanged with reduced microvascular compliance and impaired re-saturation after ischemia [17]. Reduced muscle oxygen consumption is also confirmed during stagnant ischemia [18] and correlates closely to worsening organ failure scoring (sequential organ failure assessment, SOFA). A similar outcome relationship was seen with abnormalities in mitochondrial function [19]. However, it appears that muscle mitochondrial structure and function is more protected than in other tissues such as the liver [20] and, therefore, the changes observed in muscle are likely to be more adaptive. Trying to resolve the contribution of the hypotension that arises during sepsis to force generation is clearly a challenge since no septic animal studies examining function appear to have studied this in detail [21]. Nevertheless, various forms of contractile dysfunction occur independent of the cross-section of muscle [22], some developing early within minutes to hours (possibly related to altered membrane potential and excitability), while others occur later within hours to days (possibly reflecting impairment of calcium activation or energy production). The resting membrane potential of muscle is reduced by 10–50% in the critically ill. This is sufficient to change muscle sodium and potassium content [23,24] and this will impact on contractility. In critically ill patients [25] and in animal studies [26] there is a major and rapid decrease in activity of several mitochondrial enzymes. Cytochrome C oxidase decreases to very low levels within days after arrival in the ICU, reflecting a rapid decrease in mitochondrial content.

## Neuropathy and Myopathy

Early descriptions of muscle pathology in critically ill patients focused on either electrophysiological (critical illness polyneuropathy, CIP [27]) or histological (critical illness myopathy, CIM [28]) manifestations. However, time has shown that both coexist with a spectrum of tissue involvement to various extents [29–32]. The key to appreciating these pathological changes has been the association with inflammatory states and the evidence of a vasculopathy with marked endothelial activation in both nerve [33] and muscle [34]. In the 'Leuven' study, good nutrition and strict glycemic control in the critically ill improved survival and reduced the incidence of neuropathy [6]. Subsequent investigation suggested that this was manifested through protection of the endothelium with a reduction in endothelial cell activation with lower intercellular adhesion molecule (ICAM)-1 and E-selectin levels, possibly through a more regulated induced nitric oxide (NO) synthase (iNOS) gene expression [35]. The ability to reduce the incidence of the neuropathy is encouraging. In the short, term critical illness neuropathy can compromise weaning from mechanical ventilation and prolong hospital stay with increased ICU mortality. However, once discharge from hospital occurs there is no discernable increased mortality risk [36]. Although follow-up experience suggests that in very long stay ICU patients electromyographic (EMG) evidence of chronic denervation may be detected many years later, the clinical consequences of this are usually minor, and despite initial profound weakness (probably more due to the myopathy) in these patients, only a very few show clinical weakness or limitations in the activities of daily living when followed up 1–2 years later [37]. Recovery of the myopathy with restoration of muscle bulk remains the major determinate of functional recovery.

## Muscle Loss

Muscle wasting can be extreme. Over a three week period following either severe trauma or sepsis, an average of 16% of total body protein is lost [38]. The total loss of skeletal muscle mass was estimated to be ∼ 3 kg. Such loss of lean body mass (whole body water and protein) ranging from 0.5–1.0% loss per day is far greater than that due to bed rest alone. In the very severely ill patient, the catabolic breakdown of muscle proteins shows losses approaching 2% per day [9], with a daily decrease in the fiber area of 3% to 4% [10]. Muscle biopsies show the greatest atrophy in the contractile myosin filaments with relative preservation of other structural proteins. The septic ICU patient shows increased proteosome proteolytic activity [39]. Increased expression of this ubiquitin proteolytic pathway is well characterized in sepsis and is promoted through a number of transcription factors including activator protein-1 (AP-1), nuclear factor-kappa B (NF-κB) and CCAAT/enhancer binding protein (C/EBP) [40]. The key proteolytic enzymes are the E3 ubiquitin ligases that act as the substrate recognition component. Increased calcium levels occur in muscle in sepsis [41] and this is likely to influence protein metabolism through the regulation of the calpain-calpastatin system. Increased calpain activity provides an early step in muscle wasting with degradation of Z-band associated proteins, in particular titin and alpha actinin, leading to release of myosin which is ubiquinated and degraded through the proteosome [42]. The targeted loss of mysosin, with the retention of other structural proteins, suggests that these fibers may have the potential to recover. Immobility and absence of the normal stretch and stresses, however, adds to this process, since passive stretching alone in neuromuscularly paralyzed ICU patients has been shown to reduce protein loss and maintain structure [43].

## Pathogenetic Factors in Myopathy of Critical Illness

From the above one can see that a number of factors may come together to result in muscle dysfunction. These factors include a combination of inflammatory catabolic or even toxic triggers and physiological adaptive mechanisms. During sepsis, the upregulation of several hormones and numerous pro- and anti-inflammatory mediators makes the identification of any single factor clinically worthless. Nevertheless, excess prostaglandins, tumor necrosis factor (TNF)-α, reactive oxygen species (ROS), such as NO, have all been implicated [21]. Hypercortisolemia is responsible for a significant catabolic effect on muscle after trauma or in sepsis [44] which is amplified by inactivity. In normal subjects, protein breakdown is not increased any more than during starvation. However, if cortisol is given after 14 days of bed rest, the net catabolic state is similar to a patient with 70% burn injury [45]. The effect of steroids may combine with locally produced cytokines, such as TNF-α and interleukin (IL)-6 [46], to produce a potent stimulus. It has been suggested that there is a more generalized systemic process with the identification of a low molecular weight neurotoxic factor in the serum from patients who have a neuromyopathy [47] that appears to block intracellular $Ca^{2+}$ release channels and depolarize the resting membrane potential. This combination leads to impaired force development and membrane hypoexcitability with impaired recovery from repetitive action potentials [48].

In the wear and tear of normal exercise activity and following ischemic injury, neutrophils and macrophages dominate the basic inflammatory response [49]. Superoxide-dependent mechanisms appear to be involved, though probably mediated through conversion of hydrogen peroxide to highly reactive radicals, a mechanism involving myeloperoxidase. Neutrophils, however, are also involved in repair through the eventual phagocytosis of debris. Clinically, however, the invasion of neutrophils into skeletal muscle in the critically ill patient is less apparent than occurs following exercise-related muscle damage and is seen only in the extreme necrotic stages that occur in severe MOF [28]. *In vitro*, muscle-derived NO reduces neutrophil-mediated lysis of muscle cells [50] and the leukocyte interaction with the vascular endothelium [51]. Removal of normal muscle loading by inactivity causes a decrease in the expression and activity of neuronal NO synthase (nNOS) in muscle [52]. The same authors subsequently suggested a link with muscle wasting with disuse through studies of dystrophies [53]. NO appears to modify the active site of calpains that initially cleave myosin in degradation. Reduction in NO through reduced nNOS production could contribute to muscle wasting through the loss of a regulatory role for NO on calpain-mediated proteolysis.

While the systemic inflammatory process may impact on skeletal muscle, it is also important to realize that activation of systemically released mediators from within skeletal muscle tissue can lead to disturbances in distant organ systems. During infrarenal aortic abdominal aneurysm repair, an ischemia/reperfusion injury response occurs in the lower limbs. After 30 mins of clamping, increased expression of genes for angiotensinogen, angiotensin converting enzyme (ACE) and IL-6 occur in muscle. Increased IL-6 levels were detectable systemically for 12 hours after reperfusion and were associated with impaired pulmonary function [54].

## Failed Protective Responses in Skeletal Muscle During Sepsis: A Role for Heat Shock Proteins and Glutamine in Mediating Muscle Function

The rapid increased expression of stress or heat shock proteins (HSPs) is one of the most highly conserved mechanisms of cellular protection. HSPs may be central to protect muscle against the assault from systemic inflammation and are critical for cell survival. Increased HSP expression has been reported following ischemia/reperfusion and shock. Further, enhanced HSP expression has been shown to be associated with cyto-protection in a wide variety of experimental injury models. These include models of experimental sepsis, lung injury, transplantation injury, and cardiac ischemia/reperfusion injury.

Skeletal muscle normally adapts following stress, such that it is protected against subsequent damage [55]. This adaptation occurs following a variety of insults, including exercise. The mechanism of activation of the stress response is not fully understood, but increased ROS generation has been implicated as a major signal. The adaptive responses of muscle to exercise stress are by far the most studied. In this instance, increased ROS are produced and these in turn lead to activation of redox-sensitive transcription factors, such as NF-κB, AP-1 and heat shock factor-1 (HSF1), and subsequent increases in the activity of protective enzymes, such as superoxide dismutase and catalase, and an increase in the cellular content of HSPs [57]. Only once the increased ROS production becomes excessive or chronic does failure in adaptation and subsequent damage occur. A putative model of how sepsis can affect the cellular adaptive and protective mechanisms of muscle from young and older patients is illustrated in Fig. 1.

The increase in protective enzymes and HSPs protects the tissue against subsequent exposure to damage [56]. The HSP70 family of proteins has been most studied in skeletal muscle. Major components of this family are a constitutively expressed but inducible HSP, known as HSC70, and a highly inducible HSP (HSP70

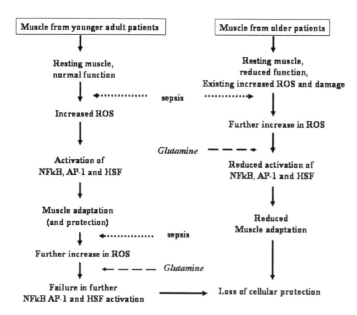

Fig. 1. A putative model of how sepsis can affect the cellular adaptive and protective mechanisms of muscle from younger and older patients. Glutamine may restore these adaptive mechanisms. ROS: reactive oxygen species; HSF: heat shock factor; AP: activator protein; NF-κB: nuclear factor-kappa B

or HSP72). Other HSPs include HSP60, primarily located within the mitochondria and the small HSPs such as αB-crystallin and HSP25/27, which appear to play a role in maintenance of cytoskeletal integrity.

All HSPs act to preserve cellular integrity. Cells stressed by a sub-lethal insult that induces the expression of HSPs are rendered more resistant to a subsequent extreme stress. One of the possible mechanisms underlying stress tolerance involves the concept that the proper folding of proteins in a cell requires an intricate set of folding machinery known as molecular chaperones, of which HSPs are members. Thus, when induced following cellular stress, HSPs appear to repair denatured/damaged proteins, when possible, or may promote degradation of these proteins following irreparable injury [57].

In addition to their local intracellular role, HSPs participate in cytokine signaling, cytokine gene expression, and enhanced antigen presentation to T lymphocytes [58]. This modification of the inflammatory response coupled with increased HSP content of cells results in an increased resistance to cytokine-mediated toxicity. Increased HSP expression has been shown to attenuate plasma concentrations of the pro-inflammatory cytokines, IL-1β and TNF-α, in both *in vitro* and *in vivo* models and this appears to correlate with improved survival from a septic insult [59].

Glutamine appears to be a potent facilitator of HSP production [60–62] with induction as early as 1 hour post-glutamine administration. This enhanced HSP expression was protective against cecal ligation and puncture-induced sepsis in the rat and markedly decreased end-organ injury and overall mortality [63]. The survival benefit from glutamine was abrogated if an inhibitor of HSP was administered. Glutamine appears to regulate protein turnover in muscle cell cultures, increasing the half-life of long-lived proteins and this may be related to an increase in HSP70 [64]. Importantly this effect of glutamine at physiological concentrations was not seen in the unstressed state, only in the myotubes exposed to heat stress.

In ICU patients, trauma or sepsis causes circulating plasma glutamine to decline by about 50%, with a 75% decline in the free glutamine pool in muscle [65]. The mechanism for depletion of muscle glutamine represents a demand for increased rates of glutamine utilization at the whole body level and a relative impairment of *de novo* synthesis in skeletal muscle leading to a deficiency [66]. A low plasma glutamine is an independent predictor for a poor ICU outcome [67] and low glutamine concentration correlates with advanced age. Further, a recent study regarding serum HSP72 concentrations after severe trauma illustrated a correlation between HSP concentrations and survival, but again low HSP concentrations correlated with advanced age [68]. This is not surprising and animal models have demonstrated an attenuated HSP response after non-damaging stress in older animals [69]. It has been suggested that glutamine substitution can induce a HSP response. Glutamine added to parenteral nutrition to meet this deficiency significantly increased serum HSP70 in critically ill patients and the magnitude of HSP70 enhancement showed a correlation with improved clinical outcomes [70]. These findings support clinical evidence that overcoming the relative deficiency of glutamine improves survival from MOF [71,72]; whether it can augment the HSP response in the elderly and act as a HSP inducing agent remains to be seen (Fig. 1).

Half of se ᵥe ᵣely ill ICU patie ᵣts are ove r 65 years of age with upwards of 25% over 75 years of age. The ability to withstand sepsis is particularly dependent upon available skeletal muscle mass. The normal age-related loss of skeletal muscle between the years of 20 to 80 produces a 40% reduction in muscle cross-sectional area [73]. Thus, in the elderly, many physical activities may be conducted at near the critical threshold of failure [74]. The rate of muscle loss in septic ICU patients with MOF is between 2 and 4% per day. This substantial rate of muscle loss, taken together with an already compromised muscle in the elderly, is catastrophic. This is seen in the inability to wean from a ventilator and becomes a determinant of survival.

## Conclusion

Skeletal muscle is a significant player in MOF, showing marked metabolic and structural changes and contributing to the metabolic and inflammatory fluxes in the body. Muscle function is severely compromised, but muscle is a resilient organ and shows an excellent ability to recovery. As a highly plastic organ, muscle shows marked adaptation to activity levels and immobility, and in situations of whole body stress provides a major store of amino acids through controlled degradation. However, muscle provision of certain, conditionally essential amino acids can become limiting. The opportunity for specific nutritional interventions is encouraging.

## References

1. Leijten FS, Harinck-de Weerd JE, Poortvliet DC, de Weerd AW (1995) The role of polyneuropathy in motor convalescence after prolonged mechanical ventilation. JAMA 274:1221–1225
2. Wagenmakers AJM (1999) Fuel utilization by skeletal muscle during rest and exercise. In: Stipanuk MH (ed) Biochemical and Physiological Aspects of Human Nutrition. Saunders, Philadelphia, pp 882–900
3. Lipman RL, Raskin P, Love T, Triebwasser J, Lecocq FR, Schnure JJ (1972) Glucose intolerance during decreased physical activity in man. Diabetes 21:101–107
4. Saltin B, Blomqvist G, Mitchell JH, Johnson RL, Wildenthal K, Chapman C (1968) Response to exercise after bedrest and training. A longitudinal study of adaptive changes in oxygen transport and body composition. Circulation 38:VII 1–78
5. Stein TP, Wade CE (2005) Metabolic consequences of Muscle disuse atrophy. J Nutr 135:1824S-1828S
6. Van den Berghe G, Wouters P, Weekers F, et al (2001) Intensive insulin therapy in the critically patient. N Engl J Med 345:1359–1367
7. Herndon DN, Tompkins RG (2004) Support of the metabolic response to burn injury. Lancet 363:1895–1902

8.  Levy B, Gibot S, Franck P, Cravoisy A, Bollaert PE (2005) Relation between muscle Na+ K+ ATPase activity and raised lactate concentrations in septic shock: a prospective study. Lancet 365:871–875
9.  Gamrin L, Andersson K, Hultman E, Nilsson E, Essen P, Wernerman J (1997) Longitudinal changes of biochemical parameters in muscle during critical illness. Metabolism 46:756–762
10. Helliwell TR, Wilkinson A, Griffiths RD, McClelland P, Palmer TEA, Bone JM (1998) Muscle fibre atrophy in critically ill patients is associated with the loss of myosin filaments and the presence of lysosomal enzymes and ubiquitin. Neuropathol Appl Neurobiol 24:507–517
11. Ruderman NB, Sha AK, Vavvas D, Witters LA (1999) Malonyl-CoA, fuel sensing, and insulin resistance. Am J Physiol 276:E1-E18
12. Sponk P, Zandstra D, Ince C (2004) Bench-to-bedside review: sepsis is a disease of the microcirculation. Crit Care 8:562–468
13. Ince C, Sinaasappel M (1999) Micocirculatory oxygenation and shunting in sepsis and shock. Crit Care Med 27:1369–1377
14. Fink MP (2002) Cytopathic hypoxia: Is oxygen use impaired in sepsis as a result of an acquired intrinsic derangement in cellular respiration? Crit Care Clin 18:165–175
15. Callahan LA, Supinski GS (2005) Sepsis induces diaphragm electron transport chain dysfunction and protein depletion. Am J Respir Crit Care Med 172: 861–868
16. Singer M, DeSantis V, Vitale D, Jeffcoate W (2004) Multiorgan failure is an adaptive, endocrine-mediated, metabolic response to overwhelming ssytemic inflammation. Lancet 364:545–547
17. De Blasi RA, Palmisani S, Alampi D, et al (2005) Microvascular dysfuntion and skeletal muscle oxygenation assessed by phase-modulation near-infrared spectrospy in patients with septic shock. Intensive Care Med 31:1661–1668
18. Pareznik R, Knezevic R, Voga G, Podbregar M (2006) Changes in muscle tissue oxygenation during stagnant ischemia in septic patients. Intensive Care Med 32:87–92
19. Brearley D, Brand M, Hargreaves I, et al (2002) Association between mitochondrial dysfunction and severity of outcome of septic shock. Lancet 360:219–223
20. Vanhorebeek I, De Vos R, Mesotten D, Wouters PJ, De Wolf-Peeters C, Van den Berghe G (2005) Protection of hepatocyte mitochondrial ultrastructure and function by strict blood glucose control with insulin in critically ill patients. Lancet 365:53–59
21. Lanone S, Taille C, Boczkowski J, Aubier M (2005) Diaphragmatic fatigue during sepsis and septic shock. Intensive Care Med 31:1611–1617
22. Rooyackers OE, Hesselink MKC, Wagenmakers AJM (1997) Energy metabolism and contractility of electrically stimulated muscle of rats recovering from critical illness. Clin Sci 92:189–195
23. Cunningham JN, Carter NW, Rector FC, Seldin DW (1971) Resting transmembrane potential difference of skeletal muscle in normal subjects and severely ill patients. J Clin Invest 50:49–50
24. Gamrin L, Andersson K, Hultman E, Essen P, Wernerman J (1997) Longitudinal changes of biochemical parameters in muscle during critical illness. Metabolism 46:756–762
25. Helliwell TR, Griffiths RD, Coakley JH, et al (1990) Muscle pathology and biochemistry in critically ill patients. J Neurol Sci 98S:329
26. Rooyackers OE, Kersten AH, Wagenmakers AJM (1996) Mitochondrial protein content and in vivo synthesis rates in skeletal muscle from critically ill rats. Clin Sci 91:475–481
27. Bolton CF, Gilbert JJ, Hahn AF, Sibbald WJ (1984) Polyneuropathy in critically ill patients. J Neurol Neurosurg Psychiatry 47:1223–1231
28. Helliwell TR, Coakley JH, Wagenmakers AJM, et al (1991) Necrotizing myopathy in critically-ill patients. J. Pathology 164:307–314
29. Coakley JH, Nagendran K, Yarwood GD, Honavar M, Hinds CJ (1998) Patterns of neurophysiological abnormality in prolonged critical illness. Intensive Care Med 24:801–807
30. Latronico N, Peli E, Botteri M (2005) Critical illness myopathy and neuropathy. Curr Opin Crit Care 11:126–132

31. 1 Andrews FJ, Griffiths RD (2003) Intensive care myopathy and neuropathy. Anaesth Intensive Care Med 4:123–125
32. Bolton CF (2005) Neuromuscular manifestations of critical illness. Muscle Nerve 32:140–163
33. Fenzi F, Latronico N, Refatti N, Rizzuto M (2003) Enhanced expression of E-selectin on the vascular endothelium of peripheral nerve in critically ill patients with neuromuscular disorders. Acta Neuropathol (Berl) 27:686–693
34. Helliwell TR, Wilkinson A, Griffiths RD, Palmer TEA, McClelland P, Bone JM (1998) Microvasculatur endothelial activation in the skeletal muscles of patients with multiple organ failure. J Neurol Sci 154:26–34
35. Langouche L, Vanhorebeek I, Vlasselaers D, et al (2005) Intensive insulin therapy protects the endothelium of critically ill patients. J Clin Invest 115:2277–2286
36. Leijten FS, Harinck-de Weerd JE, Poortvliet DC, et al (1995) The role of polyneuropathy in motor convalescence after prolonged mechanical ventilation. JAMA 274:1221–1225
37. Fletcher SN, Kennedy DD, Ghosh IR, et al (2003) Persistent neuromuscular and neurophysiologic abnormalities in lon-term survivors of prolonged critical illness. Crit Care Med 31:1012–1016
38. Finn PJ, Plank LD, Clark MA, Connolly AB, Hill GL (1996) Progressive cellular dehydration and proteolysis in critically ill patients. Lancet 347:654–656
39. Klaude M, Hammarqvist F, Wernerman J (2005) An assay of microsomal membrane-associated proteosomes demonstrates increased proteolytic activity in skeletal muscle of intensive care unit patients. Clin Nutr 24:259–265
40. Hasselgren P-O, Menconi MJ, Fareed MU, Yang H, Wei W, Evenson A (2005) Novel aspects on the regulation of muscle wasting in sepsis. Int J Biochem Cell Biol 37:2156–2168
41. Fisher DR, Sun X, Williams AB, et al (2001) Dantrolene reduces serum TNFalpha and corticosterone levels and muscle calcium, calpain gene expression, and protein breakdown in septic rats. Shock 15:200–207
42. Hasselgren PO (2002) Molecular regulation of muscle wasting. Sci Med 8:230–239
43. Griffiths RD, Palmer TEA, Helliwell T, Maclennan P, Macmillan RR (1995) Effect of passive stretching on the wasting of muscle in the critically ill. Nutrition 11:428–432
44. Bessey PQ, Lowe KA (1993) Early hormonal changes affect the catabolic responses to trauma. Ann Surg 218:476–491
45. Ferrando AA, Stuart CS, Sheffield-Moore M, Wolfe RR (1999) Inactivity amplifies the catabolic responses of skeletal muscle to cortisol. J Clin Endocrinol Metab 84:3515–3521
46. De Letter M, van Doorn P, Savelkoul H, et al (2000) Critical illness polyneuropathy and myopathy (CIPNM) evidence for local immune activation by cytokine-expression in the muscle tissue. J Neuroimmunol 106:206–213
47. Druchky A, Herkert M, Radespiel-Troger M, et al (2001) Critical illness polyneuropathy: clinical findings and cell culture assay of neurotoxicity assessed by a prospective study. Intensive Care Med 27:686–693
48. Friedrich O, Hund E, Weber C, Kacke W, Fink RHA (2004) Critical illness myopathy serum fractions affect membrane excitability and intr-cellular calcium release in mammalian skeletal muscle. J Neurol 252:53–65
49. Tidball JT (2005) Inflammatory processes in muscle injury and repair. Am J Physiol Regul Integr Comp Physiol 288:R345-R353
50. Nguyen HX, Tidball JG (2003) Interactions between neutrophils and macrophages promote macrophage killing of muscle cells in vitro. J Physiol 547:125–132
51. Niu XF, Smith CW, Kubes P (1994) Intracellualar oxidative stress induced by nitric oxide synthesis inhibition increases endothelial cell adhesion to neutrophils. Cir Res 74:1133–1140
52. Tidball JG, Lavergne E, Lau KS, Spencer MJ, Stull JT, Wehling M (1998) Mechanical loading regulates nitric oxide synthase expression and activity in developing and adult skeletal muscle. Am J Physiol Cell Physiol 275:C260-C266

53. 1 Tidball JG, Wehling-Henricks M (2004) Expression of a NOS transgene in dystrophin-deficient muscle reduces muscle membrane damage without increasing the expression of membrane-associated cytoskeletal proteins. Mol Genet Metab 82:312–320

54. Adembri C, Kastamoniti E, Bertolozzi I, et al (2004) Pulmonary injury follows systemic inflammatory reaction in infrarenal aortic surgery. Crit Care Med 32:1170–1177

55. McArdle A, Pattwell D, Vasilaki A, Griffiths RD, Jackson MJ (2001) Contractile activity-induced oxidative stress: cellular origin and adaptive responses. Am J Physiol Cell Physiol 280:C621–627

56. McArdle F, Spiers S, Aldemir H, et al (2004) Preconditioning of skeletal muscle against contraction-induced damage: the role of adaptations to oxidants in mice. J Physiol 561:233–244

57. Hightower LE (1991) Heat shock, stress proteins, chaperones, and proteotoxicity. Cell 66:191–197

58. Pockley AG (2003) Heat shock proteins as regulators of the immune response. Lancet 362:469–476

59. Chu EK, Ribeiro SP, Slutsky AS (1997) Heat stress increases survival rates in lipopolysaccharide-stimulated rats. Crit Care Med 25:1727–1732

60. Nissim I, States B, Hardy M, Pleasure J, Nissim I (1993) Effect of glutamine on heat-shock-induced mRNA and stress proteins. J Cell Physiol 157:313–318

61. Wischmeyer PE, Musch MW, Madonna MB, Thisted R, Chang EB (1997) Glutamine protects intestinal epithelial cells: role of inducible HSP 70. Am J Physiol 272:G879–884

62. Wischmeyer PE, Kahana MD, Wolfson R, Ren H, Musch M, Chang E (2001) Glutamine induces heat shock protein and protects against endotoxin shock in the rat. J Appl Physiol 90:2403–2410.

63. Singleton KD, Serkova N, Beckley VE, Wischmeyer PE (2005) Glutamine attenuates lung injury and improves survival after sepsis: Role of enhanced heat shock expression. Crit Care Med 33:1206–1213

64. Zhou Z, Thompson JR (1997) Regulation of protein turnover by glutamine in heat-shocked skeletal myotubes. Biochim Biophys Acta 1357:234–242

65. Palmer TEA, Griffiths RD, Jones C (1996) Effect of parenteral l-glutamine on muscle in the very severely ill. Nutrition 12:316–320

66. Biolo G, Zorat F, Antonione R, Ciocchi B (2005) Muscle glutamine depletion in the intensive care unit. Int J Biochem Cell Biol 37:2169–2179

67. Oudemans-van Straaten HM, Bosman RJ, Treskes M, et al (2001) Plasma glutamine depletion and patient outcome in acute ICU admissions. Intensive Care Med 27:84–90

68. Pittet JF, Lee H, Morabito D, Howard MB, Welch WJ, Mackersie RC (2002) Serum Levels of HSP 72 measured early after trauma correlate with survival. J Trauma 52:611–617

69. McArdle A, Vasilaki A, Jackson MJ (2002) Exercise and skeletal muscle ageing: cellular and molecular mechanisms. Ageing Res Rev 1:79–93

70. Ziegler TR, Ogden LG, Singleton KD, et al (2005) Parenteral glutamine increases serum heat shock protein 70 in critically ill patients. Intensive Care Med 31:1079–1086

71. Griffiths RD, Jones C, Palmer TEA (1997) Six-month outcome of critically ill patients given glutamine-supplemented parenteral nutrition. Nutrition 4:296–302

72. Griffiths RD, Allen KD, Andrews FJ, Jones C (2002) Infection, multiple organ failure, and survival in the intensive care unit: Influence of glutamine-supplemented parenteral nutrition on acquired infection. Nutrition 18:546–552

73. Lexell J, Taylor CC, Sjostrom M (1988) What is the cause of the ageing atrophy? Total number, size and proportion of different fiber types studied in whole vastus lateralis muscle from 15- to 83-year-old men. J Neurol Sci 84:275–294

74. Young A (1986) Exercise physiology in geriatric practice Acta Med Scand Suppl 711:227–232

# Subject Index

Printed in the USA
CPSIA information can be obtained
at www.ICGtesting.com
LVHW012132040324
773565LV00003B/26